THE PHYSICS OF
RADIOLOGY

THE PHYSICS OF RADIOLOGY

FOURTH EDITION

HAROLD ELFORD JOHNS, OC, Ph.D., F.R.S.C., LL.D., D.Sc., F.C.C.P.M.

University Professor Emeritus, University of Toronto
Professor Emeritus, Department of Medical Biophysics and Department of
Radiology, University of Toronto
Former Head of, and now consultant to, the Physics Division, Ontario
Cancer Institute and the Radiological Research Laboratories; University
of Toronto

and

JOHN ROBERT CUNNINGHAM, B.Eng., M.Sc., Ph.D., F.C.C.P.M.

Senior Clinical Physicist, Ontario Cancer Institute
Professor, Department of Medical Biophysics
University of Toronto

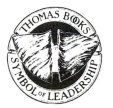

CHARLES C THOMAS • PUBLISHER
Springfield • Illinois • U.S.A.

Published and Distributed Throughout the World by

CHARLES C THOMAS • PUBLISHER
2600 South First Street
Springfield, Illinois 62717 U.S.A.

ISBN 0-398-04669-7

Library of Congress Catalog Card Number: 81-21396

First Edition, 1953
Second Edition, First Printing, 1961
Second Edition, Revised Second Printing, 1964
Second Edition, Third Printing, 1966
Third Edition, First Printing, 1969
Third Edition, Second Printing, 1971
Third Edition, Revised Third Printing, 1974
Third Edition, Fourth Printing, 1977
Third Edition, Fifth Printing, 1978
Fourth Edition, 1983

*With THOMAS BOOKS careful attention is given to all details of
manufacturing and design. It is the Publisher's desire to present books that are
satisfactory as to their physical qualities and artistic possibilities and
appropriate for their particular use. THOMAS BOOKS will be true to those
laws of quality that assure a good name and good will.*

Printed in the United States of America
CB-1

Library of Congress Cataloging in Publication Data

Johns, Harold Elford.
    The physics of radiology.

    (American lecture series; publication no. 1054)
    First published in 1953 under title: The physics of
radiation therapy.
    "A monograph in the Bannerstone Division of American
lectures in radiation therapy"—ser. t.p.
    Bibliography: p.
    Includes index.
    1. Radiology, Medical. 2. Radiology. I. Cunningham,
John Robert. II. Title. III. Series. [DNLM: 1. Health
physics. WN 110 J65p]
    R895.J6   1983   616.07'57   81-21396
    ISBN 0-398-04669-7   AACR2

PREFACE

Since the publication of the Third Edition of *The Physics of Radiology*, various international organizations have attempted to introduce SI (système international) units into their fields. Of particular interest to us are the new terms that have been defined for the radiological sciences: the *gray* has replaced the rad as the unit of absorbed dose, and the *becquerel* has replaced the curie as the unit of activity.

We are convinced of the advantages of SI and the new units are used throughout the book. We realize, however, that it will take some time before workers in the field are at ease with them and for this reason the older units are often used in parallel with the new ones.

Committees of the I.C.R.U. are attempting to deemphasize the use of the roentgen as a unit of exposure. In spite of this we have continued to use it, especially in diagnostic radiology. When patients are exposed to soft x rays, as they are in diagnostic radiology, there is no single factor which allows one to go from exposure to dose. The authors feel that the I.C.R.U. has not adequately assessed the impact of their decision on this subject. Because the roentgen remains a practical unit, the chapter on diagnostic radiology still makes extensive use of it.

The use of small electronic calculators has relieved the scientist of many of the boring arithmetical tasks of the past. We believe that all scientists now use calculators, and we have felt at greater liberty to do calculations that involve logarithms or exponentials, a procedure which was previously more difficult. In addition, we have introduced, in the first chapter, exponential growth and decay, since it is common to all aspects of radiation and since, for example, we believe the doubling time for the growth of cells is no more complicated a concept than the determination of the doubling time of invested money, a topic which everyone understands.

The emphasis in radiation therapy has shifted further towards the use of high energy beams. We therefore give less attention to cobalt 60 and more to the higher energy radiation produced by linear accelerators in the 10 to 25 MeV range.

There have been explosive developments in diagnostic radiology with the invention and exploitation of the CT scanner. In addition, other methods of imaging are rapidly becoming available. We have, therefore, more than doubled the size of the chapter on this subject. In addition, because of the general fear of radiation, we have emphasized the idea that for every risk there should be a benefit and have discussed ways of reducing this risk without loss of diagnostic information.

In the chapter on radiobiology we have removed some basic radiation chemistry and replaced it with discussions on survival curves of patients so that the reader will have ways of comparing the results of different modes of treatment.

We are especially indebted to R.J. Howerton of Lawrence Livermore Laboratory for supplying us with a library of photon interaction coefficients on magnetic tape and to Dr. M.J. Berger of the National Bureau of Standards for supplying us with his latest calculations of electron stopping powers. The helpful discussions we have had with Mr. J.H. Hubbell, Dr. R. Loevinger, and Dr. S. Domen, all of the U.S. National Bureau of Standards, on topics of radiation dosimetry are much appreciated. Similarly, helpful correspondence and discussions on stopping powers with M. Pages of Centre d'Études Nucléaires de Saclay, France, are acknowledged. In addition, our association with members of AAPM Task Group 21 on High Energy Dose Calibrations has helped to clarify many concepts dealt with in this book.

We thank Dr. P. Leung, Mr. A. Rawlinson, Mr. J. Van Dyk, and Dr. P. Shragge for many discussions on clinical radiation physics and Dr. G. Ege and Dr. M. Bronskill for their help with the chapter on Nuclear Medicine.

In preparing Chapter 15 on radiation protection we were helped by Dr. H.O. Wyckoff of the ICRU, Washington; Dr. H. Johnston and Dr. C.L. Greenstock of Atomic Energy of Canada, Whiteshell, Manitoba; Dr. G. Cowper and Dr. A.M. Marko of the Chalk River Laboratories of Atomic Energy of Canada; Dr. M. James of the Atomic Energy Control Board, Ottawa; and Dr. D. Grogan of the Health Protection Bureau, Ottawa.

We are greatly indebted to Dr. K.W. Taylor, of the Radiological Research Laboratory, University of Toronto, who worked with us over a period of three years to create the chapter on diagnostic radiology. Valuable assistance in this task was also provided by Dr. M. Yaffe, Dr. A. Fenster, and Dr. A. Holloway, all of whom are closely associated with us.

The chapter on radiobiology was created in collaboration with Dr. R.P. Hill and valuable discussions on this topic were held with Dr. G. DeBoer, Dr. R.S. Bush, Dr. G.F. Whitmore, Dr. J.W. Hunt, Dr. A.M. Rauth, and Dr. W.D. Rider of our Institute.

We thank Dr. R.S. Bush, Dr. W.D. Rider, and the late Dr. C.L. Ash for their efforts at keeping our writings relevant to clinical problems.

We also acknowledge the help of our radiation oncology residents and radiation physics students who provided criticism and worked many of the problems. In particular we mention Luis Cabeza, David Hunter, Paul Johns, Gordon Maudsley, Henriette Von Harpe, and John Wong.

The Ontario Cancer Institute continues to be a research facility in which ideas are fully exchanged and discussed and this kind of environment is essential to produce a book of this complexity. We acknowledge the leadership of its director, Dr. R.S. Bush.

We thank Mr. D. McCourt of the Ontario Cancer Institute who drafted over 200 diagrams for the book and Mr. A. Connor and his staff of our photography department who prepared them for publication. We thank Miss C. Morrison, Librarian at OCI, and her staff for helping with the references. We are most deeply indebted to and do sincerely thank our personal secretaries, Mrs. Stellis Robinson and Miss Ann Lake, for all they have done in the preparation of this manuscript.

In the thirty years that Charles C Thomas, Publisher, has been our publisher we have always been able to count on its understanding and support.

The writing of a book of this complexity, spread as it was over the past five years, needed the continuous support and encouragement of our wives and families, and this is gratefully acknowledged.

Harold E. Johns
J.R. Cunningham

CONTENTS

THE PHYSICS OF RADIOLOGY

Chapter **1**

BASIC CONCEPTS

1.01 **INTRODUCTION**

The sciences of diagnostic radiology, radiotherapy, radiobiology, and nuclear medicine continue to develop and expand. They are all based on an understanding of the underlying physics. This book is written to help a student interested in any of these fields to understand his science and to help the medical physicist who applies the science of physics to these fields of medicine. In this book we will discuss only those physical principles that are absolutely essential to an understanding of these medical applications. Some of the chapters will be of more interest to physicists than to radiologists. For a first reading of this text, the following guidelines are suggested:

• Physicists should read each chapter in order.
• Diagnostic radiologists should read chapters 1, 2, 3, 5, 15, 16, and parts of 7, 8, 9, 10, and 17.
• Radiotherapists should read chapters 1 to 5, 7 to 13, 15, 17, and parts of 14 and 16.
• Specialists in nuclear medicine should read chapters 1, 2, 3, 5, 14, 15, and parts of 7, 8, 9, and 17.
• Radiobiologists should read chapters 1, 2, 3, 5, 15, 17, and parts of 4, 7, 8, 9, and 14.
• For further study all the chapters should then be read in order.

The availability of pocket calculators has freed scientists of much of the drudgery of handling numerical calculations. Each student should therefore obtain a pocket calculator for his own personal use. It should include exponential functions (e^x and y^x) and the ability to manipulate very large or small numbers using powers of ten.

1.02 **QUANTITIES AND UNITS**

All meaningful measurements require the statement of a numerical value, which is a pure number, and the unit in which the physical quantity is measured, i.e.,

$$\text{(physical quantity)} = \text{(numerical value)} \times \text{(some unit)} \quad (1\text{-}1)$$

For example, one might say the potential across an x ray tube was 80 kilovolts. This involves the pure number 80 and the unit "the kilovolt."

3

As each science develops, there is a tendency for each to create its own special units to deal with its own special problems. This has led to confusion when a worker in one field attempts to use work arising from another. In recent years, the Comité International des Poids et Mésures (CIPM) has adopted an international system of units with the abbreviation SI (Système International). These are being officially introduced into most countries of the world.

The International Commission on Radiation Units and Measurements (ICRU) has studied the special problems of units for radiology and has created a number of special units in the past. They now recommend that these special units gradually be phased out and be replaced by SI units. To meet the needs of radiological science, the General Conference of Weights and Measures (CGPM), on the advice of the ICRU, in 1975 established two special SI units, the becquerel and the gray. For further details on these see Wyckoff et al. (W1). In this text we will use the new SI units wherever possible but continually relate these to the earlier ICRU units, which are still in common use.

Fundamental Units

Table 1-1 gives some of the important units that are dealt with in this book. Others are introduced as needed. All measurements in science are based on four basic physical quantities: mass, length, time, and electric current. These are shown in the first section of Table 1-1. The corresponding fundamental basic units are the kilogram (kg), the meter (m), the second (s), and the ampere (A), whose *magnitudes* or size are carefully preserved in standardization laboratories throughout the world. They are independent of one another since they represent different ideas and thus cannot be converted from one to another. For example, it would be meaningless to attempt to convert a time in seconds into a length in meters.

Derived Units

The next section of the table introduces a few of the *derived* physical quantities that are relevant to our field. These are based on various combinations of the four fundamental quantities.

Velocity (entry 5) is the ratio of an increment of distance, Δl, to the corresponding increment in time, Δt. It has no special name and can be expressed using *any* unit of distance and *any* unit of time, such as cm per second, meter per second, kilometer per hr, etc. The SI unit of velocity is meter per second (m/s or m s^{-1}).

Acceleration (entry 6) is the ratio of the change in velocity, Δv, to the change in time, Δt, required for this change in velocity. It may be expressed in *any* unit of velocity and *any* unit of time. For example, a car

TABLE 1-1
Fundamental Quantities and Units

	Usual Symbol for Quantity	Defining Equation	SI Unit	Relationships and Special Units
		FUNDAMENTAL UNITS		
1 mass	m	Basic physical units	kilogram (kg)	
2 length	l	defined arbitrarily	meter (m)	
3 time	t	and maintained in	second (s)	
4 current	I	standardization laboratories	ampere (A)	
		DERIVED UNITS		
5 velocity	v	$v = \Delta l / \Delta t$	m s^{-1}	
6 acceleration	a	$a = \Delta v / \Delta t$	m s^{-2}	
7 force	F	$F = m\,a$	newton (N)	1 N = 1 kg m s^{-2}
8 work or energy	E	$E = F\,l = 1/2\ m\ v^2$	joule (J)	1 J = 1 kg m^2 s^{-2}
9 power or rate of doing work	P	$P = E/t$	watt (W)	1 W = 1 J/s
10 frequency	f,ν	number per second	hertz (Hz)	1 Hz = 1 s^{-1}
		ELECTRICAL UNITS		
11 charge	Q	$Q = I\,t$	coulomb (C)	1 C = 1 A s
12 potential	V	$V = E/Q$	volt (V)	1 V = 1 J/C
13 capacity	C	$C = Q/V$	farad (F)	1 F = 1 C/V
14 resistance	R	$V = I\,R$	ohm (Ω)	1 Ω = 1 V/A
		RADIATION UNITS		
15 absorbed dose	D	energy absorbed from ionizing radiation per unit mass	gray (Gy)	1 Gy = 1 J kg^{-1} 1 Gy = 100 rads*
16 exposure	X	charge liberated by ionizing radiation per unit mass air	C kg^{-1}	roentgen (R)* 1 R = 2.58 $\times$ 10^{-4} C/kg
17 activity	A	disintegrations of radioactive material per second	becquerel (Bq)	1 Bq = 1 s^{-1} 1 curie* (Ci) = 3.7 $\times$ 10^{10} Bq

*The ICRU (W1) recommends that the special units the rad, the roentgen, and the curie be gradually abandoned over the period 1976–1986 and be replaced by the gray (Gy), the coulomb per kg (C/kg), and the becquerel (Bq). An additional unit, the sievert (Sv), has been defined for radiation protection problems and is discussed on page 533.

(Useful conversion factors are given in Appendix A-1.)

with a velocity increase of 7.2 km per hour every second would accelerate 7.2 km per hr per second. Acceleration expressed this way involves two different units of time, the hour and the second, and the unit of distance, the km. This acceleration can be expressed in any of the following ways:

$$a = 7.2\ \frac{\text{km}}{\text{hr}} \times \frac{1}{\text{s}} = 7.2 \times 1000\ \frac{\text{m}}{\text{hr}} \times \frac{1}{\text{s}}$$

$$= \frac{7.2 \times 1000\ \text{m}}{3600\ \text{s}} \times \frac{1}{\text{s}} = \frac{2.0\ \text{m}}{\text{s} \times \text{s}} = 2\ \text{m s}^{-2} = 2.0\ \text{m/s}^2$$

It is important that the student understand that numbers (such as 7.2) and units (such as km, hr, etc.) should be carried together in the equation. For example, 1 km is replaced by its equivalent 1000 m. From the above example we see that acceleration involves velocity and time, or distance and time squared. The SI unit of acceleration is meters per s² or $m/s^2 = m\ s^{-2}$. It has no special name.

The next quantity in the table (entry 7) is force, F, for which everyone has an intuitive feeling. If a ball on the level floor starts to move or accelerate, we know that a force has been applied to it. Likewise, if a car suddenly comes to rest or decelerates we know a force has been applied to it. Force is related to acceleration and is defined by Newton's law of motion, which states that F = m a. Force is measured by the product of mass and acceleration, and since mass and acceleration are already defined, the unit of force is automatically defined as $1\ kg\ m\ s^{-2}$. This unit of force is so important it is given a special name, the newton:

$$1\ newton = 1\ N = 1\ kg\ m\ s^{-2} \qquad (1\text{-}2)$$
the defining equation is F = m a

We now distinguish between mass and force. Suppose you weigh yourself on a hospital balance and obtain the reading 70 kg. This means that you have a mass 70 times the mass of the standard kilogram in Paris. Suppose you now go to the gymnasium and hang from a horizontal bar; what force do you exert on the bar? You know that if the bar breaks you will fall with the acceleration due to gravity of $9.8\ m\ s^{-2}$. Hence the pull of the earth on you will give your 70 kg mass an acceleration of $9.8\ m\ s^{-2}$ and the force exerted by gravity is $F = 70\ kg \times 9.8\ m\ s^{-2} = 686\ kg\ m\ s^{-2} = 686$ newtons. Thus, your mass is 70 kg and the force of attraction of the earth for you is 686 newtons. This force varies slightly from place to place on the earth's surface as the acceleration due to gravity changes,* but your mass is constant.

The next quantity is work or energy (entry 8), which is defined as the product of force times distance. Thus, if while hanging from the gym bar you raise your center of gravity 0.50 m, the work done by you against gravity is 686 N × 0.50 m = 343 newton meters = 343 N m. The newton meter is such an important quantity that it has been given the special name, the joule:

$$1\ joule = 1\ J = 1\ newton\ meter = 1\ N\ m = 1\ kg\ m^2\ s^{-2} \quad (1\text{-}3)$$
the defining equation is E = F l

It should be emphasized that work in the physical sense described here requires that motion take place. For example, one would get very tired in

---

*The acceleration due to gravity increases with latitude and decreases with altitude. A few values are Toronto 9.805, London 9.812, North Pole 9.832, Equator 9.780 m s⁻².

just hanging from the bar, but one does *not* work until one *raises* oneself.

The next quantity is power (entry 9 in Table 1-1), which is defined as the rate of doing work, or the work done per unit time. The unit of power is the joule per second, but this is so important a unit that it is called a watt:

$$1 \text{ watt} = 1 \text{ W} = \frac{1 \text{ joule}}{1 \text{ second}} = 1 \text{ J/s} = 1 \text{ J s}^{-1} \qquad (1\text{-}4)$$

the defining equation is $P = E/t = E \, t^{-1}$

A related unit widely used in the English speaking parts of the world is the horsepower, which equals 746 watts.

Frequency (entry 10) is used to describe a repetitive event such as the vibration of a violin string or the oscillations of a crystal. It is simply the number of oscillations per unit time and so has dimensions of 1/second = s^{-1}. This is such an important unit that is called the hertz.

$$1 \text{ hertz} = 1 \text{ Hz} = 1 \text{ oscillation per second} = s^{-1} \qquad (1\text{-}5)$$

Power line frequencies are measured in hertz; on the North American continent, for example, this frequency is usually 60 Hz.

Example 1-1. A young scientist of mass 75 kg at the Ontario Cancer Institute, in a foolish trial of endurance, ran from the basement to the seventh floor (height 25.8 m) in 23.6 s. Calculate the work done and the power developed. In Toronto the acceleration due to gravity is 9.8 m s^{-2}.

Force of attraction of the earth for scientist
$$F = 75 \text{ kg} \times 9.8 \text{ m s}^{-2} = 735 \text{ newtons}$$

Work done
$$E = 735 \text{ N} \times 25.8 \text{ m} = 19{,}000 \text{ N m}$$
$$= 19000 \text{ joules}$$

Power developed
$$P = \frac{19000 \text{ J}}{23.6 \text{ s}} = 805 \text{ J s}^{-1} = 805 \text{ watts}$$
$$= 1.08 \text{ hp}$$
$$\text{since } 746 \text{ watt} = 1 \text{ horsepower}$$

This is an impressive development of power. The experiment is not recommended, since the subject was not of much value as a scientist for a few days after the experiment.

Electrical Units

The next section of Table 1-1 involves electrical units (all items involve the fundamental unit of current, the ampere, in combination with other fundamental or derived units). Charge (entry 11) is the product of current times time and has dimensions ampere seconds (A s). Because of its fundamental importance it is given a special name, the coulomb:

$$1 \text{ coulomb} = 1 \text{ C} = 1 \text{ ampere second} = 1 \text{ A s} \qquad (1\text{-}6)$$
$$\text{the defining equation is } Q = I \text{ t}$$

Potential, or potential difference (entry 12), is a difficult concept that deals with the electrical pressure that causes a current to flow in a circuit. If we connect a dry cell to a light bulb, a current flows through the bulb producing heat and light. Work is being done by the battery, and the amount of work is proportional to the charge, Q, which passes through the bulb. Potential difference is defined by

$$\text{potential difference} = \frac{\text{work done in electrical circuit}}{\text{charge passing through circuit}} \qquad (1\text{-}7)$$

Since our unit of work is the joule and unit of charge is the coulomb, potential difference is measured in joules per coulomb. This is such an important unit it is called the volt:

$$1 \text{ volt} = 1 \text{ V} = \frac{1 \text{ joule}}{1 \text{ coulomb}} = 1 \text{ J/C} \qquad (1\text{-}8)$$

By rearranging equation 1-7 we see that the work done in an electrical circuit is

$$\text{work done} = Q \text{ V} = I \text{ t V} \qquad (1\text{-}9)$$

This leads us to a special unit of energy, the electron volt (eV), which is the energy acquired when an electron of charge e $= 1.602 \times 10^{-19}$ C falls through 1 volt. Thus,

$$\textbf{1 eV} \text{ (a unit of energy)} = 1.602 \times 10^{-19} \text{ C} \times 1 \text{ volt} \qquad (1\text{-}10)$$
$$= \mathbf{1.602 \times 10^{-19} \text{ J}}$$
$$\textbf{1 MeV} = 10^6 \text{ eV} = 10^6 \times 1.602 \times 10^{-19} \text{ J} = \mathbf{1.602 \times 10^{-13} \text{ J}}$$

The electron volt and its multiples are extensively used in radiological science.

Capacity (entry 13) describes the ability of an insulated conductor to store charge. Such an insulated conductor is called a condenser or capacitor. When a charge Q is placed on such a conductor, its potential is raised to V and the capacity C is defined by

$$\text{capacity C} = \frac{\text{charge Q stored on conductor}}{\text{potential V to which conductor is raised}} \qquad (1\text{-}11)$$
$$\text{or } Q = C \text{ V}$$

Since charge is measured in coulombs and potential in volts, the unit of capacity is coulombs per volt. This is such an important unit it is called the farad:

$$1 \text{ farad} = 1 \text{ F} = \frac{1 \text{ coulomb}}{\text{volt}} = 1 \text{ C/V} \tag{1-12}$$

The farad is an enormous capacity, and one usually deals with capacities some 10^6 to 10^{12} times smaller.

The final electrical quantity in which we are interested is resistance (entry 14). Suppose a potential difference V is applied to the ends of a wire causing a current I to flow. The size of the current will be proportional to the applied potential and will depend on the nature of the wire—its area, its length, and the material from which it is made. The resistance of the wire, R, is defined as the ratio of V to I and so is measured in volts per ampere. This unit is given a special name, the ohm:

$$1 \text{ ohm} = 1 \ \Omega = \frac{1 \text{ volt}}{1 \text{ ampere}} = 1 \text{ V/A} = 1 \text{ V A}^{-1} \tag{1-13}$$

the defining equation is $V = IR$

Example 1-2. A potential of 12 volts placed across a heating coil produces a current of 1.5 amperes. Find the resistance of the coil, the charge which passes through the coil in 1.0 min, the energy dissipated, and power developed.

Resistance $\quad R = \dfrac{V}{I} = (\text{eq. 1-13}) = \dfrac{12 \text{ volts}}{1.5 \text{ amperes}} = 8 \text{ ohms} = 8 \ \Omega$

Charge $\quad \begin{aligned} Q &= I \ t = 1.5 \text{ A} \times 1 \text{ min} = 1.5 \text{ A} \times 60 \text{ s} \\ &= 90 \text{ A s} = 90 \text{ C} \end{aligned}$

Work done (eq. 1-8) $\quad E = Q \ V = 90 \text{ C} \times 12 \text{ V} = 1080 \text{ C V} = 1080 \text{ J}$

Power $\quad P = \dfrac{E}{t} = \dfrac{1080 \text{ J}}{60 \text{ s}} = 18 \text{ J s}^{-1} = 18 \text{ W}$

or, by rearranging equation 1-9 we obtain

$$P = \frac{\text{work done}}{t} = I \ V = 1.5 \text{ A} \times 12 \text{ V} = 18 \text{ W}$$

Example 1-3. A current of 2.5×10^{-6} A flows into a 20.0×10^{-6} F condenser for 20 seconds. Find the potential to which the condenser is charged.

Charge placed on condenser (eq. 1-6) $\quad Q = I \ t = 2.5 \times 10^{-6} \text{A} \times 20 \text{ s} = 50 \times 10^{-6} \text{ C}$

Potential dif- $V = \dfrac{Q}{C} = \dfrac{50 \times 10^{-6}\,\mathrm{C}}{20.0 \times 10^{-6}\,\mathrm{F}} = 2.5\,\mathrm{C\,F^{-1}} = 2.5\,\mathrm{volts}$
ference between
plates of con-
denser (eq. 1-11)

Radiation Units

We now discuss a few of the quantities and units that are used in the field of ionizing radiation.

Absorbed dose (entry 15) is defined as the energy deposited by ionizing radiation per unit mass of material and is expressed in J/kg. This is such an important quantity in radiological science that a special SI unit, the gray (Gy) has been created (W1)*, to represent 1 J/kg. Another unit that has been used for some 20 years and will now slowly be abandoned is the rad, which is smaller by a factor of 100 (1 Gy = 100 rads = 1 J/kg).

Exposure (entry 16) is the quantity that is used to describe the output of an x ray generator. It is the charge liberated by ionizing radiation per unit mass of air and in SI units is expressed in C kg^{-1}. For many years exposure has been expressed in roentgens, where 1 roentgen = 2.58 × 10^{-4} C kg^{-1}. There is no doubt that the roentgen will continue to be used for a few years in spite of the fact that it is not accepted as an SI unit by CGPM. In this book we will often express exposures in roentgens as well as in C/kg.

Activity (entry 17) describes the number of disintegrations per unit time of a radioactive isotope. Since disintegrations have no dimensions, activity is measured in reciprocal seconds, or s^{-1}. The special unit of activity is the becquerel (Bq) = s^{-1}. For many years activities have been measured in curies (Ci); 1 Ci = 3.70 × 10^{10} Bq. The introduction of the becquerel may create some problems so throughout the book we will use the curie as well.

It should be noted that the becquerel is measured in the same fundamental unit, s^{-1}, as the hertz. This is unfortunate but will probably not create too serious a problem since the fields of radioactivity in which the becquerel is used should not often be confused with electrical engineering, where the hertz is used. One would certainly not measure activity in hertz or an electrical frequency in becquerels. There is one important distinction between the two concepts: in radioactivity disintegrations are at random, while frequencies in hertz are periodic functions with pulses evenly spaced in time.

PREFIXES: All of these units can be altered by various factors of 10 through the use of appropriate prefixes. These are summarized in Table 1-2.

---

*References are found at the end of the book.

TABLE 1-2
Prefixes to be Used to Alter Units by Powers of 10

deci (d) = 10^{-1}	deka (da) = 10^{1}
centi (c) = 10^{-2}	hecto (h) = 10^{2}
milli (m) = 10^{-3}	kilo (k) = 10^{3}
micro (μ) = 10^{-6}	mega (M) = 10^{6}
nano (n) = 10^{-9}	giga (G) = 10^{9}
pico (p) = 10^{-12}	tera (T) = 10^{12}
femto (f) = 10^{-15}	peta (P) = 10^{15}
atto (a) = 10^{-18}	exa (E) = 10^{18}

For example, one might refer to the capacity of a particular condenser as being 100 picofarads (100 pF) or 0.1 nF or 10^{-10} F. In addition the use of a double prefix should be avoided. For example, although 1 mμs = $10^{-3} \times 10^{-6}$ s = 10^{-9} s = 1 ns is correct, the use of the double prefix, mμ (milli micro), is not recommended. When a prefix is used before the symbol of a unit the combination of prefix and symbol should be considered as one new symbol. For example, cm^3 means (cm)^3 not c(m)^3. Thus, cm^3 = (0.01 m)^3 = 10^{-6} m^3, not 0.01 m^3.

The reader may well wonder why numbers such as 2.58×10^{-4} C/kg should appear in a so-called logical science and why some numbers should be so large and others so small. The answer is that once the fundamental units of mass (kg), length (m), time (s), and current (A) are defined all others follow. The coulomb is logically an ampere second and is a useful unit to measure charge in an electrical circuit, but it is far too large a unit to be useful in describing the charges liberated in an ion chamber by ionizing radiation. Now we require a unit some 10^{12} times smaller, such as the picocoulomb (pC). The curious numbers involved in the definition of the roentgen = 2.58×10^{-4} C/kg arise from the fact that roentgen was defined as the radiation required to liberate 1 electrostatic unit of charge in 1 cm^3 of air, a logical definition. To use it, however, in relation to other SI units requires a knowledge of a troublesome conversion factor between the electrostatic unit and the coulomb and more confusion results. Similarly, the curie = 3.7×10^{10} s^{-1} needs comment. This unit of activity was originally defined as the activity of 1 gm of radium, a logical but troublesome definition as with each improved measurement of the emissions of radium, a redefinition of the unit of activity would be required.

Often it is required to convert a measurement from one unit to another. For example, since 1 gray (Gy) = 100 rad, a dose of 50 Gy could be expressed:

$$\text{Dose} = 50 \text{ Gy} = 50 \times 100 \text{ rad} = 5000 \text{ rad}$$

Observe that one carries the unit along in the calculation with the numerical value; in this case we replace 1 Gy by its equivalent 100 rad. Note that the rad is a *smaller* unit of dose than the gray, hence to describe a given dose in rads, one requires a *larger* numerical value. Mistakes can often be avoided by asking if the answer seems reasonable. If the new unit is smaller, a larger number is required to describe a given quantity and vice versa.

Example 1-4. A patient is given an x ray exposure X, of 5.16×10^{-5} coulombs per kg. Convert this exposure into roentgens (R), given that $1R = 2.58 \times 10^{-4}$ coulombs per kg.

> In equations and in conversion factors, rather than use "per," it is simpler and better to use a fraction or a reciprocal:

$$X = 5.16 \times 10^{-5} \frac{C}{kg} \quad \text{or} \quad X = 5.16 \times 10^{-5} \, C \, kg^{-1}$$

$$1 \, R = 2.58 \times 10^{-4} \, C \, kg^{-1} \quad \text{or} \quad 1 \, C \, kg^{-1} = \frac{1 \, R}{2.58 \times 10^{-4}}$$

Replacing $1 \, C \, kg^{-1}$ $\quad X = 5.16 \times 10^{-5} \, C \, kg^{-1}$
by its equivalent

$$= 5.16 \times 10^{-5} \times \frac{1 \, R}{2.58 \times 10^{-4}} = .200 \, R$$

By carrying the units along with the numbers we obtain our answer with its units. We then ask, is the answer reasonable? In this case, the roentgen is a much smaller unit than the C/kg, hence our answer must be a much larger number (0.2) than the original number of 5.16×10^{-5}.

1.03   **ATOMS**

All matter is composed of atoms. Each atom consists of a small dense nucleus with a radius of about 10^{-14} m, and a surrounding "cloud" of moving planetary electrons that travel in orbits with radii of about 10^{-10} m. The electrons have a small mass compared to the nucleus but, because of their diffuse nature, occupy a great deal of space. A group of atoms then consists of a few dense spots (nuclei) while the rest of the space occupied by the electrons is virtually empty. As an illustration, if an atom were increased in size to "occupy" a room, the nucleus would occupy a space the size of a pin point placed at the center of the room. Because of this emptiness of so-called solid matter, a high energy electron or nucleus from one atom may readily penetrate many atoms before a collision results between the moving particle and any part of the atom.

Atoms differ from one another in the constitution of their nuclei and in the number and arrangement of their electrons. *The number of electrons in the atom is referred to as the atomic number and is represented by Z.* Z ranges from one for the simplest atom (hydrogen) to 105 for the most complex atom as yet discovered (hahnium). The chemical properties of an atom are determined by the atomic number. The properties of the lighter atomic species are given in Table 1-3. The first column gives the element, the second column the symbol used to represent this element, and the third column the atomic number, Z. To understand the rest of the table, we must inquire into the structure of the nucleus.

TABLE 1-3
Atomic Numbers, Atomic Weights, and Mass Numbers of a Few of the Lighter Elements

Element	Symbol	Atomic Number (Z)	Atomic Weight (amu)	Mass Numbers of Stable Isotopes (A)	Mass Numbers of Unstable Isotopes (A)
Hydrogen	H	1	1.00797	1, 2	3
Helium	He	2	4.0026	3, 4	5, 6, 8
Lithium	Li	3	6.941	6, 7	5, 8, 9, 11
Beryllium	Be	4	9.0122	9	6, 7, 8, 10, 11, 12
Boron	B	5	10.811	10, 11	8, 9, 12, 13
Carbon	C	6	12.011	12, 13	9, 10, 11, 14, 15, 16
Nitrogen	N	7	14.0067	14, 15	12, 13, 16, 17, 18
Oxygen	O	8	15.9999	16, 17, 18	13, 14, 15, 19, 20

1.04   THE NUCLEUS

A nucleus can be broken up into its constituent parts by bombarding with high speed particles. When this occurs, it becomes evident that there are two important, fundamental particles within the nucleus: *protons and neutrons*. Either particle may be referred to as a *nucleon*. Protons carry a positive charge, equal in size but opposite in sign to that carried by the electrons, while neutrons have no charge. Protons and neutrons have nearly the same mass, some 1900 times that of the electron. Since the atom as a whole is electrically neutral, there must be one proton in the nucleus for every electron outside the nucleus. Hence Z, which represents the number of electrons outside the nucleus, also represents the number of protons in the nucleus.

Mass Number, A: The total number of nucleons in the nucleus (protons plus neutrons) is called the mass number and range from 1 for hydrogen to about 250 for the heaviest nuclei. Since Z represents the number of protons in the nucleus, $(A - Z)$ gives the number of neutrons.

Isotopes: Most elements consist of a mixture of several atomic species with the *same* extranuclear structure but *different* nuclear masses, that is, different mass numbers. *Atoms composed of nuclei with the same number of protons but different number of neutrons are called isotopes.* Isotopes may be stable or unstable and a few of both types are given in Table 1-3. For example, hydrogen has two stable isotopes with mass numbers 1 and 2, and an unstable one with mass number 3. Helium has two stable isotopes, mass numbers 3 and 4, and three unstable isotopes, mass numbers 5, 6, and 8. Lithium consists of two stable isotopes, mass numbers 6 and 7, and four unstable isotopes, mass numbers 5, 8, 9, and 11. The stability of an isotope depends upon there being the right mixture of protons and neutrons. If there is an unbalance in this mixture, a particle will be ejected; this process will continue until a stable configuration is achieved. The ejection of a particle is called a disintegration and the isotope is said to be radioactive. This will be dealt with in later sections of this book.

Since *isotopes* have the same number of protons, and hence the same number of electrons, they *have the same chemical properties.* For this reason they cannot be separated chemically. They can, however, be separated in the mass spectrometer, which exploits the mass differences between the nuclei.

Atomic masses are related to the mass of one of the isotopes of carbon (mass number 12), which is arbitrarily assigned the value 12.0000. Since carbon 12 has 6 protons and 6 neutrons, and since protons and neutrons have nearly the same mass, each particle on this scale has a mass of nearly 1. This means that atomic masses are very nearly whole numbers and equal to the mass number. For example, the two isotopes of hydrogen have atomic masses of 1.007825 and 2.014102, which are very nearly equal to the mass numbers 1 and 2.

Atomic masses as used in chemistry (and usually called atomic weights) and represented by A are generally different from atomic masses since usually there are a number of isotopes involved in a naturally occurring element. For example, boron as found in nature consists of a mixture of two isotopes of mass numbers 10 and 11 in the proportions 19.8% and 80.2%, giving an atomic weight of 10.811 (see Table 1-3). Sometimes atomic masses are nearly whole numbers because one of the isotopes may be much more abundant than any of the others. For example, hydrogen in nature exists as a mixture of mass number 1 (99.985%) and mass number 2 (0.015%), giving an atomic mass of nearly 1 (1.00797).

NOTATION FOR ATOMIC SPECIES: It is usual to represent atomic species using subscripts and superscripts preceding the chemical symbol. For example, the three isotopes of hydrogen (see Table 1-4) are represented by ^1_1H, ^2_1H, and ^3_1H. The subscript gives Z, the number of protons in the nucleus, while the superscript gives the mass number, A. There is some redundancy in this notation, the subscript really being unnecessary because the chemical symbol tells the chemist the atomic number. Often then one could refer to the isotopes of hydrogen as simply ^1H, ^2H, and ^3H. In speaking, these are referred to as hydrogen 1, hydrogen 2, and hydrogen 3.

ISOTOPES OF HYDROGEN: The nucleus ^2H, containing one proton and one neutron, is important in nuclear disintegration experiments. It is called a *deuteron.* An atom composed of one deuteron and an electron is

TABLE 1-4
Isotopes of Hydrogen and Helium

Element	Symbol	Number Protons	Number Neutrons	Mass Number (A)	Properties	Name of Nucleus	Name of Corresponding Atom
Hydrogen $Z = 1$	$_1^1H$	1	0	1	Stable	Proton	Hydrogen
	$_1^2H$	1	1	2	Stable	Deuteron	Deuterium
	$_1^3H$	1	2	3	Radioactive		Tritium
Helium $Z = 2$	$_2^3He$	2	1	3	Stable		
	$_2^4He$	2	2	4	Stable	Alpha	
	$_2^5He$	2	3	5	Radioactive		
	$_2^6He$	2	4	6	Radioactive		
	$_2^8He$	2	6	8	Radioactive		

called heavy hydrogen or deuterium. The nucleus ^3H, consisting of one proton and two neutrons, is radioactive and decays into an isotope of helium ($_2^3He$). The atom formed from ^3H is called *tritium*.

ISOTOPES OF HELIUM: There are five known isotopes of helium, $_2^3He$, $_2^4He$, $_2^5He$, $_2^6He$, and $_2^8He$, of which the first two are stable and the latter three radioactive. $_2^4He$ is the major constituent of helium and is widely used in nuclear disintegration experiments. It is known as an *alpha* particle. Helium 5, 6, and 8 decay into isotopes of lithium.

ISOTOPES OF COBALT: ($_{27}^{54}Co$, $_{27}^{55}Co$, $_{27}^{56}Co$, $_{27}^{57}Co$, $_{27}^{58}Co$, $_{27}^{59}Co$, $_{27}^{60}Co$, $_{27}^{61}Co$, $_{27}^{62}Co$, $_{27}^{63}Co$, $_{27}^{64}Co$.) $_{27}^{59}Co$ is the only stable isotope of cobalt, containing 27 protons and 32 neutrons. The others disintegrate in a variety of ways to form isotopes of iron and nickel. Cobalt 60 is used as the source of radiation in many therapy units.

In general, as the atomic number is increased, the number of isotopes and the number of stable isotopes increase. For example, naturally occurring tin consists of a mixture of 10 stable isotopes and at least 15 radioactive ones may be produced artificially.

1.05 ELEMENTAL PARTICLES

In the last section, we saw that the nucleus consists of protons and neutrons. However, in nuclear disintegration experiments, a host of other "particles" have been discovered. A few of these of interest to us are briefly described in Table 1-5. In this table masses are expressed in terms of the mass of one of the isotopes of carbon = 12.0000, and charges in terms of the charge on the proton = 1.602×10^{-19} C.

1.06 EXTRANUCLEAR STRUCTURE

In discussing x rays and their effects on atoms, we are interested in their extranuclear structure, that is, the arrangement of the planetary electrons outside the nucleus.

TABLE 1-5

Properties of the Important Elemental Particles

(Masses given in atomic mass units, charges in terms of the charge on the proton)

Particle	Mass	Charge	Properties
proton p	1.007277	+1	The *proton* is the nucleus of the hydrogen atom. The hydrogen atom consists of 1 proton in the nucleus and 1 external electron. The mass of the neutral atom is 1.007277 + 0.000548 = 1.007825 mass units. The proton is one of the fundamental building blocks of all nuclei. Beams of protons are being used in radiotherapy.
neutron n	1.008665	0	The *neutron* is the other fundamental building block of all nuclei. Neutrons have nearly the same mass as protons. Since the neutron is an uncharged particle it is hard to stop and difficult to detect. Beams of neutrons are being used in radiotherapy.
electron e, e⁻ or β⁻	0.000548	−1	The *electron* has a very small mass compared with the proton. Electrons abound in nature. Every atom contains electrons outside the nucleus. The electron is easily detected. It is sometimes called a negatron or beta particle and represented by e, e⁻, or β^-. Beams of high energy electrons are extensively used in radiotherapy.
positron e⁺ or β⁺	0.000548	+1	The *positron* has the same mass as an electron but carries a positive charge. Positrons exist in nature only while they are in motion. A slowly moving or stationary positron quickly combines with an electron to form a burst of radiation in the form of two gamma rays (see below). Positrons are represented by e⁺ or β^+ and referred to as beta plus particles. They are used in nuclear medicine.
photon hν or gamma ray γ	0	0	Strictly speaking, the *photon* is not a particle, but a bundle of energy which travels at the speed of light (3×10^8 m s⁻¹). In many interactions it acts much like a particle. Photons are referred to almost interchangeably as *quanta* or *gamma rays* and are represented symbolically by hν or γ. Beams of photons account for the major part of external beam radiotherapy.
neutrino ν_e	less than 1/8000 of an electron mass	0	The *neutrino* is a very small particle with practically no mass and no charge. For this reason, it has been very difficult to detect experimentally. Its interaction with protons to form neutrons and positrons according to the reaction $$\nu_e + p \longrightarrow n + \beta^+$$ has been observed. The neutrino was introduced originally from theoretical considerations to help explain beta decay.
Mu mesons μ^+ μ^-	207m₀ 207m₀	+1 −1	Mu mesons may be either positively or negatively charged and have a mass 207 times the mass of the electron. They are produced indirectly by the interaction of very high energy particles with matter. The particles are unstable and decay spontaneously into electrons and neutrinos according to the reactions $$\mu^+ \longrightarrow e^+ + 2\nu$$ $$\mu^- \longrightarrow e^- + 2\nu$$ The mean life of the particles is 2.15×10^{-6} sec.

TABLE 1-5—cont'd.
Properties of the Important Elemental Particles
(Masses given in atomic mass units, charges in terms of the charge on the proton)

Particle	Mass	Charge	Properties
Pi mesons			Pi mesons may have a positive or a negative charge or may
π^+	$273m_0$	$+1$	be neutral. They are produced by the bombardment of mat-
π^-	$273m_0$	-1	ter with high energy protons or photons. The charged π
π^0	$265m_0$	0	mesons decay into mu mesons and neutrinos according to

$$\pi^+ \longrightarrow \mu^+ + \nu$$
$$\pi^- \longrightarrow \mu^- + \nu$$

with a mean life of 2.5×10^{-8} s. The neutral π^0 meson decays into 2 photons

$$\pi^0 \longrightarrow h\nu_1 + h\nu_2$$

with a mean life of 10^{-15} seconds. Beams of negative π mesons are being used in radiotherapy.

Hydrogen is the simplest atom, consisting of one electron moving about the nucleus (Fig. 1-1). The nucleus, with its positive charge, attracts the electron with its negative charge, constraining it to move in an orbit much the same as the earth moves about the sun. All isotopes of hydrogen have this simple arrangement of one external electron, regardless of the number of particles in the nucleus. Helium, the next simplest atom, has two electrons. These two electrons travel in the same orbit spinning in opposite directions (Fig. 1-1). This electronic configuration is very stable and, as a result, it is impossible to make helium interact chemically with any other material. Hydrogen owes its chemical activity to the fact that it would like to acquire one more electron to achieve the dynamic stability of helium.

Lithium has 3 electrons (Fig. 1-1). The third electron must be added to a new orbit outside the first one, because 2 electrons in the inner orbit completely fill this orbit or shell. The innermost orbit or shell is referred to as the K shell. The next shells are, in order, the L, M, and N shells. Since lithium has 3 electrons, the third electron is located alone in the L

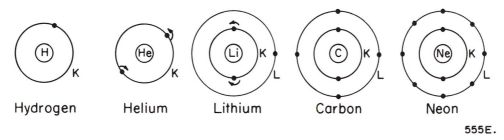

Hydrogen   Helium   Lithium   Carbon   Neon

555E.

Figure 1-1. Schematic diagram showing electron structure for hydrogen, helium, lithium, carbon, and neon.

shell, a fact that makes lithium very active chemically. Generally speaking, an atom has its greatest stability if its outermost shell is completely filled. If it is not filled, it will tend to react with any element that can supply the extra electron; or if it has an excess of electrons, it will react with any element that can take these excess electrons.

As one proceeds to higher values of Z in the periodic table, the L shell gradually fills up to form beryllium (Z = 4) with 2 electrons in the L shell, then boron (Z = 5) with 3 electrons, carbon (Z = 6) with 4, nitrogen (Z = 7) with 5, oxygen (Z = 8) with 6, fluorine (Z = 9) with 7, and finally neon (Z = 10) with 8. The L shell will not hold any more electrons.

Neon, with a completely filled outer shell, is an inert gas and cannot be made to react chemically. Carbon, on the other hand, can form many compounds since it can give up 4 electrons or take on 4 electrons to achieve stability. Oxygen is 2 electrons short of a completed shell. It will try to acquire 2 electrons. Carbon and oxygen can combine to form CO_2, in which case the carbon shares its 4 outer electrons with 2 oxygen atoms. Fluorine, with 1 electron short of a completed shell, is very active. Sodium (Z = 11) is formed with the K and L shells filled and 1 electron in the M shell. Sodium will thus react with any atom, such as fluorine, that will take up one electron to form a stable compound. Chlorine is similar in structure to fluorine with one empty place in the M shell and combines with sodium to form NaCl or salt.

With increase in the atomic number, Z, the extranuclear structure becomes more and more complicated; the M shell will be filled, then the N and so on. Chemical properties will repeat themselves as the shells fill up. For example, the inert gases (helium, neon, argon, krypton, to name a few) will occur as each shell is filled. In a similar way alkaline elements (lithium, sodium, potassium) will appear when the outermost shell is occupied by only 1 electron. In general, the chemical properties and valence will be determined by the number of electrons in the outermost incompleted shell.

1.07   **ATOMIC ENERGY LEVELS**

Although the electrons of Figure 1-1 are shown circulating and spinning in specific orbits, we know from quantum mechanical reasoning that the electron has a finite probability of being anywhere in space, but with its most probable value near the orbit. This means orbits have no real existence. A quantity that does have real existence, however, is the energy of the atom. The atom may exist in a number of discrete energy states or energy levels, which may be measured with great precision. A few of these for tungsten are represented by the horizontal lines of Figure 1-2. The corresponding orbits are shown on the left side of Figure 1-2. The energy levels for K, L, and M shells are about 70,000 eV, 11,000 eV, and

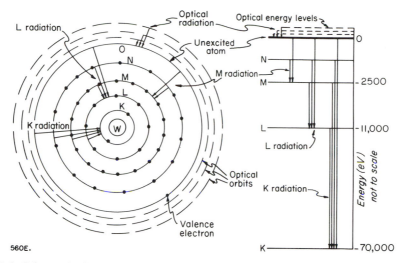

Figure 1-2. Schematic diagram of the tungsten atom showing the shells on the left and an energy level diagram on the right. The energy scale in eV is not drawn to scale. X-radiation arises through transitions of electrons to the K, L, and M shells. Optical radiation arises by transitions of the valence electron from optical orbits to the O shell.

2500 eV respectively. This means that to remove a K electron from the atom, the tungsten atom must be supplied with 70,000 eV of energy or it must be bombarded with electrons that have fallen through a potential difference of at least 70,000 volts. To remove an L electron, about 11,000 eV of energy is required. The zero for the energy scale is arbitrarily chosen to correspond to the atom in the unexcited state and is represented by the heavy horizontal line marked zero near the top of the diagram. In this unexcited state, the outermost valence electron of tungsten occupies an 0 shell. If this electron is given energy, it may be moved out to one of the optical orbits and the atom is raised on the energy scale a few electron volts to occupy one of the optical energy levels. The atom cannot remain for long in one of these energy states (or to put it another way, the electron cannot remain in one of the optical orbits) and when it falls back to its normal position energy is radiated. This is called optical radiation.

Now suppose more than 70,000 eV of energy is given the atom and an electron is ejected from the K shell to leave a hole in it. Electrons from the outer shells will try to fill this hole, giving rise to the K radiation illustrated in Figure 1-2. Radiations arising from transitions to the *inner* shells are called x radiation and will be discussed in section 1.12.

1.08   **NUCLEAR ENERGY LEVELS**

Nuclei also have energy levels. Figure 1-3 shows some of the energy levels of carbon 12, which contains 6 protons and 6 neutrons. In the ground state, carbon 12 is represented by the heavy line at the bottom of the diagram. If the nucleus is given energy it may be raised to one of the excited states at 4.4, 7.7, 9.6, 10.7, 11.8, 12.7, 16.6, 17.2, and 18.4 MeV. On returning from one of these excited states, energy is radiated corresponding to the energy difference. The return to the ground state could occur in one jump, with the release of all the excess energy at one time, or by a series of jumps in cascade, with the release of several smaller bundles of energy giving the same total energy release.

The energy levels of two related species of nuclei, $^{12}_{5}B$ and $^{12}_{7}N$, are shown in Figure 1-3. Their ground states are above $^{12}_{6}C$ by 13.4 and 17.67 MeV respectively. The nuclei $^{12}_{5}B$ and $^{12}_{7}N$ will both disintegrate into $^{12}_{6}C$ to reach the position of minimum energy. $^{12}_{5}B$ reaches the ground state by the conversion of a neutron into a proton with the ejection of an electron (β^-) while $^{12}_{7}N$ achieves stability by the conversion of a proton into a neutron with the ejection of a positive electron (β^+). Such disintegrations will be discussed in detail in Chapter 3. In general, the energy levels of nuclei are just as complex as the energy levels in atoms, and Figure 1-3 is an oversimplification. As more complex nuclei are built up, the protons and neutrons are added into a system of nuclear levels until certain shells are filled up, in much the same way that electrons are added to successive shells in the atom.

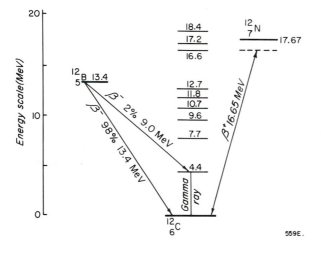

Figure 1-3. Energy level diagram for carbon 12.

1.09   ELECTROMAGNETIC RADIATION

Radio waves, heat waves, light waves, ultraviolet rays, x rays, and gamma rays are all examples of electromagnetic radiation. They all travel in a vacuum with a velocity of

$$c = 2.998 \times 10^8 \text{ m s}^{-1} \approx 3 \times 10^8 \text{ m s}^{-1}$$

Waves of all kinds have associated with them a wavelength, λ, and a frequency, ν. If a tuning fork makes ν vibrations per second and the length of each wave given off is λ, then in one second the wave disturbance will travel $\nu\lambda$ from the source and the velocity of the wave is $\nu\lambda$. For electromagnetic waves we have the important relation

$$\nu\lambda = c \tag{1-14}$$

Example 1-5. Green light has a wavelength of 500 nm in air (or in a vacuum). Find the frequency.

$$\nu = \frac{c}{\lambda} = \frac{3 \times 10^8 \text{ m s}^{-1}}{500 \text{ nm}} = \frac{3 \times 10^8 \text{ m s}^{-1}}{500 \times 10^{-9}\text{m}}$$

$$= 6 \times 10^{14} \text{ s}^{-1} = 6 \times 10^{14} \text{ Hz}$$

The wave discussed in the example can be seen and is called green light. Blue light has a shorter wavelength of 400 nm and red light a longer wavelength of 700 nm. If the wavelength is longer than 700 nm, the human eye cannot detect it and we refer to the radiation as infrared. If the wavelength is shorter than 400 nm, the radiation is again invisible to the eye and is called ultraviolet. Radiations with wavelengths less than 10 nm are called x rays.

As the wavelength becomes very short and the corresponding frequency very large, it is necessary to consider the *quantum* nature of the radiation.

1.10 QUANTUM NATURE OF RADIATION

Although often electromagnetic radiation appears to have the properties of waves, at other times it behaves more like a stream of small bullets, each traveling with velocity c and each carrying a certain amount of energy. This bundle of energy is called a quantum or photon. The amount of energy carried by the photon depends upon the frequency of the radiation. If the frequency is doubled, the energy of the photon is doubled. The actual amount of energy carried by a photon is given by the important equation

$$E = h \nu \tag{1-15}$$

where h is Planck's constant = 6.63×10^{-34} J s

Example 1-6. Calculate the energy carried by one photon of radiation produced in a diagnostic x ray generator at a wavelength of 10 pm. Using equations 1-14 and 1-15 we obtain:

$$E = h\nu = h \frac{c}{\lambda} = \frac{6.63 \times 10^{-34} \text{ J s} \times 3 \times 10^8 \text{ m s}^{-1}}{10 \text{ pm}}$$

$$= \frac{19.89 \times 10^{-26} \text{ J m}}{10 \times 10^{-12} \text{ m}} = 1.989 \times 10^{-14} \text{ J}$$

Note that the units are carried along in the calculation the same as the numbers. We can express our answer in eV using equation 1-10.

$$E = 1.989 \times 10^{-14} \, J = \frac{1.989 \times 10^{-14}}{1.60 \times 10^{-19}} \, eV$$

$$= 1.24 \times 10^5 \, eV = 124 \, keV$$

If we substitute values for c and h in $E = hc/\lambda$ and convert energy to keV we obtain, by the method of example 1-6, the important relation

$$E = \frac{1240 \, keV \, pm}{\lambda} \tag{1-16}$$

The student should note that the number 1240 is more than a number: it is in fact 1240 keV pm. Using equation 1-16, we calculate that a photon of wavelength 10 pm carries an energy

$$E = \frac{1240 \, keV \, pm}{\lambda} = \frac{1240 \, keV \, pm}{10 \, pm} = 124 \, keV$$

in agreement with the calculations of example 1-6. Equation 1-16 is a very simple useful relation since it enables one to calculate the energy of a photon from its wavelength or the wavelength of a photon from its energy.

It is readily seen from equation 1-16 that as the wavelength becomes shorter and shorter, the energy associated with one photon becomes larger and larger. In fact, the energy carried by one photon of wavelength 10 pm (124 keV) is more than enough to trigger a device such as a Geiger counter so that the passage of an *individual photon* can be recorded. If a Geiger counter is placed in the room next to an operating x ray machine, it will be observed that the photons of radiation are emitted in a discontinuous way. There will be no doubt then as to the quantum nature of radiation. In the case of radiation of long wavelength (low frequency), such as radio waves, the quantum nature is unimportant since each photon will now carry a very small amount of energy and many will be emitted per second. For example, a radio transmitter operating at a power of 10,000 watts at a frequency of 300 kHz emits about 5×10^{31} photons per second. A radio receiver many miles away would receive so many per second that the quantum nature would disappear, and the receiver would appear to receive energy continuously. The concept of quanta is indispensable when dealing with high energy x rays and gamma rays but is not pertinent when dealing with very low energy radiation.

1.11   THE ELECTROMAGNETIC SPECTRUM

The electromagnetic spectrum includes radiation from very long radio waves to the exceedingly short penetrating gamma rays, all of which travel at velocity c in a vacuum. In Table 1-6 the frequency, wavelength, photon energy, and properties of the complete spectrum are summarized. It should be emphasized that the regions of the spectrum overlap and there is no sudden change in properties in the progression from one region to the next. It is seen that the quantum of energy for high frequency (short wavelength) radiation becomes very large.

TABLE 1-6
The Electromagnetic Spectrum

Frequency (Hz)	Wavelength	Photon Energy	Properties
1.0×10^5	3 km	413 peV	Radio waves ranging from long waves through the broadcast band, to short waves and to ultra short waves in radar. These waves are produced by electrical oscillations and detected by electronic equipment. They will pass through nonconducting layers of materials but are reflected by electrical conductors.
3.0×10^{10}	0.01 m	124 μeV	
3.0×10^{12}	100 μm	12.4 meV	Infrared radiations. These are produced by molecular vibration and the excitation of the outer electrons of the atom. They are generated by heat in stoves, radiators, et cetera, and can be detected by heat devices and films. Most solid materials are opaque to infrared radiations.
3.0×10^{14}	1 μm	1.24 eV	
4.3×10^{14}	700 nm	1.77 eV	Visible light ranging from red through yellow, green and blue to violet. Produced by the excitation of the outer electrons of an atom. Generated in lamps and in gas tubes by electrical discharge. Detected by films, by photoelectric cells, and by the eye. Transmitted by materials such as glass.
7.5×10^{14}	400 nm	3.1 eV	
7.5×10^{14}	400 nm	3.1 eV	Ultraviolet light. Produced by the excitation of outer electrons in the atom. Detected by films, Geiger counters, and ionization chambers. Produces erythema of the skin; kills bacteria and is an agent in the production of vitamin D.
3.0×10^{16}	10 nm	124 eV	
3.0×10^{16}	10 nm	124 eV	Soft x rays. Produced by the excitation of the inner electrons of an atom. Detected by films, Geiger counters, and ionization chambers. Have the ability to penetrate very thin layers of material. Of little value in radiology because of their limited power of penetration.
3.0×10^{18}	100 pm	12.4 keV	
3.0×10^{18}	100 pm	12.4 keV	Diagnostic x rays and superficial therapy.
3.0×10^{19}	10 pm	124 keV	
3.0×10^{19}	10 pm	124 keV	Deep therapy x rays and gamma rays from radium decay products.
3.0×10^{20}	1 pm	1.24 MeV	
3.0×10^{21}	100 fm	12.4 MeV	Radiation from a small betatron or linear accelerator.
3.0×10^{22}	10 fm	124 MeV	Radiation from a large linear accelerator.
3.0×10^{23}	1 fm	1.24 GeV	Produced in the operation of large proton synchrotrons or linear accelerators.

In Table 1-6 the energy of the photon will also be the energy required to produce the radiation. For example, 1.24 million volts will be required on an x ray tube to produce x rays of wavelength 1 pm. No wavelength shorter than this can be produced by such a potential difference, but longer waves are produced. In general, the minimum wavelength, λ_{min}, that can be produced by the voltage V will be given by

$$\lambda_{min} = \frac{1240 \text{ kV pm}}{V} \qquad (1\text{-}17)$$

This relation comes directly from equation 1-16 and is identical to it except voltage* replaces energy in electron volts.

1-12   RADIATION OF ENERGY FROM AN ATOM

To understand the mechanism by which energy can be radiated from an atom, consider again the energy levels of tungsten (Fig. 1-2). Suppose a high speed electron impinges on an atom of tungsten and removes a K electron. This will require at least 70,000 eV of energy. In a very short time another electron from the L shell may fall down into the K shell to occupy the vacancy and when this occurs (70,000 − 11,000 =) 59,000 eV of energy will be radiated as a quantum of x rays. This radiation is called characteristic radiation since it is characteristic of the material in which it is produced.

It may happen that the high speed electron will remove an L, M, or N electron instead of the K electron. If the L electron (binding energy 11,000 eV) is removed and the space filled with an M electron (binding energy 2,500 eV), then the radiation emitted will have an energy of (11,000 − 2,500 =) 8,500 eV. In all cases the energy of the emitted quantum in electron volts is just the difference between the two binding energies.

The vacancy in any shell can be filled in many ways. If a K electron is removed, an electron may fall into this "hole" from an L shell, an M shell, or any other shell. If an electron fills the K shell from the L shell, then a hole will be left in the L shell and when it is filled, L radiation will result. This is illustrated in Figure 1-2. Actually, the energy level diagram is much more complicated than this, for the L shell is divided into 3 subshells, the M into 5, and the N into 7.

When we deal with an element of low atomic number, the binding energies of the K shell are small. For carbon this energy is 285 eV, for oxygen 528 eV, and for organic tissues we may take the average value of

---

*Note that a distinction is made between a voltage (such as the voltage on an x ray tube) expressed in volts, kilovolts, or megavolts (V, kV, MV) and the corresponding energy an electron acquires in falling through these potential differences. These energy units are the electron volt, the kiloelectron volt, and the megaelectron volt represented by eV, keV, and MeV, respectively.

500 eV. The characteristic K radiation of "tissue" is very soft and will be absorbed in a very short distance in tissue.

1.13   MASS AND ENERGY

One of the important concepts of Einstein's theory of relativity is that mass is a form of energy and the two are related by:

$$E = m\,c^2 \qquad\qquad (1\text{-}18)$$

where c is the velocity of light. Since the velocity of light squared is an enormous number, a small mass, m, will yield an enormous amount of energy, E. For example, suppose 1 gm of material is converted into energy; the energy release will be:

$$E = 1 \times 10^{-3} \text{ kg} \times (3 \times 10^8)^2 (\text{m s}^{-1})^2 = 9 \times 10^{13} \text{ kg m}^2 \text{ s}^{-2} = 9 \times 10^{13} \text{ J}$$

The answer is in joules because $1 \text{ kg m}^2 \text{ s}^{-2} = 1$ joule (see equation 1-3). This is enough energy to supply the power requirements of 4000 homes for 1 year. The conversion of mass to energy takes place in the sun, in the nuclear reactor, and when positrons (positive electrons) are stopped in matter.

The energy release corresponding to one electron mass (9.109×10^{-31} kg) is an important quantity. We calculate it thus:

$$E = 9.109 \times 10^{-31} \text{ kg } (2.998 \times 10^8)^2 \text{ m}^2 \text{ s}^{-2} = 81.87 \times 10^{-15} \text{ J}$$

$$= 81.87 \times 10^{-15} \times \frac{1}{1.602 \times 10^{-13}} \text{ MeV} = 0.511 \text{ MeV (using eq. 1-10)}$$

Example 1-7. Calculate the energy equivalent of 1 atomic mass unit (amu). For this calculation we need Avogadro's number, 6.022045×10^{23}, which gives the number of atoms in a mass equal to the atomic weight.

$$\text{mass of one carbon atom} = \frac{12.000 \text{ g}}{6.022045 \times 10^{23}} = 1.99268 \times 10^{-23} \text{ g}$$

Since carbon has a mass number of 12, it contains 12 amu. Hence the conversion of 1 amu to energy yields:

$$E = \frac{1.99268 \times 10^{-26} \text{ kg}}{12} \times (2.998 \times 10^8)^2 \text{ m}^2 \text{ s}^{-2} = 1.4925 \times 10^{-10} \text{ J}$$

$$= \frac{1.4925 \times 10^{-10}}{1.6022 \times 10^{-13}} \text{ MeV} = 931.5 \text{ MeV}$$

We thus have two important mass-to-energy conversion factors:

$$\textbf{1 electron mass} = \textbf{0.511 MeV} \qquad\qquad (1\text{-}19)$$
$$\textbf{1 amu} \qquad\quad = \textbf{931.6 MeV}$$

1.14   **MASS AND VELOCITY**

Until the advent of modern physics, mass was considered an entity that could not be created or destroyed. In the last section it was shown that mass and energy are equivalent and in later sections situations will occur in which mass is converted into energy and energy into mass. Experiments with high speed nuclear particles show that the mass of a particle depends upon its velocity and that this mass increases with velocity. We must now distinguish between the "rest mass" of the particle (the mass of the particle when it is at rest) and its mass when it is moving. The relation between mass and velocity was derived by Einstein from his theory of relativity and is given by

$$m = \frac{m_0}{\sqrt{1 - v^2/c^2}} \qquad (1\text{-}20)$$

In this expression, m_0 is the rest mass, m is the mass when the particle is traveling with velocity v, and c is the velocity of light. At the velocities encountered in everyday life, the increase in mass with velocity is completely negligible. However, when a particle travels with a velocity comparable to that of light, the effect becomes important. Substitution in equation 1-20 will show that a particle traveling at 1/10 the velocity of light suffers an increase in mass of 0.5%. As the particle approaches closer and closer to the velocity of light, the mass becomes larger and larger. If the velocity is 98% of that of light (v/c = 0.98), the mass becomes 5 times the rest mass, as shown by substitution in equation 1-20, thus:

$$m = \frac{m_0}{\sqrt{1 - (.98)^2}} = \frac{m_0}{\sqrt{.04}} = 5\ m_0$$

From section 1.13, we may consider that a particle at rest with mass m_0 has an energy $m_0 c^2$. A particle moving with velocity, v, has a mass, m, given by equation 1-20 and energy, mc^2. The difference between these two energies is the energy of motion or the kinetic energy (K.E.) of the particle; that is

$$\text{K.E.} = mc^2 - m_0 c^2 \qquad (1\text{-}21)$$

If the velocity of the particle is small compared with the velocity of light, it may be shown that this formula for the kinetic energy reduces to the simple familiar expression $1/2\ m_0 v^2$ (see problem 21).

Some data relating the kinetic energy to the total energy, velocity, and mass for electrons and protons is given in Table 1-7. The second column gives the total energy corresponding to the kinetic energy, which is given in the first column. Since an electron has a rest energy of 0.511 MeV (eq. 1-19), the total energy entered in column 2 is 0.511 MeV greater

TABLE 1-7

Velocity Relative to the Velocity of Light and Mass Relative to the Rest Mass for Electrons and Protons

Kinetic Energy	Electrons			Protons	
	Total Energy (MeV)	Velocity Relative to Vel. of Light	Mass Relative to Rest Mass	Velocity Relative to Vel. of Light	Mass Relative to Rest Mass
10 keV	0.521	0.1950	1.020	0.0046	1.0000
100 keV	0.611	0.5483	1.196	0.0147	1.0001
200 keV	0.711	0.6954	1.392	0.0208	1.0002
500 keV	1.011	0.8629	1.979	0.0326	1.0005
1 MeV	1.511	0.9411	2.957	0.0465	1.0011
2 MeV	2.511	0.9791	4.916	0.0657	1.0021
5 MeV	5.511	0.9957	10.79	0.1026	1.0053
10 MeV	10.511	0.998817	20.58	0.1451	1.0107
20 MeV	20.511	0.999689	40.16	0.2033	1.0213
50 MeV	50.511	0.999949	99.01	0.3141	1.0533
100 MeV	100.511	0.999987	192.31	0.4283	1.1066

than the values given in the first column. The third column gives the velocity of the electron relative to the velocity of light.

It is seen that a 100 keV electron—one which has fallen through 100 kV—is traveling with a velocity more than half that of light (0.5483c). Electrons with energies greater than 5 MeV are for all practical purposes traveling at the speed of light. Column 4 gives the mass of the electron relative to the rest mass. It is seen that a 5 MeV electron has a mass more than ten times its rest mass. It is evident that, for electrons, the change in mass with velocity is an important effect.

Similar data for protons is given in the last two columns. Since protons are some 1800 times as heavy as electrons, a proton with an energy equal to that of an electron will be traveling at a much smaller velocity and the change in mass with energy is not nearly as great.

1.15   EXPONENTIAL BEHAVIOR

Exponential behavior occurs in fields of study ranging from the social and economic sciences to the biological and physical sciences. It occurs whenever *the rate of change of a function is proportional to the function.* It can also be described in a slightly different way. *If a quantity changes by a certain factor in a given interval of time, then there will be exponential behavior if in any other equal interval of time it changes by the same factor.* It describes the growth of money in a bank account due to interest, the growth of populations, the growth of cells in tissue culture, the decay of radioactive isotopes, the killing of cells by radiation, and the attenuation of x ray beams in passing through matter. Since exponential behavior is so widespread, we will discuss it in detail here and develop the required mathematics using radioactive decay as our example.

**1.16   EXPONENTIAL DECAY OF A RADIOACTIVE
                    ISOTOPE—HALF-LIFE**

A radioactive source contains many atoms and there is no way to tell when a *given* atom will disintegrate. However, on the average, one can predict that in a given time, called the half-life, half the atoms will disintegrate. In the next half-life, one-half of the remaining atoms will decay. For example, if one had a source of radioactive gold (^{198}Au) with a half-life of 2.69 days, one could predict that if one started with 100×10^6 atoms, after 2.69 days there would be 50×10^6 remaining, after 5.38 days 25×10^6, after 8.07 days 12.5×10^6. The exponential decay of such a source is shown in Figure 1-4a.

The exponential decay curve of Figure 1-4a can be plotted in such a way to give a straight line. This is illustrated in Figure 1-4b, where the *same data* is plotted using semilog graph paper, in which the vertical scale is logarithmic while the horizontal scale is linear.

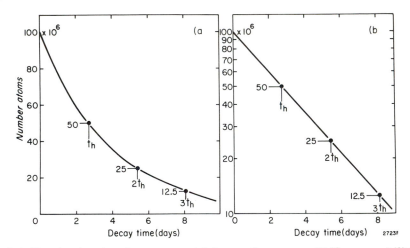

Figure 1-4. Graphs showing the exponential decay of a source of 10^8 atoms of ^{198}Au with half-life of 2.69 days. The vertical scale on the left is linear while the one on the right is logarithmic.

The student can show that on the logarithmic scale the distance from 100 to 50 is exactly the same as from 50 to 25 or, in fact, from any number N to N/2. When the decay of Figure 1-4a is plotted on semilog paper, a straight line must result because in 2.69 days the source decays from 100 to 50, in the next 2.69 days from 50 to 25. To plot such a decay on this type of paper, one merely needs to locate the 50% point at the half-life or the 25% point at two half-lives and draw in a straight line. For plotting such data, a number of types of semilog paper are available, known as single, double, triple cycle, etc. In single cycle paper the scale extends from 100 to 10 (or 10 to 1); in double cycle, from 100 to 10 to 1.0; and in triple cycle, from 100 to 10 to 1 to 0.1.

A mathematical relation between the number of atoms present and the elapsed time can be obtained as follows. Let t_h be the half-life and N_0 the number of atoms present initially. The number of atoms, N, present after any time, t, is given by:

$$N = \frac{N_0}{2^{t/t_h}} = N_0 \times 2^{-t/t_h} \qquad (1\text{-}22)$$

That this relation is correct can be verified by substituting $t = t_h$, $2t_h$, $3t_h$. The number, N, after these times is $N_0/2$, $N_0/4$, $N_0/8$ as expected. Equation 1-22 is easily evaluated for times that are integral numbers of half-lives. For other times evaluation is possible using a table of fractional powers of 2 and many calculators.

Example 1-8. Calculate the number of atoms of ^{198}Au ($t_h = 2.69$ days) after 7 days if initially there were 10^8 atoms present. Compare with the graphical solution of Figure 1-4b.

$$\text{Decay time (in units of half-lives)} = \frac{t}{t_h} = \frac{7}{2.69} = 2.60$$

We now determine with a calculator that $2^{2.60} = 6.06$

$$\therefore N = 10^8/6.06 = 1.65 \times 10^7 \text{ atoms, which checks with Figure 1-4.}$$

For the above example the graphical solution is quick and nearly as accurate, but if the decay time were very long, the mathematical method would probably be easier. As well as being able to do a precise calculation as above, it is important to be able to do approximate calculations quickly.

Example 1-9. Estimate the number of atoms present after 60 days if initially there were 10^8 gold 198 atoms in the source.

Number half-lives in 60 days $60/2.69 \approx 22$

In 10 half-lives decay factor $2^{10} = 1024 \approx 1000$
is almost exactly 1000 since

Decay factor for 22 half-lives $2 \times 2 \times 1000 \times 1000 = 4 \times 10^6$

Number atoms remaining $10^8/(4 \times 10^6) \approx 25$

There is nothing special about the use of powers of 2.0 in equation 1-22. In fact, from a mathematical point of view, there is some advantage in using powers of a special number called *e*. This number is the base of natural logarithms and has the value 2.718.

Using a calculator the student can show that $e^{0.693} = 2.00$ so that equation 1-22 can equally well be written:

$$N = N_0(2)^{-t/t_h} = N_0(e^{.693})^{-t/t_h} = N_0\, e^{-.693t/t_h} \qquad (1\text{-}23)$$

A plot of this expression will convince the reader that the two expressions, 1-22 and 1-23, are identical.

We now consider a more fundamental approach to exponential decay that introduces the base e naturally.

1-17   TRANSFORMATION CONSTANT

Suppose there are N atoms present at any time, t. In a short interval of time, Δt, a certain number, ΔN, of the atoms present will decay. The number, ΔN, that decay will be proportional to the number, N, present and to the interval of time, Δt. If twice as many atoms were present, we would expect twice the number of disintegrations. Also, if twice the interval of time were considered, we would expect twice the number of disintegrations. Symbolically these ideas may be written

$$\Delta N = -\lambda N \Delta t \quad \text{provided} \quad \lambda \Delta t \ll 1 \qquad (1\text{-}24)$$

where λ is a constant of proportionality called the transformation constant. The negative sign indicates that the number of atoms present is decreasing. Since N and ΔN have the same dimensions, λ must have dimensions of $(\text{time})^{-1}$.

This equation is strictly correct only if Δt is so small that $\lambda \Delta t \ll 1$, so that ΔN is very small compared to N, i.e. over the time interval, Δt, N remains essentially constant. If we make ΔN and Δt very small we refer to them as differentials, which are written dN and dt, and our equation becomes

$$dN = -\lambda N \, dt \qquad (1\text{-}25)$$

To solve this differential equation, using calculus, we separate the variables N and t to give $dN/N = -\lambda dt$ and then integrate to yield $\ln N = -\lambda t + C$ where $\ln N$ is the log of N to the base e and C is a constant of integration. If we assume that at $t = 0$ the number present is N_0, then substitution of these values in the above equation shows that $C = \ln N_0$. Our equation then becomes

$$\ln N - \ln N_0 = -\lambda t \qquad \text{or} \qquad \ln(N/N_0) = -\lambda t \qquad (1\text{-}26)$$

or $\qquad\qquad (N/N_0) = e^{-\lambda t} \qquad$ or $\qquad N = N_0 \, e^{-\lambda t}$

This equation is identical to equation 1-23 if

$$\lambda = \frac{0.693}{t_h} \qquad (1\text{-}27)$$

which is the important relation between the transformation constant and the half-life. A related concept we will discuss in greater detail in Chapter

3 is the mean or average lifetime of the atoms in the population. It is represented by t_a and is the reciprocal of λ.

$$t_a = \frac{1}{\lambda} = \frac{t_h}{.693} = 1.44\, t_h \qquad (1\text{-}28)$$

1.18 EXPONENTIAL GROWTH OF MONEY

The reader may feel that this mathematics has taken us a long way from reality. We will therefore discuss the exponential growth of money deposited in a bank at interest, a process everyone understands. Let V represent the value of a deposit at any time, t. The interest earned by this deposit in time, Δt, will be $+r\, V\, \Delta t$, where r is the interest rate expressed as a fraction rather than a percent. If the interest earned after each increment of time is added to the deposit, then the increase in the value of the deposit in time, Δt, will be

$$\Delta V = +r\, V\, \Delta t \qquad (1\text{-}29)$$

This equation is identical to equation 1-24 except for the positive sign, and leads to exponential growth rather than exponential decay. It is left to the reader to integrate this expression as in the last section to yield

$$V = V_o\, e^{+rt} \qquad (1\text{-}30)$$

This expression describing exponential growth is similar to equation 1-26 except for the positive sign on the exponential. The time taken for the investment to double is called the doubling time, t_d, and is simply

$$t_d = \frac{0.693}{r} \qquad (1\text{-}31)$$

exactly analogous to the relation $t_h = 0.693/\lambda$ involving the half-life.

Suppose, for example, that the interest rate were 10 percent per annum so that $r = 0.10\ \text{yr}^{-1}$. Equation 1-31 tells us that the doubling time is

$$t_d = 0.693/.10\ \text{yr}^{-1} = 6.93\ \text{yr}$$

Thus, at 10 percent per year, money will double every 6.93 years provided it is *compounded continuously.* For an investment compounded *annually,* the value of 1 after 1 year is 1.10, after 2 years $(1.10)^2$ and after 7 years $(1.10)^7 = 1.95$, so the doubling time is slightly over 7 years. Our calculation of 6.93 is based on ΔV and Δt of equation 1-29 both being very small, whereas the figure of 1.95 results from a calculation based on $\Delta t = 1$ year.

1.19   **EXPONENTIAL GROWTH OF CELLS**

Suppose a colony contains N cells at time t. The number of new cells that might be formed in time, Δt, should be proportional to N and Δt and could be expressed by

$$\Delta N = + \lambda N \Delta t \qquad (1\text{-}32)$$

where λ is a constant of proportionality. This equation is identical to equation 1-29, so its solution leads to

$$N = N_0\, e^{\lambda t} \quad \text{and} \quad \lambda = \frac{0.693}{t_d} \qquad (1\text{-}33)$$

where N_0 is the initial number of cells in the culture at time t, and t_d is the doubling time. Exponential growth is shown in Figure 1-5. After many doublings, the rate of growth of the culture usually slows down as space or the food supply is used up, and the cells eventually enter a stationary phase shown in Figure 1-5.

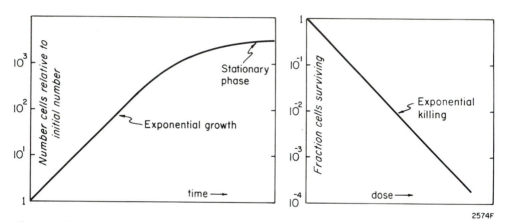

2574F

Figure 1-5. Graphs showing exponential growth of cells and exponential killing of cells.

1.20   **EXPONENTIAL KILLING OF CELLS**

Suppose a culture contains N cells. The number of cells killed, ΔN, by an increment of dose, ΔD, of radiation should be proportional to the number of cells present, N, and to ΔD, thus

$$\Delta N = - \lambda N \Delta D \qquad (1\text{-}34)$$

where λ is the constant of proportionality and the negative sign is used since cells are killed and ΔN is negative. This equation is similar to equation 1-24, and so leads to

$$N = N_0\, e^{-\lambda D} = N_0\, e^{-D/D_0} \qquad (1\text{-}35)$$

where D_0 is the mean lethal dose equal to $1/\lambda$ and analogous to the mean life described in section 1.17. Exponential killing is illustrated in Figure 1-5 and will be dealt with in greater detail in Chapter 17.

1.21   **EXPONENTIAL ATTENUATION**

Suppose a beam of N photons impinges on a thin layer, Δx, of some absorber. The change in the number of photons in the beam, ΔN, will be proportional to N and Δx and may be written

$$\Delta N = -\mu\ N\ \Delta x \tag{1-36}$$

where μ is the constant of proportionality called the *linear attenuation coefficient*. This equation is similar to equation 1-24, so the solution is

$$N = N_0 e^{-\mu x} \quad \text{where} \quad \mu = \frac{0.693}{x_h} \tag{1-37}$$

The quantity x_h is called the half-value thickness, or half-value layer. The reciprocal of μ is the mean range, x_a, which is the average distance a photon travels in the absorbing material before it interacts in a collision. The mean range, x_a, is exactly analogous to the mean lethal dose, D_0, of the last section or the mean life, t_a, of equation 1-28. Exponential attenuation will be discussed in greater detail in Chapters 5 and 6.

1.22   **SUMMARY OF EXPONENTIAL BEHAVIOR**

These examples should convince the reader of the importance of exponential behavior in nature. The ones with which we have dealt are summarized in Table 1-8. They are all described by the same differential equations of the following form:

exponential decay $dN = -\lambda N dt$
exponential growth $dN = +\lambda N dt$

Growth and decay are very different behaviors, but from a mathematical point of view, the equations describing them differ only in the sign of the proportionality constant. The integration of these equations yields $N = N_0 e^{-\lambda t}$ or $N_0 e^{+\lambda t}$ given in the last column of Table 1-8. The equations differ only in the sign of the exponent. The reciprocal of λ is given appropriate names such as mean life, mean lethal dose, and mean free path depending on the phenomena being described. A related constant, 0.693 times as large, is called the half-life, the doubling time, the lethal dose—50, or the half-value layer. Exponential growth or decay occur whenever the rate of change of a function is proportional to the function. It is left to the reader to find other examples of these phenomena.

TABLE 1-8
Examples of Exponential Behaviour

Process	Variable	Constant of Proportionality	Useful Relations		Usual Equation
Radioactive decay of atoms, N	time, t	transformation constant, λ	mean life, $t_a = 1/\lambda$	half-life, $t_h = .693/\lambda$	$N = N_0 e^{-\lambda t}$
Growth of investment, V	time, t	interest rate, r		doubling time, $t_d = .693/r$	$V = V_0 e^{+rt}$
Growth of pop. of cells, N	time, t	growth constant, λ		doubling time, $t_d = .693/\lambda$	$N = N_0 e^{+\lambda t}$
Killing of cells, N, by radiation	dose, D	killing constant, λ	mean lethal dose, $D_0 = 1/\lambda$	dose to kill 50%, $D_h = .693 D_0$	$N = N_0 e^{-D/D_0}$
Attenuation of a beam of photons, N	thickness, x	attenuation coefficient, μ	mean free path, $1/\mu$	half-value layer $x_h = .693/\mu$	$N = N_0 e^{-\mu x}$

PROBLEMS

It is essential that the student obtain a pocket calculator for this course. The calculator should be of the scientific type to allow calculations of exponentials, logarithms, and trigonometric functions. Problems marked with an asterisk (*) are more difficult.

1. A car accelerates at a rate of 5.0 km per hour per second. Express this acceleration in m s^{-2}.

2. A current of 1.0 μA flows into a condenser of capacity 100 nF for 5.0 s. Calculate the potential difference between the plates of the condenser.

3. A patient is given an x ray exposure of 200 R. Calculate this exposure in C kg^{-1}.

4. After a full course of treatment, a tumor received a dose of 4000 rads. Express this dose in grays, in MeV per g.

5. A source of cobalt 60 with half-life of 5.2 years has an activity of 1100 Ci. Express this activity in becquerels. Estimate the activity after 55 years.

6. Hydrogen in nature exists as a mixture of $^1_1$H and $^2_1$H with atomic masses of 1.007825 and 2.014102, respectively. These occur in relative abundance 99.985% and 0.015%. Calculate the atomic weight of hydrogen. Check your answer with Table 1-3.

7. Lithium in nature consists of two isotopes of atomic masses 6.01513 and 7.01601, with percentage abundances of 7.42% and 92.58%. Find the atomic weight. Check your answer with Table 1-3.

8. In the complete decay of 1000 atoms of $^{12}_5$B, how many beta particles will be released and how much energy as gamma rays? (See Fig. 1-3.)

9. A deuterium atom is made up of a proton (atomic mass 1.007276), an electron (atomic mass 0.000548), and a neutron (atomic mass 1.008665). The mass of the deuterium atom is 2.014102. Find the energy in MeV required to bring about the disintegration of the deuterium into hydrogen plus a neutron.

10. A certain radioactive material emits gamma rays with energy 1 MeV. Another sample of radioactive material emits gamma rays with energy 10 keV. If both of these emit the same amount of energy per unit time, compare their activities.

11. A radio station transmits at a frequency of 900 kHz. Find the wavelength of the radiation. Find the energy in electron volts of 1 quantum of such radiation.

12. Electromagnetic waves of length 10 cm are used in radar installations. Calculate the frequency of such radiation and the energy of 1 quantum of such radiation.

13. The eye is sensitive to yellow light with wavelength 550 nm. Find the frequency of such radiation and the energy in electron volts of 1 quantum of such radiation.

14. An x ray machine operates with a peak potential of 280,000 volts. Find the minimum wavelength of the radiation emitted by the x ray tube, and the frequency of this radiation.

15. Gamma rays from radium have energies up to 2.2 MeV. What is the wavelength in pm of 2.2 MeV radiation? The distance between adjacent atoms in a rock salt crystal is 281 pm. Can you see why the radiations from radium pass through a material such as rock salt as if it were transparent?

16. Determine the minimum wavelength of the radiation emitted from a 35 MeV linac.

17. A radio transmitter operates at 10 kW at 300 kHz. Find the number of quanta emitted per second.

18. What is the energy and wavelength of the radiation emitted from tungsten when an electron falls from the M to the K shell?

19. An antiproton is a proton with a negative charge. What energy would be emitted if a proton annihilated an antiproton?

20. An electron has a kinetic energy of 1 MeV. Find its *total* energy and hence m/m_0. Use equation 1-20 to determine its velocity relative to the velocity of light. Check your answer against Table 1-7.

*21. Show that when $v \ll c$, equation 1-21 reduces to K.E. $= m_0 v^2/2$.

22. A source of gold 198 with a half-life of 2.69 days has an initial activity of 5 Ci. Calculate the activity after 4.0 days. Express this activity in becquerels.

23. The two forms of equation 1-23 are identical. Prove this by showing that $2^{-x} = e^{-.693x}$ where x is any number.

24. The gamma rays from ^{60}Co have a half-value layer in lead of 1.1 cm. Estimate the thickness of lead required to attenuate such a beam by a factor of 10^6. What is the mean range of these photons in lead?

25. Cells grow with a doubling time of 20 hours. Assuming exponential growth, calculate the number of cells present after three days, starting with 10^3 cells. Plot on semilog paper.

26. A tumor containing 10^6 cells is inactivated by radiation with a mean lethal dose of $D_0 = 1.50$ Gy. Find the number of survivors after a dose of 45 Gy.

*27. From the definition of λ, the transformation constant, and the use of equation 1-24 calculate the *initial* number of disintegrations per second for the gold source described in Figure 1-4. Express this initial activity in bequerels and curies. Plot the decay of this activity as a function of time and show that the total number of disintegrations is 10^8.

28. Show by numerical integration that the area under the curve of Figure 1-4 is approximately 3.9×10^8 atom days. Since there were 10^8 atoms present initially this shows that the mean life is 3.9 days. This checks with $1/\lambda$.

*29. Calculate the value of one dollar compounded *monthly* at 10% per annum after 1 year. Compare this result with the value obtained when compounding is continuous.

30. What interest rate compounded continuously is required to double your money every 10 years?

31. A cell culture containing 10^8 cells has a doubling time of 10 hours. Find the number of cells "born" per s.

32. The half-life of gold 198 is 2.69 days. Calculate the transformation constant and the mean life.

*33. With your calculator determine 2^x, e^x, and 3^x for a few values of x between 0 and 4. Now determine the slope of these functions numerically. For example, the slope of e^x at x = 4 is about $(e^{4.1} - e^{3.9})/0.2$. Plot the functions and the slopes as a function of x. Observe that the slope of e^x is the same as e^x while the slope of 2^x is less than 2^x and slope of 3^x is greater than 3^x. *e^x is the only function whose derivative is equal to the function.*

34. Using the result from problem 33, differentiate the equation $N = N_0 e^{-\lambda t}$ with respect to time and show that you obtain the differential equation 1-25. This shows the integration performed in the final part of section 1.17 is correct.

35. Obtain a portable Geiger counter with speaker output so that individual pulses can be heard. Place this outside the room or down the corridor from a cobalt 60 unit. Observe the counting rate with the machine off. Turn on the cobalt unit and observe the quantum nature of radiation. By moving the detector behind wall barriers, demonstrate the extreme penetrating power of the radiations from cobalt.

36. Find at least two other examples of exponential behavior. Write down the differential equation and the integrated equation describing the phenomena.

Chapter **2**

THE PRODUCTION AND PROPERTIES
OF X RAYS

2.01　　　**THE X RAY TUBE AND SIMPLIFIED CIRCUIT**

X radiation is produced whenever a substance is bombarded by high speed electrons. All x ray tubes consist of a cathode and anode assembly (Fig. 2-1a), placed inside a glass envelope that has been evacuated. The cathode assembly consists of a filament of tungsten in the form of a coil placed in a shallow focusing cup (see Fig. 2-9). When this filament is heated to a white heat, electrons are "boiled" out of the surface of the tungsten. If, now, the anode is made positive with respect to the filament, these electrons will be attracted to the anode to constitute an electron current around the circuit in the anticlockwise direction. This is equivalent to a conventional current (the motion of positive charges) in the opposite direction. This tube current is measured by the milliammeter.

Because the space between anode and cathode is a high vacuum, the electrons do not collide with gas molecules in crossing the gap and so acquire very high velocities. When they are suddenly stopped in the anode, x rays are emitted in *all* directions as suggested by the arrows in Figure 2-1a. At least one-half of these are absorbed in the target itself; of the remaining portion, only those that emerge in the cone of the primary beam are useful. For the voltages used in diagnostic radiology, less than 1% of the energy carried by the electrons is converted to x rays and over 99% appears as heat and must be removed from the anode. The focusing cup is designed to concentrate the electrons on a small part of the anode, called the focal spot. The part of the anode where the electrons are focused is usually made of tungsten or a tungsten rhenium alloy (90% tungsten, 10% rhenium). The addition of rhenium to the tungsten makes the target tougher and less likely to crack under the severe stresses caused by heating.

To understand the operation of an x ray tube in a circuit, it is essential to know how the tube current depends upon the tube voltage for a given filament excitation. Figure 2-1b shows data for a typical diagnostic x ray tube. When a few kV are applied across the tube, the current is small due to *space charge* effects. Surrounding the filament is a cloud of electrons that tend to repel electrons back into the filament unless sufficient voltage is applied between anode and cathode to pull them away from the filament as fast as they are produced. This cloud of electrons is known as a

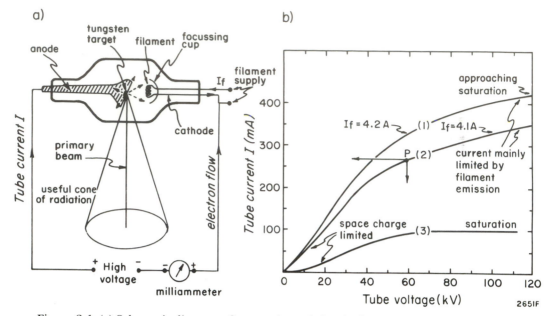

Figure 2-1. (a) Schematic diagram of x ray tube and circuit. (b) Tube current as a function of tube voltage: curves 1 and 2, Siemens B150 RGS tube. Curve 3, typical data for tube operating at a lower current.

space charge. As the kV is increased, the effects of the space charge are gradually overcome and the current increases until most of the electrons liberated in the filament are pulled to the anode. Finally, at still higher voltages the region of saturation is reached where all the liberated electrons are pulled to the anode. Most diagnostic x ray tubes operating at high currents are in the region (such as P in Fig. 2-1b) above the space charge limitations region and below the saturation region. Here the current is determined by *both* kV and filament emission. When tubes are operated at lower tube currents, as in fluoroscopy or in therapy, operation is near the saturation region and the tube current is determined only by filament emission (as illustrated by curve 3 in Fig. 2-1b).

Figure 2-1b shows that a 2.5% change in filament current (4.1 to 4.2 A) alters the tube current by 23% (325 to 410 mA) when excitation is at 100 kV. Hence, to achieve stability in the operation of an x ray tube, the current used to excite the filament must be carefully stabilized and controlled.

The shapes of the curves shown in Figure 2-1b depend upon many factors, including the distance between the anode-cathode assembly, the configuration of the focusing cup with respect to the filament, the focal spot size, and the filament temperature. These curves can be drastically altered by changing the potential of the focusing cup with respect to the filament. If the cup is made very negative with respect to the filament, the electron cloud is effectively contained in the cup, no current crosses the gap, and the tube is turned off. Some tubes are provided with an extra lead to this cup so that its potential can be altered at will. Such tubes, called grid-controlled tubes, are useful in certain procedures requiring rapid switching and short exposure times, on the order of milliseconds.

2.02   SELF-RECTIFIED X RAY CIRCUIT

The basic components of a self-rectified x ray circuit are shown in Figure 2-2. Power from a 220 V, 60 Hz line first excites an auto transformer, which consists of a single winding on an iron core. By moving the kV selector from contact point 1 to 30, any voltage between 0 and 220 V can be selected and read on the voltmeter V. When the switch (S) is closed, power from the auto transformer at the selected voltage energizes the primary of the step-up high tension transformer. The secondary of this transformer has perhaps 500 turns for each turn on the primary so that the voltage is stepped up by a factor of about 500. The secondary winding is usually broken at its center point and grounded, and a milliammeter to measure the tube current, I, is placed between the two portions of the winding. When the milliammeter is wired into the circuit this way, it is at ground potential and so can be placed at any convenient position on the control panel. The filament of the x ray tube is energized by about 10 V, which is obtained from an isolation step-down transformer. This transformer must be able to withstand a high voltage between the two windings since the primary is never more than 220 volts from ground while the secondary, which is connected to the filament, may be 100 kV or more above or below ground potential. The primary of this transformer is energized from a 220 V line through a rheostat or auto transformer, which can be adjusted to alter the temperature of the filament. Thus, the filament control determines the number of electrons "boiled" out of the filament, while the kV selector determines the maximum energy of the x rays that are generated.

Because the tube current also depends on tube voltage at high tube currents, the manufacturer usually supplies a series of kV and mA "positions" that may be selected by push-button on the control panel and that have been preset to give the selected kV and mA. For example, Figure 2-1b shows that to get 300 mA at 80 kV the filament current should be 4.1A, while to get the *same* current at 50 kV requires a filament excitation of 4.2A. Thus, for a 300 mA technique, the filament current would be automatically raised from 4.1 to 4.2 A when the kV selector is moved from 80 to 50. Tests should be carried out to insure that the controls have been set up properly so that the currents and voltages achieved correspond to the settings on the control panel.

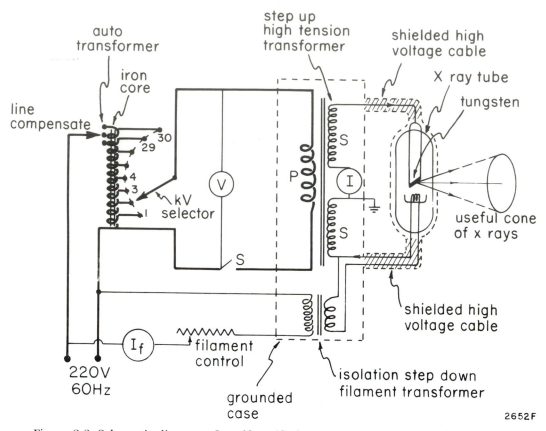

Figure 2-2. Schematic diagram of a self-rectified x ray generator connected to an x ray tube.

It is essential to make the unit independent of line voltage variations. This is done by supplying a line voltage compensator on the input of the auto transformer (as shown in Fig. 2-2). In newer units the contact point is automatically adjusted by a small motor as line fluctuations occur; in others, the adjustment must be carried out by the operator.

The high tension transformer and the isolation step-down transformer are together placed in a large grounded metal tank filled with oil. The oil prevents the electrical breakdown that would occur in or between parts of the circuit at different high voltages. The oil also acts as a heat transfer device to carry heat from the windings to the case. Power is carried from this tank to the x ray tube with high voltage shielded cables. The x ray tube is also mounted inside an oil-filled grounded container so that the whole system is surrounded by a grounded conductor (dotted line in Fig. 2-2) and so is shock proof. The x ray tube housing is made ray proof by the judicious use of lead, which allows x rays to emerge only in the direction of the useful cone of radiation.

Alternating Currents and Voltages

To understand the circuit of Figure 2-2, we must digress to discuss alternating currents and voltages. The nature of an alternating voltage is illustrated in Figure 2-3, where the voltage from a 60 Hz power line is plotted against the time. It is seen that the voltage increases from zero to

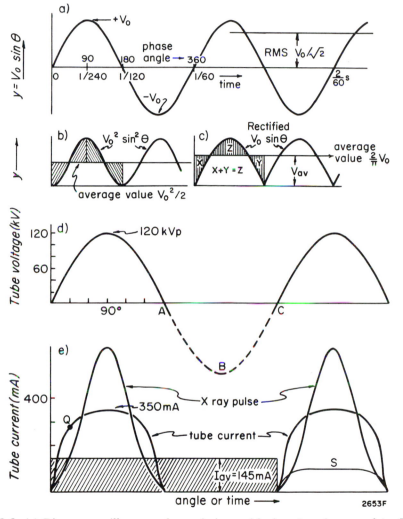

Figure 2-3. (a) Diagram to illustrate the variations with time (or phase angle) of an alternating voltage at 60 Hz. (b) Diagram to show that the RMS value is $V_0/\sqrt{2}$. (c) Diagram to illustrate that the average value of a sinusoidal rectified voltage (or current) is $2/\pi$ times the peak value. (d) High voltage from secondary of transformer with peak value of 120 kV. The inverse part of the cycle is ABC. (e) Tube current for the circuit of Figure 2-2 when the x ray tube has the characteristics of curve 2 of Figure 2-1b and the tube voltage is given by Figure 2-3d. The intensity of the resulting x ray pulse calculated assuming x ray production is proportional to IV^2 is also given. Curve S is the current pulse using the saturation curve 3 of Figure 2-1b.

the maximum value, V_0, falls to zero, increases in the negative direction to $-V_0$, and then returns to zero—all in 1/60 s. Instead of plotting the voltage as a function of time, it is sometimes convenient to use the phase angle, Θ, which increases from 0 to 360 degrees during the time for one cycle (1/60 s). Such a voltage can be represented by $V_0 \sin \Theta$. If such a voltage is applied to a D.C. voltmeter, no reading will be obtained because the moving coil of the voltmeter will first be deflected in one direction and then in the opposite direction, giving no net deflection. A reading can be obtained if the negative wave is suppressed or reversed in sign (rectified, as shown in Fig. 2-3c). The reading will now be the average value found by determining the height of the rectangle that includes the same area as the area under the pulsating curve. The reader can show either graphically or using calculus that when the negative wave is reversed in sign (as shown in Fig. 2-3c) V_{av} is given by:

$$V_{av} = \frac{2}{\pi} V_0 = 0.637\, V_0 \tag{2-1}$$

Another type of averaging gives the root mean square (RMS) value. It is found by squaring $V_0 \sin \Theta$, averaging the squared value to give $V_0^2/2$ (see Fig. 2-3b), and then taking the square root to yield $V_0/\sqrt{2}$. Thus

$$V_{RMS} = V_0/\sqrt{2} = .707\, V_0 \tag{2-2}$$

AC voltmeters or ammeters are usually calibrated to read RMS values. When one refers to a 110 volt line, this means the RMS value is 110 V, the peak value is $110 \sqrt{2} = 156$ V, and the average value is $(2/\pi) \times 156 = 99.0$ volts. RMS values are used so that 110 volts AC will produce the same energy dissipation in a resistor as 110 volts DC. This follows from the fact that since $P = VI = V^2/R$, the power developed over a cycle will be proportional to the average value of the square of the voltage.

Current Pulse in an X ray Circuit

We return now to the x ray circuit. Suppose the auto transformer is adjusted so that the maximum voltage from the high tension transformer is 120 kV_p (p refers to peak value). The variation with time is shown in Figure 2-3d. Now, although the x ray tube of Figure 2-2 is excited by an alternating voltage, the current through the tube can flow only when the anode is positive with respect to the cathode. Hence, the current through the tube will be as indicated in Figure 2-3e and will consist of a series of pulses in one direction that last for 1/120 s and that are repeated 60 times per s.

The shape of the pulse may be obtained from the tube characteristics of Figure 2-1b. We illustrate this using curve 2 of Figure 2-1b. At the phase angle of 30° the high tension transformer is producing 120 kV $\times$

sin 30° = 60 kV (see also Fig. 2-3d), which gives a current of 270 mA
(see point P on Fig. 2-1b). This locates point Q on Figure 2-3e. Calculations for a few points give the current pulse of Figure 2-3e. It should be
noted that it is *not* sinusoidal. The milliammeter in the tube circuit will
read some average value, I_{av}, chosen so that the area of the rectangle is
equal to the area under the hump-shaped curve. The reader can show
graphically that, for this example, $I_{av} \approx 145$ mA while the peak current is
350 mA. The ratio of peak-to-average current will depend in a complex
way on the tube characteristics and the wave form of the high tension
transformer. If we use in our calculations curve 3 of Figure 2-1b, which
shows saturation, then we obtain the flat-topped current pulse S of
Figure 2-3e. The shape of current pulses usually lie between these two
extremes.

Since the current through the tube occurs in pulses, x rays are also
produced in pulses. X rays are produced with greatest efficiency when a
large voltage is applied, hence the x ray pulse will tend to be sharply
peaked at the center of each conducting cycle as shown in Figure 2-3e,
which was plotted assuming that x ray production is proportional to
IV^2.

2.03   **RECTIFICATION**

Under electron bombardment, the target of an x ray tube may become
hot enough to emit electrons in the same way as does the filament. If this
happens, electrons will flow from anode to cathode during the inverse
cycle ABC of Figure 2-3d, and the delicate filament will be destroyed by
electron bombardment. To prevent this, rectifiers must be placed in the
circuit to act like a switch to block the current on the inverse cycle.

Rectifiers for x ray applications are usually made of silicon. The silicon
rectifier consists of a wafer of silicon (see insert to Fig. 2-4) into which
are introduced impurities to make p and n type silicon. The "p type"
junction is made by introducing a small amount of an impurity such as
indium into the silicon, making it into an electron acceptor, while the n
junction is made by adding an impurity such as arsenic to make the silicon into an electron donor. This device conducts electrons from n to p or
current in the conventional sense from p to n. Such a rectifier is represented by an arrow directed against a plate as indicated. The arrow indicates the direction of conventional current flow.

The electrical characteristics of the silicon rectifier are shown in Figure
2-4. When p is made positive with respect to n, the device starts to conduct quite suddenly at about 0.6 volts, the current rising rapidly to about
1000 mA at about 0.9 V. When the voltage is reversed, practically no conduction occurs until about 470 V is applied, and then a reverse current
of a few μA starts to flow. If the reverse voltage is increased beyond about

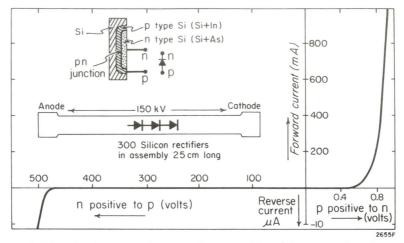

Figure 2-4. Schematic diagram of a p,n silicon rectifier. The operating characteristics are for the MR2272, a typical silicon rectifier. Note that the voltage and current scales are different for the forward and reverse directions. In the insert is shown a Machlett rectifier, which consists of some 300 rectifiers in series in a tube 25 cm long and capable of withstanding an inverse voltage of 150 kV.

550 V, the reverse current becomes excessive and would damage the device. Since each rectifier will stand a reverse voltage of about 500 V, 300 of these in series are required for 150 kV. The 300 rectifiers can be mounted in a tube some 2 cm in diameter and 25 cm long, as illustrated in Figure 2-4. They are immersed in the oil bath with the high tension transformer. They are so simple to use that circuits using up to 12 rectifier stacks (section 2.04) are feasible.

HALF-WAVE AND FULL-WAVE RECTIFICATION: Rectifiers may be used in many different configurations. The ones in most common use are shown in Figures 2-5 and 2-6. Figure 2-5a shows a half-wave rectifier circuit using two rectifier stacks with the center point of the secondary winding grounded. The anode then goes only to $+V_p/2$ at the peak of the conducting cycle and the cathode to $-V_p/2$, where V_p is the peak voltage of the transformer. In principle, one really requires only one rectifier, but with two the circuit is symmetric, and each has to withstand only half the voltage, V_p. The tube voltage, tube current, and x ray pulse are shown as a function of time in Figure 2-5a. These have exactly the same appearance as Figure 2-3d obtained using *self*-rectification, and in fact the two circuits would have identical behavior as long as the anode of the x ray tube did not get hot enough to emit electrons. The discontinuous nature of the x ray yield causes no serious trouble in a therapy machine, but in a diagnostic machine it means that the tube is inoperative at least half the time. This means that exposures must be twice as long to get the same x ray flux. This increases the chance of organ motion during the exposure with a consequent loss of diagnostic information.

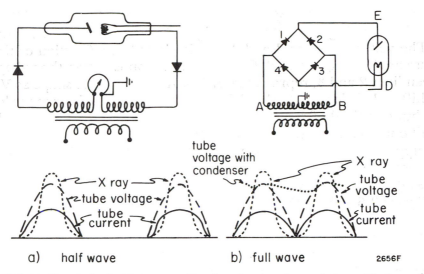

Figure 2-5. (a) Circuit for half wave rectification showing the variation with time of the current through the tube, the voltage across the tube, and the x ray flux. (b) Circuit for full wave rectification with appropriate wave forms. The dotted line in b is the tube voltage when a condenser is placed across the x ray tube between D and E.

To produce x rays *every* half cycle, four rectifiers can be connected as in Figure 2-5b. The rectifiers are arranged to conduct in the directions indicated. When the end A of the transformer swings positive, the current flows in series through rectifier 1, the x ray tube, rectifier 3, and back to the negative end B of the transformer. Rectifiers 2 and 4 do not conduct during this half cycle. On the next half cycle, when B swings positive, the current flows through rectifier 2, the x ray tube, rectifier 4, and back to A, which is now the negative end of the transformer. The current therefore flows through the x ray tube every half cycle, as illustrated in Figure 2-5b, giving an x ray pulse every 1/120 s. This is called full-wave rectification.

If a condenser C is placed across the terminals E D of the x ray tube, sufficient charge may be stored on it to maintain almost a constant voltage to the x ray tube (as illustrated in Fig. 2-5b). The charging current to this condenser only flows when the voltage of the transformer exceeds the voltage across the condenser, so the current wave is a large short pulse each half cycle (not shown in Fig. 2-5c). This situation may be present when small tube currents are used in fluoroscopy, the capacity, C, being supplied by the distributed capacity of the high voltage cables.

2.04   **THREE PHASE UNITS**

Delivering enough x ray flux in a very short time so that patient motion can be frozen requires the use of three phase power and powerful three phase x ray generators. The power line to the unit now consists of three wires, between *any two of which* there exists some 380 volts, 440 V, or 510 V depending on local supply. Figure 2-6a shows the three lines, 1, 2, 3. The voltage between 1 and 2, V_{12}, is plotted as a function of time or phase angle in Figure 2-6d. On the same graph is shown the voltage between lines 2 and 3, represented by V_{23}. It has the same shape as V_{12} but is shifted 120 degrees to the right and thus takes on the same values as V_{12} but one-third of a cycle later. Similarly, V_{31} is shifted in phase by an additional 120 degrees with respect to V_{12}.

Suppose now such a 3-phase power line is used to excite an x ray unit. We now require a step-up transformer with *three separate windings* and *three separate iron cores.* The primary of this special transformer is shown in Figure 2-6a where the three windings are labelled A, B, C; the corresponding secondary windings A', B', and C' are shown in Figure 2-6b. The configuration of the primary looks like a delta (Δ) and is called a delta connection, while the secondary configuration is called a Y or star connection. The Y connection in the secondary is convenient because the common junction point, G, can be grounded as shown. We now connect each of the "high" ends of A', B', and C' to the x ray tube with a pair of rectifiers with the polarities shown in Figure 2-6b. This completes the circuit.

If the three phases are properly matched, the peak values of V_{12}, V_{23}, and V_{31} will all be the same, and if the three transformers are identical then the voltages developed across A', B', and C' will also be the same. Since one end of each of these windings is grounded, the potentials of points D, E, and F will vary with time in exactly the same way as V_{12}, V_{23}, and V_{31} so the graphs of Figure 2-6d can equally well represent the potentials V_D, V_E, V_F. Let the peak value of these three voltages be V_p.

Consider now the instant of time when point D of Figure 2-6b reaches its first voltage maximum (point P of Fig. 2-6d). At this instant, E and F will be at the same negative potential (point Q), with a value exactly one-half that of P, so the total voltage between D and E or D and F is $V_p + V_p/2 = 1.5\ V_p$. Current will thus flow from G, through A' to D, through rectifier 1, through the x ray tube, then divide so that half goes through rectifier 5 to E and back to G and the other half through rectifier 6 to F and back to G. At a phase angle 30° later, D will have dropped to $V_p \sin 60°$ (point P') and Q will have gone more negative, to $-V_p \sin 60°$ (point Q'), so the net voltage across the tube is $2\ V_p \sin 60° = 1.73\ V_p$. At this instant current will flow from G to D, through rectifier 1, the x ray tube, through rectifier 6 to F, and through winding C' to G while no current will flow through rectifier 5 and winding B'. At instant P'', the voltage P''Q'' developed by the circuit again has the value of 1.5 V_p. Now rectifiers 1 and 2 are conducting equally and the full current is passing through rectifier 6.

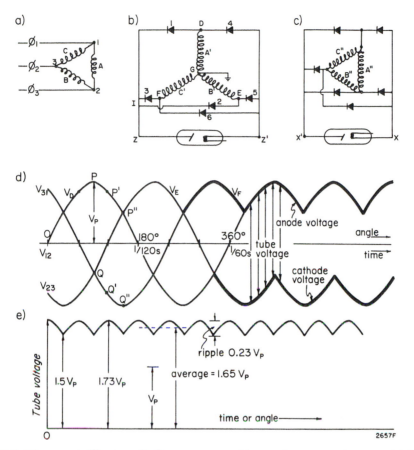

Figure 2-6. Diagram to illustrate 3 phase power and its use in x ray generators. (a) Three phase power line 1,2,3 connected to three primary windings A, B, C in a delta configuration. (b) Connections of the secondaries A', B', C' in Y configuration to an x ray tube using 6 rectifiers giving a "6 pulse" system. (c) Secondaries A'', B'', C'', connected in a delta configuration to also give a 6 pulse system. (d) Wave forms for either V_{12}, V_{23}, V_{31}, or the voltages on D, E, and F, relative to ground. (e) Tube voltage, that is the voltage across ZZ', as a function of time.

The anode voltage varies with time according to the heavy upper contour of Figure 2-6d, while the cathode voltage follows the heavy lower contour. The distance between these contours (illustrated in Fig. 2-6d and plotted in Fig. 2-6e) is the voltage applied to the tube. It varies between 1.73 V_p and 1.5 V_p, where V_p is the peak voltage generated by one of the secondary windings. The output has a ripple of .23 V_p. The student may show that the average output voltage is 1.65 V_p (see Fig. 2-6e) so that the percentage ripple is 14%. In this analysis, we have neglected the effects of any capacity. The capacity of high voltage cables will tend to smooth out some of the ripple. Because there are 6 peaks per cycle, this system is often called "6 point rectification" or a 6 pulse system. It should be noted from Figure 2-6e that that maximum values occur at phase angles of 0, 60, 120, etc. degrees and the minimum values at 30, 90, 150, etc. degrees.

SECONDARIES CONNECTED IN A DELTA CONFIGURATION: The secondaries may also be arranged in a delta connection, as shown in Figure 2-6c. The reader may show that the voltage across the tube reaches a maximum value of V_p at angles of 30, 90, 150, etc. degrees and a minimum value of $(\sqrt{3}/2)V_p = 0.866\ V_p$ at 0, 60, 120, 180, etc. degrees. The average value is $0.955\ V_p$ and the ripple $0.134\ V_p$, again about 14%. This delta arrangement yields 6 point rectification similar to the Y connection, but the phase angle at which the maxima and minima occur are now shifted 30° from where they were with the Y connection, which is important in 12 pulse systems. The Y connection is a little more convenient than the Δ connection because the common point of the secondaries may be grounded and the voltages at the tube are a little higher.

3 PHASE 12 RECTIFIER SYSTEM (12 PULSE SYSTEM): Suppose we arrange the x ray transformer with *two* independent sets of secondary windings on each of the three primaries so we are using the three circuits a, b, and c of Figure 2-6. Remove the ground from G and join x' and z' together and to ground and connect the x ray tube between z and x. The anode of the x ray tube will follow the voltage shown in Figure 2-6e, while the cathode will follow a somewhat similar voltage function with 6 pulses per second but shifted 30° in phase. The net voltage across the tube will thus exhibit 12 peaks and 12 minima per cycle and will show very little ripple. For further details see problem 13.

2.05   **ANODE AND CATHODE STRUCTURES**

X ray tubes take many different forms depending on the purpose for which they are designed. Of interest to us are diagnostic and therapy tubes.

Diagnostic X ray Tubes

Diagnostic x ray tubes are designed to produce a sharp shadow picture of a part of the patient. Even if the patient is completely immobilized, some physiological motion is always present due to respiration and heart motion. In order then that the picture be sharp, the x rays must come from a "point source" and exposure must be short enough to freeze the motion. A "point source" and "very short exposure" are, however, incompatible since they imply an infinite electron flux concentrated on zero area of the target, which would destroy it. X ray tube manufacturers have found a number of ways to spread the electrons over a large area of the target and yet make the x rays *appear* to come from a much smaller one.

In the **line focus tube** (Fig. 2-7a) the electrons are made to strike an area on the sloping target of length ab and width cd. Length cd is made

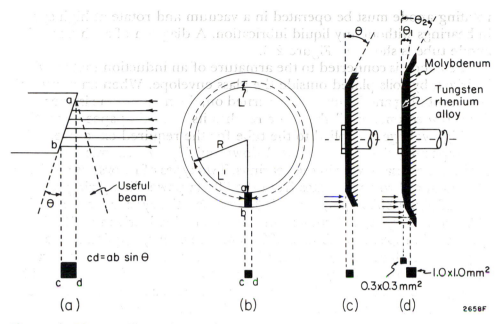

Figure 2-7. Diagrams illustrating anode construction and focal spots. (a) Line focus fixed anode. (b) Line focus rotating anode, viewed from the end. (c) Line focus rotating anode viewed from the side. (d) Alternative arrangement of rotating anode using two separate "tracks" at different angles as in the Siemens "Biangulix" series.

equal to ab sin Θ, so that when viewed from below, this area will appear as a square of dimensions cd × cd. Thus, the x rays will appear to come from a small area, whereas the electrons bombard a relatively large area of the target. The gain (actual area/apparent area) obtained in this way depends on the slope of the target. For example, if $\Theta = 16°$ and cd = 2 mm then ab = cd/sin Θ = 7.3 mm. In such a tube, the electrons bombard an area of 7.3 mm × 2 mm while the x rays appear to come from an area of 2 mm × 2 mm, yielding a gain of 3.6. If Θ is made smaller the gain may be increased but the angular width of the useful cone of radiation is correspondingly reduced. Diagnostic tubes have target angles between 16° and 6°. Targets at 6° are used for special techniques such as angiography that need a small focal spot, relatively heavy loading, but only a small field.

The **rotating anode** tube illustrated in Figure 2-7b,c, was developed to increase the possible loading still more by rapidly spinning the target during the exposure. The electrons then bombard a region of height ab and a length that may range from a value such as L′ up to L = $2\pi R$ depending on the time of the exposure, yet the x rays always *appear* to come from a focal spot of area cd × cd. With this arrangement a large increase in loading can be achieved. The construction of such a rotating anode is a remarkable technological development since the white hot rotating anode must be operated in a vacuum and rotate at high speeds in bearings without any liquid lubrication. A diagram of such a rotating anode tube is shown in Figure 2-8.

The anode is connected to the armature of an induction motor, which is driven by coils placed outside the glass envelope. When an x ray unit with a rotating anode tube is first turned on, the motor alone is energized for a few seconds until the rotor reaches its operating speed and then the high voltage is applied to the tube for the required exposure. After the exposure, the rotor is slowed down quickly by dynamic braking to avoid unnecessary wear in the bearings. Two types of rotors are available. The standard rotor operates from the 60 Hz power line giving rotation rates of about 3000 rpm, about 15% less than the synchronous speed of 3600 rpm. High speed rotors can also be obtained driven at 180 Hz to give rotation speeds of about 9,000 rpm. The energy applied to the driving coils produces eddy currents in the rotor on both the acceleration and the deceleration cycles, which causes heating of the rotor. This energy amounts to about 3×10^3 J per start-stop sequence and must be taken into account in energy dissipation calculations when many exposures are taken in sequence and the rotor is stopped between them.

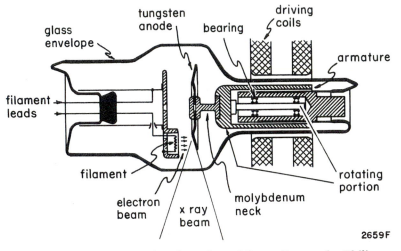

Figure 2-8. Rotating anode tube, adapted from diagram by Philips.

To increase the versatility of x ray tubes, they are usually fitted with two filaments in two cathode structures as illustrated in Figure 2-9c. One filament is designed to focus the electrons on a large area of the anode and is used when the tube must be loaded heavily. The second filament, a much finer one, is used to focus the electrons on a small part of the target and is used when high resolution is required and loading is not a problem. Both filaments should focus the electrons on the same part of

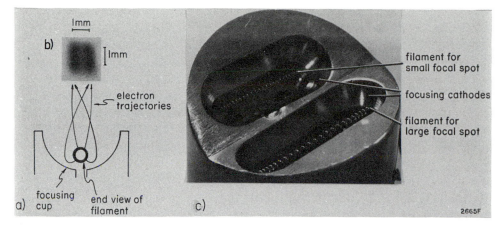

Figure 2-9. (a) Schematic diagram of filament in its focusing cup showing the electron trajectories and the way they are focused into two "lines" on the target. (b) Pinhole picture of the focal spot of a tube, which the manufacturer claimed was a 1.0×1.0 mm^2 spot. In actual fact it is ~1.5×1.7 mm^2. (c) Photograph of the cathode assembly of a double focus tube.

the anode so that the focal spot is centered at the same point in space for both modes of operation of the tube. The user usually has a choice of two possible focal spots on nearly all line focus and rotating anode tubes.

In a similar way, some manufacturers supply rotating anodes with two angles (Θ_1 and Θ_2 shown in Fig. 2-7d). The smaller angle is used with the smaller focal spot. Most anodes today are made using a tungsten rhenium alloy (90 : 10) bonded to a molybdenum disc (as shown in Fig. 2-7). Such an alloy resists electron bombardment better than pure tungsten and so has a much longer useful life. With use, all tubes deteriorate because of pitting due to the electron bombardment. This pitting reduces the x ray yield and changes the spectral distribution, for x rays produced at the bottom of a "hole" may be partially filtered and shielded from the patient by the "projections" around the "hole." The output of a tube may sometimes drop to half its initial value before failing due to other causes such as internal sparking or filament destruction. *A pitted anode will affect the electric field between cathode and anode and so alter the size of the focal spot.*

In Figure 2-7 the focal spot was pictured as being a rectangular area that uniformly emitted x radiation. This would be the situation if a uniform flux of electrons impinged on each part of the focal spot and this flux dropped to zero at the periphery of the rectangular area. In an actual situation the spot looks more like two lines, as shown in Figure 2-9b, which shows a pinhole picture of the spot of a tube taken with its own radiation (see Chapter 16). Moores and Brubacher (M1) have studied the shape of the focal spot as a function of the position of the filament in its focusing cup. If this is adjusted to make the spot as small as possible, the electron beam is focused into two lines on the target (as shown in Fig.

2-9b). The electron trajectories are shown for the optimum setting. These lines on the target can create artifacts by making a single object look double (see T1).

Stray or "nonfocal" radiation is a problem in all x ray tubes. This arises from the bombardment by stray electrons of parts of the tube other than the focal spot. To minimize this, some anodes are covered with a thin layer of carbon except for the actual target area. Since the yield of x rays depends upon Z^2 (see section 2.10) the x rays produced in the carbon areas by stray electrons will be minimized.

X ray Tubes for Radiotherapy

In a therapy tube, the instantaneous energy input is small (about 1/10) compared with a diagnostic tube but the average energy input over a long time is some 10 times as great. In a therapy tube the focal spot may be large, so there is no difficulty in designing the anode to handle the instantaneous power input without the use of a rotating anode but now heat must be removed continuously from the target through the circulation of cooled oil.

The simple anode construction of Figure 2-7a is not suitable when the bombarding electrons have energies greater than 200 keV because of the phenomenon of secondary emission. When high energy electrons hit the target, secondary electrons, some with substantial energy, are ejected and some of these may reach the glass envelope where an electrostatic charge is built up. These may produce enough field distortion to interfere with the focusing of the electrons on the target. Furthermore, when these electrons are stopped by the glass or some other part of the tube, x rays are produced. These "off target" x rays may be very troublesome because they make it difficult to define a sharp x ray beam. The problems of secondary emission may be largely overcome using a *hooded anode* tube shown in Figure 2-10. The target is now mounted at the bottom of a hollow tube in the anode. The high energy electrons enter this anode and travel without further acceleration until they strike the target, where they produce x rays. The secondary electrons produced at the target will be intercepted by the copper portion of the hooded anode and will not reach the glass envelope. On striking the copper hood, some x rays will be produced, but their intensity will be small compared with those produced in the tungsten target because of the lower atomic number (copper $Z = 29$; tungsten $Z = 74$). These x rays will be largely absorbed by a sleeve of tungsten that surrounds the copper. The useful beam emerges through a thin window in the hooded anode.

Special tubes have been designed for special purposes. In the treatment of skin conditions, use is often made of an x ray tube operating at relatively low voltage and at a very short distance from target to skin. In

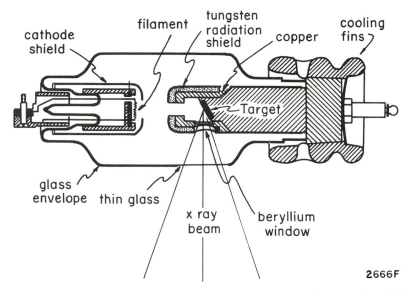

Figure 2-10. Hooded anode therapy tube, adapted from diagram by Philips.

the Chaoul tube or a contact tube, the anode is made hollow and very thin and is placed almost in contact with the skin. Electrons from the heated filament bombard the inside of this anode, producing x rays that are transmitted through the target to the skin. With such a configuration, the falling off of dose with increase in distance from the anode is very rapid, so that healthy tissues below the surface of the skin are protected. Even less penetrating radiations generated at 5 to 10 kV are sometimes used by dermatologists and are known as Grenz rays.

2.06   RATINGS OF DIAGNOSTIC TUBES

The manufacturer supplies rating charts for a given x ray tube for the common conditions (single phase, 3 phase 6 pulse, 3 phase 12 pulse, normal rotor, high speed rotor, etc.) under which it may be used. These must be understood and used if the equipment is to be employed properly. First, the focal spot must not be loaded beyond a certain power input. Second, the anode must not be loaded by successive exposures beyond a certain limit, and finally the housing must not be expected to dissipate its energy at rates beyond a certain value. We will discuss each of these limitations in turn and discuss them with reference to a Machlett Dynamax 69 rotating anode tube. Before proceeding with this it is important to get some real appreciation of the heat developed and the temperature rises that may occur in the target during an exposure.

Example 2-1. Calculate the rise in temperature of a rotating anode after an exposure of 100 mA for 2 s at constant potential of 100 kV. As-

sume the target to have a mass of 500 g and the surface area of the
bombarded region to be 30 cm² (L = 30 cm, ab = 1 cm of Fig. 2-7b); take
the density of tungsten to be 19.3 g/cm³ and specific heat 0.03 cal g⁻¹
°C⁻¹. Perform the calculations for two limiting conditions: (a) assume the
heat instantly distributes itself over the whole of the anode and none is
lost by heat transfer; (b) assume no heat escapes from the immediate area
of the bombarded region but is concentrated to a depth of 1 mm under
the bombarded area.

Energy input $= 100 \times 10^3 \text{ V} \times 0.1 \text{ A} \times 2 \text{ s}$
(Table 1-1, Eq. 1-9) $= 2 \times 10^4 \text{ J}$

Heat input to anode $= 2 \times 10^4 \text{ J} = \dfrac{2 \times 10^4}{4.18} \text{ cal} \approx 5 \times 10^3 \text{ cal}$
(4.18 J = 1 calorie)

Thermal capacity of $= 500 \text{ g} \times 0.03 \text{ cal g}^{-1} \text{ °C}^{-1}$
anode $= 15 \text{ cal °C}^{-1}$

(a) Rise in temperature $\dfrac{5 \times 10^3 \text{ cal}}{15 \text{ cal °C}^{-1}} = 330 \text{ °C}$
of anode

(b) Mass of bombarded $= 30 \times 0.1 \text{ cm}^3 \times 19.3 \text{ g cm}^{-3} = 58 \text{ g}$
volume

Rise in temperature $= \dfrac{5 \times 10^3 \text{ cal}}{58 \text{ g} \times 0.03 \text{ cal g}^{-1}\text{C}^{\circ-1}} = 2900 \text{ °C}$

This is close to the melting point of tungsten, 3400 °C, so the target
would be white hot and on the point of vaporization. Certainly such a
target would emit a copious supply of electrons, underscoring the need
for rectification.

The calculations of temperature rise just performed are very crude,
since we have taken no account of heat losses by conduction or by radiation, both of which increase rapidly as the target area starts to get hot.
They do suggest, however, that there will be a limit to the local loading
of the focal spot area.

FOCAL SPOT LOADING: For a given focal spot there is a maximum power
input that can be tolerated before the tungsten at the spot is melted. It
will depend upon the size of spot, the anode angle, the speed of rotation
of the anode, the type of rectification, and the type of power supply, i.e.
whether it is 3 phase or single phase. Figure 2-11 shows data for a Machlett Dynamax 69, selected to illustrate some of the principles involved.
The combination of current and kilovoltage in a given exposure must
lie to the left of the appropriate curve of Figure 2-11. For example, using
a tube current of 300 mA and 110 kV$_p$ any exposure up to 0.036 s (point
P) can be used with single phase or 0.2 s (point Q) with 3 phase using a
high speed rotor. If a low speed rotor is employed, the maximum voltage

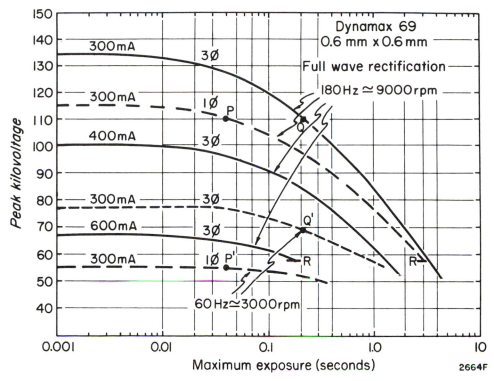

Figure 2-11. Curves giving the maximum kV_p for a given exposure for a Machlett Dynamax 69 under a number of different excitation conditions. Focal spot 0.6 mm × 0.6 mm, full wave rectification. Data for single exposures.

permissible for the above exposures at 300 mA are about 55 kV_p for single phase (point P′) and 69 kV_p for 3 phase (point Q′).

From this example we see the great advantages of 3 phase power and the improvement achieved by the use of a high speed rotor. When the exposure is less than about 0.01 s, the curves of Figure 2-11 become essentially flat—as might be expected since the time for 1 rotation at 9000 rpm is about 0.007 s. This means that for times up to 0.007 s only unheated target will come under electron bombardment during the exposure. For exposures longer than the time of rotation, the peak kilovoltage must be reduced since heated target is now bombarded for the second (or more) time. For exposures of ~0.01 s, we would expect the current and the kilovoltage would be related in such a way that the power input is constant.

That this is indeed the case can be seen from Table 2-1. In the first two columns we obtain from Figure 2-11 the current and peak voltage for short exposures at 3 phase with the high speed rotor. The product of current in mA and voltage in kV gives the power in watts as shown in the third column. It is constant and equal to 40 kW.

TABLE 2-1

Current (mA)	Peak Voltage (kV$_p$)	Power (kV$_p$A or kW)
300	134	40.2
400	100	40.0
600	67	40.2

This power rating of 40 kW is determined by the fundamental properties of the target material and its ability to get rid of its heat energy.
Energy developed in the focal spot area is lost by radiation to the walls
of the tube and by conduction to the rest of the anode. The two processes are about equally effective. The power rating will depend on the
size of the focal spot.

The curves of Figure 2-11 are somewhat confusing, since a number of
conditions are presented on the one graph. In an x ray department one
would display only one set of data for the particular generator for each
of the two focal spots available in the tube. Such a set of curves would
show some curves ending at R on horizontal lines (as shown in Fig. 2-11).
At such points there is a restriction for another reason. For example,
below 58 kV$_p$ a current of 300 mA on single phase cannot be obtained
from the tube without heating the filament beyond its allowed maximum
value.

ANODE COOLING: From the data given above, one can determine the
maximum exposure for a given set of conditions. We now inquire into
the *number* of exposures that may be given in sequence. To do this we
need an *easy* way to calculate the energy deposited in the target from the
settings on the machine. The three parameters that can be read from the
control panel are the *average tube current in mA*, the *peak voltage in kV*,
and the *exposure time in seconds*. The product of these three factors is called
a heat unit (HU) and was defined originally for a single phase full-wave
circuit. In such a circuit the current and voltage are *not* constant during
the cycle but vary with time (as shown in Fig. 2-3c). The *energy deposited
in joules will be less than HU* by some factor, f, which will depend on the
tube characteristics and the wave forms of the current and voltage pulse.
For single phase full-wave rectification the factor, f, is about 0.75,* hence

$$\text{Energy deposited for single phase, full-wave} \qquad (2\text{-}3)$$
$$= \text{f} \times \text{HU} = 0.75 \text{ HU joules}$$

Now, consider 3 phase, 6 or 12 pulse systems. In these, the current
is almost constant with time and equal to the mA setting, and the voltage
across the tube is also essentially constant and equal to the kV$_p$ setting.

---

*The reader may use the data of Figure 2-3e to calculate the product of V and I as a function of time
and by taking the area under this curve obtain the energy input. If the circuit gave full-wave rectification, the factor, f, for this example is 0.71.

Hence, the energy input in HU is about $1/0.75 \approx 1.35$ times as great as it was for single phase. For 3 phase, 6 or 12 pulse systems we calculate the heat input thus:

$$\text{HU for 3 phase, 6 or 12 pulse systems} = \qquad (2\text{-}4)$$
$$1.35 \times \text{voltage (kV)} \times \text{current (mA)} \times \text{time (s)}$$

With this rather arbitrary definition of the HU, the energy in joules is 0.75 HU for either single or 3 phase systems.

Example 2-2. A tube is given 10 exposures each for 2.0 s at 150 mA and 100 kV_p. Determine the heat units and energy deposited in the target for (a) a single phase full-wave system and (b) a three phase 6 pulse system:

(a) Energy deposited $= 100 \times 150 \times 2 \times 10 = 3 \times 10^5$ HU

$$= 0.75 \times 3 \times 10^5 \text{ HU} = 2.2 \times 10^5 \text{ J}$$

(b) Energy deposited $= 1.35 \times 100 \times 150 \times 2 \times 10 = 4 \times 10^5$ HU

$$= 0.75 \times 4 \times 10^5 \text{ HU} = 3 \times 10^5 \text{ J}$$

The heat unit is an unsatisfactory and unnecessary unit and should be replaced by the joule. Unfortunately, the practicing radiologist is forced to use it since the manufacturers give the thermal characteristics of anodes and tube housings in terms of it. The user should be sure that any heat unit calculation he may make is done in the way specified by the manufacturer, otherwise the charts may not apply. More standardization in this field is necessary.

The dissipation of energy from the anode and from the housing of the tube is a complex problem depending on many factors. Figure 2-12a shows important data dealing with heat dissipation problems related to the anode. For example, when the heat input is 1000 HU/s the energy stored in the anode after 8 minutes is about 2.1×10^5 HU. The actual input of energy is of course $1000 \times 8 \times 60 = 4.8 \times 10^5$ HU. The difference is due to the fact that the anode loses heat during the exposure. The cooling of the anode is described by the cooling curve whose maximum slope is 1250 HU/s. The maximum rate of heat loss occurs when the anode is at its maximum temperature, which will be attained when the heat *stored* in the anode is 3×10^5 HU.

Heat transfer from the tube housing is also important and is illustrated in Figure 2-12b. The housing can store 15×10^5 HU and can dissipate heat at the maximum rate of 600 HU/s with air circulation. Although the anode can in fact dissipate energy at twice the rate of the housing, in continuous operation the housing becomes the limiting component. These ideas are illustrated by an example.

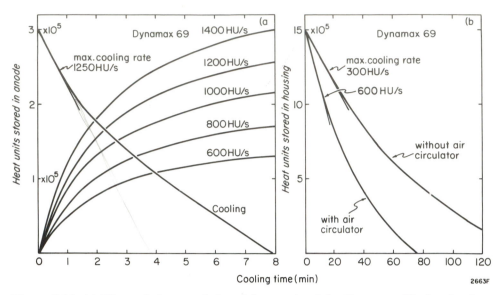

Figure 2-12. (a) Thermal characteristics of the anode of the Dynamax 69, showing heat units stored in the anode as a function of time for different heat input rates. The cooling curve is also given. (b) Cooling curve for the housing of the same tube with and without the air circulation unit.

Example 2-3. A Dynamax 69 (Machlett) with a high speed rotor (180 Hz) is energized from a 3 phase 12 pulse transformer. It is desired to give a series of exposures of 300 mA at 100 kV$_p$ lasting 0.2 s spaced 6 s apart. Is this permissible, and if so, how many such exposures can be given? Would the heating of the tube housing be a problem?

From Figure 2-11 we see that at 300 mA and 100 kV$_p$ exposures up to 0.45 s are permissible so our exposure of 0.2 s will not exceed the focal spot rating.

$$\text{Heat input/exposure (eq. 2-4)} = 1.35(300)(100)(.2) = 8.1 \times 10^3 \text{ HU}$$

$$\text{Average rate of heat input} = \frac{8.1 \times 10^3 \text{ HU}}{6 \text{ s}} = 1400 \text{ HU/s}$$

This is greater than the maximum cooling rate of 1250 HU/s (see Fig. 2-12a); hence, there is a limit to the number of exposures. For input at 1400 HU/s maximum time is 8 min = 480 s (Fig. 2-12a).

$$\text{Max. number exposures} = 480/6 = 80$$

$$\text{Energy deposited in housing} = 80 \times 8.1 \times 10^3 = 6.5 \times 10^5 \text{ HU}$$

This is less than half the energy of 15×10^5 HU, which may be stored in the housing, so heating of the housing is not a problem.

In this example it was assumed that both the anode and housing were cold initially. If they were not, then the heat stored in them would have to be taken into account. Thus, the immediate past history of the tube will determine the permissible loading for the next exposure. Some units have a photocell that "looks at" the anode and continuously monitors its temperature and the HU stored in it. In this example we have assumed the rotor was not stopped after each exposure; if it were one would have to add 4000 HU per exposure, or 3.2×10^5 HU for 80 exposures, for a total of 9.7×10^5 HU deposited in the housing.

2.07   X RAY SPECTRA

To understand the fundamental processes involved in x ray production, we first look at the properties of a typical x ray beam. Figure 2-13 shows measured spectral distributions of the photons emitted from a diagnostic x ray tube excited at 60, 80, 100, and 119 kV_p. The graphs give the relative number of photons in each energy interval as a function of photon energy. The area under the curves is proportional to the total number of photons emitted. The *same* data can be presented in a different way (as in Fig. 2-13b). Here the relative energy in each energy interval is plotted as a function of photon energy. These graphs were obtained from the first set by multiplying each ordinate by the energy of the photon at that ordinate. This tends to suppress the low energy end of the spectrum and accentuate the high energy end. The area under these curves is proportional to the energy carried by the beam. This relative

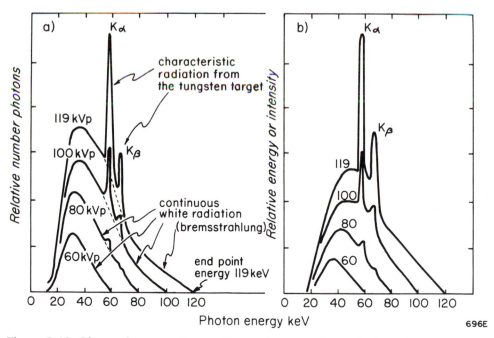

Figure 2-13. Observed spectra from a diagnostic x ray tube excited at 60, 80, 100, and 119 kV_p, due to Yaffe (Y1), added filter 2 mm Al.

energy or intensity distribution will be compared with calculated spectra
to be discussed in section 2.10.

From these measured spectra it is evident that the spectrum consists
of a continuous spectrum called *"white radiation"* or *bremsstrahlung* with
discrete sharp spikes superimposed in it. These spikes or peaks are called
characteristic radiation since their position depends upon the atomic number of the target. The continuous spectrum is called white radiation because of its similarity to the white light of the continuous spectrum
emitted by a heated filament in a light bulb. We now seek an explanation
for these spectra.

**2.08   INTERACTIONS OF ELECTRONS WITH
                 THE TARGET TO GIVE X RAYS**

When a high speed electron penetrates the surface layers of the target,
it may suffer a number of different types of encounters or collisions.
Most of the encounters involve small energy transfers leading to ionization of the target atoms. These are illustrated by track a of Figure 2-14
and are called ionizational collisions. Another class of encounter, leading
to the production of radiation and illustrated by tracks b, c, and d, are
called radiative collisions. Detailed calculations of these ionizational and
radiative energy losses will be deferred to Chapter 6; here we deal with
the matter in a qualitative manner.

Track a shows a number of collisions in which the direction of the electron's motion is altered and ionization is produced. All of these encounters transfer some energy to electrons that are knocked out of the atoms.
For example, a 100 keV electron may suffer 1000 such interactions before coming to rest and most of its energy will eventually appear as heat.
In a few of these collisions the electron that is knocked out of the atom
will have enough energy to produce a track of its own. These are called
delta rays and are also illustrated in Figure 2-14.

Of more interest to us at the moment are the much rarer events illustrated by tracks b, c, and d that produce x rays. In track b, we picture
our incident electron making a direct hit on one of the K electrons of the
tungsten atoms in the target. When the hole so created is filled by an
electron from an outer shell, characteristic K radiation will be emitted. If
the incident electron b has insufficient energy to eject the K electron of
tungsten, then no K radiation will appear, as illustrated by the spectrum
of Figure 2-13 excited by 60 kV$_p$.

Occasionally the electron will approach very close to the nucleus of the
atom and suffer a radiation loss, as represented by track c. Here the electron is made to orbit partially around the nucleus, N, by the strong attraction between the positive nucleus and the negative electron. The electron
will recede from the interaction with reduced energy. The loss in energy

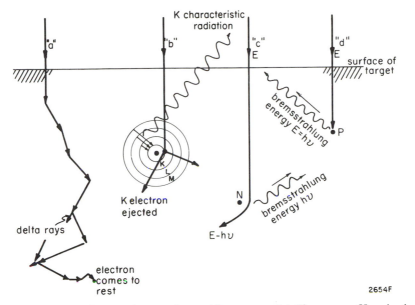

Figure 2-14. Typical electron interactions with a target. (a) Electron suffers ionizational losses, giving rise to delta rays and eventually heat. (b) The electron ejects a K electron, giving rise to characteristic radiation. (c) Collision between an electron of energy E and a nucleus, leading to bremsstrahlung of energy hν. The electron recedes from the "collision" with energy E − hν. (d) Rare collision when the electron is completely stopped in one collision, giving rise to a photon of energy E = hν.

will appear as a photon with energy hν and the primary electron will recede with energy E − hν. The sudden deceleration of the electron gives rise to the radiation described by the German word *bremsstrahlung*, or "braking radiation." At low electron energies, this process is very unlikely but at high energies becomes even more probable than the ionizational process. This radiation is responsible for the white radiation of Figure 2-13.

Finally, track d represents the unlikely type of interaction where an electron heads straight towards a nucleus and is stopped completely in one collision and the whole of its energy appears as bremsstrahlung. The number of these collisions is small but finite and gives the high energy limit shown in Figure 2-13. Thus, when a 100 keV electron bombards a target we expect to observe a few photons with 100 keV energy but none with higher energy.

Radiation events illustrated in tracks b, c, and d are very rare compared with a at the energies used in x ray machines. At 100 kV$_p$, for example, the electrons on striking the target lose over 99% of their energy in ionizational losses that lead eventually to heat. The x ray tube is a very inefficient converter of energy into x rays. At high energies such as are present in betatrons or linear accelerators, the reverse is true and now perhaps 95% of the energy appears as bremsstrahlung.

The processes illustrated in Figure 2-14 are very complex and all may occur in one track. For example, an electron could suffer many ionizational losses, then a radiation loss, then several more ionizational losses before coming to rest. Furthermore, they could occur at any depth in the target, which is less than the electron range. The radiation, once produced, must emerge before it is of any use; thus, radiation generated at point P of Figure 2-14 has a greater chance of emerging than that emitted at point N.

2.09   CHARACTERISTIC RADIATION

To understand the production of characteristic radiation, a more detailed energy level diagram is required than that given in Figure 1-2. Careful investigations have shown that the L shell is really made up of three subshells (L_I, L_{II}, and L_{III}), the M shell of 5 subshells (I to V), the N shell of 7 subshells. The energies of these shells have been measured with great precision and a few of these, taken from tables by Storm and Israel (S1), are given in Table 2-2.

The entries in the table are in keV and thus give the voltages in kilovolts required to excite the particular level. For example, in tungsten 69.525 kV is required on the tube to eject the K electron from the atom. If this voltage is supplied, all the K lines will appear.

Once the K electron is ejected, the space may be filled with an electron from the L, M, or N shells. When the electron moves in this way, we say that a *transition* has taken place. For example, when an electron moves from the L_{III} to the K shell, energy is radiated and the amount is the difference between the corresponding energy levels of Table 2-2, i.e.

TABLE 2-2
Critical X ray Absorption Energies (keV)

Shell	Oxygen Z = 8	Calcium Z = 20	Copper Z = 29	Molybdenum Z = 42	Tin Z = 50	Tungsten Z = 74	Lead Z = 82
K	.533	4.037	8.981	20.000	29.200	69.525	88.004
L_I	.024	1.438	1.096	2.867	4.465	12.098	15.861
L_{II}	.009	.350	.953	2.625	4.156	11.541	15.200
L_{III}	.009	.346	.933	2.521	3.929	10.204	13.035
M_I	—	.044	.122	.505	.884	2.820	3.851
M_{II}	not	.025	.074	.410	.756	2.575	3.554
M_{III}	filled	.025	.074	.392	.714	2.281	3.066
M_{IV}	—	—	.007	.230	.493	1.871	2.586
M_V	—	—	.007	.228	.485	1.809	2.484

From Storm and Israel (S1)

69.525 − 10.204 = 59.321 keV. We refer to this as a K-L$_{III}$ transition. The photon emitted is called the Kα_1 line, a notation that comes from the early days of x ray spectroscopy.

One might expect a K line for a transition from all of the L, M, and N shells to the K shell. Quantum mechanical reasoning shows, however, that many of the transitions are "forbidden" and only those that follow certain selection rules are allowed. For example, the Kα_1 and Kα_2 lines result from transitions between L$_{III}$ and L$_{II}$ to K, but few transitions occur from L$_I$ to K. In the K series there are four important lines appearing as a pair of close doublets. Kα_1 and Kα_2 have nearly the same energy and are separated by about 10 keV from the higher energy doublet Kβ_2 and Kβ_1. A few of the important emission lines from tungsten and molybdenum are given in Table 2-3. In addition, the relative numbers emitted are given in Table 2-3. For example, the Kα_1 line is observed nearly twice as often as the Kα_2 line. The relative numbers are determined by the "forbiddenness" of the transition.

TABLE 2-3
Principal Emission Lines in keV for Tungsten and Molybdenum

K Lines Tungsten				L Lines Tungsten			
Transition	Symbol	Energy (keV)	Relative Number	Transition	Symbol	Energy (keV)	Relative Number
K-N$_{II}$N$_{III}$	Kβ_2	69.081	7	L$_I$-N$_{III}$	Lγ_5	11.674	10
K-M$_{III}$	Kβ_1	67.244	21	L$_{II}$-N$_{IV}$	Lγ_1	11.285	24
K-M$_{II}$	Kβ_3	66.950	11	L$_{III}$-N$_V$	Lβ_2	9.962	18
K-L$_{III}$	Kα_1	59.321	100	L$_I$-M$_{III}$	Lβ_3	9.817	37
K-L$_{II}$	Kα_2	57.984	58	L$_{II}$-M$_{IV}$	Lβ_1	9.670	127
	K lines Molybdenum			L$_I$-M$_{II}$	Lβ_4	9.523	29
K-M$_{II}$M$_{III}$	Kβ_{31}	19.602	24	L$_{III}$-M$_V$	Lα_1	8.395	100
K-L$_{III}$	Kα_1	17.479	100	L$_{III}$-M$_{IV}$	Lα_2	8.333	11
K-L$_{II}$	Kα_2	17.375	52				

From Storm and Israel (S1)

The importance of characteristic radiation relative to white radiation depends upon kilovoltage and filtration. For diagnostic x rays this can be some 30%, while for therapeutic x rays at 200 kV it is only a few percent. The relative intensities of the four K lines remain the same regardless of the excitation energy, but the amount compared to the total white radiation increases rapidly as the energy is increased above the minimum value needed to eject the K-electron and then decreases slowly. No peaks are shown on this curve for 60 kV (of Fig. 2-13) although this energy is greater than the Kα lines; 60 kV cannot excite this line because there is insufficient energy to eject the K electron from the atom. When the K electron is ejected, all the K lines will appear simultaneously.

In the low energy region of Figure 2-13, the L lines of Table 2-3 are produced but are not observed because they are completely absorbed in the housing of the tube.

The discrete lines of the characteristic spectrum are usually not of great importance either in diagnosis or therapy because they contribute only a small fraction of the energy in the total spectrum. Mammography with films and screens may be an exception since tubes fitted with molybdenum targets to produce K radiation at 17 to 19 keV are frequently used. Molybdenum filters are added to reduce the bremsstrahlung spectrum. This particular arrangement improves contrast in mammography.

2.10   WHITE RADIATION, OR BREMSSTRAHLUNG

The type of electron interaction giving rise to bremsstrahlung has already been described. A theory to predict the interaction of x rays in a target would have to take into account (a) the paths of the electron into the target, (b) the change in direction at each interaction, (c) the chance of an ionizational loss and the chance of a radiation loss in each increment of path, (d) the direction of emission of the bremsstrahlung, and (e) its attenuation and scattering in emerging from the target. This is so complex a situation that no satisfactory theoretical solution to the problem has been developed.

THIN TARGET RADIATION: If one restricts the problem to a "thin target" so that *no* electron suffers more than one collision on the average in passing through the target, then the problem can be solved. Simplified theory indicates that when a beam of electrons of energy E_1 strikes a thin target, the intensity of radiation emitted in each photon energy interval from 0 to E is constant. The intensity resulting from electron energy, E_1 is shown in insert a of Figure 2-15. Since the intensity is proportional to the product of the number of photons and their energy, a photon with energy $E_1/2$ will be produced with twice the probability of a photon of energy E_1 and one with energy $E_1/10$ with 10 times the probability. If then we plot the number of photons per energy interval against energy we will obtain a curve rising to large values at small energies as illustrated by insert a' of Figure 2-15. Although this curve looks very different from a it gives exactly the same information. The area under a gives the total energy radiated; this is equal to kE_1 and is proportional to the maximum energy, E_1. It may also be shown to be proportional to the first power of the atomic number. Thus, for "thin target" radiation the energy radiated is proportional to EZ. This simplified theory agrees well with experiment for low energy electrons (up to about 100 keV) but is only approximately correct for higher energy electrons (for detailed theoretical discussions of x ray production, see E1, H1, S2).

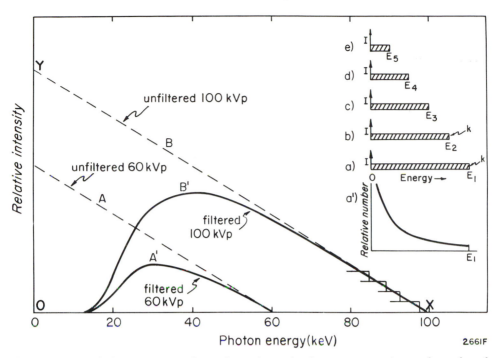

Figure 2-15. Relative energy or intensity I, in each photon energy interval produced when a beam of monoenergetic electrons of energy E_1 bombard a thin target. The distribution a′ is the data of a converted to a number distribution. Curves b, c, d, and e are thin target intensity spectra similar to a but for electron energies of E_2, E_3, E_4, and E_5. The main diagram shows *thick target* spectra (dotted lines A and B) produced by the superposition of many thin target spectra when the target is bombarded with 60 and 100 keV electrons. The solid curves A′ and B′ were obtained from A and B by taking into account the attenuation of 2 mm Al.

THICK TARGET RADIATION: A thick target may be considered as a number of thin targets superimposed. Thus, electrons with initial energy E_1 will, after passing through a thin layer of target, have energy E_2 and will then produce the spectrum corresponding to E_2 and represented by insert b. After passing through the next layer the electron will have energy E_3 and produce spectrum c, etc. The total spectrum will then be the superposition of all the thin target spectra for energies E_1, E_2, E_3, E_4, E_5, etc. This total spectrum is the dotted straight line XY of Figure 2-15 and its equation is:

$$I(E) = C Z (E_{max} - E) \qquad (2\text{-}5)$$

where I(E) is the intensity at energy E. In this equation E_{max} is the maximum energy of the photons emitted and is also equal to the energy of the bombarding electron as it enters the target. C is a constant and Z the atomic number of the target. This has its maximum value of C Z E_{max} for

E = 0 and drops linearly to zero as E is increased to E_{max}. Since the base OX and the altitude OY are both proportional to E_{max}, the area under the dotted line, which represents the energy radiated as x rays, is proportional to E_{max}^2.

The dotted lines A and B are the spectra produced by the bombardment of a thick target with 60 keV and 100 keV electrons. Before comparing it with the measured spectra of Figure 2-13b we should take into account the effects of filtration of the beam by the window of the tube and any added filter. When this is done we obtain the solid curves (Fig. 2-15), which have peaks at about 40 keV and 30 keV and are roughly the same shape as the measured continuous spectrum of Figure 2-13b, which also shows a peak at about 40 and 30 keV. Finally, we should add the appropriate amount of characteristic radiation to the theoretical curves to obtain agreement with experiment. The agreement between theory and experiment is good considering the many factors that have not been taken into consideration. For instance, no account has been taken of the absorption of the radiation produced by the overlying portions of the target or for the complex nature of the electron paths into the target. Fortunately, measured spectra are available today for most conditions of interest (Y1, M2, E2) and we need not depend upon spectra calculated using approximate theory.

Although the simple theory suggests that the thick target x ray intensity depends upon E^2, examination of Figure 2-15 will convince the reader that since filtering preferentially removes the low energy photons its effect on the 60 kV_p radiation will be proportionally greater than on the 100 kV_p curve so the intensity will depend on the kilovoltage to a higher power than 2.0. For example, increasing the kilovoltage on a typical diagnostic machine from 100 kV_p to 105 kV_p (i.e. 5%) keeping the tube current constant will increase the x ray intensity by some 15%, showing that the yield depends on the third power of E. This underscores the importance of accurate control of kV in attempting to make a series of identical x ray exposures.

2.11   THE ANGULAR DISTRIBUTION OF X RAYS

THIN TARGET: If a beam of low energy electrons is incident on a very thin target, it is found that the x rays are radiated primarily in a direction at right angles to the electron stream. This is illustrated by curve A in Figure 2-16b, which shows experimental data by Honerjäger (H2) for the angular distribution of x rays produced by bombarding a foil of aluminum 200 nm thick with 34 keV electrons. This angular distribution is for radiation at the high energy limit. The length of the arrows from the target indicate the relative intensity in the different directions. The distribution in space is found by rotating the curve about the axis of the electron beam. It is seen that the maximum intensity is at an angle of 55° with the direction of the electrons, while the intensity in the forward direction is small and the intensity in the backward direction zero. As the energy of the bombarding electrons is increased, the two lobes of curve A tip forward to yield at very high energies a distribution with all the radiation in the forward direction. Curves B and C are theoretical curves as calculated by Schiff (S2) for the angular distribution of the radiation produced by bombarding a 0.05 cm thick tungsten target with 10 and 20 MeV electrons. These distributions are in essential agreement with a number of experimental results using betatrons.

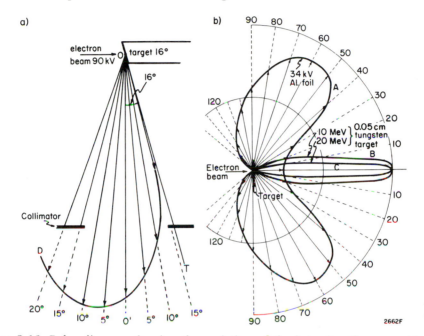

Figure 2-16. Polar diagram showing the variation of the intensity of x rays with angle produced by the electron bombardment of various targets. Curve A, 34 keV electrons bombarding a *thin* aluminum foil due to Honerjäger (H2). Curves B and C, 10 and 20 MeV electrons bombarding a *thin* 0.05 cm tungsten target as calculated by Schiff (S2). Curve D typical intensity distribution for a diagnostic x ray tube with a 16° *thick* tungsten target, with the beam taken at right angles to the electron beam and excited at 90 kV$_p$ (Courtesy of K.W. Taylor).

THICK TARGET: The distributions of Figure 2-16b are for targets so thin that most of the high speed electrons pass right through the target without deviation. In a practical x ray tube (illustrated in Fig. 2-16a), the target is thick enough to stop the electron beam. In the stopping process the electrons are deviated widely from their initial direction so that x rays are produced in all directions about 0. However, those that are produced in directions to the right of the line OT will be absorbed in the target and will not escape, so the polar distribution is as indicated. The maximum yield is usually 5 to 10° to the cathode side of the line 00' and falls slowly as the angle is increased beyond 10°. The distribution shown in Figure 2-16a is typical of a practical diagnostic tube with a target angle at 16°. Naturally, if the target angle is made smaller, the beam is even more constricted on the anode side. Decreasing the angle allows one to use greater loading for the same size focal spot but reduces the useful area of the beam. In a practical tube, the housing for a 16° target would contain a collimator, which would restrict the beam to about 12° each side of 00'. Even with this restriction, the intensity will vary with angle by some 30% over the useful beam, being lowest on the anode side. The reduced intensity on the anode side is called the *heel* effect. The beam near the heel, although of reduced intensity, is more penetrating because of self-filtration in the target.

The best configuration of the electron beam, the target, and the useful x ray beam depends on energy. For electron energies up to 400 keV, the x ray beam at right angles to the electron direction is used as illustrated in Figure 2-16a. In 4 to 30 MeV linear accelerators, the x ray beam transmitted through the target in the direction of the electrons is more useful. This beam is more intense than the beam produced at right angles because of the effect illustrated in Figure 2-16b. The target is often made of tungsten bonded to copper and cooled by water. For energies from 10 to 30 MeV the beam becomes very peaked in the forward direction and a flattening filter that reduces the intensity along the axis of the beam must be used to achieve a uniform radiation field (see Chapter 4).

PROBLEMS

Problems marked with asterisk are more difficult.

1. The high voltage transformer for an x ray machine has 500 turns on the secondary for each turn on the primary. The primary is excited by 120 volts, 60 cycle. Find the root mean square voltage and peak voltage developed across the secondary of the transformer.

2. An x ray tube requires a filament voltage of 8 volts. How would you construct a step-down transformer to excite this filament from a 230 volt line? Discuss the difficulties with insulation.

3. Find the approximate power dissipated in a diagnostic tube operating at 80 kV$_p$, 3 phase at 400 mA. If the tube is operated for 2 s at this rating, calculate the number of joules of energy and the number of calories imparted to the anode (4.18 joules = 1 calorie).

4. A therapy unit is designed to operate at 30 mA and 250 kV constant potential continuously. Find the rate of energy input to the target in joules/s and calories/s.

5. A diagnostic tube has a target that is sloped at 15°. The electrons are focused along a strip of the anode 2.5 mm wide. How long should this strip be to yield a projected focal spot 2.5 mm × 2.5 mm? What is the gain in loading that might be expected from the use of this line focus rather than a point focus?

6. If the tube described in the last problem were made into a rotating anode tube with a disc of radius 3 cm, estimate the gain in loading over the line focus tube.

7. Explain the advantage of the hooded type anode in a therapy tube. Explain why the target in a therapy tube must be placed at a larger angle than in a diagnostic tube.

*8. A Siemens B150 RGS tube with characteristics given in Figure 2-1 is used in the full-wave circuit of Figure 2-5b with 4 rectifier stacks each containing 150 silicon rectifiers with the characteristics shown in Figure 2-4. The transformer is excited to give 100 kV_p between the terminals A and B of Figure 2-5b and the tube filament is operated at 4.1 A. Plot the current through the tube, the voltage across the tube, and the voltage across one of the rectifiers as a function of time. Determine the average tube current. Plot the power dissipated in one of the rectifiers as a function of time and determine the mean power dissipated.

9. If the RMS value of an AC line is 117 volts, determine the peak value and the average value of the rectified voltage.

10. Show either graphically or by calculus that the average value of a rectified AC voltage is $(2/\pi)V_0$ and the RMS value $V_0/\sqrt{2}$, where V_0 is the peak voltage.

11. Show graphically that for the tube current wave form shown in Figure 2-3e, the average current as measured by the milliammeter is about 145 mA.

12. Show that the ripple in Figure 2-6e is $0.23 V_p$ and the average value of the voltage is $1.65 V_p$, where V_p is the peak voltage. To get the average value use a graphical method or calculus.

*13. (a) For the delta connection of Figure 2-6c, plot the voltage as a function of time (or angle). Show that it varies between $0.866 V_p$ and V_p with an average value of $0.955 V_p$ and that the maximum values occur at angles of 30, 90, 150, etc. degrees and the minimum values at 0, 60, 120, etc. degrees, where V_p is the peak voltage across one winding of the secondary.

(b) Draw the complete circuit for 12 pulse rectification. If the system is balanced so that the anode of the x ray tube goes as much positive as the cathode goes negative, what must be the ratio of turns on the secondaries of the two circuits of Figures 2-6b and 6c? When the ratios are adjusted in this way, plot the anode voltage and the cathode voltage as a function of time. Find the maximum, minimum, and average cathode to anode voltage. Determine the ripple as a percent of the average.

14. Is an exposure of 0.15 s permissible on a Dynamax 69 with focal spot 0.6 × 0.6 mm and rotor speed 180 Hz operating at 100 kV_p at 300 mA using single phase, 3 phase?

15. Why may the Dynamax tube of problem 14 not be operated at 300 mA, 3 phase and at 50 kV_p?

16. Determine the energy input in heat units for a tube operated on single phase full-wave rectification for 10 s, at 400 mA and 120 kV_p.

17. A Dynamax 69 (Machlett) with high speed rotor (180 Hz) is energized from a 3 phase, 12 pulse transformer. Is an exposure of 0.1 s at 300 mA and 100 kV_p permissible? What is the longest single exposure that may be used? If an exposure of 0.1 s is used, approximately how many of these spaced 3 s apart are permitted?

18. By estimating the areas under the 100 kV_p, 80 kV_p, and 60 kV_p curves of Figure 2-13, determine the relative numbers of photons emitted and the relative energy radiated. Plot these as a function of kilovoltage and estimate how these depend on kilovoltage.

19. In a delta connection, show that at all times the sum of the voltages across two windings is equal to the voltage across the third.

20. An x ray tube operated at 200 kV_p with a tube current of 10 mA gives an exposure rate of 30 R/min at 50 cm. Estimate the exposure rate from the same x ray tube if the tube current is increased to 12.5 mA.

PROJECTS

1. Obtain a picture of the target of a double focus x ray tube in the department. Place a lead sheet with a pin hole in it about 40 cm from the target and a "no screen film" or a film-screen combination at 120 cm from the target. (This will give an image with magnification 2.0.) Obtain pictures of both focal spots.
2. Obtain a small rectifier from the local electronic supply house and measure a set of characteristics similar to those of Figure 2-4.

Chapter **3**

THE FUNDAMENTALS OF NUCLEAR PHYSICS

3.01 **NATURAL RADIOACTIVITY**

The nuclear particles (protons and neutrons) within the nucleus are in continual motion. As a result of this motion, collisions occur and energy is transferred back and forth from one particle to another. Were it not for the strong forces of attraction that exist between the nuclear particles, such particles would escape from the nucleus and new nuclear species would be formed. In a stable nucleus, no particle ever acquires enough energy to escape; however, in a radioactive nucleus, it is possible for a particle, by a series of chance encounters, to gain enough energy to escape from the nucleus. The ejection of a nuclear particle is pure chance, and there is no way to decide when any particular nucleus will disintegrate. However, if there are many nuclei, a certain percentage will disintegrate in a given time. In the disintegration process, alpha particles, beta particles, or gamma rays may be ejected. These will be discussed in later sections of this chapter.

In most of the lighter atoms, with $Z < 82$, there is at least one configuration of nucleons that is stable. Evidently, in these, the forces of attraction between particles are sufficient to prevent their random escape. All elements with Z greater than 82 (lead) are, however, radioactive and disintegrate through long series until stable isotopes of lead are formed.

3.02 **ARTIFICIAL RADIOACTIVITY**

With the development of high energy devices—the cyclotron, the betatron, the Van de Graaff generator, the linear accelerator, and the nuclear reactor—many new radioactive isotopes have been discovered. A chart of all the stable and radioactive isotopes known to date may be obtained from a number of sources (G1, K1, M3) and should be available in every radiology department. New isotopes are produced by bombarding stable nuclei with neutrons, high energy protons, deuterons, alpha particles, or gamma rays. A few of these projectiles will make a direct collision with the nucleus and will be absorbed or will eject some particle from the nucleus to form a new substance. The probability of such a collision is very small because the cross-sectional area of the nucleus is only about 10^{-25} cm^2. It follows that to produce any appreciable amount of radioactive material from stable nuclei, that is an amount that could be separated chemically, the nuclei must be bombarded for long periods of time in an intense beam.

When a patient is treated with a 25 MeV betatron or linear accelerator, it is easy to show that the patient becomes radioactive. A few of the oxygen 16 atoms are struck by high energy photons and a neutron is ejected, giving $^{15}_{8}O$. This isotope decays to a stable isotope of nitrogen ($^{15}_{7}N$) by ejecting a positive electron, and this activity can easily be detected by a hand-held Geiger counter. However, although oxygen atoms are converted to nitrogen, it would be impossible to detect this conversion by chemical means since the amounts involved are very small. The probability of a hit on a nucleus is analogous to the probability of a marksman hitting a pinhead with a rifle shot at a range of several kilometers.

When materials are exposed to intense beams for long periods of time, as in a nuclear reactor, it is possible to produce enough new material to make a chemical separation feasible. In a large reactor (500 megawatts) about 500 g of ^{235}U are consumed per day. Within a few months, enough plutonium is produced to enable it to be separated chemically. In general, however, the new isotopes can only be detected by their activity and not by any chemical separation process.

3.03   ACTIVITY

In Figure 1-4 the number of radioactive atoms present at any given time was plotted as a function of time. Since there is no direct way to determine how many atoms are present except through the radioactivity of these atoms, the activity defined as the number of disintegrations per unit time is a more useful concept. This activity is the quantity that may be measured directly with a Geiger or scintillation counter.

The number of atoms present and the activity of the source are related by the transformation constant, λ, described in section 1.17. From equation 1-25, activity, A, expressed as number per unit time is seen to be:

$$A = \frac{\Delta N}{\Delta t} = \lambda N \qquad (3\text{-}1)$$

where the negative sign has been left off because now ΔN refers to the number that disintegrate in time, Δt, rather than the change in the number of atoms in the source. Substituting the value of N given by equation 1-26, we see that activity can be expressed as:

$$A = N_0 \lambda e^{-0.693t/t_h} = A_0 e^{-0.693t/t_h} = A_0/2^{t/t_h} \qquad (3\text{-}2)$$

where $A_0 = N_0 \lambda$ is the initial activity. Since activity is directly proportional to the number of atoms present, Figure 1-4 (which shows N as a function of time) could equally well represent, with a different scale, the decay of activity. Figure 3-1 shows the decay of activity of the ^{198}Au source described in Figure 1-4. To obtain it, we first determine the initial activity, thus:

$$\text{Initial activity} = A_o = N_o\lambda = N_o\frac{0.693}{t_h} \qquad \text{(from 1-27)}$$

$$= \frac{10^8\,(0.693)}{2.69\ \text{d}} = \frac{10^8\,(0.693)}{2.69 \times 8.64 \times 10^4\,\text{s}}$$

$$= 298\ \text{disintegrations/s} = 298\ \text{Bq}$$

We then determine the activity after an integral number of half-lives (after 6 half-lives activity = 298/64 = 4.6), and finally draw a straight line between these points. Activity may be measured in any number of units such as per s, per min, per h (s^{-1}, min^{-1}, h^{-1}). However, because it is such an important concept, a special SI unit for activity, the becquerel (Bq) has been defined (W1) thus:

$$1\ \text{becquerel (Bq)} = 1\ \text{disintegration per second} \qquad (3\text{-}3)$$

$$\text{or} \qquad \mathbf{1\ Bq = 1\ s^{-1}}$$

Another useful unit, which has been in use for many years, is the curie (Ci) defined as:

$$\mathbf{1\ curie\ (Ci) = 3.700 \times 10^{10}\ Bq} \qquad (3\text{-}4)$$

The becquerel and curie are named after two famous physicists who did much of the early work on radioactivity and radium. The curie,

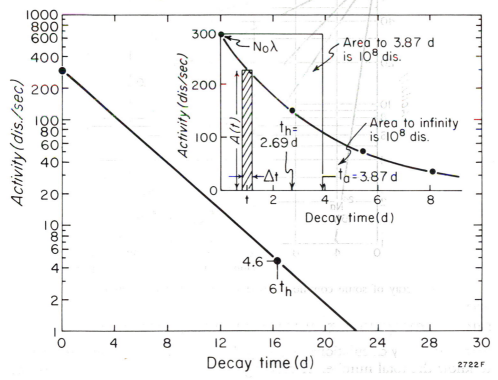

Figure 3-1. Decay of the activity of a ^{198}Au source containing 10^8 atoms.

named after Madame Curie, originally referred to the number of disintegrations per second from 1 gram of radium.

The source whose decay is shown in Figure 3-1 has an initial activity of 298 Bq or $298/(3.7 \times 10^{10}) = 8.05 \times 10^{-9}$ Ci = 8.05 nCi. This is a very weak source. Activities in thousands of curies ($\sim 10^{14}$ Bq) are used in therapy machines (Chapter 4) while activities in mCi ($\sim 10^8$ Bq) are used in diagnostic procedures (Chapter 14).

Exponential Decay of Some Commonly Used Isotopes

Isotopes decay with half-lives ranging from microseconds to millions of years. Figure 3-2 shows the decay of the activity of a number of commonly used isotopes. To plot these decay curves on semilog paper, one suitable point (50% after one half-life, 25% after 2 half-lives) is located and a straight line is drawn. Cobalt 60, having a half-life of 5.26 years, can hardly be represented on this graph, because in 28 days it decays only by 1.1%. To plot it, a much longer time scale is required. On the other hand, ^{24}Na, with a half-life of 15 hours, decays to 1% of its initial value in about four days. Graphs of this kind for isotopes in common use in the department are a convenient aid in estimating the activity at any time.

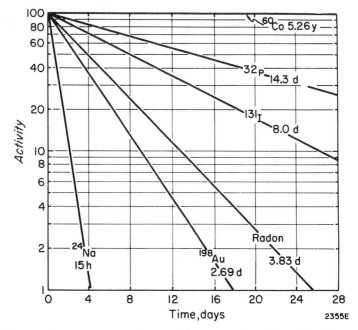

Figure 3-2. Decay of some commonly used isotopes plotted on double cycle semilog paper.

3.04   EMITTED RADIATION (AVERAGE OR MEAN LIFE)

In dosimetry calculations involving decaying isotopes, one often needs to know the total number of disintegrations that occur while the source is in or near the patient. This quantity is referred to as the "emitted radiation" and will be used in Chapters 13 and 14. A similar quantity called the "cumulated activity" (L1) is used in health physics circles to describe the radiation energy deposited in one organ from an isotope distributed in another. To calculate the "emitted radiation" consider the insert of Figure 3-1 where the activity is plotted as a function of time on a linear scale. The initial activity is $N_0\lambda = 298$ Bq. Consider the interval of time, Δt, centered about time t at which time the activity is A(t). During this interval of time the number of disintegrations is the shaded area, $A(t) \cdot \Delta t$. It follows that the total number of disintegrations from the decaying source is the complete area under the exponential from $t = 0$ to $t = \infty$. This total area must be the initial number of atoms, N_0, for after the complete decay of the source all the atoms in the source will have disintegrated. In this example the area is 10^8 atoms.

Consider now a *hypothetical* source that has a *constant* activity equal to the initial activity of the exponentially decaying source. We wish to determine how long such a source would have to remain active in order that it produce the same number of disintegrations as the exponentially decaying source. In terms of Figure 3-1 we wish to determine the width, t_a, of the rectangle of height $N_0\lambda$ that includes the same area as appears under the exponential. Clearly this width, t_a, is such that $t_a N_0\lambda = N_0$. Solving for t_a one obtains

$$t_a = \frac{1}{\lambda} = \frac{t_h}{0.693} = 1.44\, t_h \qquad (3\text{-}5)$$

The quantity t_a is called the average life or mean life. It is related to the transformation constant, λ, and the half-life, t_h, by equation 3-5. For gold 198 the half-life is 2.69 days, while the average life is 1.44 (2.69d) = 3.87 d.

This means that a source of gold that decays at a constant rate equal to its initial rate for 3.87 days would give the same number of disintegrations as a source that decays exponentially with a half-life of 2.69 days. The use of mean life in dose calculations is now illustrated.

Example 3-1. A 2.0 mCi source of Au-198 is permanently implanted into a patient. Determine the emitted radiation (1 day = 8.64×10^4 s).

Average life $= 1.44\, t_h = 1.44\ (2.69\ d) = 3.87$ d

Emitted radiation $= 2.0$ mCi $\times$ 3.87 d $= 7.74$ mCi d
$= 6.69 \times 10^5$ mCi s

$= 6.69 \times 10^5 \times 3.70 \times 10^7$ Bq s
$= 2.48 \times 10^{13}$ Bq s $= 2.48 \times 10^{13}$ dis.

"Emitted radiation" may be expressed as the product of any unit of activity and any unit of time. In a few years the most common unit will

probably be the Bq s (one disintegration) but at the time of writing it is
the mCi h or in radium dosage the mg h (see Chapter 13). The biological
effect resulting from the implant of example 3-1 will be proportional to
the emitted radiation but will also depend upon many other factors such
as the distribution of the source in the patient as well as the number
and types of particles emitted in each disintegration. If a source is removed from the patient before its complete decay, the emitted radiation
may be determined as follows.

Example 3-2. A source of Au-198 of initial activity 8×10^7 Bq is placed
in a patient for 2.9 d and then removed. Find the emitted radiation.

Activity after 2.9 d $= 8 \times 10^7 \times e^{-.693(2.9/2.69)} = 3.79 \times 10^7$ Bq d
(eq. 3-2)

Emitted radiation $= (8 \times 10^7 - 3.79 \times 10^7)$ Bq $\times 3.87$ d
$= 16.3 \times 10^7$ Bq d $= 141 \times 10^{11}$ Bq s

3.05   **CHARTS OF ISOTOPES**

Nuclei are characterized by the number of protons, Z, and the number
of neutrons (N = A − Z) in the nucleus. It is convenient to represent
each species as a square on a chart (similar to Fig. 3-3) where the vertical
scale gives the number of protons and the horizontal scale the number
of neutrons. For example, $^{60}_{27}$Co appears at the intersection of the horizontal line at Z = 27 and the vertical line at N = 60 − 27 = 33. Stable
nuclei are represented by solid squares and radioactive ones by a cross.
Complete charts of this kind can be obtained from a number of sources
(G1, M3, K1).

On such charts useful information is recorded in the square for each
species and thus the chart is a convenient reference source. It is immediately evident from Figure 3-3 that all the stable and radioactive nuclei
cluster along a line that starts out at 45° for small values of Z and rises less
steeply for the larger values of Z. For small values of Z the condition of
stability is satisfied for a nucleus in which the numbers of protons and
neutrons are equal or nearly equal. Hence, the line appears at 45°. For
large values of Z, there tend to be more neutrons than protons so the isotopes occupy squares below the 45° line. In a heavy nucleus, such as
uranium, which contains 92 protons and 146 neutrons, the protons exert
a force of repulsion upon one another so the stable mixture contains an
excess of neutrons.

Species that appear along any horizontal line of Figure 3-3 are isotopes
(same Z, different values of N) while species that appear along lines at
45° have the same mass number and are called isobars. Examination of
an isotope chart will convince the reader that there are usually several
stable species with Z even but usually only one with Z odd. For example

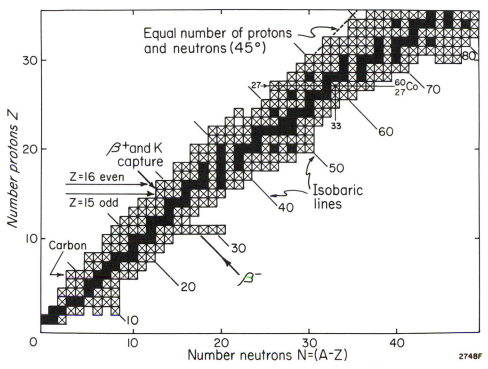

Figure 3-3. Chart showing the proportions of protons and neutrons in nuclei. Stable nuclei are represented by solid squares, radioactive nuclei by crosses. Nuclei with equal numbers of neutrons and protons lie along the line N = Z. Isotopes appear along horizontal lines and isobars along lines at 45°.

there are four stable isotopes of sulphur (Z = 16) but only one stable isotope of phosphorus (Z = 15). Study of the chart will also show that along most isobaric lines there is only one stable species, but if there are two they are almost always separated by an unstable one.

All the unstable species appearing as crosses decay in some way until some stable form is reached. The most common decay mode is along an isobaric line. Decay upwards along such a line is β^- decay, while decay downwards along such a line is β^+ decay. Other modes of decay involve α emission, electron capture, electron conversion, isomeric transition, and nuclear fission. These will be discussed in the following sections.

3.06   **ALPHA DISINTEGRATION**

Alpha disintegration occurs mainly in heavy nuclei. In such disintegration, a helium nucleus, consisting of two protons and two neutrons, is ejected. Thus, the atomic number is reduced by 2 and the neutron number by 2. On a chart such as Figure 3-3, it would appear as a transition, two places to the left and two places down. Radium is a typical alpha emitter and the reaction is represented by:

$$^{226}_{88}\text{Ra} \xrightarrow[1620 \text{ years}]{} {}^{222}_{86}\text{Rn} + {}^{4}_{2}\text{He}$$ (3-6)

$$4.78 \text{ MeV } (94.5\%)$$

$$4.60 \text{ MeV} + 0.18\,\gamma\,(5.5\%)$$

and schematically in Figure 3-4.

In this reaction the radium emits a monoenergetic alpha particle with 4.78 MeV energy in 94.5% of the disintegrations and in the other 5.5%, a lower energy alpha particle of 4.60 MeV energy. In the latter case, it disintegrates to an excited state of radon, which loses its excess energy by the emission of a photon (gamma ray) of 0.18 MeV energy. The radium nucleus is thus 4.78 MeV higher than radon on the energy scale. For each disintegration, this energy is released either as an alpha particle or as an alpha particle plus a gamma ray.

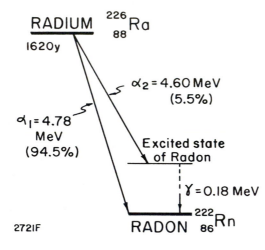

Figure 3-4. Energy level diagram for radium showing the 2 modes of disintegration into radon. (H3)

The alpha particle, on striking a fluorescent screen, can produce enough light to be made visible to the human eye; in fact, much of the original work of Rutherford was done using the eye as the detector of alpha particles. Luminous dials on watches used to contain alpha emitting material in close proximity to a scintillating material.

The alpha particle, although its energy is great, is stopped in a few cm of air or in a few thousandths of a cm in tissue. In traveling through the air the large particle, with its positive charge, removes electrons from the atoms along its path and produces intense ionization.

PARTICLE TRACKS. This intense ionization may be rendered visible in a Wilson cloud chamber (or the modern equivalent, a bubble chamber) where the particle is made to pass through air partially saturated with water vapor. Just after the passage of the particle, the air in the cloud chamber is suddenly expanded, which causes water vapor to condense on the ions. These small droplets of water may be photographed to give the tracks shown in Figure 3-5. Usually the path of an alpha particle is straight because of its large mass, but at times one will collide with a nucleus and be deflected (as shown near the end of the track in Fig. 3-5). The alpha particle produces from 3000 to 7000 ion pairs per mm of path in air, so many water droplets are formed and the track in the cloud chamber is very heavy. The ranges of alpha particles are from 2 to 10 cm in air, depending on their origin. A common range is about 4 cm in air. These particles are stopped completely by a thick sheet of paper.

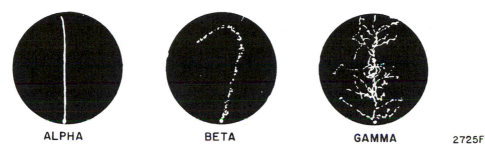

ALPHA   BETA   GAMMA   2725F

Figure 3-5. Cloud chamber photograph of alpha, beta, and gamma ray tracks. (J.B. Hoag: *Electron and Nuclear Physics,* courtesy D. Van Nostrand Co.) (H4)

When an electron or beta particle passes through air, it produces some 6 to 20 ion pairs per mm of path so only a few droplets are formed and the individual droplets may be counted (as in Fig. 3-5). The path of an electron is tortuous because the electron, with its small mass, may easily be deflected from a straight line path.

A gamma ray in passing through a cloud chamber does not leave a track itself except through the electrons that it sets in motion. In Figure 3-5 the gamma ray passed upward through the center of the treelike structure setting in motion the electrons, which appear as branches. These electron tracks originate along the path of the gamma ray and are projected slightly forward in the direction of the gamma ray.

3.07   **BETA DISINTEGRATION**

Many radioactive disintegrations are accompanied by the ejection of a positive or a negative electron from the nucleus. The nucleus that emits the electrons is called a positron (β^+) or negatron (β^-) emitter. It might well be asked how an electron may be emitted from the nucleus when there are *no* electrons in the nucleus. In a β^- emitter we consider that a neutron within the nucleus changes into a proton and a negative electron is ejected. Such a transformation will leave the mass number the same (the electron mass is negligible compared with the proton or neutron) but the atomic number Z will increase by 1 since there is now one more proton in the nucleus.

In a β^+ a proton changes into a neutron and a positive electron is ejected. In this case, Z will decrease by 1, since there is now one less proton in the nucleus. In Figure 3-3 a β^- emission appears along an isobaric line upward from the lower right while a β^+ emission appears along an isobaric line downward from the upper left. The beta particle that is ejected from a beta active nucleus may have any energy from zero up to a maximum value characteristic of the parent nucleus. This is illustrated in Figure 3-6, which gives the distribution of β^- energies from radioactive phosphorus, ^{32}P. Energies from zero to a maximum value of 1.71 MeV are possible, with a mean energy of 0.695 MeV. This means that one nucleus can disintegrate, giving a beta ray of maximum energy 1.71 MeV, whereas the next nucleus to disintegrate may give a beta particle with only 0.5 MeV energy.

Since the energies of all the nuclei in the original state are the same and all those in the final state the same, but less by 1.71 MeV, the question may well be asked, where has the rest of the energy gone when a 0.5 MeV particle is emitted? Theory and experiment show that in a beta disintegration a neutrino is also ejected, and this neutrino carries the rest of the energy. This means that each disintegration corresponds to the release of the maximum energy, but this energy may be distributed in any way between the two particles. For example, if the beta particle has an energy of 1.0 MeV, then the corresponding neutrino will have an energy of 0.71 MeV. The relations for beta decay may then be written:

$$\beta^- \text{ emission} \quad n \rightarrow p + \beta^- + \nu \quad \text{Z increases 1} \quad (3\text{-}7)$$

$$\beta^+ \text{ emission} \quad p \rightarrow n + \beta^+ + \nu \quad \text{Z decreases 1}$$

The neutrino, ν, is a neutral particle with a mass that is small compared with an electron. Since it has no charge, it produces no ionization and hence cannot be made visible in a cloud chamber. Furthermore, the neutrino has such a small mass that it cannot set other particles in motion through collision. The neutrino thus has properties that make it very difficult to observe and, as a result, many of the early attempts failed; for many years, only indirect evidence for its existence was available. In recent years, however, several unequivocal experiments have been carried out demonstrating the existence of the neutrino.

Figure 3-6 also shows the beta ray spectra (E1) for the decay of Cu-64, which can emit either a β^- or β^+ particle. The shapes of the three curves of Figure 3-6 are somewhat similar: they all show a maximum or *end point energy* and a peak at some lower energy.

Of interest to us is the mean energy, $\bar{E}$, deposited in tissue from a beta

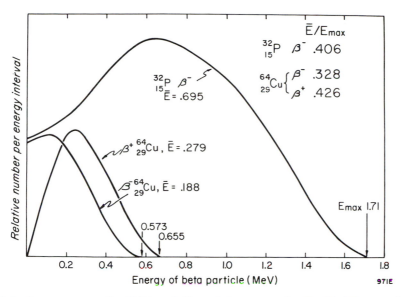

Figure 3-6. β^- ray spectra for P-32 and β^+ and β^- spectra for Cu-64. The graphs show the relative number of beta particles per energy interval as a function of energy. The maxima and mean energies of the spectra are given.

emitter and, expressed as a fraction of E_{max}, is shown in Figure 3-6. This ratio is different for each isotope. It is determined from the shape of the spectrum and is a function of the end point energy of the spectrum, the atomic number of the nucleus, whether it is β^- or β^+, and whether it is an "allowed" or "forbidden" transition. The "forbiddenness" relates to the change in nuclear spin that accompanies the beta decay and is important to the nuclear physicists. Of interest to us is the ratio $\bar{E}/E_{max}$, which may be found in tables (D1). In general, β^+ spectra tend to have more high energy beta particles than β^- emitters (compare the two Cu-64 spectra of Fig. 3-6) because during the disintegration the β^+ particle will be repelled by the positively charged nucleus while the β^- particle will be attracted.

We now inquire into the energy transformations that occur during beta decay. Now we must deal with β^- and β^+ emission as separate problems.

3.08   BETA MINUS DECAY

In dealing with disintegrations from one isotope to another, it is usual to represent the changes that occur by a disintegration scheme. Typical transformations involving beta minus particles are given in Figure 3-7. The simplest shows $^{32}_{15}P$ with a half-life of 14.3 days decaying into $^{32}_{16}S$ with the emission of a β^- with a maximum energy of 1.71 MeV. The difference in energy between the initial atom and the final atom is

1.71 MeV and this energy will be shared between the beta particle and a neutrino.

$$\ce{^{32}_{15}P} \xrightarrow[14.3 \text{ days}]{} \ce{^{32}_{16}S} + \beta^- + \nu \qquad (3\text{-}8)$$

(total K.E. of β and ν is 1.71 MeV)

We may find the K.E. released by noting the masses of each of the nuclei involved. From tables (N1) the atomic masses of P-32 and S-32 are 31.973909 and 31.972073 amu respectively. To obtain the nuclear masses we must reduce these by the mass of the appropriate number of electrons, 15 for phosphorous and 16 for sulphur. Setting up a balance for the two sides of equation 3-8 we obtain:

mass of P-32 nucleus		$31.973909 - 15\, m_0$
mass of S-32 nucleus	$31.972073 - 16\, m_0$	
mass of β^-	$1\, m_0$	
mass of neutrino (ν)	0	
total mass	$31.972073 - 15\, m_0$	$31.972073 - 15\, m_0$
energy release		$.001836$ amu
(by subtraction)		

Energy release (eq. 1-19) equals $0.001836 \times 931.5 = 1.71$ MeV in agreement with Figure 3-6. Evidently, the energy release for beta minus decay may be obtained by taking the difference in the atomic masses between the parent and product nucleus.

It should be emphasized that when phosphorus is placed in a patient, although 1.71 MeV is released per disintegration, on the average only 0.695 MeV, or less than half, will be given to the beta particle and absorbed by the patient. From a nuclear physicist's point of view, the maximum energy is the important concept, but from a medical physicist's point of view, the mean energy is the quantity of interest.

The disintegration scheme of phosphorus is the simplest type that may be observed; the beta transition is called an allowed transition. The decay of Co-60 is slightly more complicated. Most of the disintegrations (99.8%) are an allowed transition with the emission of a β_1^- with maximum energy of 0.313 MeV. This leads to an excited state of Ni-60, which gives up its energy very quickly by the emission of two gamma rays in cascade, with energies of 1.173 and 1.332 MeV. In a few of the disintegrations (0.12%) a β_2^- particle with a maximum energy of 1.486 MeV is emitted, leading to the lowest excited state of Ni-60. The two gamma rays provide the useful radiation in a Co-60 therapy unit.

The disintegration scheme for ^{137}Cs shows two β^- pathways, one leading to an excited state of barium and the more energetic one to the ground state. The excited state of barium, $^{137m}_{56}$Ba, is almost stable and decays with a half-life of 2.55 min. An excited state with a long half-life such as this is called an isomeric state. The excess energy of the excited state (.662 MeV) is mostly (85%) emitted as a gamma ray, which is the useful component when cesium is used in the form of needles as an interstitial source (Chapter 13). Part of the energy of the excited state can set electrons in motion by internal conversion in the K, L, and M shells (as shown in Fig. 3-7). Internal conversion or electron conversion as it is often called will be discussed in section 3.11.

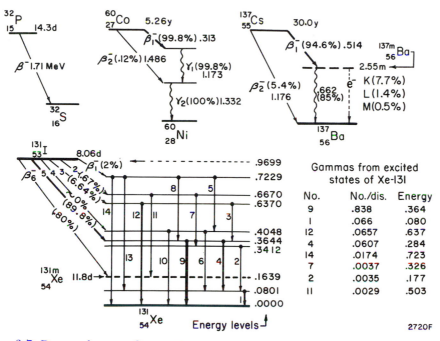

Figure 3-7. Decay schemes of some β^- emitters (D1). Only the important pathways are shown.

The decay of I-131 is complex, leading to a large number of excited states of Xe-131. The energies of these energy levels are shown in Figure 3-7. It is seen that the ground state of Xe-131 is 0.9699 MeV below I-131. Six of the excited states are reached directly from the parent material through β rays of 6 different maximum energies. The most important pathway is by β_5^-, which occurs in 89.8% of the disintegrations and has a maximum energy of 0.606 MeV (.9699 − .3644). The next most probable pathway is by β_3^- (6.64%) and the next by β_1^- (2%). All three of these are allowed transitions. The remaining βs decay by first forbidden transitions. One of these, β_6^-, goes to a metastable state of xenon (represented by Xe-131m), which has a half-life of 11.8d. The excited states of Xe-131 lose their energies by a series of gamma emissions, γ_1 to γ_{14}, which lead to lower excited states of Xe-131 or its ground state.

The relative number of each type are given in the table shown in Figure 3-7. For example, the strongest line is γ_9 with energy 0.364 MeV, which is observed in 0.838 of the disintegrations of I-131. Note that the level at 0.3644 MeV is populated by β_5 and γ_3 and is depleted by γ_4 and γ_9. The decay scheme is quite complex and only the 8 most important gammas are listed in the table. Each of these gammas has a finite probability of causing internal conversion from the K, L, and M shells of Xe-131, so the complete description of the energy deposited is very complex. This will be dealt with in Chapter 14.

3.09   **BETA PLUS DECAY**

In the production of isotopes in a nuclear reactor a neutron is usually added to a stable nucleus. For example, to produce ^{60}Co a neutron is added to ^{59}Co. When this radioactive isotope decays, the extra neutron will probably change into a proton and β^-, according to equation 3-7, giving rise to a beta minus decay. Hence, most reactor-produced isotopes show β^- activity. On the other hand, in some high energy machines a neutron is removed from the parent nucleus, and the daughter nucleus has an excess of protons, which makes it a positron emitter. Since reactor-produced isotopes are much cheaper and more readily available than those produced by particle accelerators, there are many more β^- emitters used in medicine than positron emitters. The decay schemes for a few positron emitters are given in Figure 3-8. The first scheme shows N-13 decaying by β^+ emission to C-13 according to:

$$^{13}_{7}N \rightarrow {}^{13}_{6}C + \beta^+ + \nu \quad \text{(total K.E. of } \beta^+ \text{ and } \nu \text{ is 1.20 MeV)} \quad (3\text{-}9)$$

From published tables (N1), the masses of nitrogen 13 and carbon 13 are 13.0057388 and 13.0033551 amu, respectively. Using these we record the nuclear masses and set up the balance according to equation 3-9.

mass of N-13 nucleus		$13.0057388 - 7\,m_0$
mass of C-13 nucleus	$13.0033551 - 6\,m_0$	
mass of β^+	$1\,m_0$	
mass of neutrino (ν)	0	
total	$13.0033551 - 5\,m_0$	$13.0033551 - 5\,m_0$
energy released in mass		$.0023837 - 2\,m_0$
units (subtract)		

$$\text{energy released} = .0023837 \times 931.5 \text{ MeV} - 2(.511) \text{ MeV}$$
$$= (2.220 - 1.022) \text{ MeV} = 1.198 \text{ MeV}$$

Hence, to obtain the total kinetic energy given to the positron and the neutrino or the maximum energy of the beta particle in a beta plus disintegration, we take the difference between the atomic masses of the parent and product nucleii and reduce this by 1.022 MeV ($2m_0c^2$). It is instructive to inquire into the fate of the positron. When the positron approaches close to an electron, they annihilate one another, their charges neutralize each other, and their masses are converted into 1.022 MeV of energy. This energy appears as two photons, each with energy 0.511 MeV, traveling in opposite directions from the annihilation site. In the final analysis, the total energy liberated in the above example is 2.22 MeV. This is made up of 1.198 MeV shared between the kinetic energy of the positron and the neutrino, and two gamma rays each with energy 0.511 MeV. In disintegration diagrams, it is usual to represent the starting of the β^+ particle arrow from a point $2m_0c^2$ below the parent nucleus as indicated in Figure 3-8a.

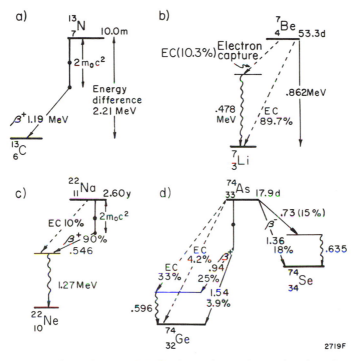

Figure 3-8. Disintegration schemes (D1) for beta plus emitters showing electron capture (EC). Only the important pathways are given.

3.10   ELECTRON CAPTURE (EC)

In the previous section, the energies involved in positron decay were discussed. It is evident that unless the nuclear energy levels of the parent and daughter nuclei differ by more than 1.02 MeV, no beta plus decay could take place since 1.02 MeV of energy is required to produce an electron positron pair. How then could such an excited nucleus get rid of its energy and achieve stability? We recall from Chapter 1 that although electrons are depicted as being in orbits outside the nucleus they are not strictly confined to these orbits and have a finite probability of being at any point in space. If then an electron came into the region of the nucleus, it could be captured by the nucleus. In the nucleus it could combine with a proton to give a neutron plus a neutrino thus:

$$p + e \text{ (usually K electron)} \rightarrow n + \nu \qquad (3\text{-}10)$$

This process is called *electron capture* (EC) and is illustrated in Figure 3-8b, by the 89.7% pathway for the decay of Be-7. In this example the neutrino would carry away $(0.861 - E_K)$ MeV where E_K is the binding energy of the K electron that was captured. Thus, in EC most of the available energy is radiated from the system as neutrinos. Often after electron capture the nucleus may still be in an excited state, as shown by the 10.3% pathway of Be-7. The excess energy of 0.478 MeV is emitted as a gamma ray.

Electron capture can occur from L and M shells but this is less likely than from the K shell. After K capture, the resulting atom has a hole in the K (or L shell). This hole can be filled in many ways, leading to all the K, L, and M lines of the spectrum as described in Chapter 2 and Auger electrons (see later section). Thus EC gives rise to the ejection of a neutrino, characteristic x rays, and at times, gamma rays from the daughter nucleus (if it is still in an excited state) and Auger electrons.

Na-22 shows two modes of decay to the excited state of neon, 90% by β^+ and 10% by electron capture. In 100 disintegrations of ^{22}Na, there will result 100 gamma rays of 1.27 MeV, x rays appropriate to the filling of 10 holes in the K shell of ^{22}Ne (.87 keV), and 90 β^+ disintegrations with 0.546 MeV of energy shared between the positron and the neutrino. When the 90 positrons are annihilated, 180 gamma rays of 0.511 MeV energy will be produced.

Finally, Figure 3-8 shows the decay scheme for As-74, an isotope that has a stable isobar on either side of it so it can decay by a β^- or a β^+ emission. The stable isotope Se-74, which lies 1.35 MeV below As-74, can be reached by two different β^- decay processes. The stable isotope Ge-74 is reached by two modes of β^+ decay and two modes of electron capture.

3.11   **INTERNAL CONVERSION**

Figure 3-9 shows the β^- spectrum of Au-198. It has the same general shape as those shown in Figure 3-6, but it has superimposed on it spectral lines at 329 and 403 keV. These electrons with precisely determined energies are called conversion electrons. Of the disintegrations of Au-198, 98.6% occur by a "first forbidden" transition to the excited state of Hg-198 (see insert of Fig. 3-9), so the observed spectrum is mainly due to this transition. The excited state may lose its energy directly by the emission of a gamma ray, γ_1, of energy 0.412 MeV. There is, however, an alternative way the excited nucleus may lose its excess energy. A bound electron may perturb the unstable nucleus and induce the transition to the lower energy state. In this process, the energy is transferred to the electron and it will leave the atom with energy $E = \gamma_1 - E_B$, where E_B is the binding energy of the electron to its atom. For example, if a K electron were ejected we would expect an electron of energy $(412 - 83) = 329$ keV; binding energy of the K electron in Hg is 83 keV (S1). Similarly, an interaction with an L or M electron will yield a group of lines at about 403 keV. This interaction of the excited nucleus and an orbital electron is known as internal conversion.

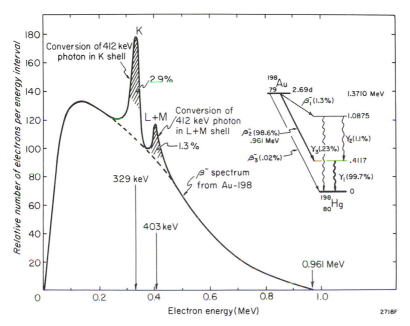

Figure 3-9. β^- spectrum of Au-198 showing electrons at the discrete energies of 329 keV and 403 keV superimposed on the continuous spectrum. Electrons with these energies arise from conversion of the 412 keV nuclear gamma ray in the K, L, and M shells.

Internal conversion is depicted schematically in Figure 3-10a, where we see a nucleus with Z protons and N neutrons ejecting a β^- by converting a neutron into a proton and creating the daughter nucleus shown in b with Z + 1 protons and N − 1 neutrons. Suppose this *daughter* has excess energy, which is emitted from the nucleus as a gamma ray of energy, γ_1. It also could interact with an electron in its K shell, ejecting it with energy $\gamma_1 - E_K$. This would leave the daughter atom with a hole in the K shell as illustrated in c. Thus, internal conversion gives rise to groups of electrons with discrete energies and corresponding "holes" in the shells from which the electrons were ejected.

The energy level diagram in the insert of Figure 3-9 is slightly mislead-ing since it is not complete. It implies that for every 100 disintegrations of Au-198 there are 99.7 gammas emitted. Although there are 99.7 *transitions* from the .4117 level, some of the transitions involve internal conversion. The number of gammas (D1) is 95.55, the number converted in the K shell 2.87, in the L shell .95, and in the M shell .31, giving a total of 99.7.

The relative probability of K electron conversion is described by the internal conversion yield α_K where:

$$\alpha_K = \frac{\text{number of conversions in K shell}}{\text{number of } \gamma \text{ rays observed}} \qquad (3\text{-}11)$$

α_K can have values ranging from 0 to 100 or more. In general, α_K in-creases with increase in Z. Similar expressions define conversion yields for the L and M shells. From the numbers given above, α_K for gold 198 is $2.87/95.55 = 0.030$.

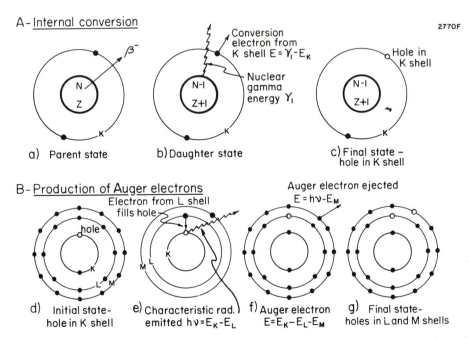

Figure 3-10. A: Schematic representation of internal conversions. B: Representation of a KLM Auger electron resulting from a hole in the K shell.

3.12   **AUGER ELECTRONS**

We now inquire into the ways the K, L, or M shell can be filled once a hole has been created. These holes can be produced by a high speed elec-tron as described in Chapter 2 or by electron capture (section 3.10) or by internal conversion described in the last section. In Chapter 2 we as-sumed that the holes in a shell were filled by electrons from outer shells with an emission of characteristic radiation. In some cases, this radiation is absent or at reduced intensity, and one observes in its place mono-energetic electrons referred to as Auger electrons. These electrons carry away the extra energy of the excited atom. Figure 3-10B shows one possible sequence of events that could occur following the creation of a hole in the K shell, as shown in d. In e we see an electron from the L shell moving to fill this hole with the emission of characteristic radiation at energy $h\nu = E_K - E_L$ and leaving a hole in the L shell as seen in f. There is an alternative way for the atom to lose its excess energy that is somewhat similar to internal conversion discussed in the previous section. The excess energy may be emitted directly in the form of an electron ejected from the M shell as indicated in Figure 3-10f. This electron, called an Auger electron, will leave the atom with energy $E = h\nu - E_M = E_K - E_L - E_M$. In the final state, represented in g, the atom has two holes, one in the L the other in the M shell. To describe Auger electrons one uses a notation involving three shells. The illustrations in Figure 3-10B describe a KLM Auger electron. The filling of the L and M holes could give rise to more Auger electrons.

The relative probability of the emission of characteristic radiation to the emission of an Auger electron is called the fluorescent yield, ω:

$$\omega_K = \frac{\text{Number K x ray photons emitted}}{\text{Number K shell vacancies}} \qquad (3\text{-}12)$$

Values for ω_K are given in Table 3-1. We see that for large Z values fluorescent radiation is favored, while for low values of Z Auger electrons tend to be produced.

From this table we see that if a nucleus with Z = 40 had a K shell hole, then on the average 0.74 fluorescent photons and 0.26 Auger electrons would be emitted.

TABLE 3-1
Fluorescent Yield

Z	ω_K	Z	ω_K	Z	ω_K
10	0	40	.74	70	.92
15	.05	45	.80	75	.93
20	.19	50	.84	80	.95
25	.30	55	.88	85	.95
30	.50	60	.89	90	.97
35	.63	65	.90		

From Evans (E1)

3.13   ISOMERIC TRANSITIONS

After beta emission the nucleus is often left in an excited state. Usually it decays very quickly to the ground state so that the lifetime in the excited state is a small fraction of a microsecond. However, in some cases the excited state may be almost stable and the nucleus may remain in it for a period of seconds, minutes, or even days. The nucleus in this state appears like a separate isotope and is called an *isomer*. The transition to the ground state is called an isomeric transition. In Figure 3-7 was shown a transition from I-131 to an excited state of Xe-131, which decays to the ground state Xe-131 with a half-life of 11.8 days. The excited state is represented by Xe-131m (m standing for metastable state) to distinguish it from the ground state Xe-131. Another example is Ba-137m, which is produced by the decay of Cs-137 (see Fig. 3-7) and decays with a half-life of **2.55** min to Ba-137. Many of the isotopes used to advantage in isotope generators, to be discussed in section 3.16 and Chapter 14, involve isomeric transitions. For example, if Ba-137 is quickly separated from Cs-137 in a generator, then the short-lived Ba-137m can be isolated and used to advantage in tracer studies.

3.14   ENERGY ABSORPTION FROM RADIOACTIVE ISOTOPES

When radioactive isotopes are used in medicine, it is necessary to calculate the energy absorbed by the patient. This may be done using the principles enunciated in the last six sections, if one bears in mind that the *neutrino* gives up *no energy* to biological material. The conclusions of the last few sections are summarized in Table 3-2. More detailed calculations will be given in Chapter 14.

TABLE 3-2
Energy Absorption from Radioactive Decay

Mode of Decay	Energy Absorption
Alpha	Total energy of the alpha particle is absorbed.
Beta minus	*Mean* energy, $\bar{E}$, of the β^- particle is absorbed. $\bar{E}$ should be obtained from tables. It is usually about 1/3 the maximum value.
Beta plus	*Mean* energy, $\bar{E}$, of the β^+ particle is absorbed. $\bar{E}$ should be obtained from tables. It is usually slightly more than 1/3 the maximum value. In addition, 2 annihilation gamma rays of 0.511 MeV are liberated and since these gammas are quite penetrating they will usually be only partially absorbed in the biological material.
Electron capture	Most of the available energy in the reaction is carried away by neutrinos. When the K or L shell holes resulting from the capture are filled, fluorescent radiation is emitted and Auger electrons are produced. Most of the energy from these two processes will be locally absorbed.
Gamma rays	When gamma rays are emitted they will be absorbed if their energy is small and the biological material large in extent. If they are of high energy only a fraction of their energy will be absorbed.
Internal conversion	A high energy electron with energy $E - E_K$ or $E - E_L$ is emitted and absorbed where E is the excess energy in the nucleus. In addition fluorescent radiation from the daughter nucleus will be emitted and usually absorbed in the biological material. Some of the fluorescent radiation may be absent and in its place will appear Auger electrons, which are absorbed.
Auger electrons	The excess energy arising from holes in the electronic shells can give rise to Auger electrons, which are locally absorbed.

3.15 <center>**DECAY SERIES**</center>

Almost all the radioactive isotopes of the *lighter elements* achieve stability by keeping their mass number constant, through beta decay or K capture. Thus, in Figure 3-3 decay is usually along an isobaric line (constant mass number) and often involves a number of successive transitions before stability is reached. Consider, for example, disintegrations along the isobaric line for mass number 90.

	$^{90}_{42}\text{Mo}$	$\rightarrow$	$^{90}_{41}\text{Nb}$	$\rightarrow$	$^{90}_{40}\text{Zr}$	$\leftarrow$	$^{90}_{39}\text{Y}$	$\leftarrow$	$^{90}_{38}\text{Sr}$	$\leftarrow$	$^{90}_{37}\text{Rb}$	$\leftarrow$	$^{90}_{36}\text{Kr}$
Activity	β^+		β^+		Stable		β^-		β^-		β^-		β^-
Half-life	5.7 hr		14.6 hr				64 hr		28 yr		2.9 min		14s
Energy	8.6 MeV		6.1		0		2.27		2.82		9.4 MeV		

In this series, only $^{90}_{40}\text{Zr}$ is stable. Elements to the left with higher Z values decay by β^+ or K capture and those to the right with lower Z values by β^-. From the atomic masses of these elements, we may calculate the energy difference between the unstable isotopes and ^{90}Zr. These show an increase as one proceeds either way from the stable species. Furthermore, in general, the larger the energy difference the more unstable the isotope and the shorter the half-life.

In a similar way, it is instructive to examine the types of activity exhibited by elements of the same Z appearing along a horizontal line in Figure 3-3. Near the lower left-hand corner of Figure 3-3, the condition of stability is most nearly satisfied by an isotope with equal numbers of protons and neutrons. The farther the isotope is from the stable species, the more unstable it will be.

Consider the case of carbon, Z = 6, for which 8 isotopes are known, 2 of which are stable.

$$^{9}_{6}\text{C} \xrightarrow{.1 \text{ s}} {}^{9}_{5}\text{B} + \beta^+ \quad 3 \text{ excess protons}$$

$$^{10}_{6}\text{C} \xrightarrow{19.4 \text{ s}} {}^{10}_{5}\text{B} + \beta^+ \quad 2 \text{ excess protons}$$

$$^{11}_{6}\text{C} \xrightarrow{20.3 \text{ m}} {}^{11}_{5}\text{B} + \beta^+ \quad 1 \text{ excess proton}$$

$$^{12}_{6}\text{C} \quad \text{stable} \quad 98.89\%$$

$$^{13}_{6}\text{C} \quad \text{stable} \quad 1.11\%$$

$$^{14}_{6}\text{C} \xrightarrow{5730 \text{ y}} {}^{14}_{7}\text{N} + \beta^- \quad 2 \text{ excess neutrons}$$

$$^{15}_{6}\text{C} \xrightarrow{2.4 \text{ s}} {}^{15}_{7}\text{N} + \beta^- \quad 3 \text{ excess neutrons}$$

$$^{16}_{6}\text{C} \xrightarrow{.74 \text{ s}} {}^{16}_{7}\text{N} + \beta^- \quad 4 \text{ excess neutrons}$$

$^{12}_{6}\text{C}$ is the most stable form of carbon and is found in nature with an abundance of 98.89%. On the one side of the stable isotope, there are nuclei with excess protons that are β^+ emitters; on the other side, there are species with excess neutrons that are β^- emitters. The heavier isotopes for a given Z are β^- active and the lighter isotopes β^+ active. They decay, keeping their mass numbers constant, until a stable species is reached.

3.16   **GROWTH OF RADIOACTIVE DAUGHTER**

In departments of nuclear medicine, extensive use is made of isotope generators. These provide an instant source of short-lived isotopes. A variety of these generators, or radioactive "cows" as they are called, are now available from radiochemical firms. The generator consists of a radioactive parent in a closed, sterile, shielded container arranged so that the user, by adding a suitable solvent, may "milk" from the parent the radioactive daughter product. A number of the useful parent-daughter combinations are dealt with in Chapter 14. To be practical, the parent should have a half-life of at least a few days while the daughter should have a half-life of a few minutes to hours and emit radiations that can be detected from outside the patient. We will now discuss the relation between the radioactive daughter and its parent, assuming the daughter has the shorter half-life.

Suppose we start with a pure sample of the parent that has a half-life t_{hl}, has a transformation constant λ_1, and contains $(N_1)_0$ atoms initially. This source will decay according to equation 1-26 so that at any later time, t:

$$N_1 = (N_1)_0\, e^{-\lambda_1 t} \qquad (3\text{-}13)$$

The radioactive daughter is *formed* at the rate at which the parent decays (i.e. $\lambda_1 N_1$), and itself *decays* at the rate $\lambda_2 N_2$, where λ_2 is the transformation constant of the daughter and N_2 is the number of atoms of the daughter present. The net rate at which the daughter product builds up is the difference between the rate of formation and the rate of decay and can be expressed mathematically as:

$$\frac{dN_2}{dt} = \lambda_1 N_1 - \lambda_2 N_2 \qquad (3\text{-}14)$$

Starting with a pure parent, the student may show that the solution of this equation is:

$$N_2 = \left(\frac{\lambda_1}{\lambda_2 - \lambda_1}\right)(N_1)_0\,(e^{-\lambda_1 t} - e^{-\lambda_2 t}) \qquad (3\text{-}15)$$

This equation may be described in terms of the activity of the parent, $A_1 = \lambda_1 N_1$, and the activity of the daughter, $A_2 = \lambda_2 N_2$, to give:

$$A_2 = A_1\left(\frac{\lambda_2}{\lambda_2 - \lambda_1}\right)\left[1 - e^{-(\lambda_2 - \lambda_1)t}\right] \qquad (3\text{-}16)$$

Of course, the equation can also be written in terms of the half-lives when one remembers that $t_{h1} = .693/\lambda_1$ and $t_{h2} = .693/\lambda_2$ where t_{h1} and t_{h2} are the half-lives of parent and daughter respectively.

To illustrate these equations, consider the isotope technetium-99m (^{99m}Tc), which is widely used in nuclear medicine. This isomer is produced from ^{99}Mo with a half-life $t_{h1} = 66.7$ h ($\lambda_1 = 0.01039$ h^{-1}) and decays to the stable form of ^{99}Tc with a half-life $t_{h2} = 6.03$ h ($\lambda_2 = 0.1149$ h^{-1}). Substituting these values in the above equations we obtain the curves shown in Figure 3-11. The parent, as expected, decays exponentially with half-life 66.7 h and appears as a straight line. The activity of the daughter Tc-99m, on the other hand, starts at zero, rises rapidly to a maximum value, and finally decays with the half-life of the parent. This behavior can be understood from equation 3-16. At $t = 0$ the exponential term is 1.0 so the term in the square bracket is zero. At very long times the exponential term is zero and the activity of the daugher becomes

$$A_2 \approx A_1 \left(\frac{\lambda_2}{\lambda_2 - \lambda_1} \right) \tag{3-17}$$

This shows that its activity is proportional to the activity of the parent but is larger by the ratio $\lambda_2/(\lambda_2 - \lambda_1)$. It is left to the student to show that the maximum activity of the daughter occurs at the time when the two curves of Figure 3-11 cross, and at this time

$$\lambda_2 N_2 = \lambda_1 N_1 \quad \text{or} \quad A_2 = A_1 \tag{3-18}$$

At this instant in time the parent and daughter have the same activity and are said to be in equilibrium.

The growth curve of Figure 3-11 shows the amount of daughter that is present in the container with the parent at any time. To be useful it is essential to separate the daughter from the parent or "milk" the parent. This can be easily achieved by a suitable chemical process since the daughter, Tc, and parent, Mo, are different chemical species. In most departments, such a radioactive cow would be "milked" every day, as illustrated in the insert, yielding activities of about 80%, 62%, 49%, and 38% on successive days. After about one week a new generator would be obtained from the radiochemical firm.

The detailed mathematics of the growth of the daughter is somewhat complicated and often an approximate calculation will suffice. If the daughter has a half-life that is small compared to the parent (the usual case), then $\lambda_2 \gg \lambda_1$ and equation 3-16 reduces to:

$$A_2 \approx A_1 [1 - e^{-\lambda_2 t}] \approx A_1 [1 - e^{-.693t/t_{h2}}] \tag{3-19}$$

This shows that after 1, 2, 3, and 4 half-lives of the daughter the activity that can be milked is approximately 50%, 75%, 87.5%, 94% of the activity of the parent.

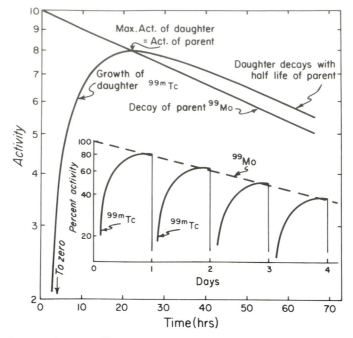

Figure 3-11. Decay of parent ^{99}Mo and growth of daughter ^{99m}Tc with time, assuming that initially we have a pure source of parent ($\lambda_1 = 0.01039$ h^{-1}, $t_{h1} = 66.7$ h; $\lambda_2 = 0.1149$ h^{-1}, $t_{h2} = 6.03$ h). The insert shows the same data when the daughter is "milked" from the parent once each day. (This diagram illustrates the principles involved. The actual situation is somewhat more complicated because only about 86% of the parent ^{99}Mo nucleii decay to the daughter ^{99m}Tc. This means that the activity of the ^{99m}Tc is at all times about 14% less than the values shown.)

Example 3-3. The isotope department receives a ^{99}Mo generator with 100 mCi activity on Monday morning at 10:00 A.M. On Thursday at 10:00 A.M. the source is milked and all the ^{99m}Tc is used in tests during the morning. In the afternoon more ^{99m}Tc is required for a new patient. Approximately what activity can be milked from the cow at 1:00 P.M.?

> The source of ^{99}Mo has decayed for 3 d 3 h and from Figure 3-11 will have an activity of about 45 mCi. The elapsed time is 3 h from the last milking or half of one half-life of the daughter. Expected activity 25% of 45 mCi = 11 mCi. The accurate solution to this problem is 14.0 mCi (see Problem 19).

3.17   **NUCLEAR FISSION**

The uranium reactor is the most important source of radioactive materials. Most isotopes can be produced more easily in it than by a cyclotron or any other high energy device. In a reactor, uranium splits into two parts with the release of neutrons and an enormous amount of energy according to the relation:

$$^{235}_{92}\text{U} + ^{1}_{0}\text{n} \longrightarrow ^{236}_{92}\text{U} \quad + 200 \text{ MeV} \qquad (3\text{-}20)$$

with the fission fragments diagram showing: n and fission fragment (up), n and fission fragment (down).

The release of 200 MeV of energy by the fission of uranium is enormous in comparison with the energy released by most nuclear reactions. In fission, 2.5 neutrons on the average are released and if these neutrons are used to initiate fission in other nuclei, a chain reaction will be set up. All the elements near the center of the periodic table can appear as fission fragments but, in particular, elements with mass numbers in the region of 140 and 90 appear most often. The uranium nucleus has many more neutrons than protons; thus when the nucleus splits up, the fragments will have a considerable excess of neutrons and be β^- emitters.

The total energy released after the complete β^- decay of the fission fragments can be calculated from mass data (N1). We will assume that the final isotopes formed are $^{90}_{40}\text{Zr}$ and $^{143}_{60}\text{Nd}$ and that 3 neutrons are liberated in the fission process.

The energy release is found as follows:

Mass of ^{235}U atom		235.043944
Mass of 1 neutron		1.008665
		236.052609
Mass of ^{90}Zr atom	89.904710	
Mass of ^{143}Nd atom	142.909856	
Mass of 3 neutrons	3.025995	
Total	235.840561	235.840561
Energy release in mass units (by subtraction)		0.212048
Energy release (931.5) (0.2120) = 198 MeV		

We would obtain very nearly the same energy release regardless of the pair of fission fragments used for the calculation. This energy release is not all immediately available but only appears after all the beta decays have taken place. In the above example the final products contain 100 protons (40 + 60), while the uranium contained only 92, hence 8 β^- decays have been included in the calculation of the energy release.

A number of heavy isotopes other than uranium are fissionable, some by slow neutrons, others by fast neutrons, others by gamma rays. In all cases, the energy release per fission is about 200 MeV.

3.18 **NUCLEAR FUSION**

Energy is released when one heavy atom disintegrates to form two lighter ones in a fission reaction. It is also possible to obtain energy by the fusion of two light atoms to form one heavier one thus:

$$_1^2H + \,_1^2H \rightarrow \,_2^3He + n + \text{Energy} \qquad (3\text{-}21)$$

This leads to the release of 3.27 MeV of energy (see problem 27). To make this reaction "go," the two deuterons must be made to approach very close to each other. This may be done by bombarding deuterium with high energy deuterons or, alternatively, by giving deuterons high energies by raising the temperature to about 150 million degrees. Once this temperature is reached, the reaction will be self-sustaining and energy will be released. There are several other possible fusion reactions that will yield energy.

Fusion is initiated in a hydrogen bomb by using the fission of uranium to produce the high temperature, at which point the fusion reaction becomes self-sustaining. To date no practical method has been found to achieve energy production from a controlled fusion reaction but much research in this field is underway. If a practical breakthrough were achieved, fusion would offer many advantages over fission for the production of energy because the amount of available fuel in the form of heavy hydrogen is almost unlimited. In addition, one would avoid the environmental problem of dealing with enormous quantities of highly radioactive fission fragments.

3.19   ACTIVATION OF ISOTOPES

When almost any material is placed in a reactor, it may become activated by neutron bombardment. The probability of activation is determined by the *cross section* for the nuclear reaction. It is usually represented by σ and is expressed in cm² per atom or in *barns* per atom where 1 barn $= 10^{-24}$ cm². If a neutron passes through this area, that is, "hits" the nucleus, then it is captured and an activation takes place. In Figure 3-12 is shown a block of target material to be activated. It contains N_t nuclei and can be of any shape or thickness. Imagine it placed in a uniform flux density of neutrons in the reactor. This neutron flux density is usually represented by ϕ and is expressed in neutrons per cm² per sec. The flux density will depend upon the type of reactor, ranging from 10^{10} for a small reactor to 10^{14} for a large reactor. Imagine that all parts of the target are bathed in this flux of neutrons. To calculate the number of activated atoms produced we project each nuclear area, σ, onto the front plane, ABCD, of the target. The total area covered by all the nuclei will be $N_t\,\sigma$. The total number of neutrons that will intercept this area in time, Δt, will be:

$$\Delta N = N_t\,\sigma\,\phi\,\Delta t \qquad (3\text{-}22)$$

and this will be the number of activations (ΔN) produced.

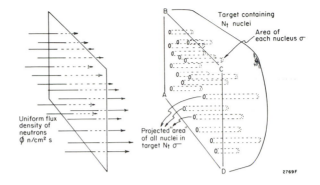

Figure 3-12. Diagram to illustrate the activation of target containing N_t nuclei bombarded by a neutron flux density ϕ. The cross section for activation is σ.

This relation is illustrated by a simple example.

Example 3-4. Find the number of active atoms of ^{60}Co produced in a 1 g sample of ^{59}Co that is placed in a neutron flux density of 10^{13} cm^{-2} s^{-1} for 1 y (3.16×10^7 s). The atomic weight of cobalt is 58.94, and the activation cross section is 37 barns per atom.

$$\text{number atoms in target} = \frac{6.02 \times 10^{23}}{58.94} \text{ g}^{-1} \times 1 \text{ g} = 1.02 \times 10^{22}$$

$$\text{no. activated} = 1.02 \times 10^{22} \times 37 \times 10^{-24} \text{ cm}^2 \times \frac{10^{13}}{\text{cm}^2 \text{ s}}$$

$$\times 3.16 \times 10^7 \text{ s} = 1.19 \times 10^{20}$$

It should be noted that in doing this calculation the shape of the target is *not* involved. The same answer would be obtained using equation 3-22 if the target were in the form of a foil of large area or in a block of small area. In deriving the equation the implicit assumption has been made that nuclei at the front of the target do not shield those at the back and this is often the case. For example, if the 1 g target of example 3-4 were 2 cm^2 in area, then the total projected area of all the nuclei onto the front plane would be $1.02 \times 10^{22} \times 37 \times 10^{-24}$ cm^2 = 0.38 cm^2, which is only 1/5 of the 2 cm^2 so shielding would not be a serious problem. If however, the *target* covered an area 1/10 as large, that is 0.2 cm^2, shielding would be a problem and a more refined calculation would be necessary.

Another assumption we have made is that in the activation process the number of target atoms remains constant during the irradiation. In example 3-4 this is essentially true since only a little over 1 percent of the atoms present initially are activated in the one year's irradiation.

NEUTRON CROSS SECTIONS: The interaction of neutrons with nuclei is a very complex phenomena. The neutron may be absorbed by the nucleus and then reemitted either with the same or different energy; this is called neutron scattering. Alternatively, a nucleus may capture a neutron to produce a new species that is stable; we then refer to a capture cross section. Many other types of reactions such as (n,γ), (n,p), (n,α), and (n,F) may take place in which a neutron is absorbed followed by the ejection of a gamma ray, a proton, or an α particle, or by fission. Each of these processes has an appropriate cross section. Further, these cross sections depend in a complex way on the energy of the neutron. The probability of a neutron being captured by a nucleus is proportional to the time the neutron spends in the vicinity of the nucleus; hence the cross section varies as 1/v where v is the velocity of the neutron. In addition, there are often narrow energy regions showing very strong selective absorption of slow neutrons. These resonance absorptions are superimposed on the 1/v variation. Since most of the neutrons present in a reactor are slow or "thermal neutrons," these are the ones that are important in the activation of isotopes. Table 3-3 gives the cross section for a few reactions by these thermal neutrons.

The cross sections given in the table vary from a fraction of a barn up to 20,000 barns for Cd-113. The cross section may be less than the "area" of the nucleus to several thousand times the area as if the neutrons in passing by were sucked into the nucleus. Further, the nucleus can have a very large cross section for one reaction and very small cross section for another.

Table 3-3 gives the cross section for specific isotopes rather than for the mixture as they appear in nature. For example, K-41 (which exists in nature with an abundance of 6.9%) has a thermal neutron cross section of 1.46 barns. If, however, we irradiate potassium as it exists in nature, the yield of K-42 will correspond to a cross section of 6.9% of 1.46 barns, or 0.101 barns. The cross sections for boron and cadmium are very large, so these materials are used to absorb neutrons in a reactor and thus control the reaction.

TABLE 3-3
Cross Sections for the Activation of a Few Isotopes by Thermal Neutrons

Isotope that is Activated	Abundance %	Isotope Produced	Half-life	Cross Section in Barns/Atom
Na-23	100	Na-24	15 h	.93
P-31	100	P-32	14.3 d	.18
K-41	6.9	K-42	12.4 h	1.46
Fe-58	.33	Fe-59	45.1 d	1.15
Co-59	100	Co-60	5.26 y	37
Au-197	100	Au-198	2.69 d	99
B-10	19.8	Li-7	stable	3837
B-all isotopes				759
Cd-113	12.3	Cd-114	stable	20,000
Cd-all isotopes				2,450

From Brookhaven National Laboratory (B1)

3.20   ACTIVITY PRODUCED BY NEUTRON IRRADIATION

In the activation of isotopes, one is usually not interested in the number of active atoms produced but in the activity of the sample that results from an irradiation. Let ΔA represent the activity resulting from the production of ΔN activated nuclei according to equation 3-22. If λ is the transformation constant of the isotope that is produced then:

$$\Delta A = \lambda \, \Delta N = \lambda \, N_t \sigma \, \phi \, \Delta t = \frac{.693}{t_h} \, N_t \, \sigma \, \phi \, \Delta t \qquad (3\text{-}23)$$

To illustrate this we calculate the activity produced in example 3-4:

$$\Delta A = \frac{0.693}{5.26 \text{ y}} \times 1.19 \times 10^{20} = 1.57 \times 10^{19} \text{ y}^{-1}$$

$$= \frac{1.57 \times 10^{19}}{3.16 \times 10^7 \text{s}} = 4.96 \times 10^{11} \text{ Bq} = 13.4 \text{ Ci}$$

In this calculation we have taken no account of the decay of the isotope during the irradiation. To take this into account we may proceed as follows. At any time t during the irradiation, let the number of activated atoms be N. In the interval of time, Δt, a number $N_t \sigma \, \phi \, \Delta t$ will be produced (eq. 3-22) and a number $\lambda \, N \, \Delta t$ will decay, hence the increase in number of active atoms ΔN will be:

$$\Delta N = N_t \sigma \, \phi \, \Delta t - \lambda \, N \, \Delta t \qquad (3\text{-}24)$$

The number of active atoms will increase initially linearly with time according to the first term but the growth rate will gradually slow down as the second term builds up as more active atoms are produced. The number will reach a maximum or saturation value (N_s) when the rate of production equals the rate of decay, so that ΔN of equation 3-24 is zero. From equation 3-24 we see that:

$$N_s = \frac{N_t \, \sigma \, \phi}{\lambda} \qquad \text{or} \qquad A_s = N_t \, \sigma \, \phi \qquad (3\text{-}25)$$

The growth of activity described by the differential equation 3-24 is plotted in Figure 3-13, where the time scale is in units of the half-life. It is seen that the growth of activity increases less rapidly as the irradiation proceeds and finally approaches the saturation activity after 4 to 5 half-lives. The graph also shows that if the growth continued at its initial rate for the mean life (1.44 t_h), the activity would reach the saturation value. It is left as an exercise for the student to show (see problem 28) that the curve of Figure 3-13 is represented by:

$$A = A_s \, (1 - e^{-.693t/t_h}) \qquad (3\text{-}26)$$

In this expression the exponential term is 1/2, 1/4, and 1/8 after 1, 2, and 3 half-lives so that A reaches 50%, 75%, and 87.5% of the saturation value after these times. These points are shown in Figure 3-13.

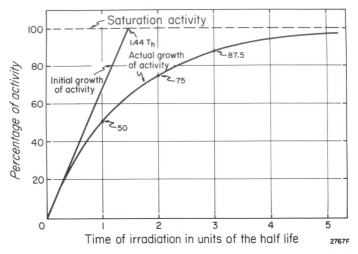

Figure 3-13. Graph showing the growth of activity as a function of irradiation time. The time is expressed in half-lives and the activity as a percentage of the saturation activity.

In any actual irradiation procedure, there are many other considerations involved in the determination of the activity to be expected. These involve variations of neutron flux with time and with position in the reactor and the shielding effects of one atom by another, especially when the atom has a large capture cross section. However, this discussion and these examples should illustrate the basic ideas involved in an irradiation procedure.

PROBLEMS

Asterisk indicates more difficult problems.

1. Plot the decay curve for Au-198 as a function of time on linear paper starting with an initial activity of 298 Bq. Show that the area under the curve to ∞ is 10^8 dis.

2. Radium has a half-life of 1620 y. A radium needle contains 1 mg of radium. The mass number is 226, and Avogadro's number is 6.02×10^{23}. Find the transformation constant for radium and the activity in Bq and mCi. (1 y = 3.16×10^7 s).

3. P-32 has a half-life of 14.3 d and emits beta particles with mean energy 0.695 MeV. Find the number of phosphorus atoms present in a 1 mCi source. Find the energy liberated per sec when such a source is placed in biological material (1 d = 8.64×10^4 s.)

4. I-131 has a half-life of 8.06 d. Find the mean life and the transformation constant. A source of iodine has an activity of 2.5 mCi. Find the activity after 12 days. Check your answer against Figure 3-2. Express your answer in mCi and Bq.

5. A source of I-131 with half-life 8.06 d has an initial strength of 1.20×10^8 Bq. Find the mean life and determine the total number of disintegrations from the source.

*6. A source of Au-198 with initial activity 10.0×10^8 Bq is used on a mold and worn by a patient for 5 days. Find the emitted radiation.

7. 1 mg of radium decays for 1 day. How many 0.18 MeV gamma rays will be emitted?

8. The mass of $^{64}_{29}$Cu is 63.9297568 amu. In a β^+ decay it is converted into $^{64}_{28}$Ni with mass 63.927956. Find the maximum energy of the β^+ particle and compare with Figure 3-6.

9. When Cu-64 emits a β^- particle it is converted into $^{64}_{30}$Zn with mass 63.9291400 amu. Determine the maximum energy of the β^- particle emitted and compare with Figure 3-6.

10. Determine the mean energy of the neutrinos emitted from the decay of P-32.

11. Numerically integrate under the curve for P-32 given in Figure 3-6 and show the mean energy is 0.7 MeV.

12. A small source of Cs-137 is embedded in a small sample of tissue. Estimate the energy absorbed after 100 disintegrations assuming fluorescent radiation is absorbed but the gammas escape. Assume the mean energy of the betas is 1/3 the maximum.

13. Repeat the calculations of problem 12 assuming all gammas are absorbed.

14. After 100 disintegrations of a source of Na-22 embedded in a small sample of tissue, estimate the energy deposited assuming all gammas escape and that the fluorescent yield is zero. Assume the mean energy of the β^+ is 1/3 the maximum.

15. Repeat the calculations of problem 14 assuming all gammas are absorbed.

16. Determine the internal conversion yield in the L shell for the 0.4117 MeV transition in Au-198.

17. Describe a KMM Auger electron. Is a KML Auger electron possible?

18. $^{90}_{37}$Rb is a fission fragment with mass 89.91487 amu. Determine the total energy released in the decay of 1 mCi of this isotope into $^{90}_{40}$Zr whose mass is 89.9047105 amu.

19. Obtain an accurate solution to example 3-3.

20. A source of Tc-99m arrives in the department at 10 A.M. on Monday, at which time the daughter is separated. The parent is found to have an activity of 5.0×10^9 Bq. Determine the activity of the parent after 3.0 d and determine the amount of daughter that may be eluted.

21. Estimate the power in megawatts which can be obtained from a reactor that consumes 50 g of U-235 per day.

22. One gram of Na-23 is placed in a reactor at a flux density of 5×10^{12} cm^{-2} s^{-1} for 30 h. Estimate the activity produced.

23. 10 g of gold is to be activated. Find the time required in a reactor to produce an activity of 200 mCi of ^{198}Au if the flux is 10^{12} cm^{-2} s^{-1}.

24. 15 g of gold is to be activated in a flux of 5×10^{12} cm^{-2} s^{-1}. Find the saturation activity. Determine the activity after 4.0 d. What fraction of the gold atoms have been activated in 4.0 days?

*25. Differentiate equation 3-15 and show that it satisfies equation 3-14.

*26. Show that the time at which the daughter (Fig. 3-11) attains its maximum value is given by $t_m = \ln(\lambda_2/\lambda_1)/(\lambda_2 - \lambda_1)$.

27. Determine the energy release from the fusion reaction of equation 3-21, given the following masses: $^2_1$H = 2.014102, $^3_1$H = 3.01602970, n = 1.00866522.

*28. Rearrange equation 3-24 so the variables N and t are separated. Then integrate the equation and obtain equation 3-26.

*29. The mean life can be considered as the average length of time an atom lives. The number of atoms present as a function of time is given by $N(t) = N_0 e^{-\lambda t}$. Sketch this exponential and break it up into a series of horizontal slices of equal height k and lengths t_1, t_2, t_3, t_4, etc. All the atoms in the first slice live time t_1, the second slice t_2, etc. so the total life of all the atoms is $k(t_1 + t_2 + t_3 + . . .)$ and this is the area under the curve. Integrate under $N_0 e^{-\lambda t}$ and thus show that the mean life is $1/\lambda$.

30. If the student adds up the number of gammas shown in the table of Figure 3-7, it will be noted that the total is greater than 1.0. How is this possible?

Chapter 4

HIGH ENERGY MACHINES

4.01 INTRODUCTION

Since 1945, the development of supervoltage machines and isotope teletherapy units has produced a dramatic change in the practice of radiotherapy. Consensus among leading radiotherapists throughout the world is that many types of cancer can be better controlled today using high energy radiations than was formerly possible (K2, P1). Further improvements in cure rate can be expected with refinements in present day machines and with greater precision in their use.

As technical developments have taken place, machines that were popular in one period have become less popular and so are replaced by new and improved units. For 20 years, cobalt 60 units, which were first installed in 1951, were the major source of radiation for radiotherapy. Cobalt units are to be found in hundreds of centers throughout the world. They are gradually being replaced by linear accelerators (linacs). In the same 20 year period (1951-1971) betatrons have found an important place in radiotherapy; however, these units suffer from low output and are now being seriously challenged by high energy linear accelerators. An isotope machine that has essentially come and gone is the cesium unit, although special units for the irradiation of mice are still in use (C1). Schultz has published an interesting historical review of the developments of high energy machines for radiotherapy (S3).

While sources of radiation were being developed specifically for radiotherapy, nuclear physicists have been building large and powerful machines for nuclear investigations. These include new types of cyclotrons and enormous linear accelerators, such as the one at Los Alamos that is one-half mile long. These machines can produce intense beams of neutrons, protons, deuterons, stripped nuclei (atoms from which the electrons have been removed), and mesons. Beams of some of these particles may be of use in radiotherapy, and so will be discussed.

Before embarking on a detailed discussion of these high energy machines, we will describe some of the properties that high energy beams in general should have to be useful in radiotherapy. We will then discuss in detail the betatron, the linear accelerator, and cobalt units and compare the beams that can be obtained from them. We will then describe the cyclotron and its use in producing high energy particles such as neutrons and protons for radiotherapy.

4.02   **CONSIDERATIONS IN THE DESIGN OF
                      HIGH ENERGY BEAMS**

In this chapter we will be discussing methods by which high energy
x ray and electron beams can be produced. Before dealing with these in
detail, it is instructive to consider some of the problems that must be
solved in order that such beams may be used correctly in the treatment
of a patient. In Chapter 10 we will describe in detail how high energy
beams are absorbed and scattered as they enter the patient. Here we give
a few of the results so that the design of high energy machines can be
properly understood.

DEPTH DOSE: Curve 1 of Figure 4-1 shows how the dose changes with
depth as a beam from a 25 MeV* betatron enters a patient. The dose at
the surface is small (20%), rises to a maximum at a depth of 5 cm, and
then falls exponentially with further increase in depth. With an ideal
high energy photon beam, uncontaminated with electrons, the entrance
dose would be nearly zero. Since these machines are almost always used
to treat tumors at least 5 cm below the skin, it is an advantage to use a
beam with *skin dose approaching zero*, and *with the peak dose as far below the
surface as possible*. The depth of the peak depends on energy but also on
other factors as illustrated by curve 2, which was obtained from a linac
operating at the *same nominal* energy as the betatron. This curve has its
peak dose at a depth of about 3 cm and is equivalent to a 16 MeV betatron. Clearly the beam from *this* linac is inferior to that from the betatron.
By altering the filters and target design of the linac, it can yield a distribution identical to curve 2 (P3, P4).

ELECTRON CONTAMINATION: The initial rising part of the depth dose
curve is called the buildup region. This region is particularly sensitive to
the design of the beam-defining collimating system. Unless care is taken,
the collimator may introduce low energy electrons into the beam and
spoil the buildup. This idea is illustrated by curves 3 and 4 of Figure 4-1.
Curve 4 is for a well-designed cobalt unit: the surface dose is small and
the peak dose occurs at a depth of 5 mm at Q. This is an inferior distribution to curves 1 or 2 but is the best that can be achieved with a cobalt
unit because the photon energy is 1.25 MeV compared to a *mean* energy
of about 8 MeV from a 25 MeV betatron or linac. The dose distribution
may, however, be a lot worse as illustrated by curve 3, which was obtained
from a badly designed cobalt unit. This curve has a high surface dose,
reaches a sharp peak at P, at 2 mm depth, and then a secondary peak at
point Q. Clearly curve 3 is very inferior to 4. The sharp peak at P is due
to low energy electrons from the collimator of the unit. These can be

---

*Imagine a betatron or linac that accelerates electrons to 25 MeV. We seek a notation to describe
the beam from such a machine. We will refer to it as a 25 MV beam, which means it contains photons
of all energy from 0 to 25 MeV. This is consistent with the terminology used for lower energy x rays.

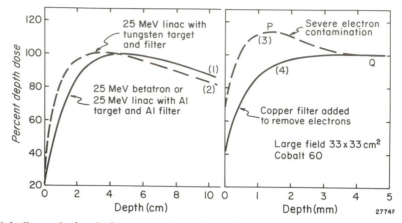

Figure 4-1. Curve 1, depth dose curve for a 25 MeV betatron or a 25 MeV linac using an Al target and Al filter. Curve 2, depth dose from a 25 MeV linac using a tungsten target and tungsten filter (P3). Curve 3, buildup curve for a large field from a Co-60 unit showing severe electron contamination, which can be removed with a copper filter to yield curve 4 (L2).

removed from the beam by the addition of an electron filter of copper to yield 4. It should be pointed out that the electron contamination illustrated in 3 is particularly severe because a large field (33×33 cm^2) was used. A similar problem arises when large fields from a linac are used. The electron contamination can be at least partially overcome with a filter. More work on this subject is required.

From these two examples we see that care should be exercised in designing the beam control devices so that the optimum distributions may be achieved from each type of machine.

FIELD FLATNESS: Another problem that must be considered is field flatness (illustrated in Fig. 4-2). A cobalt source emits the same number of photons in each direction about the axis of the beam so that the field produced by such a source is essentially uniform from the center of the field out to the edge of the beam (as illustrated in Fig. 4-2a). (There is a slight reduction in dose as one proceeds to the edge of the field, due to both increase of distance and loss of scatter, as discussed in Chapter 10). In contrast, when high energy electrons are used to produce x rays in either a betatron or a linac, photons are emitted primarily in the forward direction of the electrons (see Fig. 2-16) and so one obtains a circular distribution on the patient's skin as shown in Figure 4-2b. Such a beam would be quite useless for radiotherapy. This problem can be overcome by placing a flattening filter in the beam as illustrated in Figure 4-2c. If this flattening filter is correctly positioned and is of the proper design, it will yield a dose distribution essentially constant from the center of the field to the edge.

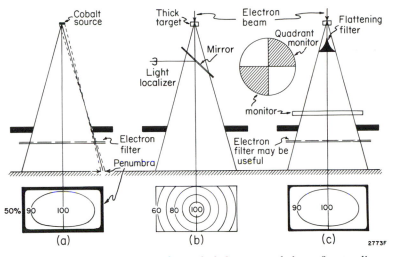

Figure 4-2. Schematic diagram comparing cobalt beams and those from a linac or beta-tron. (a) Uniform distribution from cobalt source with penumbra around the edge of the field. (b) Non-uniform dose distribution from high energy x ray beam. (c) Uniform field obtained with flattening filter. A light localizer and quadrant monitor are illustrated.

PENUMBRA: All radiation sources give a beam with unsharp edges due to penumbra arising from the finite size of the source (Fig. 4-2a). In the early days of cobalt 60 use (1951-1960), this tended to be a problem in some units because the sources were sometimes quite large (3 cm in diameter) and the beam-defining aperture was often a large distance from the patient's skin. Today penumbra, which is discussed in more detail in Chapter 10, is seldom a problem in either cobalt units or linacs.

MONITOR: Because the output of a linac or betatron is not constant, we require a very sophisticated dependable monitor system that can sense the amount of radiation that has been delivered to the patient and shut off the machine at a predetermined value. A monitor is often made with four separate quadrants so that it can also sense the alignment of the beam and alter the beam transport system to keep the beam centered on the flattening filter.

LIGHT LOCALIZER: A device is required that will show the technician the area of the field being treated. This is usually accomplished using a light and mirror combination, as illustrated in Figure 4-2b. Naturally, the light field and the radiation field should correspond.

ELECTRON FILTER: For large fields in particular, the beam is often contaminated with low energy electrons and photons. These can be partially removed by an electron filter. Good methods for introducing such filters into a beam have not yet been developed.

DESIGN PROBLEMS: A little thought will convince the reader that incorporation of all these features at the same time in a machine may create engineering problems, involving the sliding of various components in and out of the beam for the set-up and treatment sequence. For example, the light localizer must be placed below the monitor, otherwise the light will not emerge from the unit. The electron filter must be either transparent or removable when the patient is being set up for treatment so that the field size can be seen. Because of the complex interaction of all these problems, there is no ideal machine. It is essential that the reader understand these problems so that he can use the machines intelligently and, when possible, improve them. Attention to this kind of detail will improve the cure rate from high energy radiation equipment.

4.03   **BETATRONS**

The betatron, developed first by Kerst (K3), is a device for accelerating electrons. These electrons can be extracted from the machine to produce an electron beam for therapy or may be directed against a target inside the machine to produce an x ray beam. Betatrons in the energy range from 13 to 45 MeV are in use in many centers.

The essential components of a betatron are illustrated in Figure 4-3a. Acceleration of the electrons takes place in an evacuated doughnut-shaped porcelain tube placed between specially shaped poles of a magnet excited by alternating voltage. Electrons liberated by a heated tungsten filament are injected into the doughnut. The electrons are bent into a circular path by the magnetic field and spiral inwards until they reach the equilibrium orbit with radius r_0 (Fig. 4-3b). As the electrons travel around in this circle, they are continuously accelerated. This will be understood by consideration of Figure 4-3c. When the magnetic flux through a closed loop of wire is changed, an electric field is established around the loop and a reading will be obtained on a voltmeter, V, placed in the circuit. If an electron were released at some point A (Fig. 4-3c) on this copper wire, it would travel around the loop with increasing velocity were it not for the resistance of the copper, which acts as friction. In the betatron a "frictionless" path is provided inside the evacuated doughnut. As the electron acquires energy from the changing field *within* the orbit, the increasing field *at* the orbit keeps the electron moving in a circular path of constant radius. The changing magnetic field both accelerates the electron and holds it in its circular path. In order for this to happen, certain conditions must be satisfied between the field at the orbit and the flux enclosed by it. If the magnetic field at the orbit is too high the electrons will spiral in; if it is too low, the electrons will spiral out.

As the magnetic field starts to increase from 0 (Fig. 4-3d), electrons are injected and caused to spiral inward until they reach the equilibrium orbit. As the flux increases, the electrons acquire energy and at C will have their maximum energy. If they were left in the orbit, they would be

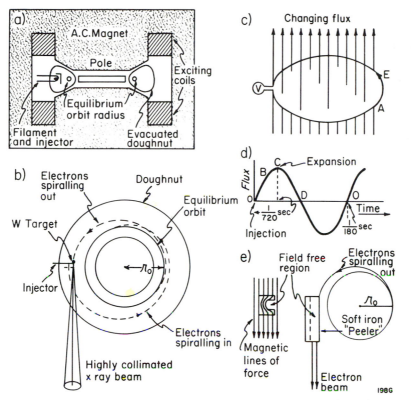

Figure 4-3. Diagrams illustrating the construction and operation of the betatron. (a) Cross-sectional diagram showing the AC magnet, the poles, the doughnut, and injector. (b) The paths of the electrons within the doughnut and the method of production of the x rays. (c) How an electric field is produced by a changing magnetic flux. (d) The cycle of operation of the betatron showing the time of injection and expansion. (e) The operation of the electron "peeler" for obtaining an electron beam. The sketch showing the magnetic lines of force is a cross-sectional view of the "peeler" device taken at right angles to the diagram through the center of the "peeler."

decelerated and brought to rest at D. However, if at C the equilibrium conditions are suddenly altered by decreasing the field at the orbit, the electron will spiral outward to strike the back of the injector where x rays are produced.

If a lower energy beam is required, the equilibrium conditions can be upset earlier in the cycle at some point, such as B (Fig. 4-3d), causing the electrons to spiral out before attaining their maximum energy. The betatron is idle for the next three-quarters of a cycle until the point 0 (Fig. 4-3d) is reached, at which time electrons are again injected to repeat the cycle. Thus radiation from the betatron is produced in pulses 1/180 of a second apart and lasting about a microsecond.

The efficiency of x ray production is very high and no cooling mechanism is required since almost all the energy lost by the electrons in passing through the target is changed into x rays. The x ray beam is highly concentrated in the forward direction (see Fig. 2-16) so a flattening filter is required (A1, J1). A filter of low atomic number material such as carbon or aluminum is most suitable since it will remove low energy photons preferentially over high energy ones (see Fig. 5-11). The optimum energy for betatron therapy is about 25 MeV. A photograph of a 25 MeV medical betatron in the Ontario Cancer Institute is shown in Figure 4-4.

The betatron may also be used to produce a beam of electrons. The electrons are removed from the doughnut by an ingenious "peeler" device illustrated in Figure 4-3e. It (S4) consists of a laminated soft iron channel placed tangentially to the equilibrium orbit and just outside it. The magnetic lines of force are conducted through the iron, leaving a field free space at the center of the channel. When the electrons are expanded into this region, they are no longer acted on by the magnetic field and so travel in a straight line, until they emerge from the betatron through a thin window in the doughnut. The electrons are not nearly as penetrating as the x ray beam and produce quite a different dose distribution, which will be discussed in Chapter 10.

The major limitation of the betatron is its low dose rate, which results from an inefficient injection mechanism of electrons into the doughnut. To increase the yield, repetition rates higher than line frequency are used. For example, in the Allis-Chalmers machine the repetition rate is 180 pulses per second, three times the line frequency. Betatrons and linacs will be compared later in this chapter.

4.04   THE LINEAR ACCELERATOR (LINAC)

Since 1960 there has been continual development of linacs for nuclear physics, radiotherapy, and radiation chemistry. Their technology grew from extensive research during World War II to produce high power, high frequency electromagnetic waves required for radar. Most modern linacs use power sources at 3000 MHz, giving a wavelength in vacuum of:

$$\lambda = \frac{c}{\nu} = \frac{3 \times 10^{10} \text{ cm/s}}{3000 \times 10^6/\text{s}} = 10 \text{ cm}$$

The time, T, for one oscillation of this power is $1/(3000 \times 10^6 \text{ s}^{-1}) =$ 333 ps. Linacs can be either of the traveling wave variety or of the standing wave type, both of which are illustrated in Figure 4-5.

Traveling Wave Linac: Suppose an electromagnetic wave at 3000 MHz is transmitted down a tube having a series of evenly spaced discs 1/4 of a wavelength (2.5 cm) apart as illustrated in Figure 4-5a. Along the axis of the tube will be an electric field whose distribution at time 0 will be as indicated. In the center of the first section the field is E to the right, in the second section zero, in the third section E to the left, in the fourth

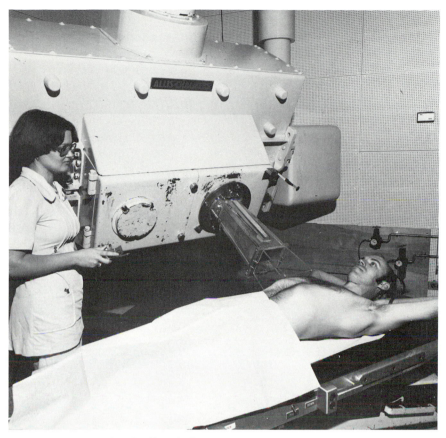

Figure 4-4. Photograph of Allis-Chalmers 25 MeV betatron installed in the Ontario Cancer Institute.

zero, and then the pattern repeats itself. At a time T/4 later, the whole pattern will be shifted λ/4 to the right as indicated. After one more quarter period the electric field will be shifted down the tube still another λ/4.

Suppose now an electron could be introduced into the wave guide at P with a velocity close to that of light. It would find itself continually in an electric field E, which would give it energy as it traveled down the tube. Since the electron already has a velocity near c, the added energy would appear as an increase in the mass of the electron. The electron would thus find itself carried along with the traveling wave, as illustrated in Figure 4-5c, a process somewhat analogous to a surf rider carried on the crest of a wave. In the traveling wave accelerator, the electric field can be as high as 80 kV/cm so that a tube 1 meter long can give an electron an energy of about 8000 keV = 8 MeV.

To capture electrons into the wave guide we require some method of reducing the velocity of the electromagnetic wave to correspond to the

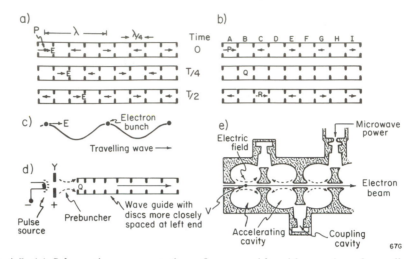

Figure 4-5. (a) Schematic representation of wave guide with a series of equally spaced discs λ/4 apart. The electric field E at various positions in the wave guide is shown at times of 0, T/4, T/2, etc. when a *traveling* wave is passing down the guide from left to right. (b) Same as a except the electric field configuration is now shown for a *standing* wave. (c) Schematic representation of electron bunch being carried on the crest of a traveling wave. (d) Diagram of buncher showing how electrons are captured into the wave guide. (e) Details of one type of wave guide used to create standing waves.

velocity of the electron at time of injection so that it will stay on the crest of the wave. The way this is done is illustrated in Figure 4-5d. The aperture Y is pulsed at 3000 MHz to about 70 kV thus producing bunches of electrons, each traveling at 0.48 c (see Table 1-7). The electromagnetic wave in the left hand end of the wave guide is matched to this velocity by suitable loading through the reduction of the spacing between the discs in this portion of the wave guide. This disc spacing is gradually increased to correspond to velocity c as one proceeds down the guide. The buncher may be a separate section directly coupled to the uniformly loaded wave guide, or it may be a few sections at the left hand end of the guide. For this traveling wave system to operate properly, the wave, on reaching the end of the wave guide, must be absorbed in a dummy load and thus be prevented from being reflected back to interfere with the incoming wave.

STANDING WAVE LINAC: Electrons can also be accelerated in a wave guide in which a standing wave is achieved (as illustrated in Fig. 4-5b). A standing wave is set up when two waves of equal amplitude and period travel through the same wave guide in *opposite* directions. The reader may show (see problem 10) that at positions, B, D, F, and H the electric field is always zero while halfway between these planes the electric field oscillates, being first to the right, then to the left, etc. The electric field configuration is shown at time T = 0; in sections A, E, and I the electric field is to the right while at C and G it is to the left. At a time T/4 later the electric field is everywhere zero while at T/4 still later all fields are reversed from their original configuration. Suppose an electron could be introduced into this wave guide with a velocity c. At P it would find itself in a field to the right, at Q in zero field, and at R once again in a field to the right, so that it would always be accelerated to the right and so receive energy as it traveled down the tube.

One way of setting up these standing waves is illustrated in Figure 4-5e. Adjacent accelerating cavities are coupled together by the coupling cavity. The diagram shows the electric field in the accelerating cavities at one instant in time. An electron at V will experience a force to the right. If it reaches the next cavity 1/2 a cycle later, it will again find itself experiencing a force to the right and so acquire energy from the standing wave. In a wave guide using standing waves, energy transfers of 150 keV per cm are possible. Most linacs today employ standing waves.

The main advantage of linacs over betatrons arises from the efficient way in which energy can be given to the electron as it moves down the axis of the wave guide. Linacs several kilometers long have been made, yielding very high energies. Betatrons of energies much greater than 100 MeV are not feasible, because of energy losses. When electrons move in a circular path they are continually accelerated towards the center and so radiate energy. When the energy loss by this mechanism is equal to the rate at which energy is transferred to the electron by the changing magnetic field, then no further increase in energy is possible. The only upper limit to the energy achievable in a linac is related to cost.

Linacs have one other important advantage over betatrons and this is related to yield. Many more electrons can be injected and captured into the wave guide in a linac than is possible in a betatron, so dose rates 10 to 100 times as great can be achieved. Further, since the linac is a linear device, there is no difficulty in extracting the electrons from the machine as a useful beam and no special peeler device (see last section) is required. Compared with betatrons, linacs also have some serious disadvantages, which will be discussed in the next section. For further details on linacs the reader is referred to review articles (K4, H5, K2).

4.05   MEDICAL LINACS

Because of the growth of linacs from World War II radar research, it is not surprising that the first practical medical machines were developed in Great Britain (M4), followed closely by developments in the United States (H6). Here we will discuss briefly some of the types of linacs now available for medical use.

Most medical linacs make use of isocentric mounts (illustrated in Fig. 4-6), where the source S is 80 to 100 cm from the axis of rotation. For treatment the patient is first positioned with the center of the tumor on the axis of rotation. After this adjustment has been made accurately, the machine is turned on to deliver a prescribed dose to the tumor from one direction. If more fields of the same size but from different directions are required, these treatments can be given without realignment of the patient simply by rotating the unit from the control room. Alternately, the machine may be rotated continuously during the treatment.

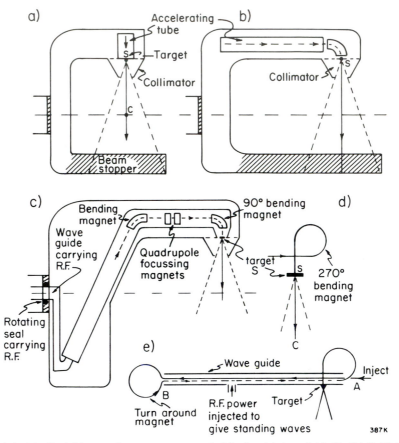

Figure 4-6. Medical Linacs: Arrangements suitable for (a) 4 to 6 MeV, (b) 8-12 MeV, (c) 30 to 35 MeV. (d) A method of bending the electron beam through 90° by using a 270° bending magnet. (e) The "turn around," or "two pass," linac.

Linacs are available with energies ranging from 4 to 35 MeV and this energy determines which of the configurations illustrated in Figure 4-6 is likely to be used. For energies from 4 to 6 MeV the accelerating tube can be made short enough (50-100 cm) to allow the arrangement of Figure 4-6a. This is the simplest design possible. Electrons travel down the tube, strike a target at S, and produce an x ray beam symmetrical about the line SC. If the electron beam is required, the target is moved to the side allowing the electrons to emerge through a thin window and be directed towards the patient.

If a higher energy beam is required, the accelerating tube must be made longer, necessitating the configuration of Figure 4-6b or c. Configuration b is useful for energies of about 12 MeV, while c is convenient for a linac with energy 25-35 MeV. In configuration c the radio frequency power from the klystron is brought to the wave guide through the axis of the machine using a rotating vacuum seal. The beam of electrons is bent through an angle of about 60°, passes through quadrupole focusing magnets, and is then bent through 90° in the head to hit a target or emerge through a thin window as an electron beam. An alternative design to c is one in which the whole accelerator is external to the unit and the electrons themselves are brought through the rotating seal and into the head by a series of bending and focusing magnets.

A variation on c is shown in d where the electrons are bent through 270° to hit the target at S and produce a beam along the axis SC. The use of a 270° bending magnet gives the beam increased stability over the 90° magnet.

A promising new development is the "turn-around" linac developed by AECL and illustrated schematically in Figure 4-6e. Electrons are injected at A and accelerated to energy E_0 in the wave guide A-B. They emerge from the wave guide at B and are turned around with a suitable magnet and are reinjected into the wave guide in the right phase to be accelerated from B back to A to attain a total energy of 2 E_0. A feature of the turn-around linac is that it allows the energy to be varied from 0.5 to 2.0 E_0. At A they are removed to produce an electron or photon beam. With this interesting new design a 24 MeV machine can be made almost as small as a 12 MeV unit. The RF power unit can be placed on the gantry, thus avoiding the need for "piping" RF from an external modulator through rotating seals as required in the design of Figure 4-6c.

PHOTON ENERGY AND ELECTRON ENERGY: After the electron has been accelerated the full length of the wave guide, its energy will naturally depend upon the design of the guide and the power applied to it. It will also depend on the current in the wave guide: the larger this current, the *lower* the energy. For a traveling wave system the final kinetic energy of the electron decreases linearly as the tube current is increased. When one buys a linac it is important to realize that the energy often quoted is the unloaded value. For example, in the Varian "clinac 35" the "35" refers to the energy given the electrons when the wave guide is essentially unloaded. When this machine is loaded to give a useful x ray output, its energy drops to about 25 MeV. In the photon mode the energy is usually about 1/3 less than the maximum value. In a similar way a Varian "12" is really about 8 MeV when used to produce x rays.

We must now draw a distinction between the electron and photon mode. In the electron mode, very high and in fact dangerously high dose rates would be achieved if the same number of electrons were accelerated as in the photon mode, so safety interlocks are used to limit the number of electrons captured into the wave guide. Since the wave guide in the electron mode is essentially unloaded, the energy of the electron beam is close to the unloaded energy of the machine. Since the photon mode is the one generally used, the nomenclature is misleading. Beams from high energy machines should be described in terms of their depth dose properties (see Chapter 10) and not in terms of some nominal electron energy.

CONFIGURATION OF COMPONENTS: Figure 4-7a shows the important components required to shape and control the beam from a linac used in both the photon and electron mode. High energy electrons from the wave guide are focused at S on the target, which is thick enough to stop the electrons. The angular distribution of the photons is determined by the direction the electrons had *before* they hit the target so the beam optics must maintain the angle α constant as well as maintain S at the same point in space. When electrons are required, the tungsten target, which is mounted on a slide, is moved to the right allowing the electrons to pass through an open port. Just below the target a second slide is located that contains a selection of electron scattering foils for each electron energy as well as an open port used for the photon mode. The beams then pass through a conical hole in the primary collimator made of heavy metal. Just below this collimator is a slide containing the flattening filter made of tungsten or an open section for electrons. Next is positioned a fixed ion chamber to monitor the dose and a quadrant section connected to a servo mechanism to control the beam optics. Just below the ion chamber is the light localizer, which is retracted from the beam after the patient has been correctly positioned in the beam. The adjustable pairs of collimators at right angles can be rotated about the axis and are designed to give any rectangular field size. All these components are mounted in the head in a space that reaches about 50 cm from the source and half way to the isocenter at 100 cm.

In most commercially produced linacs the flattening filter has been made of tungsten to save space in the head. This produces the deleterious effects on the beam illustrated in Figure 4-1. For example, 25 MeV electrons in a linac produce a beam with properties equivalent to a 16 MeV betatron (P3, P4). Part of this effect is due to the badly designed flattening filter, but part is also due to the nature of the targets in the two machines. In the betatron the target is "thin" and each interaction that gives rise to a photon is one involving the full electron energy, E_{max}. In the linac, photons are produced by electrons with all energies from E_{max} down to zero. A thin target could be used in a linac if the electrons that

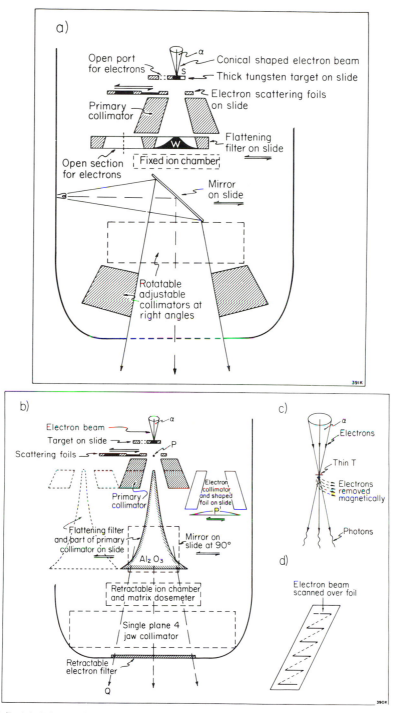

Figure 4-7. (a) Schematic representation of the components generally used by manufacturers of 20-25 MeV linacs. (b) Alternative arrangement of components for high energy linacs allowing use of an Al_2O_3 flattening filter to yield better depth dose distribution. Also included is an improved method for obtaining a uniform electron flux density with minimum bremsstrahlung (R1). (c) Diagram to show how a thin target could be used if the electrons are removed magnetically. (d) Alternative scanning arrangement to produce a uniform electron flux density.

pass through it could be swept from the beam by a magnetic field (as in Fig. 4-7c). It is hoped that linac manufacturers will take some of these ideas into consideration in improving the design of their photon mode capability. A number of configurations could be used but one possible arrangement is illustrated in Figure 4-7b. The flattening filter, now made of Al_2O_3, must be about 25 cm high. It is mounted on a sliding platform with part of the primary collimator in such a way that it can be moved to the left when electron operation is required. The mirror for the light localizer is arranged to slide in and out of the page to occupy the same position as the flattening filter. Next is arranged the ion chamber with its quadrant sections for servo control and some 49 dosemeters (J2), which give continuous read-out on a television monitor so that the flatness of the beam is under continual observation during treatment. The ion chamber must be retractable and moved out of the beam during patient positioning and back in during treatment. To save the extra space used by the flattening filter, the beam-shaping collimator can be made from 4 blocks of heavy metal moving on the surface of a sphere and coupled together much the same as the beam-defining system created by AECL (G2). Finally, just below the head would be mounted a retractable electron filter that would be used to improve the buildup characteristics of the beam when large fields are used.

BEAM CONTROL FOR ELECTRON MODE IN LINACS: Figure 4-7b shows one arrangement of the components we have found useful in achieving an optimum electron beam. The electron beam as it emerges from the accelerating tube through a thin window is so strongly peaked in the forward direction that it would be quite useless in radiotherapy. The beam can be scattered laterally by passing it through a foil of metal but this will contaminate the electron beam with x rays produced by bremsstrahlung in the foil. The thicker the foil the worse this contamination becomes. One therefore should attempt to flatten the beam with the *minimum* thickness of foil. This can be done using two relatively thin foils (J3) at P and P'.

Consider a point Q at the edge of the largest required field. With no primary electron scatterer in the beam at P, the reading of an ion chamber placed at Q would be zero. As the foil at P is increased in thickness this reading will increase as electrons are scattered to Q. Finally, with further increase in this foil thickness the reading will start to decrease as more electrons are scattered outside Q and increasing numbers are absorbed in the primary scatterer. The foil thickness that gives the maximum reading at Q should be chosen. Having selected this thickness, one then adds a *shaped* secondary scatterer at P' to give a flat field. We have found (R1) that to flatten a 20 MeV beam over a 35 cm diameter at 1 m, the primary filter should be about 3 mm of lead and the shaped filter should vary from 0 at the edge to about 3 mm of lead at the center.

Another practical way to spread the electron beam is to use a scanning magnet (illustrated in Fig. 4-7d) to move the electrons over the field area in a precise and controlled manner to yield a flat field.

A photograph of a 35 MeV linac at the Ontario Cancer Institute is shown in Figure 4-8.

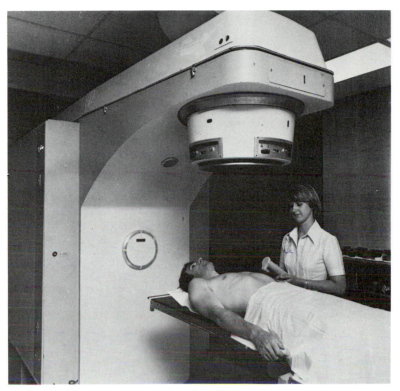

Figure 4-8. A Varian "35" MeV linac installed at the Ontario Cancer Institute.

SUPERCONDUCTING LINACS: Conventional linacs operating at room temperature suffer from power losses in the cavities. These losses amount to about 3 megawatts per meter and arise through currents in the surface layers of the microwave cavities. If one cooled these microwave cavities to liquid helium temperatures, it is conceivable that a linac could be built with power losses of about 3 watts per meter, yielding a much more compact device, which could be readily mounted on a gantry to yield a unit no larger than a cobalt unit. We look forward to developments in this direction (K4).

MICROTRONS: A microtron is an electron accelerator that may be useful in radiotherapy. Electrons are passed through a microcavity similar to one section of a linac and given a burst of energy. They then move into a region where there is a magnetic field that carries them in a circle to reenter the cavity. If they return to the cavity after one cycle, they will be

in phase with the electric field in the cavity and will be accelerated once
more. By proper design it is possible to have them take a time corresponding to one extra cycle after each transit through the microwave
cavity. A microtron has some potential advantages over a linear accelerator because higher energies can be achieved in a given volume. It may
be possible to install a 25 MeV microtron in a small compact head like a
cobalt unit. We look forward to developments in this field also (B2).

4.06   **ISOTOPE MACHINES**

Until 1951, all isotope machines made use of radium in what were
known as teleradium units. These contained from 4 to 10 g of radium. At
the time these units were being used, radium cost about 20 dollars per
mg so that a 10 g source was worth about 200 thousand dollars. This fact
alone made large sources of radium prohibitive. However, aside from
economics, large sources of radium are impractical because the front
layers of the source effectively filter out the radiation from the back
layers of the source. All this was changed in 1951 when two strong
sources of cobalt 60 were produced in Canada's high flux nuclear reactor
and made available for teletherapy (D2, G2, J4, J5, J6). Each source contained approximately 1000 Ci in a volume of 5 cm^3 with a mass of about
40 g and hence a specific activity of about 25 Ci/g. To obtain the same
radiation output from radium would require a source some 60 times as
large containing 1500 g of radium, and this source would suffer from
the self-filtration discussed above. For the first time it became feasible to
place this small source at a large distance from the patient and so emulate
the operation of a high energy x ray machine. Since 1951 the production
of cobalt 60 sources and cobalt units has been expanded to such an extent
that for many years more radiotherapy was carried out with cobalt 60
than with all other types of radiation combined.

SOURCE ARRANGEMENT: Isotope machines consist of a lead-filled steel
container, near the center of which is placed the radioactive source, and a
device for bringing this source into a position opposite an opening in the
head so that the useful beam of radiation may emerge. To facilitate inter-
change of sources from one unit to another and from one isotope production facility to another, standard source capsules have been developed. One such capsule is shown in Figure 4-9. The active material in the
form of pellets is in a stainless steel container, and this container is in
turn placed inside another and sealed by welding. To accommodate different amounts of active material, spacing wafers can be inserted to fill
the unused space. In addition, to make possible the fabrication of sources
of different diameter, sleeves, all with the same external diameter but
with the appropriate inner diameter, can be placed in the inner capsule.

A number of methods of moving the source so that the useful beam
may emerge from the unit have been developed. In one of the simplest

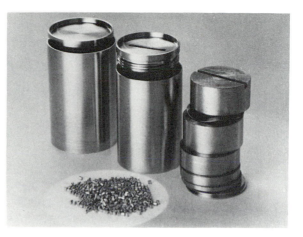

Figure 4-9. Photograph of a
cobalt source capsule.

arrangements (shown in Fig. 4-10a), the source is mounted on a heavy
metal wheel that may be rotated through 180° to carry the source from
the "off" position to the "on" position (J4). Another arrangement is
shown in Figure 4-10b where the source, mounted on a heavy metal
drawer, slides horizontally from the "off" to the "on" position (J7). All
machines are arranged so that they fail "safe"; that is, if the power fails,
the source automatically goes to the "off" position. This is essential, because these machines make no noise in their operation and every pre-
caution must be taken to insure that personnel are not near the machine
if the machine is inadvertently "on."

FIELD SIZE: To be practical a collimator should be designed to permit
all possible rectangular fields from 4 by 4 cm to 35 by 35 cm. In addition,
complex fields shaped for the individual patient by the use of additional
shielding blocks placed on a tray under the collimator are also needed.

PENUMBRA: (See Fig. 4-2.) Penumbra may be reduced by the use of a
small source. However, when the source is made small, the activity and
hence the radiation output is reduced. This may be overcome partially
by the use of very high specific activity cobalt, and today, activities up to
200 Ci/g are available, yielding sources 1.0 cm in diameter or less. In
linacs or betatrons, one usually considers the penumbra to be very small
since the electrons are focused to a very small point in the target. However, the flattening filter is a strong source of scattered radiation so that
the apparent focal spot located somewhere between the target and the
flattening filter is larger than one might assume. In most units in use
today penumbra is not a problem.

ELECTRON CONTAMINATION: One of the important clinical advantages
of a cobalt 60 beam derives from the dose in the superficial layers of the
skin being small and the maximum dose occurring at a depth below the
skin (see Chapter 10). This advantageous situation may be completely
reversed by electrons scattered from the diaphragm or treatment cone

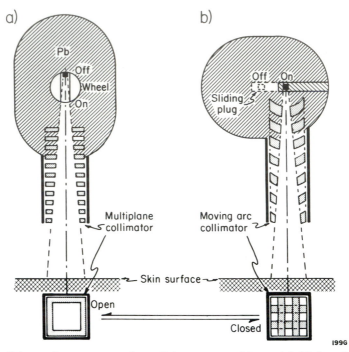

Figure 4-10. Schematic representation of isotope machines. (a) Unit using rotating wheel to carry the source from the "off" to the "on" position and a multiplane collimator to control the size of the beam. (b) Sliding drawer-type mechanism with moving arc collimator.

system as shown in Figure 4-2. Experiments have shown that this contamination is particularly bad if the diaphragm system extends right down to the skin. However, if a space of some 15 or 20 cm is left between the diaphragm and the skin and the field is not larger than about 20 by 20, these electrons are stopped or scattered in the air and do not reach the skin (J5). This factor puts a practical lower limit on the distance between the diaphragm and skin. In some cases, space does not permit this separation, and then a partial solution may be achieved with electron filters placed between the diaphragm and the skin. When large fields (35 by 35 cm²) are used, electron contamination becomes very severe. These electrons can be eliminated (L2) partially by covering the treatment port with a filter of copper or other medium atomic number material (as illustrated in Fig. 4-1). The addition of such a filter will interfere with the light localizer, and methods must then be provided to remove the filter when the patient is being set up and returned to proper position at the start of the treatment.

4.07   TYPICAL COBALT 60 UNITS

Figure 4-11 shows a Picker ceiling-mounted cobalt 60 unit installed in the Ontario Cancer Institute. The unit is essentially the same as the original one developed in Saskatoon (J4, J6). Such a unit mounted on the ceiling provides complete flexibility of beam direction and enables the patient to be moved readily to any point below the machine, thus facilitating the patient setup. It uses the popular multiplane collimator illustrated in Figure 4-10a.

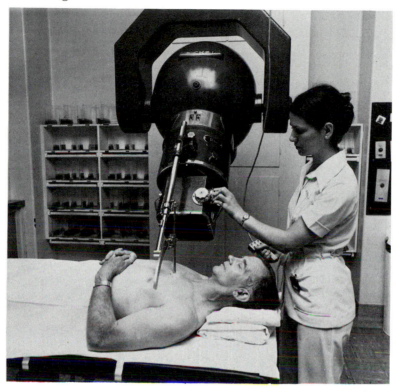

Figure 4-11. Photograph of a Picker ceiling-mounted cobalt unit installed at the Ontario Cancer Institute in Toronto. The unit uses the multiplane collimator illustrated in Figure 4-10a.

ROTATIONAL COBALT UNITS: Most cobalt units in use today are arranged on a gantry so they may be used either as fixed field machines or rotation units. A unit of this type developed by AECL is shown in Figure 4-12. This unit is a precision machine featuring many of the ideas developed by the authors (J7). The unit may be used with an x ray source so that a "placement film" may be taken to insure the tumor is centered in the beam. Some units also include a focusing transit dose meter to measure the radiation transmitted through the patient to enable one to correct the dosimetry for the effects of air and bone on the beam (F1, J7).

SPECIAL UNITS FOR LARGE FIELDS: During the 1970s there has been a gradual trend towards the use of larger and more complex radiation fields in the treatment of certain types of tumors. To produce these large fields, new types of units have been designed and built. Figure 4-13 shows

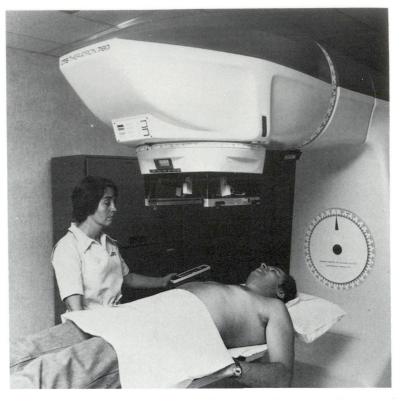

Figure 4-12. Isocentric mounted cobalt 60 unit produced by Atomic Energy of Canada and installed at the Ontario Cancer Institute.

a unit made by Atomic Energy of Canada and mounted on a vertical gantry; in our institute it is devoted almost exclusively to the treatment of large, complex-shaped fields. The field to be treated is cut out of a piece of Styrofoam® to correspond exactly to the anatomy of the particular patient. This Styrofoam mold is placed in a rectangular tray that may be swung from the wall to a *reproducible* spot over the patient. The mold is moved in the tray until the mold is accurately aligned with the patient, using various light-localizing devices. It is then clamped in this position in the tray and the whole tray unit is swung over to the wall position under a hopper filled with lead shot, where the space around the mold is filled. The tray is then swung back over the patient to its initial position and the treatment carried out. At the end of the treatment, the tray carrying the lead shot is swung back into position over a second hopper fastened to the wall and the lead shot dumped. With this device no lifting by the technician is required and treatment can be reproduced accurately from day to day (V1).

HALF BODY IRRADIATOR: Another type of special unit newly installed in the Ontario Cancer Institute is a half body irradiator. Fitzpatrick and

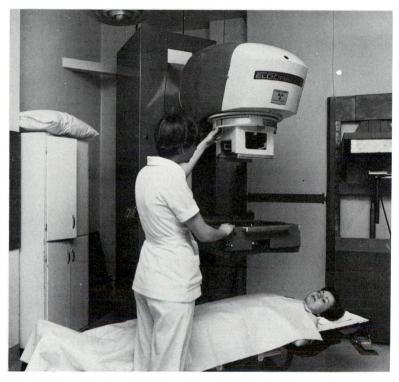

Figure 4-13. AECL pedestal cobalt 60 unit installed at the Ontario Cancer Institute and used almost exclusively for the irradiation of large complex shaped fields. The device for obtaining complex shaped fields is illustrated.

Rider (F2) have shown that for certain advanced types of cancer, involving multiple metastases, patients can be treated using the following technique. One-half of the patient is irradiated to a dose of 700 to 800 rads, a month is allowed to elapse, then the other half of the patient is treated to about the same dose. These doses are very large and would certainly kill the patient if the whole body were treated to this dose level at one time. However, with the one month interval between the two treatments, the bone marrow cells in the unirradiated area can repopulate the bone marrow in the treated area. 800 rads to half the body is still a very large dose and will cause nausea in many patients. This may interrupt the treatment unless it is carried out quickly. To carry out this kind of treatment we have developed a half body irradiator, shown in Figure 4-14. With this unit, fields up to 150 cm long and 50 cm wide can be obtained. The device is fitted with a compensating filter so that a uniform dose through the patient is achieved after treatment in the prone and supine positions with opposing fields.

DOUBLE HEADED COBALT UNIT: In a large radiotherapy department such as the Ontario Cancer Institute, many cobalt units are in operation.

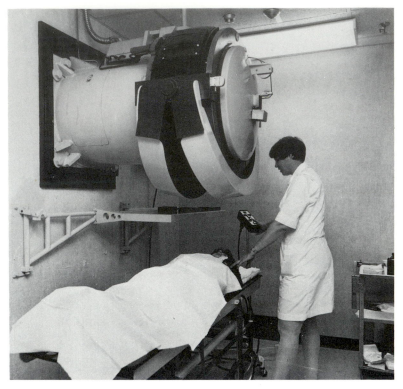

Figure 4-14. Half body irradiator at the Ontario Cancer Institute.

The sources for these units are replaced every six years or so, so that in a very short time a surplus of half expended sources are available. We therefore developed a doubleheaded unit to take two half-expended sources. These are mounted in opposite ends of a "U" shaped structure. Such a unit gives two opposing fields, which are useful in many types of treatment (C2).

HEAD AND NECK CESIUM 137 UNITS: In the period 1955 to 1960 many types of cesium units, which emit 662 keV radiation, were developed. In general these have not proved very useful, primarily because of low output. It can be shown that a specific activity of more than 79 Ci/g cannot be achieved and that the dose rate from a cesium unit is about 1/16 that of a cobalt unit with the same activity.

A head and neck unit is one type of machine that should use a short treatment distance (to give a small depth dose) and employ penetrating radiation to avoid damage to bone (see Chapter 11). In addition, it should be easily shielded so that it can be made small, making possible easy manipulation in the head and neck region. A small source of cesium 137 meets all these requirements and practical cesium units of this kind have been developed (W2).

CESIUM 137 RADIOBIOLOGY UNITS: For radiobiological studies involving small animals such as mice, the cesium irradiator developed at the Ontario Cancer Institute is ideal (C1). The unit contains two sources of cesium 50 cm apart mounted in a single lead housing. The biological material is placed in an enclosed plastic drawer halfway between the sources. The mice are loaded into the drawer outside the unit and then slid into place for the irradiation. The unit gives a uniform dose to material anywhere in the drawer at a rate of 1 to 2 Gy/min. For this type of application cesium is much better than cobalt since the shielding requirements are less and the half-life is six times longer. Adequate dose rates are achieved by using two sources at a short treatment distance.

4.08   **THE CYCLOTRON**

For many years one of the major tools of nuclear physics has been the cyclotron. Today there is renewed interest in such machines because of the possibilities of using them to produce beams of protons or neutrons for clinical use. Further, with present technological developments it may be feasible to make such machines small enough to allow them to be mounted on a gantry so that the beam may be conveniently directed toward any site in the patient.

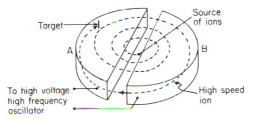

Figure 4-15. Diagram illustrating the operation of the cyclotron.

The principle of the cyclotron is shown in Figure 4-15. A and B are two hollow conducting semicircular structures (known as D's) with a short insulating gap between them. These D's are placed between the poles of a large direct current magnet (not shown) and are connected to a high frequency (10 MHz), high voltage (20 keV) oscillator. If protons are to be accelerated, a small amount of hydrogen is liberated at the center and bombarded with electrons from a tungsten filament to produce a source of positive ions or protons. These positive ions find themselves in the electric field between the edges of the two D's and will be attracted by the negative one and repelled by the positive one. Once inside the negative D, they would travel in a straight line with a uniform velocity were it not for the strong magnetic field. This magnetic field will cause the particles to move in the arc of a circle at a constant speed until they again emerge between the D's. If they reach the gap just as the direction of the electric field changes, they will be accelerated and drawn into the other D.

They are now traveling faster and so will move on a larger circle, to reach the next gap just as the electric field changes again, and so on. The operation of the cyclotron depends upon the fact that a slow moving particle will take the same length of time to travel through the D as will a higher speed particle, since the latter will travel on a larger circle. This may be seen from the following analysis.

A particle of charge e moving with velocity v at right angles to a magnetic field B experiences a force F at right angles to both B and v, given by

$$F = Bev \qquad (4\text{-}1)$$

If e is in coulombs, v in m/s, and B in tesla, then F is in newtons. Since the force F is at right angles to v, it will cause the charged particle to move in a circle. The radius of the circle, r, will be such that the centrifugal force, mv^2/r, is balanced by the force due to the magnetic field so that

$$\frac{mv^2}{r} = Bev \quad \text{or} \quad r = \frac{mv}{Be} \qquad (4\text{-}2)$$

Now the time of transit of the charged particle through the semicircular D is $\pi r/v$. Hence, using equation 4-2, we obtain the transit time, t_t:

$$t_t = \frac{\pi r}{v} = \frac{\pi m}{Be} \qquad (4\text{-}3)$$

This transit time is independent of velocity and so will be the same for all orbits provided the mass of the particle, m, remains constant.

In Chapter 1, we saw that the mass of a particle depends upon its velocity, according to equation 1-20. For an electron this increase in mass with velocity is very important even for a relatively low energy electron. We saw that an electron with only 100 keV energy has a mass that is 1.196 times its rest mass. *This means that electrons cannot be accelerated in a cyclotron* for they would very quickly get out of step with the changing electric field. Although the change of mass of a heavy particle such as a proton, deuteron, or alpha particle is not nearly so great as that of an electron, this change of mass does limit the energy of the particle that can be produced, for as the mass increases the particle gets out of step and reaches the gap between the D's too late. This can be overcome partly by increasing the field B near the periphery of the magnet in order to keep the particles in step. Unfortunately, this increase in field causes a defocusing effect on the beam; to overcome this a variation in the field with angle is introduced by changing the shape of the poles so that the particles find themselves alternatively in a high and low magnetic field region as they go around in their circular path. Accelerators with such poles are called sector focused cyclotrons. Most cyclotrons in use today are of this type.

Alternatively, the change in mass with velocity can be dealt with using a synchrocyclotron in which the frequency of the oscillator is reduced automatically as the particle acquires energy. The slight increase in time between oscillations can be made to compensate exactly for the longer time required for the particle to move through the D's.

Cyclotrons have two major potential uses in a hospital environment. A dedicated cyclotron may be used to produce an intense high energy neutron or proton beam for radiotherapy, or it may be used to activate materials for tracer studies and diagnostic procedures. Samples to be activated are placed inside the vacuum chamber where they are bombarded by the high energy particle. A hospital-based machine allows one to produce and use isotopes with very short lives.

4.09   PARTICLES FOR RADIOTHERAPY

In the mid-1970s there has been much interest in the possible use of high energy particles in radiotherapy. These particles include neutrons, protons, deuterons, stripped nuclei, and negative π mesons. These will be discussed briefly; for further details the reader is referred to two international workshops on the subject (P1, P2).

NEUTRONS: Fast neutrons were first used in radiotherapy by Stone (S5) in 1938, only six years after the neutron had been discovered. After five years' experience in their use Stone began to see some very severe late effects and came to the conclusion that neutrons were *not* a useful particle in radiotherapy. It should be remembered that at this time there was very little information concerning the biological effects of neutrons on tissue, and their mode of action was not understood. There are, however, some logical reasons why neutrons should be a useful form of radiotherapy (see Chapter 17). For these reasons a new trial was started in 1966 by the group at Hammersmith Hospital, London. Since that time many other trials have started for which the final results are not yet available. The evidence to date suggests, however, that if they have an advantage it is minimal. It should be pointed out that, although intense beams of neutrons are produced in nuclear reactors, these are thermal neutrons and do not have a high enough energy to be useful in radiotherapy. High energy neutron beams can be produced by D-T generators, cyclotrons, or linacs. These machines are expensive, and none is ideal (B3).

DEUTERIUM TRITIUM (D-T) GENERATORS: The simplest way to produce a high energy neutron beam is to bombard a tritium target with a beam of deuterons that have been accelerated by a D.C. voltage of about 200 kV. Neutrons are produced by the following reaction.

$$\underset{\text{(deuteron)}}{{}^2_1\text{H}} + \underset{\text{(tritium)}}{{}^3_1\text{H}} \rightarrow {}^4_2\text{He} + {}^1_0\text{n} + 17.6 \text{ MeV} \qquad (4\text{-}4)$$

The available energy—17.6 MeV—is distributed between the helium nucleus and the neutron, with 14.1 MeV going to the neutron. This is an interesting reaction since it yields 14 MeV neutrons from *low* energy deuterons. The neutrons are ejected isotropically *so the yield in any one direction is small*. This is the major problem with the reaction; attempts to increase the yield by increase in the deuteron current bring about the rapid deterioration of the expensive tritium target. The highest yield being discussed to date is about 5×10^{12} s^{-1} into the total solid angle of 4π about the target. Of these a fraction, $1/(4\pi \times 10^4)$, would emerge through 1 cm^2 at 1 meter, which gives a flux density of 4×10^7 cm^{-2} s^{-1} for a treatment field at this distance. This is equivalent to a dose rate of about 0.15 Gy/min, a marginally useful dose rate. D-T generators can be made small enough to allow them to be mounted on a gantry in an isocentric configuration, a major advantage. If the yield problem could be solved there is no doubt that many more D-T generators would be placed in clinical use.

CYCLOTRON PRODUCED NEUTRONS: When *high* energy deuterons from a cyclotron bombard a low atomic number material such as beryllium, neutrons are produced according to:

$$\text{}^2_1\text{H} + \text{}^9_4\text{Be} \rightarrow \text{}^{10}_5\text{B} + \text{}^1_0\text{n} + 4.36 \text{ MeV} \qquad (4\text{-}5)$$

The neutrons emerge from the target primarily in the direction the deuterons had before the collision, so a true beam emerges and intensity is not a problem as it was for the D-T generator. The reaction produces a spectrum of neutrons ranging from near zero to near the maximum energy of the deuterons, as illustrated in Figure 4-16. These curves give the neutron flux density at 1 meter, in the forward direction, per MeV interval for a deuteron beam current of 50 μA. This flux density is expressed in cm^{-2} s^{-1} MeV^{-1}. If we integrate under these curves we obtain the total flux density, cm^{-2} s^{-1}, given in the insert of Figure 4-16. These flux densities are large compared with the value of 4×10^7 cm^{-2} obtainable from the D-T generator, so intensity is not a problem. With these flux densities available, larger treatment distances can be used and flattening filters may be employed to flatten and shape the field.

The fact that cyclotron-produced neutrons are not monoenergetic complicates dosimetry somewhat but otherwise is not a disadvantage. The main disadvantage arises from the size of the cyclotron, which to date has prevented it from being mounted on a gantry, although several companies are attempting such a design. In the few centers where cyclotrons are in use the cyclotron is fixed with a horizontal beam and the high energy deuterons are "piped" into a fixed horizontal treatment head to bombard the target in the head to produce a fixed horizontal neutron beam. In a few centers such as the GLANTA facility in Cleveland, two deuteron beams are available in two separate rooms, one giving a horizontal and the other a vertical neutron beam. Further developments along these lines are expected.

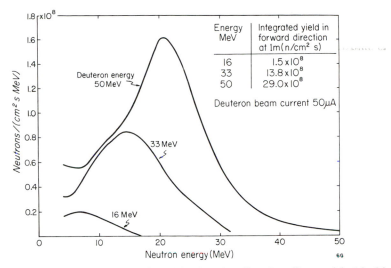

Figure 4-16. Spectra of neutrons produced by bombarding beryllium with 16, 33, and 50 MeV deuterons (adapted from Meulders et al., M5). The ordinate is the neutron flux density in the forward direction, per MeV interval expressed in $cm^{-2} \, s^{-1} \, MeV^{-1}$. It was calculated from Meulders, assuming a deuteron beam current of 50 μA.

COLLIMATION OF NEUTRONS: Neutrons are very difficult to stop because they do not have a charge and so do not interact with electrons as they pass through material. They give up their energy by collision with nuclei. When a collision occurs between a neutron and a heavy atom such as lead, the neutron merely bounces off the lead nuclei with very little transfer of energy. Thus, a beam of neutrons readily passes through lead. When a neutron collides with a particle whose mass is nearly the same as its own, a large transfer of energy may take place. For example, in a collision with a hydrogen atom the neutron can lose any energy, from all of it with a direct hit to zero for a glancing collision. The mean energy of a neutron after a collision with hydrogen is 37% of its original value. For heavy hydrogen, the mean energy after the collision is 48% while from carbon it is 85%. Thus, to stop neutrons we require an absorber rich in hydrogen and carbon. There is another important way neutrons can be absorbed, particularly at low energies: by capture. When this occurs a new nucleus is formed and often penetrating gamma rays are emitted. We thus require combinations of low atomic number materials to slow down the neutrons and high atomic number materials to absorb the gammas emitted after neutron capture. Collimators are often made with a series of layers of wax, borated wood, or plastic separated with layers of steel. Neutron facilities using cyclotrons are large and expensive. (For a review of the subject see P1, P2.)

PROTONS AND DEUTERONS: High energy charged particles from a linac or cyclotron have properties that may be useful in radiotherapy. Figure

10-27 shows the depth dose distribution from 190 MeV deuterons. They produce an almost constant dose to a depth of about 10 cm, followed by a region of high dose from 10 to 13 cm, after which the dose falls quickly to zero. The high dose at the end of the particle range is called the Bragg peak. These particles have been used in Berkeley and Harvard (P2) for a number of years to treat small inaccessible organs of the body, such as the pituitary. They are also being evaluated for more generalized radiotherapy.

STRIPPED NUCLEII: To produce high energy stripped nucleii, the group in Berkeley used their HILAC linear accelerator as a preaccelerator and the betatron as a booster. The two machines are connected by a 500 foot beam transfer line. With such a machine, energies up to 1000 MeV per nucleon are possible (P2). Most of their current experiments are carried out with 9000 MeV neon nucleii [neon has a mass number of 20 so each particle (nucleon) has an energy of about 450 MeV], 6400 MeV oxygen [400 MeV per nucleon], or 3120 MeV carbon nucleii [260 MeV per nucleon]. Stripped nucleii produce a very intense Bragg peak and have attractive radiobiological properties. The production of these high energy particles is a massive undertaking.

π MESONS: Beams of negative π mesons can be produced in a very large spiral ridge cyclotron or a very large linac. The particles produce an even more pronounced Bragg peak at the end of their range than do stripped nucleii because a nuclear reaction occurs as the π meson disappears. π meson beams suffer from low intensity so that one cannot afford to throw away any of the particles in designing the beam transport system. This means complex magnetic systems must be used to collimate the beam into a useful shape. Further, the beams are always contaminated with electrons and neutrons and their effects must be minimized. If a practical system could be designed to control π mesons, they might be useful particles since they have some very attractive radiobiological properties (Chapter 17).

Summary

1. Linear accelerators and cobalt 60 units will be the basic tools for radiotherapy during the next ten years, with linear accelerators finally dominating the market. Betatrons will gradually disappear.

2. Cobalt 60 units and 4 MeV linear accelerators produce similar distributions of radiation and so they can be used interchangeably. The cobalt unit has the advantage of being simpler and of requiring less service. It is advantageous to have at least one cobalt unit in every large radiotherapy department, since such a unit provides a predictable dose rate which may be used for calibration purposes.

3. Linear accelerators in the 6 to 10 MeV range are only marginally

better than cobalt units. Linear accelerators used in the photon mode at 18 to 30 MeV are the machines of choice.

4. Before any machine is purchased, very clear precise specifications should be laid down and the purchaser should make sure that the manufacturer meets these specifications before he accepts delivery and makes the final payment. Enough acceptance tests have been performed to indicate how such tests should be carried out (see Chapter 10).

5. The user should be alert to the following ways in which the beam may not be optimized:

(a) Low energy electrons may contaminate the beam, especially when large fields are used. These may often be removed with a proper filter.

(b) The maximum dose may not be as far below the surface as it should be, indicating low energy photon contamination. These may be removed with a change in the flattening filter design or the addition of an appropriate filter.

(c) The beam may not be uniform. A technique should be available in the department to ensure that the beam is indeed uniform. A matrix dosemeter (J2) is an ideal way to carry out this test. If the beam flatness changes with time then it may mean the beam transfer system is unstable. Ways to stabilize it should be found.

6. High energy protons, deuterons, stripped nucleii, and negative π mesons are still particles of the future and can be considered only in very large centers. They will not become a common tool of radiotherapy in the next ten years. Neutrons *may* become useful in this period. This possibility will be increased if dependable compact D-T generators can be produced.

7. Sophisticated control systems should be present in every department to insure that these complicated machines are maintained at their peak efficiency. Careful quality control will increase the cure rate.

PROBLEMS

1. In a typical betatron, the electron acquires an energy of about 100 eV per turn. The radius of the orbit is about 20 cm. Find the approximate distance in km the electron travels in acquiring an energy of 25 MeV. Assume the electron is traveling at the speed of light for the whole of the acceleration period.

2. Using data from Table 1-7, calculate the radius of the orbit of a 20 MeV electron moving in a magnetic field of 1.50 tesla (rest mass electron = 9.1×10^{-31} kg, charge 1.60×10^{-19} C.

3. Show that two waves of the same amplitude and frequency, traveling in opposite directions in a wave guide, give rise to standing waves.

4. The source in a cobalt 60 unit is 2.0 cm in diameter. The treatment distance is 80 cm and the distance from the source to the final diaphragm is 60 cm. Find the size of the penumbra on the skin surface and at a depth of 10 cm below the skin.

5. In a collision between a neutron and a proton, the neutron on the average is left with 37% of its original energy. A beam of 2 MeV neutrons bombards a hydrogen moderator. Find the mean energy of these neutrons after 5 collisions.

6. When neutrons bombard carbon, the mean energy after the collision is 85% of its original value. Find the number of collisions with carbon required to reduce the neutrons energy from 20 MeV to 0.2 MeV.

7. The magnetic field in a cyclotron is 1.00 tesla. Find the radius of the orbit of a 20 MeV proton moving in this magnetic field. Use data supplied in Table 1-7. From the radius of the orbit, calculate the time required for the particle to move through a semicircle. From this, calculate the frequency of the oscillator that must be applied between the 2 D's of the cyclotron (rest mass proton = 1.67×10^{-27} kg, charge on proton 1.60×10^{-19} C).

8. A stripped nucleus of carbon with energy 3120 MeV (mass 12, charge 6) is to be bent through 90° with a magnetic field of 2.5 tesla. Find the mass of the moving particle and the radius of curvature of the circular path. This calculation should convince the student as to the size of accelerators needed to produce energetic stripped nuclei.

9. Prove that to achieve a stable orbit in the betatron, the magnetic field at the orbit must be half the average magnetic field within the orbit.

Chapter **5**

THE INTERACTION OF IONIZING RADIATION WITH MATTER

A general discussion of the processes by which an x ray beam interacts with tissue is of interest to the radiologist and will be presented in this chapter. The more detailed calculations primarily of interest to the radiation physicist will be dealt with in Chapter 6. Many radiologists and radiobiologists will wish to study Chapter 6 after reading the rest of the book. Radiation physicists should read Chapter 5 before Chapter 6, as the concepts introduced in it are necessary for an understanding of Chapter 6.

5.01   **ABSORPTION OF ENERGY**

When a x ray beam (i.e. a beam of photons) passes into an absorbing medium such as body tissues, some of the energy carried by the beam is transferred to the medium where it may produce biological damage. The energy deposited per unit mass of the medium is known as the absorbed dose and is a very useful quantity for the prediction of biological effects. The events that result in this absorbed dose and subsequent biological damage are quite complicated. They are illustrated in a simplified way in Figure 5-1. The initial step in the process usually involves the collision between a photon and some electron in the body, resulting in the scattering of some radiation and the setting in motion of a high speed electron (represented by A in Fig. 5-1). In traveling through the tissue, the high speed electron produces a track along which ionizations occur, excitation of atoms takes place, and molecular bonds are broken (represented by B in Fig. 5-1). All of these result in biological damage. Most of the energy, however, is converted into heat, producing no biological effect. Some of the high speed electrons may suffer a collision with a nucleus and produce bremsstrahlung. This bremsstrahlung, as well as the scattered radiation, can then undergo interactions in the same way as the original photon. Usually, some 30 interactions are required before all the energy of the photon is converted into electronic motion.

In this chapter, we will discuss *A*, the first step in the series of events that constitute the interaction of the radiation with matter in the production of scattered radiation and absorbed energy. In Chapter 6 we will deal with *A* in more detail and with *B*, the types of electron tracks produced. Finally, in Chapter 17, some aspects of chemical change, *C*, and biological damage, *D*, will be discussed. At the present time, our basic understanding of process *A* is good, although the multiple interactions often complicate the process so much that a detailed analysis is difficult. Step *B* is less well understood, and the final steps, *C* and *D*, are imperfectly understood.

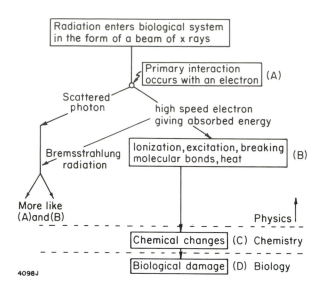

Figure 5-1. Schematic diagram illustrating the absorption of energy from radiation resulting in biological damage.

X ray photons may interact with the absorber to produce high speed electrons by three important mechanisms known as the *photoelectric* process, *Compton incoherent scattering*, and *pair production*. A less important process called *coherent scattering* also takes place. Often all four processes take place simultaneously. Before considering each process in detail, we shall define the attenuation coefficient. The reader should review the sections on exponential behavior discussed in Chapter 1.

5.02   LINEAR ATTENUATION COEFFICIENT AND EXPONENTIAL ATTENUATION

Suppose a detector that can record the number of photons that pass through it is placed in an x ray beam at point P (Fig. 5-2). Let the number of photons recorded be N. If a slab of material of thickness Δx is placed in the path of the x rays, a number, n, of the photons will interact with the attenuator and be removed from the beam. A photon cannot be partially stopped by the atoms in the slab of material. It will either come close enough to the atom to interact and thus be removed from the beam or it will not be affected at all. Hence, the number, n, removed will depend directly on the number of photons present. If N is doubled, then the chances of an interaction will also be doubled. Further, if Δx is doubled, the number of atoms placed in the beam is doubled, and so the chance of interaction is doubled. Thus, n varies as the product of N and Δx, and so may be written

$$n = \mu \, N \, \Delta x \qquad (5\text{-}1a)$$

where μ, the constant of proportionality, is called the *linear attenuation coefficient*. The equation is valid provided N remains essentially constant as we pass into the attenuator, i.e. n must be small compared to N, which means that $\mu \Delta x$ must be small compared to one.

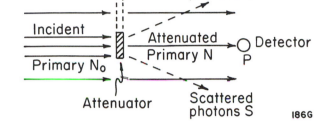

Figure 5-2. Diagram illustrating how an attenuator of thickness Δx reduces the number of photons reaching P, and how scattered radiation is produced.

Equation 5-1a may be written in a slightly different way. Let ΔN represent the change in the number of photons in the beam in passing through Δx. Then since N is reduced by one for each interaction, $\Delta N = - n$ and equation 5-1a becomes

$$\Delta N = -\mu \, N \, \Delta x \qquad (5\text{-}1b)$$

This equation describes how N changes as we pass through the attenuator, whereas equation 5-1a gives the number of interactions in a slab of thickness Δx bombarded by N photons.

From either equation 5-1a or b we may determine the dimensions in which μ is expressed. Since N, ΔN, and n are all pure numbers, $\mu \, \Delta x$ must be dimensionless and μ must have dimensions of 1 divided by length. If x is expressed in cm, μ must be measured in cm^{-1}. μ depends in a complicated way on the nature of the attenuator and the energy of the radiation. This will be discussed later; for the moment, μ should be considered a constant.

It is important for the student to have an intuitive feeling for the meaning of μ. Equation 5-1a can be rearranged to read

$$\mu = \frac{(n/N)}{\Delta x} = \frac{\text{fraction of photons that interact in } \Delta x}{\Delta x} \qquad (5\text{-}1c)$$

showing that *μ is the fraction of photons that interact per unit thickness of attenuator.* Of course, the unit thickness, Δx, must be chosen small enough so that (n/N) is small compared with 1.0. For example, if $\mu = 0.01 \ cm^{-1}$

then 1% of the photons in the beam will interact in each 1 cm layer. If μ were 100 times as large (1.0 cm^{-1}), it would be incorrect to say that 100% of the photons would interact in a 1 cm layer but we could say that 1% would interact in a layer 0.01 cm thick. In using equations 5-1, always remember that for any given μ, Δx must be chosen so that n or $\Delta N \ll N$.

To illustrate the linear attenuation coefficient, let us determine how the number of photons in the beam is reduced as successive layers of material 1 cm thick are placed in it. Suppose $\mu = 0.10$ cm^{-1} and the original number of photons in the beam is 100. Equation 5-1a tells us that in the first 1 cm slab the number of interactions will be n = 0.1 cm$^{-1} \times 100 \times 1$ cm = 10, leaving 90 photons in the beam. The next 1 cm layer will remove 10% of 90, leaving 81. Proceeding in this way we can enter the numbers shown in the first 3 columns of Table 5-1.

TABLE 5-1
Attenuation of a Beam when $\mu = 0.10$ cm^{-1}

Thickness of Attenuator x (cm)	Number of Interactions in 1 cm Slab (Eq. 5-1a)	Number of Photons Left in Beam By Step-Wise Calculation	By Eq. 5-2a
0	0	100.0	100.0
1	10	90.0	90.5
2	9	81.0	81.9
3	8.1	72.9	74.1
4	7.3	65.6	67.0
5	6.6	59.0	60.7
6	5.9	53.1	54.9
7	5.3	47.8	49.7
8	4.8	43.0	44.9
9	4.3	38.7	40.6
10	3.9	34.8	36.8
11	3.5	31.3	33.3
12	3.1	28.2	30.1
13	2.8	25.4	27.2
14	2.5	22.9	24.7
15	2.3	20.6	22.3
16	2.1	18.5	20.2

From column 2, it is seen that, as layers of attenuator are added, the number of interactions per layer gets smaller and smaller, although the number of interactions expressed as a percent of the number of photons present is always 10%. The calculations shown in the first three columns of Table 5-1 are only approximately correct, for it is assumed that the number of photons in the beam is 100 from the *front* face of the first 1 cm slab to the *back* of the slab, whereas the number at the back of the slab is really only 90. Hence the attenuation will be less than the value 10 given in column 2 and the transmitted number will be greater than the value 90 given in column 3. To obtain the correct solution, many layers, each very thin, should be considered. That is, Δx in equation 5-1a should be made very small and the calculations carried through for very many of these very thin layers. Such a task would be formidable and fortunately need not be done since equation 5-1b can be solved by calculus as discussed in Chapter 1 to yield:

$$N = N_0 \, e^{-\mu x} \tag{5-2a}$$

where N is the number transmitted by any thickness x, N_0 is the number incident, and *e* is the *base of the natural logarithms* with the value 2.718. This equation may be used to calculate the attenuation by *any* thickness of material, whereas equation 5-1 is only applicable when the fractional reduction by a layer of material is very small.

Example 5-1. A beam containing 10^3 photons is incident on a 16 cm slab of material for which $\mu = 0.10$ cm^{-1}. Determine the number transmitted.

$$\mu x = 0.10 \text{ cm}^{-1} \times 16 \text{ cm} = 1.60$$

Number transmitted $= N = N_0 \, e^{-\mu x} = 10^3 \times e^{-1.60} = 202$

Accurate calculations of the percent transmitted using equation 5-2a are given in column 4 of Table 5-1, and the last entry is 20.2, in agreement with the calculation of example 5-1. Comparison of the last 2 columns shows that the agreement is fair, indicating that equation 5-1 is reasonably satisfactory even when the fraction attenuated by each layer is as great as 10%.

5.03   **HALF-VALUE LAYER**

From Table 5-1 we see that 5 cm of material attenuates the beam by 60.7%. The next 5 cm of material will reduce this number to 0.607 of $60.7 = 36.8$ as seen by the entry in the table for 10 cm. In fact, in exponential behavior any given thickness will attenuate the beam by the *same factor* regardless of the intensity of the beam. The *special thickness that attenuates the beam to 50% is called the half-value layer* or HVL. Substituting $N = .5 \, N_0$ in equation 5-2a the reader can show that:

$$\text{HVL} = x_h = \frac{0.693}{\mu} \tag{5-3}$$

This was also derived in Chapter 1. Thus equation 5-2 can be written in any of the following ways

$$N = N_0 \, e^{-\mu x} = N_0 \, e^{-.693 \, x/x_h} = N_0 \, 2^{-x/x_h} \tag{5-2b}$$

For the example of Table 5-1, with $\mu = 0.10$ cm^{-1}, the half-value layer is $.693/\mu = 6.93$ cm.

Exponential decrease is conveniently plotted on semilog graph paper because a straight line is obtained (as illustrated in Fig 5-3). It should be noted that the scale goes from 100 to 10. This is called a cycle. Note also that 6.93, 13.9, 20.8 cm are required to reduce the transmitted number from 100 to 50 to 25 to 12.5%. If a greater range of values is to be represented, double cycle paper going from 100 to 10 and then from 10 to 1 should be used. In the insert of Figure 5-3 is shown the data plotted on triple cycle paper. It is seen that 23, 46, and 69 cm are required to reduce the number from 100 to 10, to 1 and to 0.1 respectively. *Note that 10 half-value layers gives an attenuation factor of almost exactly 1000 ($2^{10} = 1024 \approx 1000$).*

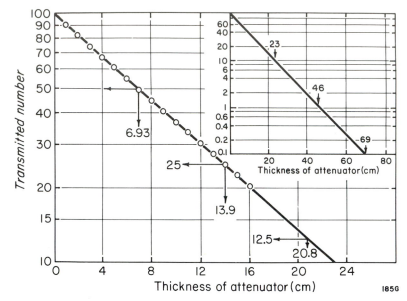

Figure 5-3. Graph showing how the number of photons is reduced by an attenuator whose linear attenuation coefficient is $\mu = 0.10$ cm^{-1}. The transmitted number is plotted on a logarithmic scale.

Example 5-2. A cobalt 60 unit gives an exposure rate of 80 R/min at 1 meter when the source is "on." Protection regulations require that, when the source is "off," the radiation level at 1 meter distance be less than 2 mR/h (0.002 R/h). Estimate the thickness of lead shielding required if the attenuation coefficient is 66.0 m^{-1}.

$$\text{HVL (eq. 5-3)} = \frac{.693}{66.0 \text{ m}^{-1}} = 0.0105 \text{ m}$$

$$\text{Attenuation factor required} = \frac{80 \times 60 \text{ R/h}}{2 \times 10^{-3} \text{ R/h}} = 2{,}400{,}000$$

Attenuation of 1000 requires 10 HVL or	.105 m
Another attenuation of 1000 requires 10 HVL or	.105 m
An attenuation of 2.4 requires more than 1 HVL, allow 2	.021 m
Total attenuation of 2,400,000 requires about	.231 m

Thus about .23 m of Pb would be required. In this problem we have taken no account of scattered radiation (see next section) and so have underestimated the protection (we actually would need about 4 more HVLs or a total barrier of .27 m); however, an approximate calculation of this kind is often all that is required.

5.04 NARROW AND BROAD BEAMS

Equation 5-2 is valid only if the attenuation coefficient is actually a constant and this is only true if the photons in the incident beam all have the same energy (a monoenergetic beam) and if the beam is narrow. The need for a narrow beam can be understood by referring to Figure 5-4, which is a modified version of Figure 5-2. The attenuator, still of thickness Δx, has been extended in the plane of its cross section and now some photons may be scattered by it so that they reach the detector, with the result that the transmitted number of photons will appear to be larger than before. Although one could still define an attenuation coefficient by equation 5-1c, it will no longer be a constant and its value will depend on the thickness of the attenuator, on its area and shape, and on the distance between the attenuator and the detector, as well as on the photon energy. The attenuation curve (such as in Fig. 5-3) will no longer be exponential. It could be described by an equation such as:

$$N = N_0\, e^{-\mu x}\, B\,(x,\, h\nu,\, A,\, L) \tag{5-4}$$

where B is a rather complicated factor, sometimes called a photon build-up factor, that takes account of the photons scattered by the attenuator. The symbols in parentheses indicate the dependence on thickness, energy, area, and distance. B can range in magnitude from 1 to over 100. It is usually obtained experimentally. It is important in shielding calculations; for example, in the problem solved in example 5-2, B could be as much as 10 to 20 and would indicate that some 4 additional half-value layers would be required to provide the full protection desired. Values for B can be found in the literature (G3, R2).

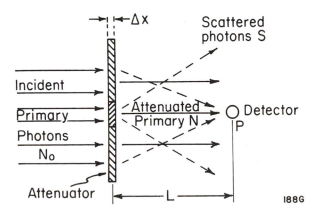

Figure 5-4. Figure 5-2 has been altered to illustrate the effect of a broad beam on a transmission measurement.

It can also be seen from Figure 5-4 that when one is measuring a μ or a half-value layer it is very important that the beam be collimated so that scattered radiation is excluded and a narrow beam is produced (see also Chapter 8).

5.05   **MASS, ELECTRONIC, AND ATOMIC ATTENUATION COEFFICIENTS**

The attenuation produced by a layer, Δx, will depend upon the number of electrons and atoms present in the layer. If the layer were compressed to half the thickness, it would still have the same number of electrons and still attenuate the x rays by the same fraction, but of course, its linear attenuation coefficient (attenuation per unit length) would be twice as great. Linear attenuation coefficients will, therefore, depend upon the density of the material. A more fundamental attenuation coefficient is the mass coefficient, which is obtained from the linear coefficient by dividing by the density, ρ. This coefficient, represented by (μ/ρ), is independent of the density. It is left to the student to show that it has dimensions m²/kg. When dealing with mass attenuation coefficients, it is often convenient to measure the thickness of an absorber in g/cm² or kg/m². To determine the thickness of a foil in these units one would cut out a square piece of foil, say 10 cm by 10 cm, and weigh it. If it weighed 30 g, then its thickness could be expressed as 30 g/100 cm² or 0.3 g/cm² or 3.0 kg/m². If one wishes to measure thickness in kg/m² then the appropriate attenuation coefficient would be the mass attenuation coefficient measured in m²/kg. As an example, suppose lead ($\rho = 11.3$ g/cm³) has a linear coefficient of 0.12 cm⁻¹, then the corresponding mass attenuation coefficient is

(margin note: MASS COEFFICIENT μ/ρ)

$$\frac{0.12 \text{ cm}^{-1}}{11.3 \text{ g cm}^{-3}} = 0.0106 \text{ cm}^2/\text{g} = \frac{0.0106 \, (.01 \text{ m})^2}{0.001 \text{ kg}} = 0.00106 \text{ m}^2/\text{kg}$$

In the same way, one could compute the number of electrons in unit area of a foil and express the thickness of the foil in electrons per cm². The corresponding attenuation coefficient would now be the electronic one, often represented by $_e\mu$, with dimensions cm² per electron or m² per electron. The electronic coefficient is very small compared with the mass coefficient because there are an enormous number of electrons in a slab of thickness 1 g/cm². Just as the mass coefficient was obtained from the linear coefficient by dividing by the density, the electronic one may be obtained from the mass coefficient by dividing it by N_e, the number of electrons per g.

(margin note: $\frac{\mu}{e}$)

In a similar way one may compute the number of atoms in a foil and express the thickness of the foil in atoms per cm² or atoms per m². The corresponding attenuation coefficient is now the atomic one with dimensions cm^2 per atom or m^2 per atom. The atomic coefficient is Z times as large as the electronic one, since there are Z electrons in each atom. The relations between these coefficients are summarized in Table 5-2. Since the mass, electronic, and atomic coefficients are measured in units of *area* per g, or *area* per electron or *area* per atom, the coefficients are often called *cross sections* as described in Chapter 3.

TABLE 5-2
Relation Between Attenuation Coefficients

Coefficient	Symbol	Relation Between Coefficients	Units of Coefficients	Units in Which Thickness is Measured
linear	μ		m^{-1}	m
mass	$\left(\dfrac{\mu}{\rho}\right)$	$\dfrac{\mu}{\rho}$	m^2/kg	kg/m^2
electronic	$_e\mu$	$\dfrac{\mu}{\rho} \cdot \dfrac{1}{1000\,N_e}$	m^2/el	el/m^2
atomic	$_a\mu$	$\dfrac{\mu}{\rho} \cdot \dfrac{Z}{1000\,N_e}$	m^2/at	at/m^2

ρ = density
N_e = number of electrons per g
Z = atomic number of material.

The number of electrons or atoms per gram can be obtained from Avogadro's number, which is represented by N_A and has the value 6.02205×10^{23}. This is the number of atoms in a mass of material in grams numerically equal to its atomic weight A. For example, since the atomic weight of carbon is 12.00, it follows that 12.00 g of carbon contains 6.02×10^{23} atoms. Consider a material with atomic weight A and atomic number Z. From the definition of Avogadro's number we have:

$$\text{Number atoms per g} = N_A/A$$

$$\text{Number electrons per g} = N_A Z/A = N_e \qquad (5\text{-}5)$$

$$\text{Number electrons per kg} = 1000\,N_e$$

The number of electrons per g is an important quantity that enters into many calculations. We will use N_e to represent this number. Values of N_e are given in Table 5-3. It is evident from the table that all materials except hydrogen have essentially the same number of electrons per g (about 3×10^{23}). This follows from the fact that all materials have about the same number of protons as neutrons (see Chapter 3) so Z/A is nearly 0.5, hence N_e is approximately one-half Avogadro's number.

Table 5-3 also gives the density, ρ, and the *effective* atomic number, $\overline{Z}$. For elements, $\overline{Z}$ is the same as the atomic number Z, but for materials containing several kinds of atoms it is a weighted average atomic number defined in section 7.10.

TABLE 5-3
Data for Absorbing Materials

Material	ρ-Density (kg/m³)	Effective Atomic Number³, $\bar{Z}$	N_e (electrons per g)
Hydrogen (at STP)¹	.08988	1	5.97×10^{23}
Carbon	2250	6	3.01×10^{23}
Oxygen (at STP)¹	1.429	8	3.01×10^{23}
Aluminum	2699	13	2.90×10^{23}
Copper	8960	29	2.75×10^{23}
Lead	11360	82	2.38×10^{23}
Air² (at STP)¹	1.293	7.78	3.01×10^{23}
Water²	1000	7.51	3.34×10^{23}
Muscle²	1040	7.64	3.31×10^{23}
Fat²	916	6.46	3.34×10^{23}
Bone²	1650	12.31	3.19×10^{23}

(1) STP, or standard temperature and pressure: 0° C, 101.3 kPa.
(2) Composition of air, water, muscle, bone, and fat are given in Appendix A.
(3) For the calculation of $\bar{Z}$ see section 7.10.

The relation between these coefficients is now illustrated.
Example 5-3. The mass attenuation coefficient for carbon at 1.0 MeV is .00636 m²/kg. (See Table A-4b in the appendix.) Calculate the linear, the electronic, and the atomic coefficients using data from Table 5-3.

$$\left(\frac{\mu}{\rho}\right) = .00636 \text{ m}^2 \text{ kg}^{-1}$$

$$\mu = .00636 \frac{\text{m}^2}{\text{kg}} \times 2250 \frac{\text{kg}}{\text{m}^3} = 14.3 \text{ m}^{-1} = .143 \text{ cm}^{-1}$$

$$_e\mu = .00636 \frac{\text{m}^2}{\text{kg}} \frac{1}{3.01 \times 10^{26} \text{ el kg}^{-1}} = 2.11 \times 10^{-29} \text{ m}^2/\text{el*}$$

$$_a\mu = 6 \frac{\text{el}}{\text{at}} \times 2.11 \times 10^{-29} \frac{\text{m}^2}{\text{el}} = 12.7 \times 10^{-29} \text{ m}^2/\text{at}$$

Another example will illustrate the attenuation of a slab of material.
Example 5-4. A beam of 1 MeV photons impinges on a slab of carbon of thickness 50 kg/m². Find the fraction of photons transmitted through the slab.

$$\left(\frac{\mu}{\rho}\right) = 6.36 \times 10^{-3} \text{ m}^2 \text{ kg}^{-1} \text{ (see Table A-4b)}$$

$$\left(\frac{\mu}{\rho}\right) x = 6.36 \times 10^{-3} \frac{\text{m}^2}{\text{kg}} \times 50 \frac{\text{kg}}{\text{m}^2} = 0.318$$

fraction transmitted $\quad e^{-.318} = 0.728$

Alternative solution using HVL (eq. 5-3) $\quad \text{HVL} = \dfrac{.693}{6.36 \times 10^{-3} \text{ m}^2 \text{ kg}^{-1}} = 109 \text{ kg m}^{-2}$

Now using single cycle semilog paper like that of Figure 5-3, one may locate the 50% point at a depth of 109 kg/m² and read a transmitted fraction of 0.728 for a thickness of 50 kg/m².

It should be noted that equation 5-3 uses a linear coefficient, in which case the HVL will be in meters. However, it may be used with a mass coefficient, in which case the HVL is a thickness measured in kg/m². The HVL thickness may also be expressed in atoms per m² or electrons per m².

5.06   ENERGY TRANSFER AND ENERGY ABSORPTION

When a photon interacts with an absorber, a complicated series of events takes place as illustrated in Figure 5-1. In general, part of the energy of the photon is radiated from the absorber as scattered radiation and part is converted into kinetic energy of high speed electrons or positrons. Once these particles have been set in motion, they can lose energy by collisional losses or by emitting bremsstrahlung radiation as described in Chapter 2 and 6. In any *one* interaction it is impossible to state exactly what will happen, but after many interactions, one can calculate the average energy transferred ($\overline{E}_{tr}$) and the average energy absorbed ($\overline{E}_{ab}$). Table 5-4 shows typical data for carbon taken from the appendix. We see, for example, that when a 10 MeV photon interacts with carbon, $\overline{E}_{tr}$ = 7.30 MeV and $\overline{E}_{ab}$ = 7.04 MeV. This means that on the average 7.30 MeV is transferred into kinetic energy of electrons and 7.04 MeV of it is absorbed. The difference, 0.26 MeV, is radiated away as bremsstrahlung. Since 7.30 MeV is transferred into K.E. the rest of the 10 MeV, i.e. 2.70 MeV, is scattered from the beam.

TABLE 5-4

Energy Transfer, Energy Absorption, and Related Interaction Coefficients for Carbon—taken from Table A-4b in Appendix

Photon Energy (MeV)	$\overline{E}_{tr}$ (MeV)	$\overline{E}_{ab}$ (MeV)	(μ/ρ)	(μ_{tr}/ρ)*	(μ_{ab}/ρ)*
				m² per kg	
.01	.00865	.00865	.2187	.1891	.1891
.1	.0141	.0141	.01512	.00213	.00213
1.0	.440	.440	.00636	.00280	.00280
10	7.30	7.04	.00196	.00143	.00138
100	95.62	71.9	.00145	.00139	.00105

*The mass transfer coefficient (μ_{tr}/ρ) and the mass absorption coefficient (μ_{ab}/ρ) are derived from (μ/ρ) using $\overline{E}_{tr}$ and $\overline{E}_{ab}$ (see eq. 5-6, 5-8).

---

*In this example we have written the electronic coefficient as 2.11 × 10⁻²⁹ m²/el. Since "el" has no units, it would be more correct to write it as merely 2.11 × 10⁻²⁹ m². We would have to know from the context that it referred to an electron. To avoid ambiguity, however, it is useful to include "el" and "at" with the units. We will do this in the example calculations that follow.

In a low atomic number material such as carbon, Table 5-4 shows that the energy emitted as bremsstrahlung is negligible for photon energies up to 1.0 MeV so $\overline{E}_{tr} \approx \overline{E}_{ab}$. As the photon energy is increased above 10 MeV an increasing portion of this K.E. is radiated as bremsstrahlung. Since most of the interactions of interest in radiology occur in low Z materials, below 10 MeV, we may often consider $\overline{E}_{ab} = \overline{E}_{tr}$.

Table 5-4 also gives us some inkling as to the importance of the scattered radiation depicted in Figure 5-2. When a low energy photon (.01 MeV) interacts in carbon, $\overline{E}_{ab} = \overline{E}_{tr} = 0.00865$ MeV, which is nearly equal to the energy of the incident photon (0.01), hence scattered radiation is *not* important. In contrast, when a photon of energy 0.1 MeV interacts, the energy absorbed is only .0141 MeV, so most of the energy is scattered. At 1 MeV about half the energy is absorbed and half scattered. For still higher energies (10 MeV), about 70% is absorbed. At extremely high energies (100 MeV) nearly all the energy is transferred to electronic motion but much of it is radiated away so that about 72% is absorbed.

This complex behavior will be explained in later sections of this and the succeeding chapter. These ideas will now be illustrated by an example.

Example 5-5. A well-collimated beam containing 10^4, 10 MeV photons impinges on a large block of carbon 20 cm thick. Determine the energy absorbed in a layer of carbon 1 mm thick at a depth of 10 cm in the block.

To do this problem we must first calculate the number of photons that reach a depth of 10 cm in the carbon block, thus:

thickness of carbon over-lying 1 mm layer at 10 cm	$0.10 \text{ m} \times 2250 \dfrac{\text{kg}}{\text{m}^3} = 225.0 \dfrac{\text{kg}}{\text{m}^2}$
using mass attenuation coef. (from Table 5-4b)	$\mu x = 0.00196 \dfrac{\text{m}^2}{\text{kg}} \times 225 \dfrac{\text{kg}}{\text{m}^2} = 0.441$
number photons reaching 10 cm depth (eq. 5-2)	$N = N_o\, e^{-\mu x} = 10^4 \times e^{-.441} = 6434$

Number of interactions in 1 mm slab (eq. 5-1):

$$= 6434 \times 0.00196 \frac{\text{m}^2}{\text{kg}} \times 10^{-3}\,\text{m} \times 2250 \frac{\text{kg}}{\text{m}^3} = 28.37$$

energy transferred (Table 5-4b)	$= 28.37 \times 7.30$ MeV	$= 207.1$ MeV
energy absorbed (Table 5-4b)	$= 28.37 \times 7.02$ MeV	$= 199.7$ MeV
energy radiated as bremsstrahlung	$= (207.1 - 199.7)$	$= 7.4$ MeV
energy scattered	$= 28.37\ (10.0 \text{ MeV} - 7.30 \text{ MeV}) =$	76.6 MeV

It should be noted that the high speed electrons set in motion will travel forward several cm before coming to rest, so the electrons set in motion in the layer will deposit their energy at a greater depth. This depletion will be mainly compensated for by particles set in motion above the layer, so the calculations are nearly correct. The rather large range of high speed electrons produces problems that will be discussed under electron equilibrium in Chapter 7. The other problem we have avoided in this solution is scattered photons. We specified the beam area to be small to minimize their effect, but some of the photons scattered above the 1 mm layer would contribute to energy absorption in the layer. To take scattered photons into account in a precise way is very difficult.

ENERGY TRANSFER COEFFICIENT: To calculate the energy transferred to a block of tissue, as in the last example, it is often convenient to use the transfer coefficient, μ_{tr}. Imagine a beam of photons incident on a block of scattering material in which N photons reach the layer Δx. From equation 5-1a the number of interactions that occur in this layer is given by

$$n = \mu N \Delta x$$

where μ is the *linear attenuation* coefficient. If now the *average* energy transferred per interaction is $\overline{E}_{tr}$ then the energy transferred is

$$\Delta E_{tr} = \overline{E}_{tr} \, \mu \, N \Delta x = \left(\mu \, \frac{\overline{E}_{tr}}{h\nu} \right) N \, h\nu \, \Delta x$$

where the last expression is obtained from the previous one by multiplying numerator and denominator by $h\nu$. The quantity in brackets has the same dimensions as μ and is called the transfer coefficient, μ_{tr}, thus:

$$\mu_{tr} = \mu \cdot (\overline{E}_{tr}/h\nu) \tag{5-6}$$

and the energy transferred in Δx is

$$\Delta E_{tr} = \mu_{tr} \cdot N \, h\nu \, \Delta x \tag{5-7}$$

Since $Nh\nu$ is the energy carried by the beam, we see that to calculate the energy transferred we merely take the product of the transfer coefficient, the energy carried by the beam at the position of the slab, and the thickness of the slab Δx.

ENERGY ABSORPTION COEFFICIENT: In an analogous way we define the energy absorption coefficient μ_{ab} thus:

$$\mu_{ab} = \mu \, (\overline{E}_{ab}/h\nu) \tag{5-8}$$

where $\overline{E}_{ab}$ is the average energy absorbed per interaction. The energy absorbed in Δx is simply

$$\Delta E_{ab} = \mu_{ab} \, N \, h\nu \, \Delta x \tag{5-9}$$

Example 5-6: Calculate the energy absorbed in the 1 mm slab of example 5-5, using the appropriate energy absorption coefficient.

From Table A-4b: $\left(\dfrac{\mu_{ab}}{\rho}\right) = .00138 \dfrac{m^2}{kg}$

1 mm has a "thickness" of $2250 \dfrac{kg}{m^3} \times 10^{-3} m = 2.25 \dfrac{kg}{m^2}$

$\Delta E_{ab} = .00138 \dfrac{m^2}{kg} \times 6434 \times 10 \text{ MeV} \times 2.25 \dfrac{kg}{m^2} = 199.8 \text{ MeV}$

in agreement with our former calculation.

When the energy loss to bremsstrahlung is small, i.e. $\overline{E}_{tr} \approx \overline{E}_{ab}$, and $\mu_{tr} \approx \mu_{ab}$, only one value for each is presented in Tables A-3 and A-4 (of the Appendix). See for example Table A-4b for carbon where, for certain energies, column 7 is combined with 8, and 9 is combined with 10.

5.07   PHOTOELECTRIC ABSORPTION

The complex variation of $\overline{E}_{tr}$ or $\overline{E}_{ab}$ with energy as illustrated in Table 5-4 can only be understood if one examines in detail the various ways by which a photon can interact with an atom or its components. In following sections we discuss in some detail the main interaction processes, which are the photoelectric effect, coherent and incoherent scattering, and pair production.

In the photoelectric process, illustrated in Figure 5-5, a photon of energy $h\nu$ collides with an atom and ejects one of the bound electrons from the K, L, M, or N shells. The ejected electron is called a photoelectron and emerges with energy $h\nu - E_s$ where E_s is the binding energy of the shell from which the electron is ejected. The atom is left in an excited state and emits characteristic radiation and Auger electrons as it returns to the ground state.

Variation of the Photoelectric Process with Photon Energy

The linear attenuation coefficient for the photoelectric process is usually represented by the Greek letter τ, and the mass coefficient by τ/ρ. The mass coefficients are plotted in Figure 5-5 as a function of photon energy for water, representing a low atomic number material, and for lead representing a high Z material. For water, there is a linear relation between τ/ρ and energy $h\nu$ on a log log plot showing that τ/ρ varies as $1/(h\nu)^n$ where n is the slope of the line. From the graph it is seen that (τ/ρ) rises by just over 3 cycles on the vertical scale for each cycle on the energy scale, showing that n is a little more than 3.

The curve for lead, between the breaks, consists of straight portions with a slope about 3; so again the variation with energy is about $1/(h\nu)^3$.

At very high energies (above 1 MeV), the curve for lead gradually changes slope, finally attaining a value of about 1.0. In this high energy region, the coefficient varies inversely as hν; doubling the energy reduces the coefficient by a factor of about 2.0.

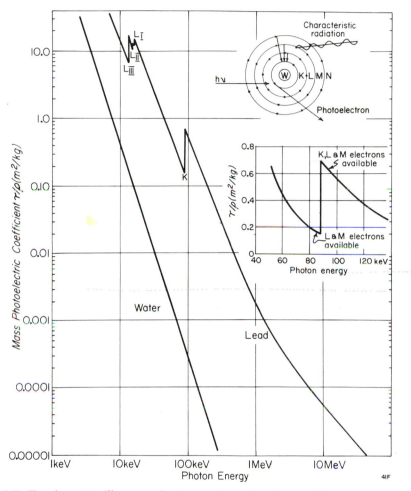

Figure 5-5. Top insert to illustrate the interaction of a photon with an atom to eject an electron from the K shell to produce a photoelectron. When the hole in the K shell is filled, characteristic radiation is emitted. Main graph—Photoelectric attenuation coefficients for water and lead plotted on a log-log scale. The second insert shows in greater detail the change in the photoelectric attenuation coefficient at the K absorption edge for lead. On the high energy side of this edge, K, L, and M electrons may be involved in photoelectric absorption, while on the low energy side, only the L and M are involved. Plotted from data in appendix, based on tables by Hubbell (H7) and Plechaty et al. (P5).

The graph for lead is more complicated, consisting of a series of straight portions with vertical "breaks" between them. Starting at the high energy end the first "break" occurs at 88 keV, which is the binding energy of the K shell in lead. Below 88 keV the photon has insufficient energy to eject a K electron and photoelectric emission is thus limited to the L and M shells. Just above 88 keV, the K electrons may be ejected and the absorption increases by a factor of about 5. On the log log plot the K break does not appear large because the scale is very condensed, so this portion has been replotted in the insert on a linear scale. At 88 keV the coefficient increases from 0.184 m²/kg to 0.748 m²/kg. This increase is all due to the *sudden* participation of the two K electrons. Thus, just above the discontinuity, all the L and M electrons give an absorption of 0.184 m²/kg, while the two K electrons contribute $0.748 - 0.184 = 0.564$ m²/kg. The 2 K electrons are more than 5 times as effective as the 8 L electrons. We may conclude *that the more tightly bound electrons are the important ones in bringing about photoelectric absorption and that the maximum absorption occurs when the photon has just enough energy to eject the bound electron.* Since, at the K break, the 2 K electrons are some 5 times as important in the absorption process as all the L and M electrons, it follows by similar reasoning that most of the absorption below the K break is due to the L electrons.

From 16 to 13 keV three more breaks appear, due to the L_I, L_{II}, and L_{III} shells. Below this energy only M electrons are involved. If the curves were continued to lower energies, 5 breaks corresponding to the 5 M shells would appear in the region from 2 to 4 keV.

In the photoelectric process the atom as a whole absorbs the photon so it is usual to record the coefficient per atom. These are given in the fourth column of Table A-4. This table shows that at each of the edges, two values appear. The first cross section is the value just *below* the edge while the second one is for an energy just above the edge. For example, in Pb (Table A-4i) double entries occur at the K edge (88.0 keV), at the three L edges at 15.8, 15.2, and 13.0 keV, and at the five M edges at 3.85, 3.55, 3.07, 2.59, and 2.48 keV.

Variation of the Photoelectric Process with Atomic Number

The cross section per atom depends upon approximately Z^4 for high atomic number materials and on $Z^{4.8}$ for low Z materials. Since each atom contains Z electrons, the coefficient per electron depends upon Z^3 and $Z^{3.8}$ for high and low Z materials respectively. Since the number of electrons per gram is more or less independent of Z, we would expect the mass coefficients to vary as Z^3 and $Z^{3.8}$ for the two classes of materials. These statements are at best rough guides. That the variation of the mass coefficient depends roughly on Z^3 can be seen from Figure 5-5. Above the K edge in lead, the coefficient is one thousand times as large as it is in water (slightly over 3 cycles on the vertical scale), while their atomic numbers of 82 and 7.5 are in the ratio of about 10:1.

Photoelectric Transfer and Absorption Coefficients in Tissue-like Materials

We have already seen (Fig. 5-5) that in a photoelectric process the photoelectron acquires an energy of $h\nu - E_s$ where E_s is the binding energy of the shell from which the electron is ejected. In the filling of the shell, part of the energy, E_s, is emitted as characteristic radiation and part is deposited through Auger electrons. For this reason, the mean energy transfer in the photoelectric process $_\tau\bar{E}_{tr}$ is greater than $h\nu - E_s$ and less than $h\nu$. For high Z materials this is a complex problem that will be discussed in section 6.01. For tissue-like materials of interest in radiology the situation is much simpler since for these materials the binding energies of the K shells are very small, being about 500 eV; hence, the photoelectron acquires essentially all the energy of the photon, so $_\tau\bar{E}_{tr} = h\nu$ and the transfer and photoelectric coefficients may be considered equal. Since the photoelectric process is only important at low energies, the electrons that are set in motion produce negligible bremsstrahlung, hence the energy absorption and energy transfer coefficients are also equal. Thus, for tissue, $\tau \approx \tau_{tr} \approx \tau_{ab}$.

Summary Concerning the Photoelectric Effect

- The photoelectric process involves bound electrons.
- The probability of ejection is maximum if the photon has just enough energy to knock the electron from its shell.
- The photoelectric cross section varies with photon energy approximately as $1/(h\nu)^3$.
- The coefficient per electron or per gram varies with atomic number— approximately as Z^3 for high Z materials and more nearly as $Z^{3.8}$ for low Z materials.
- The coefficient per atom for low Z materials varies at $Z^{4.8}$.
- In tissue $\bar{E}_{tr} = \bar{E}_{ab} \approx h\nu$ and the transfer, absorption, and the attenuation coefficients are nearly equal.

5.08   SCATTERING—COHERENT AND INCOHERENT

Coherent Scattering

In the last section we saw that a photoelectric process involved a collision between a photon of energy $h\nu$ and an atom, which results in the ejection of a bound electron. In the photoelectric process most of the energy of the photon was converted into kinetic energy and only a very little appeared as scattered characteristic radiation. Here we deal with a scattering process in which *no* energy is converted into kinetic energy and all is scattered. The process is represented schematically in Figure 5-6a, where we show an electromagnetic wave of wavelength λ passing over the atom. The electromagnetic wave has an oscillating electric field associated with it that sets the electrons in the atom into momentary vibration. These oscillating electrons emit radiation of the same wavelength, λ, as the incident radiation. This is exactly the same process as occurs in the transmitter of a radio station where electrons are forced to oscillate and energy is radiated as a radio wave. The scattered waves from electrons within the atom combine with each other to form the scattered wave. The scattering is a cooperative phenomenon and is hence called coherent scattering.

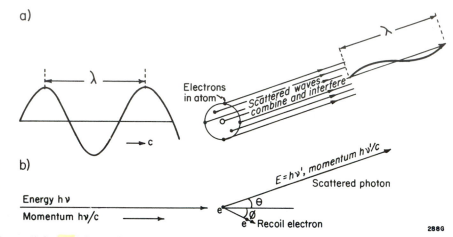

Figure 5-6. (a) Schematic representation of coherent scattering, a cooperative scattering process involving all the electrons of the atom in which no energy is transferred to the medium. (b) Incoherent scattering, or Compton scattering from an individual electron. Some energy is scattered as the scattered photon and some is given the recoil electron and absorbed.

Cross sections for coherent scattering (σ_{coh}) are given in the second column of Tables A-4a to A-4i in the appendix. They decrease rapidly with increase in photon energy and are negligibly small for energies greater than about 100 keV in low atomic number materials. Coherent scattering occurs mainly in the forward direction, so the effect of the process is to broaden the angular width of a beam slightly. Since no energy is transferred to kinetic energy, the process is of limited interest to the radiologist and will not be discussed further here. It will be dealt with in Chapter 6.

Incoherent Scattering—Compton Process

Under certain circumstances electrons can scatter independently; this is called incoherent scattering, or Compton scattering. *Some energy is scattered and some is transferred to kinetic energy. It is the most important interaction mechanism in tissue-like materials,* and so will be dealt with in some detail here and in even more detail in Chapter 6. For this type of interaction we must consider the quantum nature of the radiation and think of the electromagnetic wave as a stream of photons with energy $h\nu$ and momentum $h\nu/c$. The process is illustrated in Figure 5-6b, where we see the photon in collision with a free electron. This sets the electron in motion with energy E at an angle ϕ carrying away part of the energy while the rest of the energy is carried away by a photon with energy $h\nu'$ at angle θ. In the collision energy is conserved so

$$h\nu = h\nu' + E \qquad (5\text{-}10)$$

This equation shows that ν' must be less than ν (and the scattered waves must be of longer wavelength, λ', than the incident radiation, λ). In a Compton collision some energy is absorbed (recoil electron energy) and some scattered in every collision. Because momentum is also conserved, the recoil angle, ϕ, of the electron is determined uniquely if the angle of photon scattering, θ, is known. This will be dealt with in Chapter 6. Here we describe the process in a qualitative manner.

If the photon, $h\nu$, makes a direct hit on the electron, the electron will travel straight forward ($\phi = 0$), and the scattered photon will be scattered straight back, with $\theta = 180°$. In this type of collision the electron will obtain its maximum energy, and the scattered photon its minimum energy. If, on the other hand, the photon makes a grazing hit with the electron, the electron will emerge nearly at right angles ($\phi \approx 90°$) and the scattered photon will go almost straight forward ($\theta \approx 0$). For this collision the electron receives almost no energy and the scattered photon has essentially the full energy of the incident photon. All manner of intermediate collisions are possible.

The Compton process depicted in Figure 5-6b was illustrated assuming the electron is free or unbound. Strictly speaking, no electron is free since even the outer electrons of the atom are bound by a few electron volts. If however, these binding energies are a small fraction of the photon energy, as is often the case for tissues, the electron may be considered free. We will therefore first assume the electron is free and finally briefly show how binding can be taken into account.

5.09   **COMPTON CROSS SECTIONS**

The probability of a photon interacting in a Compton collision with a *free* electron may be evaluated by the Klein-Nishina formula to be discussed in Chapter 6. Here we summarize the phenomenon. Figure 5-7 shows that the Compton cross section per electron, usually represented by σ, falls from 66.3×10^{-30} m²/el at 1 keV to 0.82×10^{-30} m²/el at 100 MeV. This cross section is so important that values for it are given in Table A-2a. We now illustrate its use.

Example 5-6. Calculate the mass Compton coefficient at 100 keV for carbon, assuming all its electrons are free.

$\sigma = 49.27 \times 10^{-30}$ m²/el (Fig. 5-7, or Table A-2a, column 2)

Carbon contains 3.01×10^{26} electrons per kg (Table 5-3 or A-4b)

$$\frac{\sigma}{\rho} = 49.27 \times 10^{-30} \frac{m^2}{el} \times 3.01 \times 10^{26} \frac{el}{kg} = 148 \times 10^{-4} \frac{m^2}{kg}$$

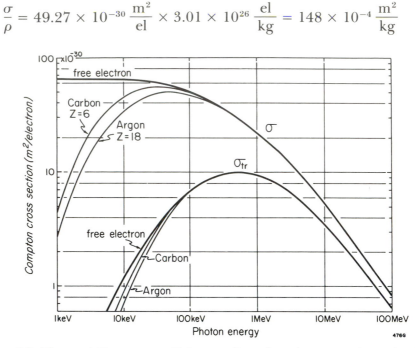

Figure 5-7. The total Compton coefficient, σ, for a free electron as determined by the Klein-Nishina formula. The curves for carbon and argon were obtained from Hubbell (H7), who made corrections for the effect of binding on the Compton cross section. The lower graphs are the Compton transfer coefficient, σ_{tr}, with curves for carbon and argon to take into account binding. Coefficients for free electrons are also given in Table A-2a.

Mean Energy Transferred in Compton Process

The energy given the recoil electron may range from zero, when the electron is ejected at right angles, to a maximum value when the electron is knocked straight forward. Using the Klein-Nishina formula, one can determine the relative probability of each energy transfer and so determine the average fraction of the incident energy given the electron (see Chapter 6). The results of such calculations are given in Figure 5-8. We see, for example, that 1 MeV photons can produce electrons with any energy from 0 to $0.8 \times 1.0 = 0.8$ MeV and that the mean energy of the electron set in motion is $_\sigma\bar{E}_{tr} = 0.44 \times 1.0 = 0.44$ MeV. The mean energy, $_\sigma\bar{E}_{tr}$, is the important parameter since it gives the energy transferred to kinetic energy in the Compton process, and so made available for absorption. Figure 5-8 shows that when the photon energy is small (0.01 MeV), the mean recoil energy is only 0.019 of the incident photon energy. *This means that when low energy photons interact in a Compton process, very little energy is transferred to the medium and most of the energy is merely scattered.* Thus, many interactions will be required to absorb the beam. On the other hand, *when the energy of the photon is large,* 10 to 100 MeV, *most of the available energy is transferred to the recoil electron and very little is scattered.* The mean energy transferred is so important that values for it are given in column 5 of Table A-2a.

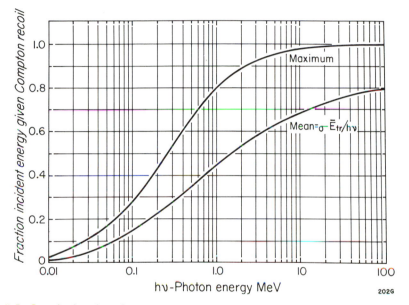

Figure 5-8. Graph showing the mean energy and the maximum energy (expressed as a fraction of the incident energy), which is given the recoil electron in a Compton collision.

COMPTON ENERGY TRANSFER COEFFICIENT: In an analogy with equation 5-6 we define the transfer coefficient for the Compton process, σ_{tr}, as

$$\sigma_{tr} = \sigma \, (_\sigma E_{tr}/h\nu) \qquad (5\text{-}11)$$

To evaluate it we take the product of the Compton cross section, σ, of Figure 5-7 for the free electron and the ratio $(_\sigma \bar{E}_{tr}/h\nu)$ of Figure 5-8. Figure 5-7 shows that σ_{tr} is a small fraction of σ for photon energies less than 10 keV, increases to a maximum value at 0.5 MeV, and then decreases slowly with increasing energy to approach the value for σ at 100 MeV. The Compton transfer coefficient is so important that values for it are given in column 4 of Table A-2a. This table also contains values for the Compton scatter coefficient, σ_s, which is simply $\sigma - \sigma_{tr}$.

Compton Coefficients Including the Effects of Binding

Figure 5-7 shows that below 10 keV substantial errors are made in the calculation of both σ and σ_{tr} if binding is ignored and the electrons are considered free. This statement is, however, somewhat misleading since in the energy range below 10 keV the photoelectric process is much more important than the Compton so that the net error in using an incorrect Compton coefficient is much reduced. For example, the reader can show that at 10 keV in carbon neglecting the binding energy alters the total attenuation coefficient by only 2.9%. Where possible, one should use the corrected Compton coefficient; these are given for a few elements in the third column of Table A-4 and are represented by σ_{inc} where the subscript refers to the incoherent Compton process. The following examples should clarify some of these concepts.

Example 5-7. A beam of 10^5 photons, each of energy 0.1 MeV, impinges on a layer of carbon of thickness 10^{26} atom per m². Calculate the number of coherent events and the number of Compton processes, first assuming all electrons are free and then taking the binding into account.

From Table A-4b $\qquad \sigma_{coh} = 0.0742 \times 10^{-28}$ m²/at

No. coherent events $= \mu N \Delta x = .0742 \times 10^{-28} \dfrac{m^2}{at} \times 10^5 \times 10^{26} \dfrac{at}{m^2} = 74.2$

Assuming electrons are free, $\quad \sigma = .4927 \times 10^{-28}$ m²/el
use Table A-2a

No. Compton events $= .4927 \times 10^{-28} \dfrac{m^2}{el} \times 10^5 \times 10^{26} \dfrac{at}{m^2} \times 6 \dfrac{el}{at} = 2956$

To take binding into account, $\quad \sigma_c = \sigma_{inc} = 2.924 \times 10^{-28}$ m²/at
use Table A-4b

No. Compton events $= 2.924 \times 10^{-28} \dfrac{m^2}{at} \times 10^5 \times 10^{26} \dfrac{at}{m^2} = 2924$

This is the correct answer and is about 1% less than 2956, which was obtained assuming all electrons to be free.

Example 5-8. Calculate the energy transferred to the carbon of example 5-7 by the Compton process.

From Table A-4b, $\overline{E}_{tr} = 14.1$ keV but this includes the contribution from photoelectric effect.
From Table A-2, $_\sigma\overline{E}_{tr} = 13.8$ keV, but this is for a free electron.
Using $_\sigma\overline{E}_{tr}$ we get energy transf. $= 2924 \times 13.8$ keV $= 40.35$ MeV

Because of effects of binding energy (Fig. 5-7), this value overestimates the energy transferred by Compton effect.

The 74.2 photons scattered coherently will have the same energy as the beam (100 keV), so no energy is transferred. These photons will be scattered into small angles around the original direction. The 2924 Compton events will give rise to 2924 recoil electrons with energies from 0 to 28 keV (see Fig. 5-8) with an average energy of 13.8 keV. There will be 2924 scattered photons with energies from 100 keV down to 72 keV at angles from 0 to 180°.

Summary of Compton Process

- It involves an interaction between a photon and an electron.
- It is almost independent of atomic number.
- It decreases with increase in energy.
- In each collision some energy is scattered and some transferred to an electron, the amount depending on the angle of emission of the scattered photon and the energy of the photon.
- On the average, the fraction of the energy transferred to K.E. per collision increases with increase in photon energy. For low energy photons $\sigma_{tr} \ll \sigma$, for high energy photons $\sigma_{tr} \approx \sigma$.
- In soft tissue the Compton process is much more important than either the photoelectric or pair process for photons in the range 100 keV to 10 MeV.

5.10   PAIR PRODUCTION

When the energy of the incident photon is greater than 1.02 MeV the photon may be absorbed through the mechanism of pair production. When the photon passes near the nucleus of the atom and is subjected to the strong field of the nucleus, it may suddenly disappear as a photon and become a positive and negative electron pair as illustrated in Figure 5-9a. This is an example of the conversion of energy into mass discussed in Chapter 3. The energy equivalent of one electronic mass is 0.511 MeV; since two particles are formed, the photon must have an energy of at least 2(0.511) = 1.022 MeV. In the process, no net electronic charge is created since the positron and the electron carry opposite charges. If the photon has energy in excess of 1.022 MeV, this excess energy would be shared between the positron and electron thus

$$h\nu - 1.022 = E_+ + E_- \tag{5-12}$$

where E_+ and E_- are the kinetic energies of the positron and the electron respectively. The process must be considered as a collision between the photon and the nucleus, and in the collision, the nucleus recoils with some momentum. It also acquires a little energy, but the energy involved is so small as to be negligible in comparison with the energies given the positron and the electron and so is neglected in equation 5-12. Because the nucleus acquires some momentum, momentum is *not* conserved between the *three* particles (photon, positron, and electron). Hence we cannot analyze the collision in detail as with the Compton process and so predict the angular deviation of the positron when the deviation of the electron is known. The total energy given to the charged particles ($E_+ + E_-$) can be divided between the two particles in many ways with one getting nearly all the energy and the other none or with both particles getting half the energy or in fact any distribution between these extremes (see Chapter 6).

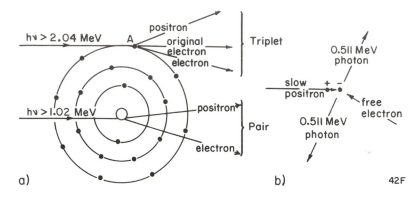

Figure 5-9. (a) The absorption of photons by pair and triplet production. (b) The annihilation of a positron and an electron to form two photons of radiation, each with an energy of 0.511 MeV.

FATE OF THE POSITRON: The positron in traveling through matter excites and ionizes atoms just the same as an electron until it is finally brought to rest. It is then annihilated as illustrated in Figure 5-9b. It combines with one of the free electrons (which are abundant in matter) to produce two photons of radiation. This is an example of mass being converted into energy. Since two electron masses are converted, the total energy release is 1.022 MeV. In order to conserve momentum, two photons, each with 0.511 MeV, are ejected in opposite directions from the scene of the annihilation. Electric charge is also conserved, since no net charge is created or destroyed. The positron is unlikely to be captured by an electron until it is nearly at rest, but if this does happen its kinetic energy will be added to the radiation energy released.

TRIPLET PRODUCTION: Illustrated in Figure 5-9, triplet production is the same as pair production except that the interaction occurs in the field of the electron rather than in the field of the nucleus. Thus, three particles appear—the positron, the created electron, and the original electron—hence the term triplet. The threshold for triplet production may be shown to occur at twice the threshold for pair production, or 2.04 MeV. Triplet production is usually small compared with pair production and will be included with it in further discussions.

VARIATION OF PAIR PRODUCTION WITH ENERGY: The cross section for pair production is usually represented by κ with suitable subscripts for the energy transfer and energy absorption coefficients. The pair production cross section increases rapidly with increase in energy above the threshold of 1.02 MeV (as illustrated in Fig. 5-10). Thus, a high energy photon is more easily stopped in a pair process than a lower energy photon and a high energy beam is *less* penetrating than a low energy beam when the main attenuation process is by pair production. This behavior is in contrast with either the photoelectric or Compton process, since the probability of their occurring *decreases* as the energy of the photon is increased.

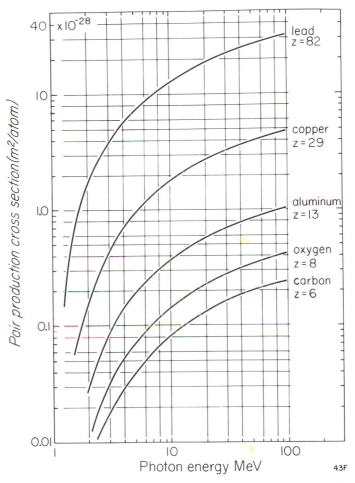

Figure 5-10. Total of pair and triplet cross sections in m² per atom for a few typical elements as a function of energy. Data taken from Plechaty et al. (P5). These values may also be found in column 5 of Table A-4 in the appendix.

VARIATION OF PAIR PRODUCTION WITH ATOMIC NUMBER: Pair production occurs in the field of the nucleus, which depends upon Z^2. Hence, the pair coefficient κ depends upon Z^2 per atom and on Z per electron or per gram. Thus 1 gram of lead will absorb about 10 times as much energy

K pair

by pair production as 1 gm of oxygen. The sum of pair and triplet coefficients per atom are given in the fifth column of Table A-4.

ENERGY TRANSFER AND ENERGY TRANSFER COEFFICIENTS FOR PAIR PRODUCTION: For each pair process the energy transferred to K.E. is $h\nu - 1.022$. Hence

$$\kappa \bar{E}_{tr} = h\nu - 1.022 \tag{5-13}$$

and in analogy with equation 5-6,

$$\kappa_{tr} = \kappa \left(\frac{h\nu - 1.022}{h\nu} \right) \text{ where } h\nu \text{ is in MeV} \tag{5-14}$$

The high energy electrons and positrons produced in a pair process have sufficient energy that some of it is converted back into radiation by bremsstrahlung and so escapes. Thus, the energy absorbed is less than the energy transferred. For carbon at 10 MeV, $\bar{E}_{ab}$ is about 3% less than $\bar{E}_{tr}$ (see Table 5-4). An example will illustrate these ideas.

Example 5-9. A beam of 10^6 photons, each of energy 10 MeV, bombards a slab of carbon containing 10^{26} atom per m². Find the number of photons that are removed from the beam by pair and triplet processes. Calculate the energy transferred to K.E.

From Table A-4b in the appendix or Figure 5-10 $\kappa = 0.0840 \times 10^{-28}$ m² per atom

No. pair interactions (eq. 5-1) $= .0840 \times 10^{-28} \dfrac{m^2}{at} \times 10^{26} \dfrac{at}{m^2} \times 10^6 = 840$

Energy transferred to K.E. $= 840 \times (10.0 - 1.022) \text{ MeV} = 7542 \text{ MeV}$

Summary for Pair Production

- It involves an interaction between a photon and the nucleus.
- The threshold for the process is 1.02 MeV.
- It increases rapidly with energy above this threshold.
- The coefficient per atom varies approximately as Z^2.
- The coefficient per unit mass depends approximately on Z^1.
- The energy transferred to K.E. is $h\nu - 1.022$ MeV.
- Two annihilation photons, each of 0.511 MeV, are produced per interaction and radiated from the absorber.

5.11   TOTAL ATTENUATION COEFFICIENT

In previous sections, the photoelectric scattering, coherent scattering, Compton incoherent scattering, and pair production were discussed in detail. In general, when a single photon interacts with matter, any of the four processes may occur. In any *one* interaction only *one* process can take place, but in many interactions all of them may occur. The relative probability of each type of interaction is proportional to the cross section for that process. The probability of an interaction is proportional to the sum of the cross sections. The total attenuation coefficient, μ, is thus the sum of the four components:

$$\underset{\text{total}}{\mu} = \underset{\text{photoelectric}}{\tau} + \underset{\text{coherent}}{\sigma_{\text{coh}}} + \underset{\text{Compton}}{\sigma_{\text{inc}}} + \underset{\text{pair}}{\kappa} \qquad (5\text{-}15)$$

In low Z materials, σ_{coh} is usually negligible except at very low energies (< 10 kev) and is often omitted from the sum.

This equation, with suitable subscripts, applies equally well to the mass, the electronic, or the atomic coefficient. The total mass coefficient is plotted in Figure 5-11 for air, copper, and lead. For all materials, the curves fall rapidly with increase in energy due to the rapid decrease with energy of the photoeffect. Then, the curves decrease more slowly in the region from 200 keV to 5 MeV (where the Compton effect is important).

In this region all materials have nearly the same mass attenuation coefficient so the three curves for (μ/ρ) almost coincide. Above 10 MeV the total coefficient for air is almost constant because the decrease in the Compton coefficient almost matches the increase due to pair production. For lead, the contribution from pair production at high energies more than offsets the decrease in the Compton process, so the coefficient increases with increase in energy.

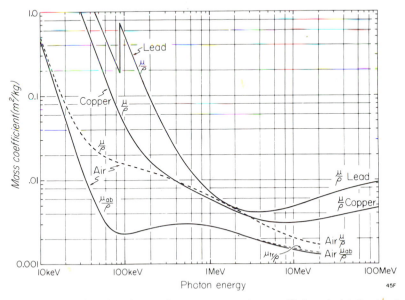

Figure 5-11. Graphs showing the total mass attenuation coefficient (μ/ρ) for lead, copper, and air. Also shown are the mass energy absorption coefficient (μ_{ab}/ρ) and the mass energy transfer coefficient (μ_{tr}/ρ) for air.

It is important to recognize that in lead the minimum absorption coefficient occurs at about 2 to 3 MeV and in copper at 5 to 10 MeV. In the 200 to 400 keV energy region, it is common practice to filter out the "soft" low energy components from an x-ray beam, using filters of high atomic number material. However, the radiation produced in a betatron or linear accelerator cannot be filtered in this way since *the more energetic components are more readily stopped in lead than the less energetic ones.* If one filters a 20 MeV linear accelerator beam with Pb, the beam that emerges will contain mainly photons in the 2 to 3 MeV region and not the most energetic components, since these components will be removed by the pair process. *To usefully filter the beam from such a machine, low atomic number filters of carbon or aluminum should be used.*

Total attenuation coefficients for a number of materials are given in Tables A-3 and A-4.

Example 5-10. Find the total mass coefficient for lead at 10 MeV from data given for the separate components in columns 2, 3, 4, and 5 of Table A-4i. Lead contains 2.9066×10^{24} atoms per kg.

$$
\begin{array}{ll}
\sigma_{coh} & 0.0093 \times 10^{-28} \text{ m}^2/\text{at} \\
\sigma_{inc} \text{ (Compton)} & 4.193 \;\; \times 10^{-28} \text{ m}^2/\text{at} \\
\tau \text{ (photoelectric)} & .168 \;\;\; \times 10^{-28} \text{ m}^2/\text{at} \\
\kappa \text{ (pair plus triplet)} & \underline{12.40 \;\;\;\; \times 10^{-28} \text{ m}^2/\text{at}} \\
\text{Total} & 16.77 \;\;\; \times 10^{-28} \text{ m}^2/\text{at}
\end{array}
$$

$$
\text{Total mass coef.} \left(\frac{\mu}{\rho}\right) = 16.77 \times 10^{-28} \frac{\text{m}^2}{\text{at}} \times 2.907 \times 10^{24} \frac{\text{at}}{\text{kg}}
$$

$$
= .004875 \frac{\text{m}^2}{\text{kg}}
$$

Total Coefficients for Compounds or Mixtures

To calculate the attenuation of x rays by compounds such as H_2O, or mixtures such as air, muscle, fat, or bone, the absorption coefficients can be determined by simply adding the individual coefficients for the atoms involved. We illustrate this by a simple example.

Example 5-11. Find the total mass coefficient for water at 1.25 MeV from the data in the appendix for hydrogen and oxygen.

For hydrogen (Table A-4a) $\mu/\rho = .1129$ cm^2/g

For oxygen (Table A-4d) $\mu/\rho = .0570$ cm^2/g

Since 18 g water contains 16 g of O_2 and 2 g of H_2:

$$
\left(\frac{\mu}{\rho}\right)_{water} = \frac{2}{18} (.1129) + \frac{16}{18} (.0570) = .0632 \text{ cm}^2/\text{g}
$$

This value appears in the second column of Table A-3b.   (5-16)

5.12   **TOTAL ENERGY TRANSFER AND**
ABSORPTION COEFFICIENTS

The total energy transfer and absorption coefficients are obtained by adding the three separate components due to photoelectric interaction, Compton incoherent scattering, and the pair process. Coherent scattering is excluded because in this process no energy is transferred or absorbed. Thus, we have:

$$\mu_{tr} = \tau_{tr} + \sigma_{tr} + \kappa_{tr} \tag{5-17}$$

$$\mu_{ab} = \tau_{ab} + \sigma_{ab} + \kappa_{ab} \tag{5-18}$$

Total mass energy transfer and mass absorption coefficients for a few elements are given in columns 7 and 8 of Table A-4 in the appendix. For low energies, $(\mu_{tr}/\rho) = (\mu_{ab}/\rho)$ and only one column of numbers appears in the table while at higher energies where (μ_{tr}/ρ) and (μ_{ab}/ρ) differ, both values are entered. Values for (μ_{ab}/ρ) for air are given in column 3 of Table A-3. The variation of (μ_{ab}/ρ) for air is also known in Figure 5-11. The energy absorption curve shows 2 minima, at 100 keV and 20 MeV, with a broad maximum at 500 keV. This maximum is due to the peak in the energy transfer coefficient for the Compton effect (see Fig. 5-7).

5.13   **THE RELATIVE IMPORTANCE OF DIFFERENT**
TYPES OF INTERACTIONS

The percentage of interactions that arise from each process can be easily calculated and are given in Table 5-5. For example, the percentage of the interactions that are photoelectric is:

$$100 \ \tau/(\tau + \sigma_{coh} + \sigma_{inc} + \kappa) = 100 \ \tau/\mu \tag{5-19}$$

with similar expressions for the other processes. These percentages are given in part 1 of Table 5-5, where we see, for example, that at 30 keV, 36.3% of the interactions are photoelectric, 50.7% are Compton, and the rest coherent. Of more importance is the percent of the energy transferred by each process. For example, the percentage of energy transfer to photoelectrons is

$$100 \ \tau_{tr}/(\tau_{tr} + \sigma_{tr} + \kappa_{tr}) \tag{5-20}$$

with similar expressions for the other processes. These values are given in the second part of the table. We see, for example, that at 30 keV although only 36% of the events are photoelectric, they account for 93% of the energy transferred. This behavior is, of course, due to the fact that in a photoelectric collision much more energy is transferred than in a Compton collision.

The last column of Table 5-5 gives the percent of the transferred energy radiated from the system by bremsstrahlung. It is calculated from

$$\text{percent of transferred energy which is radiated} \qquad (5\text{-}21)$$
$$\text{as bremsstrahlung} = 100\,(1 - \overline{E}_{ab}/\overline{E}_{tr})$$

This fraction becomes important only above 10 MeV.

Although Table 5-5 is for water, it may be used with little error for soft tissue. It may be summarized as follows:

Up to 50 keV	Photoelectric absorption is important.
60 keV to 90 keV	Photoelectric and Compton are both important.
200 keV to 2 MeV	Compton absorption alone is present.
5 MeV to 10 MeV	Pair production begins to be important.
50 MeV to 100 MeV	Pair production is most important.

It is important to distinguish between the three types of absorption because of the differences in the way energy is absorbed in bone and soft tissue. For example, if photoelectric absorption alone is present, the bone will absorb several times as much energy, mass for mass, as soft tissue.

When patients are placed in a photon beam, they are exposed to a spectrum of radiations from zero up to a maximum value, E. For the purposes of the above table, and in rough calculations, one may consider that an x ray machine operating at a peak voltage E is equivalent to a monoenergetic beam of energy E/3. Thus, a 250 kV machine is equivalent to about 85 keV, while a 22 MeV betatron is equivalent to about 7 MeV. Of course, with cobalt 60, the energy is 1.25 MeV.

• X ray tubes operating at 60 to 140 kV produce beams that give very high absorption in bone as compared with soft tissue.

• X ray beams operating at 200 to 250 kV produce some extra absorption in bone.

• Cobalt 60 (1.25 MeV), and 2 to 10 MeV x ray machines, produce beams that produce equal absorption mass for mass in bone and soft tissue.

• Betatrons and linacs operating with peak energies of 20 to 25 MeV produce beams that give slightly more absorption in bone than soft tissue.

ABSORPTION OF RADIATION BY TISSUES: In concluding this chapter, the important ideas presented in the last section are illustrated visually. Figure 5-12 shows two chest x rays of the same patient, the one on the left being taken by a standard diagnostic machine (80 kV) and the one on the right by a 2 MV machine.

The photographs show little resemblance. In one case, the ribs and bone structures are clearly shown; while in the other, the air cavities, including the trachea, appear clearly outlined. These films show a record of what comes through the patient and are of interest diagnostically. The therapeutic radiologist is interested in what is absorbed at each site in the

TABLE 5-5
Types of Photon Interactions in Water

hν (keV)	% Interactions by Each Process				% Energy Transferred			% Energy Lost to Bremsstrahlung
	a Coh	**b** Compton	**c** Photo	**d** Pair	**e** Compton	**f** Photo	**g** Pair	**h**
10.0	4.5	3.1	92.4	0.0	0.1	99.9	0.0	0.0
15.0	8.5	10.8	80.7	0.0	0.4	99.6	0.0	0.0
20.0	11.6	23.3	65.1	0.0	1.3	98.7	0.0	0.0
30.0	13.0	50.7	36.3	0.0	6.8	93.2	0.0	0.0
40.0	11.0	69.6	19.4	0.0	19.3	80.7	0.0	0.0
50.0	8.6	80.4	11.0	0.0	37.2	62.8	0.0	0.0
60.0	6.8	86.6	6.6	0.0	55.0	45.0	0.0	0.0
80.0	4.5	92.6	2.9	0.0	78.8	21.2	0.0	0.0
100.0	3.1	95.3	1.5	0.0	89.6	10.4	0.0	0.0
150.0	1.6	97.9	0.5	0.0	97.4	2.6	0.0	0.0
200.0	1.0	98.8	0.2	0.0	99.0	1.0	0.0	0.0
300.0	0.5	99.4	0.1	0.0	99.7	0.3	0.0	0.1
400.0	0.4	99.6	0.0	0.0	99.9	0.1	0.0	0.1
500.0	0.3	99.7	0.0	0.0	99.9	0.1	0.0	0.1
600.0	0.2	99.8	0.0	0.0	100.0	0.0	0.0	0.1
800.0	0.1	99.9	0.0	0.0	100.0	0.0	0.0	0.2
(MeV)								
1.0	0.1	99.9	0.0	0.0	100.0	0.0	0.0	0.2
1.5	0.0	99.8	0.0	0.2	99.9	0.0	0.1	0.4
2.0	0.0	99.2	0.0	0.8	99.3	0.0	0.7	0.5
3.0	0.0	97.1	0.0	2.9	96.7	0.0	3.3	0.8
4.0	0.0	94.5	0.0	5.5	93.3	0.0	6.7	1.1
5.0	0.0	91.6	0.0	8.4	89.6	0.0	10.4	1.4
6.0	0.0	88.9	0.0	11.1	86.2	0.0	13.8	1.6
8.0	0.0	83.1	0.0	16.9	79.0	0.0	21.0	2.3
10.0	0.0	77.0	0.0	23.0	71.9	0.0	28.1	2.9
15.0	0.0	65.6	0.0	34.4	59.3	0.0	40.7	4.6
20.0	0.0	56.0	0.0	44.0	49.3	0.0	50.7	6.5
30.0	0.0	43.2	0.0	56.8	37.1	0.0	62.9	10.0
40.0	0.0	35.1	0.0	64.9	29.7	0.0	70.3	13.6
50.0	0.0	29.3	0.0	70.7	24.6	0.0	75.4	16.8
60.0	0.0	25.3	0.0	74.7	21.1	0.0	78.9	19.8
80.0	0.0	19.7	0.0	80.3	16.4	0.0	83.6	25.3
100.0	0.0	16.0	0.0	84.0	13.3	0.0	86.7	30.1

a. $100 \, \sigma_{coh}/\mu$
b. $100 \, \sigma_{inc}/\mu$
c. $100 \, \tau/\mu$
d. $100 \, \pi/\mu$
e. $100 \, \sigma_{tr}/\mu_{tr}$
f. $100 \, \tau_{tr}/\mu_{tr}$
g. $100 \, \pi_{tr}/\mu_{tr}$
h. $100 \, (1 - \overline{E}_{ab}/\overline{E}_{tr})$

patient. The two points of view are related, for if a bone shows as a shadow, this means that radiation has been absorbed in it. The low voltage technique involves much more bone absorption than the high voltage one because of the importance of photoelectric absorption in bone.

In the high voltage technique all materials, mass for mass, absorb nearly the same amount of radiation because the main interaction process is
Compton. The trachea is clearly visible because it is filled with air.

The clavicle absorbs the same amount of radiation mass for mass as
soft tissue, but because of its higher density it still casts a shadow. The
shadows in the high voltage technique are due only to differences in
density and not to differences in atomic number.

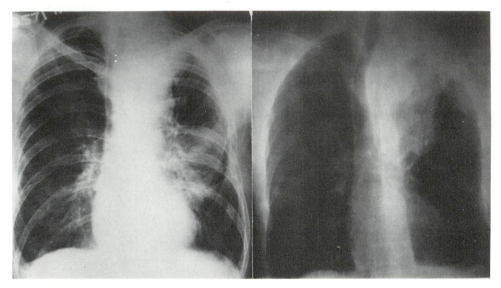

Figure 5-12. Chest x rays taken on standard diagnostic machine (80 kV), left, and 2 MV
x ray machine, right. (Courtesy Milton Friedman.)

PROBLEMS

One problem in this set cannot be solved without additional assumptions. Can you
find it? Problems marked with an asterisk are more difficult.

1. A beam of photons has a linear attenuation coefficient of 0.03 cm^{-1}. Calculate the
   fraction transmitted through layers of material 5 mm, 1.5 cm, and 20 cm thick, using
   equations 5-1b and 5-2a. Account for the differences in your answer.

2. For the beam of Problem 1 calculate the HVL and plot on semilog paper the percent
   transmitted as a function of thickness. Determine the percent transmitted for the
   thickness of 20 cm and compare with problem 1.

3. The mass attenuation coefficient for an x ray beam is .003 m^2/kg and the material has
   a density of 3000 kg/m^3. Using equations 5-1b and 5-2a, calculate the percentage
   transmitted through layers of 1 mm, 0.5 cm, and 5 cm thick.

4. For Problem 3 calculate the HVL in kg/m^2. Plot the percent transmitted as a function of thickness expressed in kg/m^2 and check the answer obtained for Problem 3
   for thickness 5 cm.

5. Find the HVL (in kg/m^2) of 100 keV photons in aluminum, copper, lead, and water.
   (Use the coefficients given in Tables A-3 and A-4 in the appendix.)

6. A linear accelerator produces a spectrum of radiation with photons from 0 to 24
   MeV. Assuming this is equivalent to photons at 8 MeV find the thickness of lead
   required to reduce the radiation from 2 Gy/min to 10^{-5} Gy/h.

7. Aluminum has a density of 2699 kg/m³. The Compton coefficient per atom is given in Table A-4e for 1.5 MeV photons as 2.232×10^{-28} m²/atom. Express this coefficient in m²/electron, cm²/g, m⁻¹. (Use Table 5-3 or top of Table A-4e.)

8. The photoelectric attenuation coefficient in lead at 150 keV is 620×10^{-28} m²/atom. Assuming that all of this coefficient arises from the K electrons, calculate the energy transfer coefficient, τ_{tr}. Determine as well τ_{tr}/ρ expressed in m²/kg.

*9. From the insert of Figure 5-5 or Table A-4i determine the number of K electrons and the number of L + M electrons ejected from a thin foil of lead of thickness 0.5×10^{20} atoms/cm², when it is bombarded by 10^4 photons each with an energy just greater than 88 keV.

10. A beam of photons with energy 100 keV suffers Compton collisions. Find the minimum energy of the scattered radiation, the maximum energy the recoil electron may acquire, and the mean energy of the recoil electron.

11. Given that $\overline{E}_{tr}$ and $\overline{E}_{ab}$ for 1 MeV photons interacting with carbon are 0.4399 MeV and .4392 MeV respectively, determine μ_{tr}/ρ given that $\mu/\rho = .00636$ m²/kg. Check your answer with Table 5-4.

12. A slab of carbon of thickness 3×10^{23} electrons per cm² is bombarded by 10^6, 1.0 MeV photons. Calculate the number of Compton interactions, the energy diverted from the beam, the energy transferred to K.E. of charged particles, and the energy scattered. Make an energy balance.

13. Determine the Compton and pair cross section at 10 MeV for water using the data of Table A-4 for hydrogen and oxygen. Find the relative number of Compton and pair processes and check with Table 5-5.

14. A large beam having 1000 photons per cm², each with energy 50 keV, is incident on a 10 g mass of carbon. Find the number of Compton electrons and photoelectrons set in motion.

15. A 10 MeV photon interacts in a pair process. Calculate the energy of the positron if the electron emerges from the interaction with an energy of 2.0 MeV.

16. A 2.0 MeV positron is annihilated by a stationary electron. What is the total energy radiated?

17. Explain why the total attenuation coefficient in lead passes through a minimum at about 3 MeV.

18. The pair process in lead has a cross section of 12.4×10^{-28} m²/at at 10 MeV. Find the energy converted into K.E. of charged particles when a beam containing 10^4 photons passes through a block of lead of thickness 1 cm. Assume only pair interactions.

19. In carbon at 10 MeV, Compton and pair processes take place. The cross sections are given in columns 3 and 5 of Table A-4b. Calculate μ/ρ and check your answer with the value given in column 6. Using the mean energies of columns 9 and 10 calculate μ_{tr}/ρ and μ_{ab}/ρ. Compare with columns 7 and 8.

*20. From the conservation of momentum and energy between the three particles involved in triplet production, show that the threshold is 2.04 MeV.

*21. At 5 MeV in lead coherent, Compton, photoelectric, and pair processes all occur. The cross sections in m²/at are given in columns 2, 3, 4, and 5 of Table A-4i. 10^6 photons each with energy 5 MeV pass through a foil of lead of thickness 10^{21} atoms/cm². Find the number of coherent, Compton, photoelectric, and pair processes. Find the mean energy converted to K.E. by each process and so determine $\overline{E}_{tr}$. Compare with the value in the table.

22. The Klein-Nishina Compton cross sections for free electrons are given in column 2 of Table A-2a. Assuming all the electrons in carbon are free, calculate the incoherent cross section at 5 keV and compare with the value in Table A-4b. Discuss.

*23. A small pencil-like beam with cross-sectional area about 10 mm^2 containing 10^6 photons each of 1.0 MeV energy passes lengthwise through a cylinder of carbon of area 2.0 cm^2 and length 10 cm. Carbon has a density of 2.25 g/cm^3 and contains 3.01×10^{23} electrons/g. Calculate the number of Compton interactions, the energy diverted from the beam, the energy transferred to K.E. of charged particles, and the energy scattered. Make an energy balance. Discuss how this answer might be altered if the absorber were made much larger in area.

24. Find the rise in temperature of the cylinder of carbon irradiated in Problem 23. Specific heat of carbon is 0.17 cal/g°C.

25. Use the department's linac or betatron or cobalt unit to obtain a chest picture like Figure 5-12. Compare with a conventional radiograph.

Chapter **6**

THE BASIC INTERACTIONS BETWEEN PHOTONS AND CHARGED PARTICLES WITH MATTER

In Chapter 5 the simpler aspects of the interaction of photons with matter were discussed. In the earlier parts of this chapter we shall deal with this topic again but in greater detail. In the latter sections we will deal with the interactions of charged particles with matter.

6.01   **PHOTOELECTRIC EFFECT**

In the photoelectric process (represented in Fig. 5-5), there is a collision between a photon and an atom resulting in the ejection of a bound electron. The process is most likely to occur if the energy of the photon is *just* greater than the binding energy of the electron. Energies just less than this cannot eject the electron and therefore the cross section varies with energy in a complicated way with discontinuities at the energy corresponding to each shell or subshell (see Fig. 5-5). Typical values for the photoelectric cross section are given in column 4 of Tables A-4 in the Appendix.

The energy transferred to K.E. in the photoelectric process can be calculated if one knows the binding energy of the shell from which the electron is ejected and the cross section for this event. One also requires a knowledge of how the hole in the shell is subsequently filled. If an Auger electron is ejected (see sec. 3.12) then all of the binding energy appears as K.E. If on the other hand fluorescent radiation is produced, all of the available binding energy will escape. Since both processes can occur, the calculations of energy transfer involve a knowledge of the fluorescent yield for each subshell (see also sec. 3.12). The calculations of energy transfer, taking all these possibilities into account, are discussed by Hubbell (H7, H8) and Plechaty (P5).

Although the principles of how these calculations should be carried out are straightforward, there is a conceptual difficulty, for even if a photon of fluorescent radiation is emitted it may often have so little energy that it will be effectively reabsorbed in the cell near its origin. For this reason, the fluorescent radiation from low atomic number materials is often considered as being converted into K.E. at the site of interaction. In the tables by Plechaty two columns for energy transfer to K.E. are given—one assuming *none* of the fluorescent radiation is converted and the other assuming *all* is converted and so locally absorbed. The true situation will lie between these extremes. *For photoelectric collisions in tissue one can usually assume that all energy is locally absorbed.*

The photoelectrons set in motion by low energy photons tend to be ejected at right angles to the beam in lobes similar to those shown in Figure 2-16. With increase in the energy of the photon, the lobes tip forward and the photoelectrons are ejected more in the forward direction. Fluorescent radiation is emitted isotropically.

6.02   THOMSON SCATTERING (CLASSICAL SCATTERING)

Coherent and incoherent scattering were illustrated in Figure 5-6. When a beam of photons (that is an electromagnetic wave in the classical sense) passes near an electron, this electron is momentarily accelerated by the electric field of the wave and so radiates energy. This process is called Thompson scattering and the cross section for it may be derived from classical physics. We think of the wave nature of a beam of photons and represent the electromagnetic wave by its electric vector E at right angles to its magnetic vector B traveling with velocity c as illustrated in Figure 6-1a. We can represent an unpolarized beam by two equal electric vectors, E_1 and E_2, at right angles as shown in Figure 6-1b. These will have a pair of magnetic vectors as well, but since these are not involved in our calculation they are not shown. Consider what happens when these two electric field components pass over the free electron at P (Fig. 6-1c). The electron, finding itself in electric field E_1 will have a force, $F_1 = keE_1$, exerted on it and will be given an acceleration, $a_1 = k E_1 e/m_0$. An accelerated charge, according to classical theory, will radiate energy in the form of an electromagnetic wave and at point Q (Fig. 6-1c) the electric vector of this wave will be:

$$E_1' = \frac{a_1 e \sin \psi}{c^2 r} = \frac{k e^2}{m_0 c^2} \frac{E_1}{r} \sin \psi \qquad (6\text{-}1)$$

where $k = 8.9875 \times 10^9$ N m^2/C^2*, c is the speed of light, r is the distance PQ, and ψ is the angle between the electric vector E_1 and the direction PQ. The quantity ke^2/m_0c^2 is called the classical electron radius, r_0, and the student may show that its value is:

$$r_0 = \frac{k e^2}{m_0 c^2} = 2.81794 \times 10^{-15} \text{ m} \qquad (6\text{-}2)$$

---

*The constant k arises from Coulomb's law, which states that the force between charges Q_1 and Q_2 distance r apart is given by $F = k\ Q_1\ Q_2/r^2$. In SI units, $k = 8.9875 \times 10^9$ newton meter^2/coulomb^2.

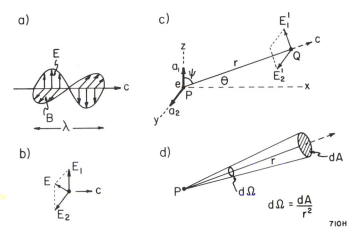

710H

Figure 6-1. (a) Representation of electromagnetic wave with E and B vectors at right angles moving at velocity c. (b) Representation of electromagnetic wave showing only the electric vectors, for an unpolarized beam $E_1 = E_2$. (c) Showing how the electric vectors E_1 and E_2 set the free electron at P into oscillation with accelerations a_1 and a_2, causing an electromagnetic wave to be emitted in direction PQ. (d) Diagram to illustrate the meaning of solid angle.

Equation (6-1) can now be written in the convenient form:

$$E_1' = \frac{r_0}{r} E_1 \sin \psi \qquad (6\text{-}3a)$$

This equation is obviously dimensionally correct and since r_0/r is very small for any reasonable distance r, it shows that the electric vector of the radiated wave is a small fraction of the electric vector of the incident wave.

Similarly the component E_2 will give rise to an electric field component:

$$E_2' = \frac{r_0}{r} E_2 \sin 90° = \frac{r_0}{r} E_2 \qquad (6\text{-}3b)$$

Now, the intensity of an electromagnetic wave, i.e. the rate of energy flow across unit area at right angles to the direction of flow, is equal to $c/4\pi$ times the square of the electric vector. Hence, the intensity at point Q of the scattered beam due to both components is:

$$I_s = \frac{(E_1'^2 + E_2'^2)}{4\pi} c = \frac{c}{4\pi} \frac{r_0^2}{r^2} (E_2^2 + E_1^2 \sin^2 \psi) \qquad (6\text{-}3c)$$

while the intensity of the original wave at point P due to the two components is:

$$I_p = \frac{c}{4\pi} (E_2^2 + E_1^2) \qquad (6\text{-}3d)$$

For an unpolarized beam $E_1 = E_2$ and the fraction of the incident energy scattered into unit area at Q is the ratio of these, which reduces to:

$$\frac{I_s}{I_p} = \frac{r_0^2}{2r^2} (1 + \sin^2 \psi) = \frac{r_0^2}{2r^2} (1 + \cos^2 \theta) \qquad (6\text{-}4a)$$

where θ is the complement to angle ψ (see Fig. 6-1). The quantity I_s/I_p is the fraction of the incident energy that is scattered by the electron into the solid angle* $d\Omega = 1/r^2$. It is convenient to represent this fraction by:

$$d\sigma_0 = \frac{r_0^2}{2} (1 + \cos^2 \theta) \, d\Omega \qquad (6\text{-}4b)$$

which may equally well be written:

$$\frac{d\sigma_0}{d\Omega} = \frac{r_0^2}{2} (1 + \cos^2 \theta) \qquad (6\text{-}4c)$$

The quantity $d\sigma_0/d\Omega$ is called the classical scattering coefficient per electron and per unit solid angle. It correctly gives the amount scattered for zero energy photons, hence the subscript zero. It is also often referred to as the Thomson coefficient in honor of the scientist who first derived it. In this process, no energy is given to the electron and the frequency and wavelength of the scattered radiation is the same as that of the incident radiation. It can, therefore, be thought of either as the fractional energy scattered or the fractional number of photons scattered into unit solid angle at angle θ.

The differential cross section $d\sigma_0/d\Omega$ is plotted as a function of angle in Figure 6-2. At $\theta = 0$ and 180° this cross section is $r_0^2 = 7.94 \times 10^{-30}$ m² while at 90° it is half this value. This means an electron will scatter twice as much energy either forwards or backwards as it does at 90°. It should also be noted that the cross section has the dimensions of an area.

To obtain the total cross section, σ_0, from the differential cross section we must integrate equation 6-4c over all values of θ from zero to 180°. Before doing this we determine the solid angle between the cones of angles θ and $\theta + d\theta$ (see Fig. 6-2). This solid angle $d\Omega = 2 \pi \sin \theta \, d\theta$. Equation 6-4c may be rewritten as:

$$\frac{d\sigma_0}{d\theta} = \left(\frac{r_0^2}{2}\right) (1 + \cos^2 \theta) \, 2 \pi \sin \theta \qquad (6\text{-}5)$$

---

*A solid angle defines a certain portion of space. In Figure 6-1d is shown a small cone that encloses a certain portion of space. This solid angle $d\Omega$ is determined by the ratio dA/r^2 where dA is the area cut out by the cone on a sphere of radius r centered at P. It is clear that the solid angle defined in this way is independent of r since doubling r will increase dA by a factor of 4. Solid angles are measured in steradians (sr). The reader may easily show that the total solid angle about a point is 4π sr and the corner of a room $\pi/2$ sr.

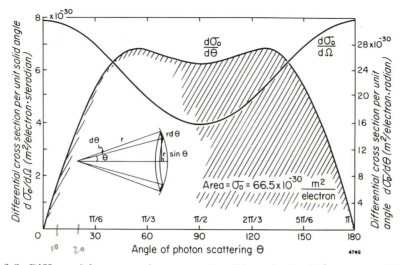

Figure 6-2. Differential cross section per unit solid angle, $d\sigma_0/d\Omega$ and the differential cross section per unit angle, $d\sigma_0/d\Theta$, as a function of the angle of photon scattering, according to Thomson's classical theory.

$d\sigma_0/d\theta$ is called the differential cross section *per unit angle* and gives the fraction of the incident energy that is scattered into the cone contained between θ and $\theta + d\theta$. This is plotted in Figure 6-2 and is zero for $\theta = 0$ or 180° and reaches maxima at about 55 and 125° and a shallow minimum at 90°. The area under this curve gives the total fraction of energy scattered by an electron. The student may determine this area by integrating equation 6-5 or graphically from Figure 6-2 to yield:

$$\sigma_0 = \frac{8}{3}\,\pi\,r_0^2 = \frac{8}{3}\,\pi\,\frac{k^2 e^4}{m_0^2 c^4} = 66.525 \times 10^{-30}\ \text{m}^2 \qquad (6\text{-}6)$$

This total cross section, σ_0, is called the Thomson classical scattering coefficient for a free electron and has the same value for all photon energies. In this type of scattering, the electron is given no energy and so no energy is absorbed; it is merely scattered from the beam. At very low energies the scattering is correctly given by equation 6-6, but as the photon energy is increased, the electron recoils and the amount of radiation scattered is less than that calculated from equation 6-6.

Example 6-1. An x ray beam is incident on a block of carbon of thickness 0.5 g/cm². Find the fraction of the energy of the beam that is scattered at an angle of 90° to impinge on a detector having a cross-sectional area of 2.0 cm² and placed 10 cm from the scattering block.*

(Fig. 6-2 or eq. 6-4c)

$$\frac{d\sigma_0}{d\Omega}(90°) = 3.97 \times 10^{-30}\ \frac{\text{m}^2}{\text{el sr}}$$

---

*For brevity we use "el" to represent "electron" and "sr" to represent "steradian," the unit of solid angle.

$$\text{Number el in 1 cm}^2 = \frac{0.5 \text{ g}}{\text{cm}^2} \times 3.0 \times 10^{23} \frac{\text{el}}{\text{g}} = 1.5 \times 10^{23} \frac{\text{el}}{\text{cm}^2}$$
of target

$$= 1.5 \times 10^{27} \frac{\text{el}}{\text{m}^2}$$

Solid angle subtended $= 2.0/10^2 = 0.02 \text{ sr}$

Fraction scattered to detector $= 3.97 \times 10^{-30} \frac{\text{m}^2}{\text{el sr}} \times 1.5 \times 10^{27} \frac{\text{el}}{\text{m}^2}$

$$\times 0.02 \text{ sr} = 1.19 \times 10^{-4}$$

Example 6-2. If the beam of example 6-1 contained 10^6 photons, calculate the number of photons reaching the detector. Determine also the total number of photons scattered by the target.

Number photons scattered to detector $= 10^6 \times 1.19 \times 10^{-4} = 119$

Total number photons scattered $= 66.5 \times 10^{-30} \frac{\text{m}^2}{\text{el}} \times 1.5 \times 10^{27} \frac{\text{el}}{\text{m}^2} \times 10^6$

$$= 9.97 \times 10^4 \text{ (eq. 6-6)}$$

It should be noted that according to classical theory the results of examples 6-1 and 6-2 are independent of photon energy. In a following section we shall see that this classical solution is not correct and the energy of the photon is involved. The correct solution involves the addition of extra modifying factors to equation 6-4c.

6.03   COHERENT SCATTERING (RAYLEIGH SCATTERING)

In Chapter 5 we saw that coherent scattering is a cooperative phenomena involving all the electrons in the atom. Photons are scattered by bound electrons in a process where the atom is neither excited nor ionized. The scattering from different parts of the atomic cloud combine to give coherent scattering. This is often called Rayleigh scattering, after the scientist who discussed it. The process mainly occurs at low energies for large Z values where the electron binding energies influence the Compton effect. The process can be described in terms of the parameter $x = (\sin \theta/2)/\lambda$ and the coefficient is given by:

$$\frac{d\sigma_{coh}}{d\theta} = \frac{r_0^2}{2} (1 + \cos^2 \theta) [F(x,Z)]^2 2\pi \sin \theta \qquad (6-7)$$

where $F(x,Z)$ is called the atomic form factor. This factor is tabulated by Hubbell (H9) and Plechaty et al. (P5)*. For small values of θ it ap-

*In the tables by Plechaty, multiply table values by Z to obtain $F(x,Z)$ to be used in equation 6-7.

proaches Z while for large values of θ it tends towards zero. Equation 6-7 is plotted as curve 4 in Figure 6-6. It is strongly peaked in the forward direction and the area under this curve is the total coherent coefficient. For the example illustrated in Figure 6-6, the area under the curve is 3.25×10^{-28} m² per atom. This value is found in the second column of Table A-4b.

Example 6-3. A layer of carbon of thickness 3.0×10^{26} at/m² is placed in a beam of 10^5 photons each with 10 keV energy. Calculate the number of photons scattered coherently. Estimate the number of these that would be scattered into a cone of half angle 10° around the forward direction.

No. coherent events
(Fig. 6-6, or Table
A-4b)
$$= 3.25 \times 10^{-28} \frac{m^2}{at} \times 10^5 \times 3.0 \times 10^{26} \frac{at}{m^2}$$
$$= 9750$$

Scattering in the forward direction is Z^2 times the value for one electron.

The classical value
per electron for the
forward direction
$$= 7.94 \times 10^{-30} \text{ m}^2/\text{sr (see Fig. 6-2)}.$$

Hence cross section
$d\sigma_{coh}/d\Omega$ (in
forward direction)
$$= 7.94 \times 10^{-30} \times 6^2 = 2.85 \times 10^{-28} \frac{m^2}{at\ sr}$$

solid angle
$$= \int_0^{10°} 2\pi \sin\theta\ d\theta = [-2\pi \cos\theta]_0^{10°}$$
$$= 2\pi(1 - .9848) = .0955$$

No. scattered into
this cone
$$= 2.85 \times 10^{-28} \frac{m^2}{at\ sr} \times .0955\ sr$$
$$\times 3.0 \times 10^{26} \frac{at}{m^2} \times 10^5 = 816$$

Thus about 9% of the coherently scattered photons will be directed into the 10° cone.

Detailed calculations similar to this show that in carbon half the coherently scattered photons are scattered into cones of half angles of 38°, 29°, 23°, 19°, 15°, 12°, and 9.5° at energies of 10, 20, 30, 40, 60, 80, and 100 keV respectively (see Hubbell H9).

6.04 ENERGY-ANGLE RELATIONS IN A COMPTON COLLISION

In classical (Thompson and Rayleigh) scattering, the scattered radiation has the same wavelength as the incident radiation and no energy is transferred. In a Compton collision or an incoherent scattering event energy is transferred to an electron, which recoils from the collision. Since energy and momentum are conserved, we may analyze the process in detail using Figure 6-3. Let $h\nu$ and p represent the energy and momentum of the incident photon, $h\nu'$ and p' the corresponding parameters for the scattered photon. The momentum, p, of a photon of energy $h\nu$ is simply $h\nu/c$. Let the electron recede from the collision with energy E, momentum q, and velocity v. Since the electron may have velocity comparable with c it is necessary to use the relativistic expressions for its kinetic energy and momentum (see Chapter 2), thus:

$$h\nu - h\nu' = E = m_0 c^2 \left\{ \frac{1}{\sqrt{1 - v^2/c^2}} - 1 \right\} \qquad (6\text{-}8a)$$

Since momentum is also conserved, the sum of the vectors p' and q must equal p; this means p, q, and p' form the sides of a triangle, so that

$$q^2 = p^2 + (p')^2 - 2\,pp'\cos\theta \qquad (6\text{-}8b)$$

or we can write down expressions for conservation of momentum in the forward direction

$$\frac{h\nu}{c} = \frac{h\nu'}{c} \cos\theta + \frac{m_0 v}{\sqrt{1 - v^2/c^2}} \times \cos\phi \qquad (6\text{-}8c)$$

and in the direction at right angles to give

$$\frac{h\nu'}{c} \sin\theta = \frac{m_0 v}{\sqrt{1 - v^2/c^2}} \times \sin\phi \qquad (6\text{-}8d)$$

By eliminating v and ϕ from 6-8a, c, and d the reader may show that:

$$E = h\nu \cdot \frac{\alpha(1 - \cos\theta)}{1 + \alpha(1 - \cos\theta)} \qquad (6\text{-}9a)$$

$$h\nu' = h\nu \cdot \frac{1}{1 + \alpha(1 - \cos\theta)} \qquad (6\text{-}9b)$$

$$\text{where } \alpha = \frac{h\nu}{m_0 c^2} = \frac{h\nu \text{ (expressed in MeV)}}{0.511} \qquad (6\text{-}9c)$$

The parameter α is the ratio of the energy of the photon to the rest energy of the electron ($m_0 c^2$). If the energy of the photon is expressed in MeV, then $m_0 c^2 = .511$ MeV. By adding the electron energy, E (eq. 6-9a), to the energy of the scattered photon, $h\nu'$ (eq. 6-9b), one obtains the incident energy $h\nu$ in agreement with equation 6-8a. Some discussion of these two equations is in order.

If the photon $h\nu$ makes a direct hit on the electron, the electron will travel straight forward (see Fig. 6-3), and the scattered photon will be scattered straight back with $\theta = 180°$. In this type of collision the electron

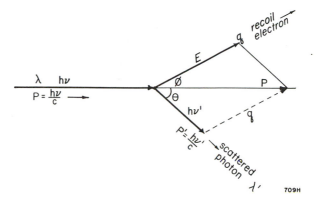

Figure 6-3. Compton collision between a photon of energy $h\nu$ and momentum $p = h\nu/c$, with a free electron. The recoil electron acquires momentum q and energy E.

will acquire the maximum energy, E_{max}, and the scattered photon its minimum energy, $h\nu'_{min}$. Substituting $\theta = 180°$ in equation 6-9a and noting that $\cos 180° = -1$, one obtains

$$E_{max} = h\nu \cdot \frac{2\alpha}{1 + 2\alpha} \qquad (6\text{-}10a)$$

$$h\nu'_{min} = h\nu \cdot \frac{1}{1 + 2\alpha} \qquad (6\text{-}10b)$$

If, on the other hand, the photon makes a grazing hit with the electron, the electron will emerge nearly at right angles ($\phi \approx 90°$) and the scattered photon will go almost straight forward ($\theta \approx 0$). Under these circumstances $\cos \theta = 1$, and $1 - \cos \theta = 0$. From equations 6-9, it is evident that $E = 0$ and $h\nu = h\nu'$. For this collision the electron receives no energy and the scattered photon acquires the full energy of the incident photon.

Any number of intermediate collisions are possible. For example, if $\theta = 90°$ (i.e. the photon is scattered at right angles to its original direction) the scattered photon acquires an energy $h\nu/(1 + \alpha)$ since $\cos \theta = 0$.

Consider a few examples in the use of these equations.

Example 6-4. Determine the maximum energy of the recoil electron and the minimum energy of the scattered photon for (a) $h\nu = 5.11$ keV and (b) $h\nu = 5.11$ MeV.

(a) $\quad \alpha = \dfrac{5.11 \text{ keV}}{.511 \text{ MeV}} = 0.010$

$\quad E_{max} = 5.11 \text{ keV} \times \dfrac{2 \times 0.01}{1.02} = 0.10 \text{ keV}$

$\quad (h\nu')_{min} = 5.11 \text{ keV} \times \dfrac{1}{1.02} = \underline{5.01 \text{ keV}}$

$\qquad\qquad\qquad\qquad\quad \text{Total} \quad \underline{5.11 \text{ keV}}$

Thus, in a collision with a low energy photon (5.11 keV), the electron can acquire at most only 2% of the energy while the scattered photon acquires at least 98% of the energy. Compton scattering at low energies results in very little deposition of energy.

(b) High energy photon (5.11 MeV): $\alpha = 10$

$$E_{max} = 5.11 \text{ MeV} \frac{2 \times 10}{21} = 4.87 \text{ MeV}$$

$$(h\nu')_{min} = 5.11 \text{ MeV} \left(\frac{1}{21}\right) = \underline{0.24 \text{ MeV}}$$

Total   5.11 MeV

Thus in a collision between a high energy photon and an electron, the electron recoils with most of the energy and the scattered photon gets very little.

Example 6-5. In a Compton collision between a very high energy photon and an electron, show that the photon scattered at right angles is approximately 0.511 MeV and the photon scattered backward is 0.255 MeV.

For $\theta = 90°$ equation 6-9b becomes

$$h\nu' = \frac{h\nu}{1 + \alpha}$$

For a high energy photon $\alpha \gg 1$ so

$$h\nu' \approx \frac{h\nu}{\alpha} = 0.511 \text{ MeV}$$

For $\theta = 180°$ equation 6-9b becomes

$$h\nu = \frac{h\nu}{1 + 2\alpha} \approx \frac{h\nu}{2\alpha} = 0.255 \text{ MeV}$$

**6.05   PROBABILITY OF COMPTON COLLISION
(Klein-Nishina Coefficients)**

In the last section we saw that one could analyze the collision between a photon and electron in detail. We now inquire into the relative probability of this type of collision. This may be determined by quantum mechanical reasoning. Initially our system involves an electron at rest and a photon with energy $h\nu$ and momentum $h\nu/c$. In the final state the electron has an energy E and momentum q at angle ϕ, and the photon an energy $h\nu'$ and momentum $h\nu'/c$ at angle θ. To evaluate the probability of this transition, one describes the initial state of the system and the final state by suitable wave functions. The probability of the transition from one to the other can then be determined by quantum mechanics. By a complex analysis of this type, Klein and Nishina (H1) showed that the differential cross section per unit solid angle is given by the product of the Thomson scattering expression from equation 6-4c and the factor F_{KN}, thus:

$$\frac{d\sigma}{d\Omega} = \frac{d\sigma_0}{d\Omega} \cdot F_{KN} = \frac{r_0^2}{2}(1 + \cos^2\theta) \quad F_{KN} \qquad (6\text{-}11)$$

where

$$F_{KN} = \left\{\frac{1}{1 + \alpha(1 - \cos\theta)}\right\}^2 \left\{1 + \frac{\alpha^2(1 - \cos\theta)^2}{[1 + \alpha(1 - \cos\theta)](1 + \cos^2\theta)}\right\}$$

F_{KN} is always less than 1.0 so that when the recoil is taken into account the scatter is reduced. When α is small the reader may show that $F_{KN} = 1$ and equation 6-11 reduces to the classical expression. Further when $\theta = 0$ and the recoil electron gets no energy, $F_{KN} = 1$ so that the scatter is again given by the classical value. Equation 6-11 is plotted in Figure 6-4 for photon energies of 0, 0.1, 1.0, and 10 MeV. For zero energy the same curve is obtained as was shown in Figure 6-2. For high energies and large angles of scattering, where the recoil electron gets most of the energy, $d\sigma/d\Omega$ is much smaller than the classical value.

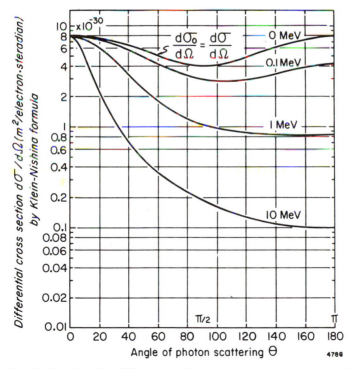

Figure 6-4. Graph showing the differential Compton cross section per unit solid angle, $d\sigma/d\Omega$, as a function of the angle of photon scattering for photon energies of 0, 0.1, 1.0, and 10.0 MeV as calculated by the Klein-Nishina formula.

Example 6-6. Repeat the calculation of example 6-1 for 0.1 MeV.

$$\frac{d\sigma}{d\Omega} \text{ for } \theta = 90° \text{ is } 2.9 \times 10^{-30} \text{ m}^2/\text{el} \quad \text{(Fig. 6-4)}$$

$$\begin{aligned}
\text{No. scattered into} \atop \text{2 cm}^2 \text{ at 10 cm} &= 10^6 \times 1.5 \times 10^{27} \frac{\text{el}}{\text{m}^2} \times 2.9 \times 10^{-30} \frac{\text{m}^2}{\text{el}} \times \frac{2}{10^2} \\
&= 87.0
\end{aligned}$$

This value is about 25% smaller than the value of 119 obtained in example 6-1, using classical theory.

Total Coefficient for Compton Process

To find the total probability that a photon will interact with a free electron in a Compton process, equation 6-11 must be multiplied by the element of solid angle, $d\Omega = 2\pi \sin\theta \, d\theta$, and integrated over all angles of θ. When this is done, the total Compton coefficient is obtained and is given by

$$\sigma = \frac{3}{4}\sigma_0 \left\{ \left(\frac{1+\alpha}{\alpha^2}\right)\left(\frac{2(1+\alpha)}{1+2\alpha} - \frac{\ln(1+2\alpha)}{\alpha}\right) + \frac{\ln(1+2\alpha)}{2\alpha} - \frac{1+3\alpha}{(1+2\alpha)^2} \right\}$$

$$(6\text{-}12)$$

For $\alpha = 0$ the reader may show that this reduces to the classical Thomson coefficient, σ_0. The total coefficient σ given by equation 6-12 is tabulated in column 2 of Table A-2a of the appendix. It is also plotted in Figure 5-7. It is seen to decrease continually with increase in energy from 64.0×10^{-30} m^2 at 0.01 MeV to $.82 \times 10^{-30}$ m^2 at 100 MeV. The value at 0.01 MeV is close to the classical value of 66.5×10^{-30} m^2 given by equation 6-6.

Energy Transfer Coefficient for Compton Process

To find the fraction of energy transferred to K.E. of charged particles in each Compton interaction, we multiply the differential cross section, $d\sigma/d\Omega$, of equation 6-11 by the fraction of the energy given the recoil electron, which may be obtained from equation 6-9a, to yield

$$\frac{d\sigma_{\text{tr}}}{d\Omega} = \frac{r_0^2}{2}(1 + \cos^2\theta) \times F_{\text{KN}} \times \left(\frac{\alpha(1 - \cos\theta)}{1 + \alpha(1 - \cos\theta)}\right) \quad (6\text{-}13a)$$

When this is integrated over all angles, we obtain the energy transfer coefficient, σ_{tr}, thus

$$\sigma_{\text{tr}} = \frac{3}{4}\sigma_0 \left\{ \frac{2(1+\alpha)^2}{\alpha^2(1+2\alpha)} - \frac{(1+3\alpha)}{(1+2\alpha)^2} + \frac{(1+\alpha)(1+2\alpha-2\alpha^2)}{\alpha^2(1+2\alpha)^2} \right.$$

$$(6\text{-}13)$$

$$\left. - \frac{4\alpha^2}{3(1+2\alpha)^3} - \left(\frac{1+\alpha}{\alpha^3} - \frac{1}{2\alpha} + \frac{1}{2\alpha^3}\right)\ln(1+2\alpha) \right\}$$

Values for σ_{tr} are given in column 4 of Table A-2a and plotted in Figure 5-7. The energy transfer cross section is seen to increase with increase in energy from a low value at low energies to a maximum value of 9.87×10^{-30} cm² at 0.5 MeV, after which it decreases slowly with increase in energy.

Scatter Coefficient for the Compton Process

This may be evaluated as the difference between the total and the transfer coefficient thus:

$$\sigma_s = \sigma - \sigma_{tr} \qquad (6\text{-}14)$$

At low energies it is nearly equal to the total coefficient, since at these energies, the recoil electron gets practically no energy. At high energies it is a small fraction of the total. It is given in Table A-2a.

Mean Energy of Compton Recoil Electrons

In the last chapter we saw that a recoil electron could have any value from 0 up to a maximum value. The *mean* energy transferred, $\overline{E}_{tr}$, to K.E. per interaction was plotted in Figure 5-8. We are now in a position to calculate $_\sigma\overline{E}_{tr}$ since it is simply:

$$_\sigma\overline{E}_{tr} = h\nu \times \sigma_{tr}/\sigma \qquad (6\text{-}15)$$

Values for $_\sigma\overline{E}_{tr}$ are given in the last column of Table A-2a.

6.06   ENERGY DISTRIBUTION OF COMPTON ELECTRONS

By a suitable manipulation, equation 6-11 may be written to yield the differential cross section for the production of an electron with energy in the range between E and E + dE. (See problem 35.) Such an expression has been plotted in Figure 6-5 for photon energies ranging from 0.2 to 1.2 MeV. Thus, for example, we see that for a photon energy of 0.5 MeV, all electron energies from 0 to 0.331 MeV are possible. The curves all show the same form with peaks, at the maximum energy and at zero energy with a shallow minimum between. Thus, in a Compton collision, low energy and high energy electrons are more likely to be produced than medium energy ones.

The vertical scale of Figure 6-5 is actually a differential cross section measured in m²/MeV. The area under the curves gives the total Compton cross sections. For example, the average height of the 1 MeV curve of Figure 6-5 is about 28×10^{-30} m²/MeV, and the horizontal distance 0.796 MeV. Hence, the area under this curve is about:

$$28 \times 10^{-30} \frac{m^2}{el\ MeV} \times 0.796\ MeV = 22 \times 10^{-30} \frac{m^3}{el}$$

From Figure 5-7 the total Klein-Nishina coefficient for 1 MeV photons is 21×10^{-30} m² per electron, in agreement with this.

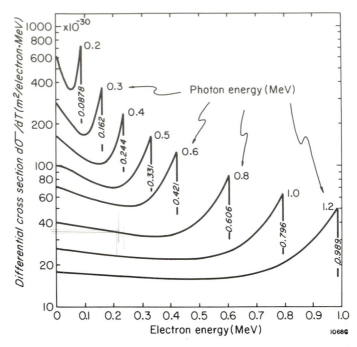

Figure 6-5. Differential cross section per unit kinetic energy interval, dσ/dE, as calculated by the Klein-Nishina coefficient for a free electron (N2). The areas under the curves give the total cross section for that photon energy. The curves give the distribution of electron energies produced by monoenergetic photons of energies 0.2 to 1.2 MeV. The numbers appearing along vertical lines at the ends of each curve are the maximum energy the recoil electron may acquire.

Example 6-7. Determine the number of Compton interactions and the number of electrons set in motion with energies between 0.15 and 0.25 MeV when a slab of bone 0.6 cm thick is bombarded by 10^4 photons each with energy 0.5 MeV.

$$\text{No. el/m}^2 \text{ in slab} = 3.19 \times 10^{26} \frac{\text{el}}{\text{kg}} \times 1650 \frac{\text{kg}}{\text{m}^3} \times 0.6 \times 10^{-2} \text{ m}$$
(Table 5-3)

$$= 3.16 \times 10^{27} \frac{\text{el}}{\text{m}^2}$$

For 0.5 MeV photons interacting with bone only the Compton process is involved and all electrons may be considered free so we use either Figure 5-6 or Table A-2a column 2 to yield $\sigma = 28.9 \times 10^{-30}$ m²/el

$$\text{No. interactions} = 10^4 \times 28.9 \times 10^{-30} \frac{\text{m}^2}{\text{el}} \times 3.16 \times 10^{27} \frac{\text{el}}{\text{m}^2} = 913$$

To obtain the number of electrons with energies in the range 0.15 to 0.25 MeV we use the data of Figure 6-5. The interval 0.15 to 0.25

MeV has a width of 0.1 MeV and is centered at 0.20 MeV, where the differential cross section is $7.0 \times 10^{-29} \dfrac{m^2}{el\ MeV}$

No. el in interval $= 10^4 \times 3.16 \times 10^{27} \dfrac{el}{m^2} \times 7.0 \times 10^{-29} \dfrac{m^2}{el\ MeV} \times$

$0.1\ MeV = 221$

Thus of the 913 photons that underwent Compton collisions in the slab of bone, 221 of them produced electrons with energies in the range 0.15 to 0.25 MeV.

6.07   EFFECT OF BINDING ENERGY ON COMPTON (INCOHERENT) SCATTERING

In all of the above discussion we have tacitly assumed that the electrons involved in the process are free and are stationary. To deal with the real situation we must take into account the fact that the electrons in the atom are in motion and that energy is required to eject them from the atom. Clearly the position and velocities of electrons in the atom are both involved, so an accurate solution would require a detailed knowledge of the wave functions of all the electrons in the atom. To do this precisely would be a formidable task, especially when one realizes that accurate wave functions for only the simplest atoms are available.

An approximate solution may be obtained as follows. We represent the probability of a Compton scattering by an atomic electron as the product of two factors, A and B. The first factor, A, is given by the Klein-Nishina cross section for a free electron. It gives the probability that the photon will be deflected through angle θ and the electron acquires a momentum, q, as if it were free. The second factor, B, is the probability that the electron, having received a momentum q, will actually leave the atom with energy E. Clearly, the second factor does involve the properties of the atom. This second factor will be important for collisions in which q is small enough that the atomic electron has a finite probability of not escaping. The momentum q is given by equation 6-8b, which we rewrite thus:

$$q = \sqrt{\frac{(h\nu)^2}{c^2} + \frac{(h\nu')^2}{c^2} - \frac{2h\nu\ h\nu'}{c^2} \cos\theta} \qquad (6\text{-}16)$$

Now from example 6-4 we saw that for low energy photons (α small), the electron acquired very little energy and hence $h\nu \approx h\nu'$. If we make this approximation then q becomes

$$q \approx \frac{h\nu}{c} \sqrt{2(1 - \cos\theta)} = \frac{h\nu}{c} \sqrt{4 \sin^2 (\theta/2)} = \frac{2h\nu}{c} \sin\left(\frac{\theta}{2}\right) \qquad (6\text{-}17)$$

$$= 2h \frac{\sin (\theta/2)}{\lambda} = 2hx \qquad \text{where} \qquad x = \sin (\theta/2)/\lambda$$

Thus the momentum transferred to the electron is proportional to the parameter x, which depends on θ and λ. The factor B may be calculated using quantum mechanics to determine the probability of an electron with a momentum q escaping. The factor is usually represented by $S(x,Z)$ where S is called the incoherent scattering function, which depends upon x and atomic number Z. Extensive tables of $S(x, Z)$, one table for each atomic number, have been derived by Hubbell (H9).* The differential cross section becomes

$$\frac{d\sigma_{inc}}{d\theta} = \frac{d\sigma}{d\theta} \times S(x,Z) \qquad (6\text{-}18)$$

The total cross section is

$$\sigma_{inc} = \int_{\theta=0}^{\pi} \frac{r_0^2}{2} (1 + \cos^2 \theta) \times F_{KN} \times S(x,Z) \times 2\pi \sin \theta \, d\theta \qquad (6\text{-}19)$$

We use the subscript inc to represent the Compton cross section, taking into account the fact that electrons are bound. Equation 6-19 cannot be integrated in closed form as we did with equation 6-11 but can be determined graphically or by numerical integration. Hubbell (H9) has carried out this type of calculation for elements with $Z = 1$ to 100 and Plechaty et al. (P5) for a number of other materials yielding σ_{inc} the Compton coefficients per *atom*. Values for this quantity appear in the appendix in the third column of Tables A-4.

To illustrate these ideas we have plotted data for carbon at 10 keV in Figure 6-6. Four curves are shown: Curve 1 is simply 6 times the classical Thomson scattering coefficient. The area under this curve is $6 \times 0.665 \times 10^{-28}$ m²/el $= 3.99 \times 10^{-28}$ m²/at. Curve 2 is the next approximation, where we take into account the recoil of the electron. It is 6 times equation 6-11 and the area under it is 6 times the value for the free electron given in Table A-2a, or $6 \times 0.6405 \times 10^{-28}$ m²/el $= 3.84 \times 10^{-28}$ m²/at. Finally curve 3 is a plot of equation 6-19 using the tabulated values (H9) for $S(x,Z)$. At small values of θ where the momentum transfer is small, $S(x,Z) \approx 0$ and the curve is much smaller than curves 1 or 2. At large values of θ ($\approx 180°$), $S(x,Z)$ approaches Z, and curve 3 approaches 6 times the Klein-Nishina coefficient per electron. The area under this curve is 2.70×10^{-18} m²/at and is found as σ_{inc} in Table A-4b. This is the correct value. Curve 4 is the coherent or Rayleigh scattering coefficient described in section 6.03.

The data presented in Figure 6-6 summarizes the material discussed so far for a sample material and a sample photon energy. Curve 1 describes classical scattering by a single, free electron with no energy transferred to

---

*Plechaty et al. (P5) also give values for $S(x,Z)$, which they call the incoherent form factor. Their form factors should be multiplied by Z to be used in equation 6-18.

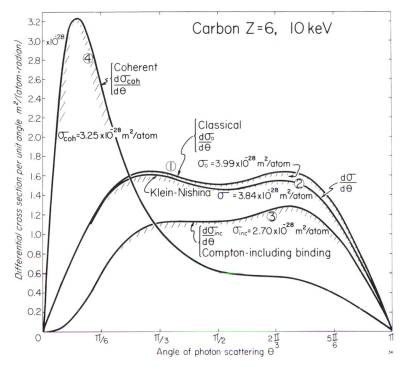

Figure 6-6. Scattering coefficients for carbon at 10 keV. Curve 1 is calculated by classical theory, as given by equation 6.5. Curve 2 is calculated by the Klein-Nishina equation, as given by equation 6-11. Curve 3 uses the Klein-Nishina derivation but takes into account the momentum and binding energy of the electrons within the atom, according to equation 6-17. Curve 4 is the coherent coefficient as given by equation 6-7, taking into account the constructive interference between the electrons of the atom.

the electron. When we consider the way electrons are bound to an atom we get Rayleigh or coherent scattering depicted by curve 4. Curve 2 describes Compton scattering by a free electron and when again the binding is taken into consideration we get curve 3 describing incoherent scattering. In an actual irradiation situation, both coherent and incoherent scattering might occur, as described by curves 4 and 3.

At small photon energies, σ_{coh} is usually much larger than σ_{inc}. This is especially true for high Z materials since coherent scattering depends on Z^2 while the incoherent process depends upon Z^1; for example in lead at 0.01 MeV: $\sigma_{coh} = 1686 \times 10^{-28}$ m²/at while $\sigma_{inc} = 15.75 \times 10^{-28}$ m²/at. Coherent scattering is neglected in most calculations of radiological interest because it gives rise to no absorbed energy. It is often neglected for another reason. Examination of Tables A-4 will show that at no energy is σ_{coh} more than about 10% of the total. At certain energies it may be large compared with σ_{inc} but at these energies the photoelectric cross section is very much larger than either σ_{coh} or σ_{inc}. For example, in lead at 0.01 MeV, the photoelectric cross section $(43960 \times 10^{-28}$ m^2/at) is 26 times σ_{coh}. Furthermore, since coherent scattering is predominantly in the forward direction (see example 6-3) the event hardly alters the properties of the beam. It is, however, included in the total attenuation coefficient data given in Tables A-3 and 4.

6.08   **PAIR AND TRIPLET COEFFICIENTS**

The mechanisms of pair and triplet production were illustrated in Figure 5-9. The calculation of pair and triplet cross sections is complicated, involving quantum mechanics.

Heitler (H1) shows that the process is almost the reverse of the production of radiation by the slowing down of a charged particle described in section 6.12 and exhibits a similar dependence on atomic number. The differential cross section for the creation of an electron-positron pair in the field of a nucleus is given by:

$$\frac{d\kappa}{d\Omega} = \frac{Z^2}{137} \frac{r_0^2}{2\pi} m_0^2 c^4 \, F_{pair} \qquad (6\text{-}20)$$

where F_{pair} is a rather complicated function of the momentum, energy, and angle of projection of both the positron and the electron. $d\Omega$ is the solid angle into which the positron is projected. This equation is analogous to equation 6-11 for the Compton effect. The total pair coefficient is obtained by integrating this expression over 2π. The total of the pair and triplet coefficient per atom is given in the fifth column of Tables A-4. The variation with energy is illustrated in Figure 5-10.

6.09   **ENERGY DISTRIBUTION OF ELECTRONS AND**
               POSITRONS PRODUCED IN PAIR PRODUCTION

The exact energy distribution of electrons and positrons in pair production is a complex function of hν and Z; see Heitler (H1) and Evans (E1). To a fairly good first approximation one can assume that all distributions of the available energy are equally probable except for the extreme one where one particle gets all the energy and the other one none. This latter probability is zero. For example, suppose hν = 20 MeV, then the available kinetic energy is $20 - 2(.511) \approx 19$ MeV and we would expect nearly equal numbers of the following pairs: 4 MeV electron and 15 MeV positron; 1 MeV electron and 18 MeV positron, etc. If a more accurate calculation is required the data of Figure 6-7 adapted from Evans (E1) may be used. The horizontal scale shows the fraction f of the energy given the electron, while the vertical scale gives the probability per fractional kinetic energy interval. Its use is illustrated in the following example.

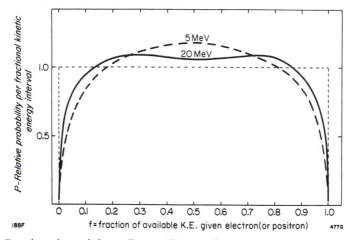

Figure 6-7. Graphs adapted from Evans (E1) to allow one to determine the number of electrons (or positrons) with a given energy produced in pair production.

Example 6-8. Determine the number of positrons with energies between 6.9 and 7.1 MeV set in motion when a layer of carbon of thickness 3×10^{26} atoms/m² is placed in a 20 MeV beam of 10^6 photons.

Number pair processes $= 0.1321 \times 10^{-28} \dfrac{m^2}{at} \times 10^6$
(Table A-4b)

$$\times 3 \times 10^{26} \frac{at}{m^2} = 3963$$

Range of possible energies $= 20 - 1 = 19$ MeV
for the positron

Approx. number positrons in range 6.9 to 7.1 MeV $= \dfrac{0.2}{19} \times 3963 = 41.7$

To a first approximation we would expect this same number in any 0.2 MeV energy range. If we want a better answer we proceed as follows:

fraction energy given positron is f $= \dfrac{19.0 - 7.0}{19.0} = .63$

For f $= .63$, Figure 6-7 shows p $= 1.09$

∴ corrected number positrons is $41.7 \times 1.09 = 45.5$.

This answer depends on the photon energy and on the way the energy is split between the two particles. For most purposes the approximate answer is all that is required.

The curves of Figure 6-7 vary only slightly with energy. For photon energies a few MeV above the threshold (1.02 MeV), the curves are peaked slightly in the middle, indicating that an equal split of the energy between the positron and electron is most probable. At energies well above the threshold the curves become slightly dished at the middle and the most probable collision is one in which one particle gets about 1/4 and the other 3/4 of the energy.

Detailed calculations show a very slight dependence on Z, which will not be discussed here. Further, if one takes into account the attractive force between the positively charged nucleus and the electron, and the repulsion between the nucleus and the positron, one would expect the mean energy of the positrons to be greater than the electrons. This is observed; for example detailed calculations by Evans (E1) for $h\nu = 2.62$ MeV in lead show that the average energy of the positron is 0.28 MeV greater than the electron.

ENERGY TRANSFER IN PAIR PRODUCTION. The energy, $_\kappa\overline{E}_{tr}$, that is transferred to electrons is $h\nu - 1.02$ (MeV) but since this energy is shared almost symmetrically between the two electrons the average energy received by each of them is $_\kappa\overline{E}_{tr}/2$.

6.11   MULTIPLE PROCESSES,
MONTE CARLO CALCULATIONS, CASE HISTORY

In this and the previous chapter, the primary processes involved in the absorption and scattering of x rays have been dealt with. In section 5.01, it was stated that some 30 interactions were required on the average to turn all the energy of an x ray beam into electronic motion. The complexity of the scattering and absorption process will be illustrated by a simple case history in which all the processes discussed so far will be illustrated.

Consider what might happen to a 20 MeV photon on entering a phantom of water-like material. One cannot tell how far it will travel before it undergoes an interaction, for it might collide with an atom on the surface or at any depth below. However, for simplicity in the example, we will assume that it travels a distance equal to the mean range. The mean range or mean free path (see section 1.22) is given by

$$\text{Mean range} = \frac{1}{\mu} = \frac{\text{HVL}}{0.693} = 1.44\,(\text{HVL})$$

For a 20 MeV photon in water $\mu = 0.0182$ cm^{-1} and the mean range is $1/.0182$ cm$^{-1} = 55$ cm. The interactions that take place are shown in Table 6-1. Interactions occur at points A, B, C, . . . X. At the interaction, electrons produced are shown as horizontal arrows while photons that are scattered appear as vertical arrows. Each of the interactions will be considered in detail.

Interaction A

At A the interaction occurs after a mean penetration of 55 cm. From Table 5-5 we find that on the average, in water, for 100 photons 44 pair processes and 56 Compton processes take place. The 44 pair processes will produce 44 positrons and 44 electrons each with an average energy of 19.0/2 = 9.5 MeV. After the 44 positrons are slowed down, they will be annihilated, giving rise to 88 annihilation quanta of energy 511 keV. The 56 Compton interactions will give rise to 56 scattered electrons of mean energy $\bar{E}_{tr}$ = 14.5 MeV (see Table A-2a) and 56 scattered photons with the rest of the energy, 5.5 MeV. In this case history we shall, for simplicity, follow only the fate of the 0.511 MeV gamma rays, but the same type of analysis would apply to the 5.5 MeV Compton scattered photons.

Interaction B

The 88 annihilation quanta will travel on the average to point B at a distance of 10.3 cm where they will undergo a Compton interaction. The pair cross sections and the photoelectric cross sections are zero for this energy photon, so only a Compton interaction is possible. $\bar{E}_{tr}$ = 175 keV, so there will be produced on the average 88 Compton electrons with 175 keV, and 88 scattered photons with energy (511 − 175) = 336 keV. These will travel a mean distance of 9.1 cm to the next point of interaction C.

Interaction C

Interactions C, D, E, and F are similar to that at B, each interaction resulting in one scattered photon and one recoil electron with a continual degradation in energy.

Interaction G

At G the photon, with energy 120 keV, has a small probability of being absorbed photoelectrically (Table 5-5). The ratio of $\tau/(\sigma + \tau)$ at this energy is about 0.01, so at G we will have 87 Compton interactions and 1 photoelectric interaction. The photoelectric interaction will give rise to one 120 keV electron, whereas the Compton will yield 87, 19 keV electrons and 87, 101 keV scattered photons.

Interactions H to X

Interactions H to X are all similar to that at G with increasing numbers of photoelectrons set in motion and a corresponding decrease in the number of Compton scattered photons until at X there is only 1 photon left and the beam has for all practical purposes been completely absorbed.

TABLE 6-1

Case History for One Hundred 20 MeV Photons

Interactions occur at the points labeled A, B . . . to X. At these points the horizontal arrows indicate the number and energy of the electrons set in motion. Arrows to the left are Compton electrons and those to the right photoelectrons for all but interaction A. The vertical lines indicate the scattered photon for each interaction. On the vertical lines, the number, energy and distance the photon travels before the next interaction are marked. The energy of the recoil electron at each interaction is taken as the mean energy and the scattered photon has the rest of the energy. In all cases, the mean range was obtained from the reciprocal of the linear absorption coefficient. For interactions from G to X the number of photoelectrons was obtained from $N\tau/(\sigma + \tau)$, where N was the number of photons involved in the interaction. Because average interactions have been considered throughout, this case history is an oversimplification of the true state of affairs. The whole process requires a very small fraction of a second to complete.

$$\ggg\to$$

If we added up all the energy given the electrons from B down, we would obtain $(.511)(88) = 44.97$ MeV indicating that all the energy of the annihilation quanta had been absorbed. It is readily seen from this example that the first 3 interactions produce a rapid degradation in the energy of the beam (20 MeV to 240 keV in 3 collisions) while the next 3 collisions only reduce the energy from 240 keV to 120 keV. Below 100 keV, the loss in energy per collision by the Compton process becomes smaller and smaller and the photon would suffer hundreds of collisions before being absorbed completely were it not for the photoelectric effect, which gradually removes the photons by complete absorption.

Any part of the case history shown in Table 6-1 may be used. For example, the history from interaction C down to X applies to a beam of 88 photons each of energy 241 keV. The example given is really that of a beam of 511 keV photons since the fate of the 56 energetic Compton photons of energy 5.5 MeV has not been followed. Also, we have neglected the possibility of radiative collisions in the slowing down of all the electrons. These will produce radiation, which must in turn be changed back into electronic motion.

Although this example appears complicated, it is in reality a gross oversimplification, for throughout we have assumed that the average *effect is the one that occurs.* The average range and the *average* energy transfer has been used. In reality any energy transfer from 0 to E_{max} can occur at each interaction and any distance of penetration from zero to infinity may take place. Case histories can be prepared similar to this, taking into account all these factors using Monte Carlo methods (B4). In this technique the operator makes a random selection to see how far the photon will go (somewhat similar to tossing a coin); then a second random selection to see what energy transfer will take place, which also determines the energy of the scattered photon; and finally a random selection of the angle in space into which the scattered photon will travel. After the operator has

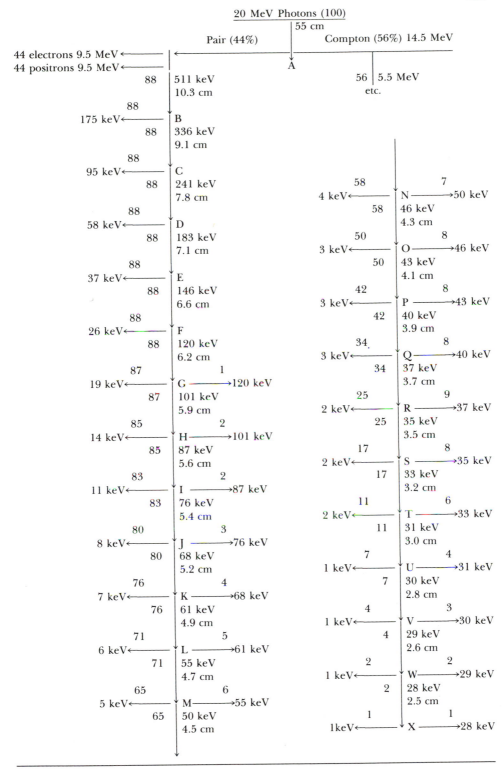

20 MeV Photons (100)

| 55 cm

Pair (44%)   Compton (56%) 14.5 MeV

44 electrons 9.5 MeV ←
44 positrons 9.5 MeV ←   A

88 | 511 keV   56 | 5.5 MeV
   | 10.3 cm   etc.

88
175 keV ←   B
      88   336 keV
            9.1 cm

88
95 keV ←   C
     88   241 keV   58   7
           7.8 cm   4 keV ←   N ——→ 50 keV
                            58   46 keV
88   4.3 cm
58 keV ←   D
     88   183 keV   50   8
           7.1 cm   3 keV ←   O ——→ 46 keV
                            50   43 keV
88   4.1 cm
37 keV ←   E
     88   146 keV   42   8
           6.6 cm   3 keV ←   P ——→ 43 keV
                            42   40 keV
88   3.9 cm
26 keV ←   F
     88   120 keV   34   8
           6.2 cm   3 keV ←   Q ——→ 40 keV
                            34   37 keV
87   1   3.7 cm
19 keV ←   G ——→ 120 keV
     87   101 keV   25   9
           5.9 cm   2 keV ←   R ——→ 37 keV
                            25   35 keV
85   2   3.5 cm
14 keV ←   H ——→ 101 keV
     85   87 keV   17   8
           5.6 cm   2 keV ←   S ——→ 35 keV
                            17   33 keV
83   2   3.2 cm
11 keV ←   I ——→ 87 keV
     83   76 keV   11   6
           5.4 cm   2 keV ←   T ——→ 33 keV
                            11   31 keV
80   3   3.0 cm
8 keV ←   J ——→ 76 keV
    80   68 keV   7   4
          5.2 cm   1 keV ←   U ——→ 31 keV
                             7   30 keV
76   4   2.8 cm
7 keV ←   K ——→ 68 keV
    76   61 keV   4   3
          4.9 cm   1 keV ←   V ——→ 30 keV
                             4   29 keV
71   5   2.6 cm
6 keV ←   L ——→ 61 keV
    71   55 keV   2   2
          4.7 cm   1 keV ←   W ——→ 29 keV
                             2   28 keV
65   6   2.5 cm
5 keV ←   M ——→ 55 keV
    65   50 keV   1   1
          4.5 cm   1keV ←   X ——→ 28 keV

followed some 50,000 of these case histories, the average may be taken to determine the actual state of affairs that will occur in the physical case. These techniques require the use of electronic computers to obtain sufficient data in a reasonable time to be practical. It is a powerful technique, allowing one to handle complex situations that arise in the absorption and scattering of radiation, provided the basic processes are understood and can be expressed mathematically. Unfortunately, to achieve any precision requires enormous numbers of case histories and much computer time.

6.11   INTERACTION OF HEAVY CHARGED PARTICLES WITH MATTER

In preceding sections it has been shown that when a photon interacts with matter, by a photoelectric, Compton, or pair production process, one or more electrons are set into motion and that these electrons carry away some of the energy of the photon. The energy given to the electrons is in the form of energy of motion and it is subsequently transferred to the medium by a multitude of relatively small interactions with the electrons and atoms of the medium through which the electron is traveling. In this section we will examine the way in which this energy transfer takes place.

All *charged* particles (electrons, protons, alpha particles, and nuclei) lose kinetic energy, chiefly through interactions between the electric field of the particle and electric fields of electrons in the material through which the particle is traveling. The basic principles involved can be seen most easily by considering heavy particles, so these will be dealt with first, followed by a detailed consideration of electron interactions.

Imagine a particle of mass M, which is large compared to m_0, the mass of an electron, moving with velocity v along the line MQ' of Figure 6-8. An electron situated at Q will experience a force towards M of value $k(ze^2/r^2)$.* This force can be considered as having two components, F_x and F_y. When the particle passes Q', the component F_x will reverse so that there will be no net motion of the electron along the X direction but the component F_y will always be in the same direction and give the electron a net impulse along the Y direction. If the mass M is large compared to m_0 the heavy particle will be deflected only very slightly from its original path along MQ', but the energy ΔE given the electron will be taken from the heavy particle. We now calculate the loss in energy of the heavy particle.

The momentum imparted to the electron, Δp, is given by

$$\Delta p = \int_{-\infty}^{+\infty} F_y \, dt = \int_{-\infty}^{+\infty} z \frac{ke^2}{r^2} \cos\theta \, dt \qquad (6\text{-}21a)$$

---

*The value of k is 8.9875×10^9 N m²/C². (see section 6.02)

Figure 6-8. Schematic diagram to illustrate the loss in
energy of a heavy charged
particle of mass M and charge
+ze moving with velocity v
past an electron at Q. The
electron is given an increment of energy ΔE by an impulse along QQ' and the
heavy particle loses this energy.

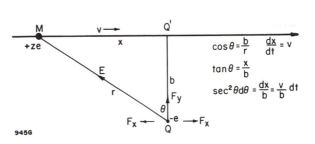

Writing all variables in terms of θ, using the equations given in Figure
6-8, this reduces to

$$\Delta p = \frac{zke^2}{bv} \int_{-\pi/2}^{\pi/2} \cos\theta \, d\theta = \frac{2zke^2}{vb} = \frac{2zr_0m_0c^2}{vb} \qquad (6\text{-}21b)$$

where we have replaced ke^2 by $r_0m_0c^2$ from equation 6-2. This expression
has dimensions of energy/velocity (m_0c^2/v) and so is dimensionally correct. Δp is the momentum transferred to the electron. The energy taken
from the heavy particle is given by

$$\Delta E(b) = \frac{(\Delta p)^2}{2\,m_0} = \frac{2z^2r_0^2m_0c^4}{v^2b^2} = \frac{z^2r_0^2m_0c^4}{b^2}\frac{M}{E} \qquad (6\text{-}22)$$

where $E = 1/2\,Mv^2$ is the kinetic energy of the heavy particle.

It should be noted that the *energy transfer is inversely proportional to the
kinetic energy of the heavy particle.* If the particle has a large energy and
hence a large velocity, it will be in the region of the electron only a short
time and so transfer little energy to it. It should also be noted that the
energy loss, ΔE, is inversely proportional to b^2, where b is the impact
parameter (the distance by which the charged particle misses making a
direct hit on the electron, see Fig. 6-8). This means close encounters will
involve large energy transfers and distant encounters small energy exchanges.

Now in any real situation electrons will be scattered throughout the
material and all types of impacts from near to far will be encountered as
the particle passes through the material. We now calculate the total
energy transfer to all the electrons and thus the energy loss of the
charged particle.

If the electrons in an absorbing material are distributed randomly in
the space around the path of the incident particle the number that will
be located in a cylindrical shell between radii b and b + db and length
Δx will be:

$$\Delta n = N_e\, 2\pi\rho b\, db\, \Delta x \qquad (6\text{-}23)$$

where N_e is the number of electrons per g ($N_e = N_0 Z/A$) (see eq. 5-5).
Δn depends upon the first power of b, showing that the number of large
energy exchanges involving a small b is small, while the number of exchanges involving small energy transfers is large. To find the total energy
loss, $\Delta E(b)$, in distance Δx we take the product of $\Delta E(b)$ and Δn from the
last two equations and integrate over all impact parameters from b_{min}
to b_{max} thus:

$$\frac{dE}{dx} = \int_{b_{min}}^{b_{max}} \Delta E(b) \times \frac{\Delta n}{\Delta x} = 4\pi N_e \rho \times \frac{z^2 r_0^2 m_0 c^4}{v^2} \int_{b_{min}}^{b_{max}} \frac{db}{b}$$

$$= 4\pi N_e \rho \times \frac{z^2 r_0^2 m_0 c^2}{\beta^2} [\ln(b_{max}/b_{min})] \qquad (6\text{-}24)$$

where β is the ratio v/c for the charged particle. The quantity dE/dx is
called stopping power and describes the amount of energy that is lost per
unit length along the track of the particle.

In deriving this expression we have taken no account of the binding
energy of the electrons in the material. Clearly at some large value for b,
i.e. b_{max}, the energy exchange will be insufficient to overcome the binding energy, and the electron will *not* be removed from the atom. It will be
momentarily pulled from its equilibrium position and then return to it.
To handle this problem, a semiempirical quantity, I, called the mean excitation energy of the atom is introduced. The larger its value, the smaller
is b_{max}. We also must take into account that the electron may be given
very large velocities, so that relativistic effects occur. When these ideas
are taken into account (H1), using quantum mechanics equation 6-24
becomes:

$$S_{ion} = \frac{1}{\rho}\left(\frac{dE}{dx}\right) = 4\pi r_0^2 N_e \frac{z^2 m_0 c^2}{\beta^2} \left[\ln\frac{2m_0 c^2 \beta^2}{I(1-\beta^2)} - \beta^2 - \sum_i \frac{c_i}{Z}\right] \quad (6\text{-}25)$$

The quantity dE/dx is the energy loss per unit thickness of medium.
A more useful quantity is the mass stopping power, which is obtained
by dividing by the density and gives the energy loss per unit thickness
measured in g/cm^2. The quantity $(1/\rho)(dE/dx)$ is usually expressed in
MeV/(g/cm²) or MeV cm²/g and is often represented by S_{ion}. The subscript "ion" indicates that this is the energy loss by the charged particle
in producing ionization in the absorbing medium.*

The last term is called a shell correction and adjusts for the way in
which the electrons are bound to their atoms. The first term in the
bracket involves the logarithm of I so its numerical value will not be
strongly affected by the value chosen for I, the average excitation energy.

---

*The subscript "col" is frequently used in the literature, representing energy loss by collisions. In
this book we will use "ion" rather than "col" to emphasize that we are describing energy exchanges
that result in ionizations.

The whole term in square brackets is a slowly increasing function of the particle energy and, for example, varies only by about a factor of two for protons over the energy range 0.5 to 100 MeV. The term outside the square bracket is the same as equation 6-24 and gives the main dependence of the energy loss on energy. This shows that the classical approach used in the derivation and illustrated by Figure 6-8 is substantially correct. The energy lost by the charged particle will appear as ionization and excitation and to a small degree as chemical change in the absorbing medium. It will ultimately be dissipated as heat.

6.12   INTERACTION OF ELECTRONS WITH MATTER

Electrons, in passing through matter, undergo interactions that are quite similar to those of heavy particles but at the same time differ in two important respects, both due to the relatively small mass of the electron. Relativistic effects are important even at quite low energies and since the collisions are with other electrons, with the same mass, they may result in quite large energy losses with marked changes in directions. In any given collision it is assumed that the electron which emerges with the most energy is the original electron so that the maximum energy exchange is one involving half the original energy. In addition, again because of the small mass of the electron, it may interact with the electric field of a nucleus and be decelerated so rapidly that some of its energy may be radiated away as bremsstrahlung. This will be discussed later. We first discuss the ionizational losses.

Ionizational Losses

The mass stopping power for heavy particles colliding with atomic electrons was given by equation 6-25. In deriving the equation for electron energy losses, however, both relativity and quantum mechanics must be used and the result is more complicated.

$$S_{ion} = \frac{1}{\rho}\left(\frac{dE}{dx}\right)_{ion} = 2\pi r_0^2 N_e \frac{\mu_0}{\beta^2} \qquad (6\text{-}26)$$

$$\left[\ln \frac{E^2(E + 2\mu_0)}{2\mu_0 I^2} + \frac{E^2/8 - (2E + \mu_0)\mu_0 \ln 2}{(E + \mu_0)^2} + 1 - \beta^2 - \delta\right]$$

This equation is originally due to Bethe (see E1 and P6). The factor in front of the square bracket is the same as the corresponding factor for heavy particles except for the factor of 2, arising because the collision is between particles of equal mass rather than one of them being very much heavier than the other. The quantity N_e is, as before, the number of electrons per g, E is the kinetic energy of the electron, and I is again the mean excitation energy for the atoms of the absorbing material. E, I, and μ_0 ($\mu_0 = m_0 c^2$) should be expressed in the same energy unit, a convenient one being MeV. The last term, δ, is the "density correction" and is needed because interactions with distant electrons will be influenced by the electrons in the intervening atoms. These atoms become polarized by the electric field and this polarization reduces the effect of the electric field of the incident electron at distant points. The result is that the energy losses will be reduced. Sternheimer (S6, W3) showed that this effect could be allowed for by calculations that take account of the density of the material and the energy levels of each of the electrons in the atoms of material. The density effect is small in all materials for electron energies below about 1 MeV but gradually increases with energy until at 100 MeV it may be as great as 20%.

The ionizational losses for carbon and lead are shown in Figure 6-9. In the low energy region, 10 to 100 keV, the important term in equation 6-26 is the one outside the bracket involving $1/\beta^2$ and the stopping power is essentially inversely proportional to the energy (doubling the energy reduces S by a factor of nearly two). At energies above 100 keV, β is close to 1.0 and the term in front of the bracket becomes essentially constant. Since the terms inside the bracket slowly increase with energy, S passes through a minimum value at about 1 MeV. The stopping power for lead is less than carbon because Z/A is less and because more of the electrons in lead are bound and so contribute less to the ionizational losses. The effect of Z on the stopping power can also be understood by noting that the excitation energy appears in the denominator of the terms in the square bracket so that S is less for higher atomic number materials, which have larger values for I. A few values for I, the average excitation energy (from Berger and Seltzer, B5) are given in Table 6-2. Ionizational stopping powers calculated by them (B5) using these values are given in Appendix A-5 for a number of materials.

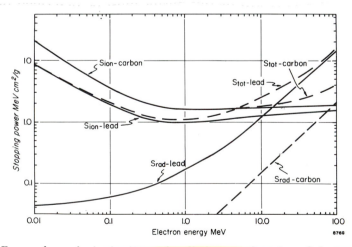

Figure 6-9. Energy losses by ionization and radiation as a function of electron energy for carbon and lead.

TABLE 6-2
Average Excitation Energies in eV

Material	I (eV)	Material	I (eV)	Material	I (eV)
hydrogen	19.0	aluminum	167.0	air	86.1
carbon	78.0	calcium	196.0	water	75.0
nitrogen	82.0	copper	322.0	bone	94.1
oxygen	97.0	tin	485.0	muscle	75.9

Energy Loss by Radiation—Bremsstrahlung

When a swiftly moving charged particle of mass M and charge ze passes close to a *nucleus* of mass M_N and charge Ze, it will also experience an electrostatic force. (In Fig. 6-8 we think of a nucleus with charge Ze replacing the electron at Q.) The force between the two particles will be $kzZe^2/r^2$ and the moving charged particle will experience an acceleration of $kzZe^2/r^2M$. If $M \ll M_N$ the nucleus at Q will not move much but the charged particle moving along MQ′ will be deflected from its path to orbit momentarily about Q. Now an accelerated charge radiates energy at a rate proportional to the square of the acceleration, in this case $(zZe^2/M)^2$. We can now predict that loss of energy by radiation should be much more important in high atomic number materials (because of the Z^2) and should be much greater for light particles such as electrons than for heavy particles such as protons (because of the $1/M^2$). Electrons, in fact, radiate energy more than a million times more strongly than protons and this type of energy loss from heavy particles is not important. Since the radiation is emitted as a result of the deceleration or slowing down of the electron, the process is known by the German word bremsstrahlung meaning "braking radiation." This was discussed in Chapter 2.

The rate of energy loss by this means must be described by quantum mechanical reasoning. For electron energies less than a 100 MeV the energy loss by radiation is:

$$S_{rad} = \frac{1}{\rho}\left(\frac{dE}{dx}\right) = 4r_0^2\frac{N_eZE}{137}\left[\ln\frac{2(E + \mu_0)}{\mu_0} - \frac{1}{3}\right] \qquad (6\text{-}27)$$

where all the symbols have the same meaning as for equation 6-26. This solution is given by Heitler (H1) and summarized by Evans (E1). It is only approximately correct. For a more detailed discussion of other approximate solutions valid under different conditions see Pages et al. (P6).

From equation 6-27 it can be seen that the energy loss by radiation (and therefore the production of x rays) increases directly with the atomic number of the material and somewhat more slowly with the energy of the electron.

Figure 6-9 shows the radiation stopping power for carbon and lead as a function of energy. In carbon, this energy loss is small compared with the ionizational loss at all energies less than 10 MeV and the two become equal at about 100 MeV. For lead the radiation losses are small compared to ionizational losses below 1.0 MeV, the two processes become equally probable at about 10 MeV, and radiation losses are some 10 times as large as ionizational losses at 100 MeV. Figure 6-9 also shows the sum of the radiation and ionizational stopping powers.

Because of the importance of the stopping power in dose calculations, values for water are given in the first four columns of Table 6-3. The results for water are quite similar to those of carbon given in Figure 6-9.

TABLE 6-3
Stopping Powers, Ranges, Radiation Yields and Average Stopping Powers for Electrons in Water

Energy E_0	S_{ion}	S_{rad} MeV cm²/g	S_{tot}	Range R g/cm² (eq. 6-28)	B-Fraction Energy Radiated (eq. 6-31)	$\bar{S}$, Average Ionizational Stopping Power (eq. 6-41)
keV						
10	22.56	.0039	22.56	.0003		39.8
20	13.17	.0040	13.18	.0009	.0001	23.4
40	7.777	.0040	7.781	.0029	.0003	13.7
80	4.757	.0041	4.762	.0098	.0005	8.19
100	4.115	.0042	4.120	.0143	.0006	6.99
200	2.793	.0048	2.798	.0447	.0010	4.47
400	2.148	.0063	2.154	.1282	.0017	3.12
800	1.886	.0104	1.897	.3294	.0029	2.42
MeV						
1	1.852	.0128	1.865	.4359	.0036	2.29
2	1.839	.0268	1.866	.9720	.0071	2.04
4	1.896	.0608	1.957	2.019	.0149	1.95
8	1.970	.1398	2.110	3.984	.0317	1.94
10	1.994	.1823	2.176	4.917	.0404	1.95
20	2.063	.4097	2.472	9.237	.0826	1.99
40	2.125	.8962	3.021	16.55	.1582	2.03
80	2.184	1.914	4.099	27.88	.2736	2.08
100	2.204	2.434	4.637	32.47	.3183	2.10

Example 6-9. A monoenergetic beam of 20 MeV electrons with a fluence of 10^4 electrons per cm² is incident on a water phantom. Find the energy deposited as ionization and radiated as bremsstrahlung in the first 1 mm layer.

From Table 6-3 $S_{ion} = 2.063$ MeV/cm

$S_{rad} = .4097$ MeV/cm

Energy converted to ionization $= 10^4 \frac{el}{cm^2} \times 2.063 \frac{MeV}{cm} \times 0.1 \text{ cm} = 2063 \frac{MeV}{cm^2}$

Energy radiated $= 10^4 \frac{el}{cm^2} \times .4097 \frac{MeV}{cm} \times .1 \text{ cm} = 409.7 \frac{MeV}{cm^2}$

Example 6-10. Electrons of energy 2 MeV strike a target of lead. Determine the fraction of the incident energy radiated as bremsstrahlung in a thin layer of the target.

From Figure 6-9

$$S_{ion} = 1.0 \frac{MeV\ cm^2}{g}$$

$$S_{rad} = 0.28 \frac{MeV\ cm^2}{g}$$

$$S_{tot} = 1.28 \frac{MeV\ cm^2}{g}$$

Fraction energy radiated $\frac{.28}{1.28} = 0.22$

6.13   RANGE OF ELECTRONS AND BREMSSTRAHLUNG YIELD

As a beam of charged particles passes through matter, the interactions cause the particles to slow down and change their directions. Eventually, a particle will lose all of its kinetic energy and come to rest. There will be a finite distance beyond which there will be no particles, and this distance is called the range of the particle. This behavior should be contrasted with that of photons, which are absorbed exponentially so that for them there is no thickness that stops a photon beam completely.

Figure 6-10 shows a plot of absorbed dose versus depth for an electron beam in a water phantom. Two ways of specifying the range of the electrons are indicated. R_{50} is the distance traveled by one-half of the electrons and is sometimes called the average range. R_P is determined by extrapolating the straight descending part of the curve to meet the background due to x rays. It is called the practical, or extrapolated, range and is the easiest to measure.

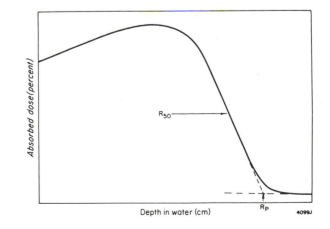

Figure 6-10. Plot of absorbed dose as a function of depth for monoenergetic electrons incident on water. R_{50} is the "half-value depth," or mean range, and R_P is the "extrapolated" or practical range.

A range can also be calculated from stopping power data as follows. Table 6-3 column 4 gives the total stopping power in MeV per unit thickness of water measured in g/cm^2 or cm. Consider a 2 MeV electron. Table 6-3 shows that the initial rate of energy loss of this electron in water is 1.866 MeV/cm. If then this electron were slowed down at this rate until it was brought to rest, it would travel a distance 2 MeV/(1.866 MeV/cm) = 1.07 cm. In actual fact, we know the electron would *not* travel this far because as it slows down it starts to lose energy more quickly. To obtain the actual range taking into account the variation of S_{tot} with respect to energy, we proceed as follows: We calculate how far the electron goes as its energy drops from 2.0 to 1.9, 1.9 to 1.8, ... 1 to 0 and add up all these increments of length to get the range. If we did the calculation numerically, the first increment would be

$$\frac{0.1 \text{ MeV}}{S_{tot}(1.95)} = \frac{0.1 \text{ MeV}}{1.866 \text{ MeV/cm}} = 0.0537 \text{ cm}$$

and the last one

$$\frac{0.1 \text{ MeV}}{S_{tot}(0.05)} = \frac{0.1 \text{ MeV}}{6.607 \text{ MeV/cm}} = 0.0151 \text{ cm}$$

These and all the intermediate values would be added together to get the range.

The range calculated in this way is called the **csda** range, or continuous slowing down approximation range. All the collisions in the slowing down process are assumed to involve very small energy exchanges and it is an integration along the actual path followed by the electron.

To do the calculation graphically, we plot $S_{tot}(E)$ versus energy as shown in Figure 6-11. The area under the curve out to 2 MeV is 0.96 cm, and this is the range of a 2 MeV electron in water. It is less than the rough estimate obtained above. Ranges for electrons in water are plotted in Figure 6-11. These values also appear as column 5 of Table 6-3. This table illustrates a convenient rule of thumb that for electron energies of about 0.5 MeV or more, the range in unit density material is, in cm, about half the energy in MeV.

Mathematically, the procedure of taking the area under Figure 6-11 is the same as calculating the integral.

$$R = \int_0^{E_o} \frac{dE}{S_{tot}(E)} \tag{6-28}$$

where R is the range of an electron with initial energy E_o. Ranges determined from equation 6-28 are given in Table A-6.

Example 6-11. Estimate the range of a 20 MeV electron in aluminum

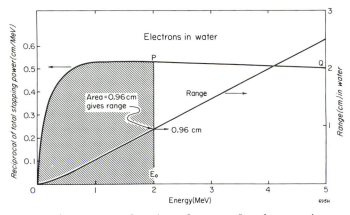

Figure 6-11. Plot of $1/s_{tot}$ (E) as a function of energy for electrons in water of density 1.0 g/cm^3. The area under this curve out to any energy E_0 is the range of an electron of energy E_0. This range is plotted (right scale) as a function of electron energy.

of density 2.7 g/cm^3 and compare with Table A-6.

$$\text{From rule of thumb given above, R} = \frac{20(.5)\text{cm}}{2.7} = 3.7 \text{ cm}$$

$$\text{From Table A-6, R} = 10.66\frac{g}{cm^2} \times \frac{1}{2.7 \text{ g/cm}^3} = 3.9 \text{ cm}$$

BREMSSTRAHLUNG YIELD: Suppose an electron of initial energy E_0 is set in motion in the medium and subsequently is brought to rest by ionization and radiation processes. Imagine that at some point in the slowing down process this electron has an instantaneous energy E. In traveling a distance Δx, it will lose an energy ΔE of which ΔE_{rad} is due to radiation losses and ΔE_{ion} is due to ionizational losses. These energy losses are:

$$\Delta E_{rad} = \frac{S_{rad}(E)}{S_{tot}(E)} \times \Delta E \quad \text{and} \quad \Delta E_{ion} = \frac{S_{ion}(E)}{S_{tot}(E)} \times \Delta E \quad (6\text{-}29)$$

Clearly their sum is ΔE, as it should be. To obtain the *total energy radiated* we integrate the first expression from 0 to E_0 thus:

$$\text{Energy radiated} = \int_0^{E_o} \frac{S_{rad}(E)}{S_{tot}(E)} \, dE \quad (6\text{-}30)$$

and the fraction of the energy radiated that we call the bremsstrahlung yield B is

$$B = \frac{1}{E_o} \int_0^{E_o} \frac{S_{rad}(E)}{S_{tot}(E)} \, dE \quad (6\text{-}31)$$

B is a function of the initial energy E_o of the electron and the atomic number Z of the material in which the electron is losing its energy. It is a very important quantity and so has been determined by numerical integration, and a few values are given in Table 6-3 and Table A-6. We illustrate these ideas with an example.

Example 6-12. Find the energy radiated and absorbed when a 10 MeV electron is brought to rest in water and in bone.

> From Table A-6 (also Table 6-3) B(water) = .0404
> B(bone) = .0527

> In water: energy radiated = .404 MeV
> energy absorbed = 9.596 MeV

> In bone: energy radiated = .527 MeV
> energy absorbed = 9.473 MeV

Extensive tables of stopping power data for electrons and positrons have been produced by Berger and Seltzer (B5) and by Pages et al. (P6). In this book we have used data kindly supplied by Berger.

6.14 ENERGY DISTRIBUTION OF ELECTRONS SET IN MOTION IN A MEDIUM EXPOSED TO MONOENERGETIC PHOTONS

In the preceding sections of this chapter we have seen how monoenergetic photons of energy $h\nu$ can set electrons in motion by the photoelectric process, by Compton scattering, and by pair production. In general, all of these processes can occur at once. The photoelectric process is easily handled since when such an event occurs all the electrons have the same energy, which is equal to $h\nu$ less the binding energy of the shell. The other two processes yield a spectrum of electrons as illustrated in Figure 6-5 and 6-7. To illustrate how such calculations may be carried out, we will determine the spectrum of electrons produced when 10 MeV photons interact with water. For this energy Table A-4d shows that the photoelectric cross section in oxygen (the major constituent of water) is negligibly small, so we need to consider only Compton and pair processes. In general, of course, we would also consider photoelectrons.

Let the fluence of the (10 MeV) photons be Φ. The number of electrons, per unit mass of water, that are given an energy E_i by the Compton process will be $\Phi (N_e/\rho)[d\sigma(E_i)/dE_i]$, where N_e is the electron density (electrons per cm^3 of water), ρ is the physical density (in g/cm^3), and the term in brackets is the differential Klein-Nishina coefficient for the production of electrons of initial energy E_i (in cm^2/MeV per electron). Curve A of Figure 6-12 shows this quantity plotted against energy, E. For this diagram the fluence, Φ, has been set equal to 1.0 (cm^{-2}). The curve goes to very high values (note the broken scale) when the electron is given an energy near its maximum value of 9.751 MeV. (See eq. 6-9a.) The area under this curve is numerically equal to the mass Compton coefficient $(\sigma/\rho) = 0.01705$ cm²/g.

For each pair process that takes place, two electrons are set into motion and so the number of pair electrons that are given energy E_i by a fluence of Φ would be $2\Phi (N_a/\rho) [d\kappa(E_i)/dE_i]$, where N_a is the number of atoms per unit volume, ρ is again the density, and the term in brackets is the probability, per atom, of producing an electron with energy E_i. This yields a symmetrical curve, similar to that shown in Figure 6-7. This is plotted as curve B in Figure 6-12, again with Φ set equal to 1.0 cm⁻². The area under this curve is $2(\kappa/\rho) = 2(0.00515$ cm²/g$) = 0.0103$ cm²/g. Curve C is the sum of curves A and B. The area under it is $[(\sigma/\rho) + 2(\kappa/\rho)] = 0.0222$ cm²/g (see Table A-3b).

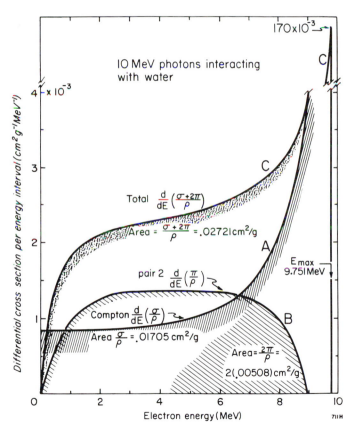

Figure 6-12. Plot of differential mass cross sections per MeV interval for 10 MeV photons interacting with ꜣater. Curve A is the differential Compton cross section and the area under it is: $\sigma = .01705$ cm²/g. Curve B is twice the differential pair cross section and the area under it is .01030 cm²/g. Curve C is A + B.

Curve C of Figure 6-12 has been replotted as curve 1 of Figure 6-13. The ordinate has been changed to a logarithmic scale so that the high energy region can be seen in more detail. It has also been relabelled $dN(E_i)/dE_i$ but retains the dimensions cm^2/g MeV.

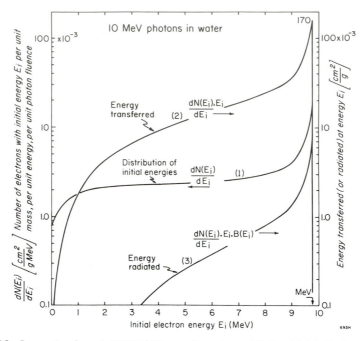

Figure 6-13. Curve 1: plot of $dN(E_i)/dE_i$ as a function of E_i for 10 MeV photons interacting with water. Curve 2: plot of $[dN(E_i)/dE_i] \cdot E_i$ against E_i. Curve 3: plot of $[dN(E_i)/dE_i] \cdot E_i \cdot B(E_i)$ against E_i.

The meaning of $dN(E_i)/dE_i$ may be further clarified by an example.

Example 6-13. Determine the number of electrons that are set in motion with energies from 4.9 to 5.1 MeV in 1.5 g of water by 10 MeV photons with a fluence of $10^4/cm^2$.

$$\frac{dN(E_i)}{dE_i} \text{ for 5 MeV electrons (Fig. 6-13)} = 2.38 \times 10^{-3} \frac{cm^2}{g \text{ MeV}}$$

$$\text{number of electrons} = 2.38 \times 10^{-3} \frac{cm^2}{g \text{ MeV}} \times 0.2 \text{ MeV} \times \frac{10^4}{cm^2}$$

$$\times 1.5 \text{ g} = 7.14$$

MEAN ENERGY TRANSFERRED: If we multiply the ordinate, $dN(E_i)/dE_i$, by E_i we obtain curve 2. This now gives the energy transferred per MeV interval to 1 g of water exposed to a photon fluence of 1 per cm^2 and the area under this curve gives the total energy transferred. If we divide this energy by the number of photon interactions per g we obtain $\overline{E}_{tr}$, given by:

$$\overline{E}_{tr} = \frac{1}{\left(\dfrac{\sigma + \kappa}{\rho}\right)} \int_0^{E_{max}} \frac{dN(E_i)}{dE_i} \times E_i \, dE_i \qquad (6\text{-}32)$$

This is the mean energy transferred per photon interaction and is given in Tables A-3 and A-4 (in the appendix). For this sample it is 7.37 MeV.

Another concept, which should not be confused with $\overline{E}_{tr}$, is the average of the initial energies acquired by the electrons that are set in motion. It is less than $\overline{E}_{tr}$ because in the pair process two electrons are set in motion per interaction. The average initial energy is the integral of equation 6-32 divided by $(\sigma + 2\kappa)$, or $\overline{E}_{tr} (\sigma + \kappa)/(\sigma + 2\kappa)$. In our example it is 7.37 (.02213)/(.02721) = 5.99 MeV. When pair production is not involved, the mean energy transferred and the average energy of the electrons set in motion are equal.

ENERGY LOSS TO BREMSSTRAHLUNG: In the last section we defined the bremsstrahlung yield, which gives the fraction of energy that an electron of initial energy E_i radiates as it is brought to rest in the medium. To deal with the distribution of initial energies, $dN(E_i)/dE_i$, we form the product of curve 2 and $B(E_i)$ to yield curve 3. This gives the energy radiated per MeV interval for the distribution. The area under curve 3 is the total energy radiated:

$$\begin{matrix}\text{Energy radiated} \\ \text{as bremsstrahlung}\end{matrix} = \int_0^{E_{max}} \frac{dN(E_i)}{dE_i} \cdot E_i \cdot B(E_i) dE_i \qquad (6\text{-}33)$$

If we divide this by $(\sigma + \kappa)/\rho$, the number of photon interactions per g of medium per photon, we obtain the mean energy radiated (in this case .28 MeV), which we represent by $\overline{E}_B$, thus:

$$\overline{E}_B = \frac{1}{\left(\dfrac{\sigma + \kappa}{\rho}\right)} \int_0^{E_{max}} \frac{dN(E_i)}{dE} \cdot E_i \cdot B(E_i) dE_i \qquad (6\text{-}34)$$

The mean energy absorbed by the medium per interaction is therefore:

$$\overline{E}_{ab} = \overline{E}_{tr} - \overline{E}_B = \overline{E}_{tr} \cdot (1 - g) \qquad (6\text{-}35)$$

In this example, $\overline{E}_{ab} = 7.37$ MeV $- .28$ MeV $= 7.09$ MeV.

In deriving these expressions we have illustrated the ideas using graphs. The areas under these curves are not easily obtained graphically because of the exceedingly sharp peak at the high energy limit. With a modern computer, however, the task is easy using numerical integration. The values for $\overline{E}_{ab}$ given in the appendix were obtained in this way.

Energy Absorption Coefficient

The energy absorption coefficient (μ_{ab}/ρ) is derived from μ/ρ using:

$$\left(\frac{\mu_{ab}}{\rho}\right) = \left(\frac{\mu}{\rho}\right) \left(\frac{\overline{E}_{ab}}{h\nu}\right) \qquad (6\text{-}36)$$

6.15   **ENERGY SPECTRUM OF ELECTRONS**
"SEEN" IN THE MEDIUM

In the last section we were concerned with the distribution of initial electron energies set in motion in the medium by monoenergetic photons. In this section we direct our attention to the medium and ask ourselves what electron energies would be observed at a point in the medium, first (a) when monoenergetic electrons are generated in the medium and (b) when monoenergetic photons interact with the medium?

Electron Spectra Resulting from Monoenergetic Electrons

In order to determine the spectrum of electron energies that result from electrons which start with initial energy E_i, consider the insert in Figure 6-14. This shows, schematically, a number of electron tracks that result from the *uniform* generation in a medium of electrons, all of which start with an energy E_i. For diagrammatic purposes the tracks are assumed straight, all in the same direction, and each with range R. A plane has been set up at right angles to the tracks and a unit area is indicated. The electron fluence is the number of electrons that pass through this area. There will be electrons passing through it with all energies from E_i down to zero. For example the electron causing track a would be seen by an observer in the plane as having an energy near zero while electron track b has energy near E_i.

We wish now to calculate the spectrum of energies that the electrons would have as they pass through such an area. Let $d\Phi(E)/dE$ represent this electron fluence spectrum. It gives the number of electrons per MeV interval with energy E passing through unit area. It can be derived by calculating the energy lost by the electrons in two different ways and equating them.

First note that if there are $d\Phi(E)/dE$ electrons per MeV interval of energy E crossing unit area then the energy lost by them in a thickness Δx (measured in g/cm^2), would be $[d\Phi(E)/dE] \cdot S_{tot}(E) \cdot \Delta x$ where $S_{tot}(E)$ is the total mass stopping power (MeV cm^2/g) given in Table 6-3. The total energy lost is found by integrating over the electron spectrum to give:

$$\text{energy lost} = \Delta x \int_0^{E_i} \frac{d\Phi(E)}{dE} \cdot S_{tot}(E)\, dE \qquad (6\text{-}37)$$

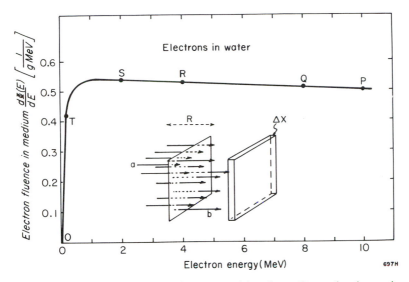

Figure 6-14. Electron fluence spectrum in water arising from the setting in motion of one 10 MeV electron in each gram of water.

Now consider this calculation from the point of view of the energies given to the electrons. Let us assume that N electrons are set in motion per gram. The energy deposited would then be $N \cdot \Delta x \cdot E_i$, if we also assume as many electrons start in any unit mass as stop in it. (The condition of as many electrons stopping per unit mass as starting is called electronic equilibrium and will be discussed in Chapter 7.) The energy given would then equal the energy lost and so:

$$N \cdot E_i = \int_0^{E_i} \frac{d\Phi(E)}{dE} \cdot S_{tot}(E) \cdot dE \qquad (6\text{-}38)$$

This is an integral equation and if it is to be true for all values of E_i then we must have:

$$\frac{d\Phi(E)}{dE} S_{tot}(E) = N \qquad \text{and} \qquad \frac{d\Phi(E)}{dE} = \frac{N}{S_{tot}(E)} \qquad (6\text{-}39)$$

Since N has dimensions g^{-1}, $d\Phi(E)/dE$ has dimensions $g^{-1}/(MeV\ cm^2/g)$ = $1/(MeV\ cm^2)$, i.e., a number per MeV interval per cm^2. Equation 6-39 is plotted in Figure 6-14 using the data from Table 6-3 for N = 1 electron set in motion per gram. Thus, if one electron of 10 MeV energy is set in motion in each gram, electrons of all energies from 10 MeV to 0 will be found in the medium with the distribution PQRSTO. If electrons of 8 MeV are generated, then $d\Phi(E)/dE$ will be given by curve QRSTO etc.

The student should note that when one deals with electron energies greater than 1–2 MeV the stopping power is nearly constant with energy, so the distribution of Figure 6-14 is nearly rectangular, i.e., if 10 MeV electrons are generated uniformly in each unit volume then an observer in the medium will see nearly equal numbers of 1, 2, 5, etc. MeV electrons, but very few electrons with energies less than 100 keV. These latter lose energy very rapidly in the slowing down process and so will be rarely "seen."

Example 6-14. Determine the number of electrons with energies between 1.9 and 2.1 MeV passing through unit area in water in which 10^3 electrons are being uniformly generated per g each with 5 MeV energy. Although Figure 6-14 was drawn for 10 MeV electrons it applies equally well to electrons of all energies less than 10 MeV.

$$\frac{d\Phi(E)}{dE} \text{ for 2 MeV electrons} = 0.54 \text{ MeV}^{-1} \text{ cm}^{-2}$$

$$\begin{array}{l} \text{Number of electrons in} \\ \text{interval 1.9–2.1 MeV} \end{array} = \frac{0.54}{\text{MeV cm}^2} \times 0.2 \text{ MeV} \times 10^3 = \frac{108}{\text{cm}^2}$$

Observe that the 5 MeV does not come into the calculation except to note that it is greater than 2 MeV.

This example is somewhat artificial because it is very difficult to uniformly generate monoenergetic electrons in a medium. It does, however, show us how to handle a situation involving the production of a distribution of initial electron energies. For example, suppose there were *generated* in the medium 10^3 electrons in each MeV interval from 10 MeV down to zero and we wished to calculate the number "seen" crossing the plane of observation in the energy interval 1.9-2.1 MeV. We first determine the number of electrons set in motion with energies *greater* than 2.0 MeV—this number is 8×10^3. These will contribute to this part of the spectrum but the rest will not. The number seen in the energy interval 1.9 to 2.1 MeV is therefore 0.54/MeV cm^2 × 0.2 MeV × 8 × 10^3 = 864/cm^2.

Electron Spectra in the Medium Resulting from the Generation of a Distribution of Initial Electron Energies

We now wish to determine the electron spectrum, $d\Phi(E)/dE$, "seen" in the medium when the distribution $dN(E_i)/dE_i$ of electrons is set in motion in the medium. Remember $dN(E_i)/dE_i$ was normalized so as to give the number of electrons generated per unit mass of medium for unit photon fluence.

As a first step, we determine the total number (per unit photon fluence) of electrons generated with energies greater than, say, E. This will be

$$\int_E^{E_{max}} \frac{dN(E_i)}{dE_i}\, dE_i$$

where E_{max} is the maximum electron energy produced. To get $d\Phi(E)/dE$, we divide by the stopping power for energy E, as in equation 6-39 and multiply by the photon fluence, $\Phi(h\nu)$, to give:

$$\frac{d\Phi(E)}{dE} = \frac{\Phi(h\nu)}{S_{tot}(E)} \int_E^{E_{max}} \frac{dN(E_i)}{dE_i} \cdot dE_i \qquad (6\text{-}40)$$

This has dimensions $\dfrac{cm^{-2}}{cm^2\, MeV\, g^{-1}} \times \dfrac{cm^2}{g\, MeV} \times MeV = \dfrac{1}{cm^2\, MeV}$

These are the correct dimensions for the electron fluence spectrum in the medium. We now evaluate $d\Phi(E)/dE$ for a photon fluence equal to 1 per cm^2. This process is illustrated in Figure 6-15 where $dN(E_i)/dE_i$ from Figure 6-13 has been reproduced and the area under this curve from E_i to E_{max} determined. This area multiplied by the ordinate at energy E_i from Figure 6-14 gives one point on the electron fluence distribution curve. By continuing the stepwise integration from right to left and dividing the cumulated "area" by S_{tot} (E), one obtains the distribution $d\Phi(E)/dE$ given in Figure 6-15. $d\Phi(E)/dE$ is zero at E_{max}, increases rapid-

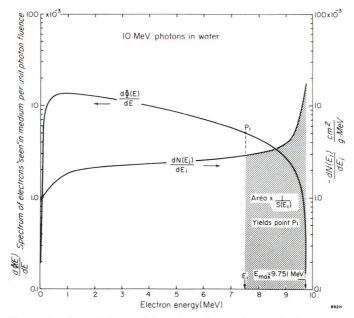

Figure 6-15. Curve 1: Plot of $dN(E_i)/dE_i$ taken from Figure 6-13; use the right scale. Curve 2: plot of $d\Phi(E)/dE$ versus electron energy for the distribution $dN(E_i)/dE_i$.

ly with decrease in energy to reach a peak value at about 1 MeV, and then decreases rapidly to zero. Since the biological effects of radiation depend to some extent on the energies of the electrons producing the damage, the quantity $d\Phi(E)/dE$ is of considerable fundamental interest since it tells us the number and energy of the electrons "seen" by the biological target in the medium. It is important to clearly distinguish between $dN(E_i)/dE_i$ and $d\Phi(E)/dE$. The difference is illustrated in the example.

Example 6-15. Water is exposed to a beam of 10 MeV photons with fluence $10^4/cm^2$. Find the number of electrons set in motion per g of water with energies in the range .95 to 1.05 MeV. Find also the number of electrons in this energy range seen crossing unit area in the medium.

From Figure 6-15
$$\frac{dN(E_i)}{dE_i} = 1.8 \times 10^{-3} \frac{cm^2}{g\ MeV}$$

$$\frac{d\Phi(E)}{dE} = 13.7 \times 10^{-3}\ MeV^{-1}\ cm^{-2}$$

No. electrons set in motion between .95 and 1.05 MeV
$$= 1.8 \times 10^{-3} \frac{cm^2}{g\ MeV} \times 0.1\ MeV \times \frac{10^4}{cm^2}$$

$$= 1.8 \text{ per g}$$

Electron fluence in energy range 0.95 to 1.05 MeV
$$= \frac{13.7 \times 10^{-3}}{MeV cm^2} \times 0.1\ MeV \times 10^4$$

$$= 13.7\ cm^{-2}$$

Note that in the last line the photon fluence of 10^4 was entered without its dimensions (cm^{-2}) because $d\Phi(E)/dE$ as presented in Figure 6-15 is the spectrum of electrons for a photon fluence of 1 cm^{-2} and thus already contains the dimensions of unit fluence. Note also that there are several times as many electrons with energy 1 MeV than are initially set into motion with that energy.

6.16   MEAN STOPPING POWERS

For dosimetry problems, to be discussed in Chapter 7, it would be convenient if one could characterize a given radiation by specifying that in the medium there were present electrons of only one energy with a *mean ionizational stopping power,* which we would refer to as $\bar{S}$. We wish to define and evaluate such an $\bar{S}$ for a number of conditions.

Monoenergetic Electrons Set in Motion in Medium

Imagine a 10 MeV electron set in motion in a water medium. From Table 6-3 we note that this electron will lose energy initially at the rate of 2.176 MeV/cm. As it slows down this rate of energy loss will increase and by the time its energy has decreased to 10 keV it will be losing energy at the rate of 22.6 MeV/cm. The mean stopping power will be some average value between these two extremes. To arrive at the average we note that the electron with initial energy E_i has a range R. In traveling the distance R, it loses $E_i B$ energy to bremsstrahlung and so deposits an energy $E_i(1 - B)$ in the medium. This is the energy deposited as ionization in distance R so the mean stopping power is:

$$\bar{S}(E_i) = \frac{E_i (1 - B)}{R} \tag{6-41}$$

This is a mean mass stopping power and R is given in g/cm². B and R are both functions of E_i and are given in Table A-6. Values for $\bar{S}$ are given in Table 6-3.

Example 6-15. Determine $\bar{S}$ for a 10 MeV electron set in motion in water.

From Table 6-3: B = .0404   and   R = 4.917 g/cm²

$$\bar{S} = \frac{10(1.0 - .0404)}{4.917} = \frac{9.596 \text{ MeV}}{4.917 \text{ g/cm}^2} = 1.952 \frac{\text{MeV cm}^2}{\text{g}}$$

This value appears in Table 6-3.

It is instructive to think of this problem also from the point of view of the electrons "seen" in the medium. This spectrum was represented by $d\Phi(E)/dE$ and was plotted in Figure 6-14. Clearly an average stopping power could also be defined by:

$$\bar{S}(E_i) = \frac{\displaystyle\int_0^{E_i} \frac{d\Phi(E)}{dE} \cdot S_{ion}(E) \cdot dE}{\displaystyle\int_0^{E_i} \frac{d\Phi(E)}{dE} \cdot dE} \tag{6-42}$$

Although this equation superficially looks very different from equation 6-41, the student may show that they are identical (see problem 32).

Mean Stopping Powers for Electrons with a Distribution of Initial Energies such as are Produced by Monoenergetic Photons

When a photon of energy $h\nu$ interacts with a medium we produce a distribution of electron energies $dN(E_i)/dE_i$ as discussed in section 6.14 and illustrated in Figure 6-13. As *each* of these electrons slows down, we observe a sequence of stopping powers whose mean value is given by $\bar{S}(E_i)$ of equation 6-42. The average stopping power for the whole spectrum, which we refer to as $\bar{\bar{S}}(h\nu)$, would be;

$$\bar{\bar{S}}(h\nu) = \frac{\displaystyle\int_0^{E_{max}} \frac{dN(E_i)}{dE_i} \cdot \bar{S}(E_i) \cdot R(E_i) \cdot dE_i}{\displaystyle\int_0^{E_{max}} \frac{dN(E_i)}{dE_i} \cdot R(E_i) \cdot dE_i} \tag{6-43}$$

where $R(E_i)$ is the range of an electron with initial energy E_i.

$\overline{\overline{S}}$ is a function of $dN(E_i)/dE_i$ and the medium in which the electrons are produced. Since $dN(E_i)/dE_i$ depends upon the energy of the photon, $\overline{\overline{S}}$ is really a function of $h\nu$ and the medium. It is given in Tables A-3 and A-4.

$\overline{\overline{S}}(h\nu)$ may also be derived from the electron fluence spectrum produced in the medium and illustrated in Figure 6-15. It is given by:

$$\overline{\overline{S}}(h\nu) = \frac{\int_0^{E_{max}} \dfrac{d\Phi(E)}{dE} \cdot S_{ion}(E) \cdot dE}{\int_0^{E_{max}} \dfrac{d\Phi(E)}{dE} \cdot dE} \qquad (6\text{-}44)$$

It is left as an exercise for the student to show that these two expressions for $\overline{\overline{S}}(h\nu)$ are identical.

It is essential to distinguish clearly between $\overline{S}$ and $\overline{\overline{S}}$. Table 6-3 shows that a 100 keV electron in water has a mean ionizational stopping power of 6.99 MeV cm²/g. Table A-3b shows that when *photons* of energy 100 keV interact with water, the mean stopping power of the electrons produced and slowed down in the water is $\overline{\overline{S}} = 18.3$ MeV cm²/g. This value is larger than the former because there are many low energy electrons set in motion by the photons.

Mean Stopping Powers for Electrons with a Distribution of Initial Energies such as are Produced by a Spectrum of Photon Energies

Inside an irradiated medium there will inevitably be a spectrum of photon energies. This will clearly be true if the incident beam consists of a photon spectrum (see Chapter 8). Even if the incident beam is monoenergetic, there will be a buildup of lower energy scattered photons within the medium itself. Let this photon spectrum be given by $d\Phi(h\nu)/dh\nu$. The average stopping power is then given by summing $\overline{\overline{S}}(h\nu)$ over all the components of the photon spectrum, thus:

$$\overline{\overline{\overline{S}}} = \frac{\int_0^{h\nu_{max}} \dfrac{d\Phi(h\nu)}{d\,h\nu} \cdot \overline{\overline{S}}(h\nu) \cdot d\,h\nu}{\int_0^{h\nu_{max}} \dfrac{d\Phi(h\nu)}{d\,h\nu} \, d\,h\nu} \qquad (6\text{-}45)$$

It is not easy to measure the photon spectrum at a point in a medium. Bruce and Johns have made Monte Carlo calculations of spectra for a wide range of photon spectra (B4), and measurements of photon spectra for cobalt x rays (B6). Comparisons between calculations and measurements were made by Bruce et al. (B7) for a very wide range of energies and Epp and Weiss (E2, E4) made measurements of photon spectra in a water phantom for diagnostic x rays.

If the electron fluence spectrum is known, the average stopping power, $\bar{\bar{S}}$, can be calculated from equation 6-45. In fact equation 6-45 is a general relation, because if the electron fluence spectrum can be determined it is not necessary to have a knowledge of the photon spectrum that produced it nor indeed even if it resulted from a photon beam at all. Equation 6-45 could also apply to electron beams.

In the last 3 sections we have discussed in depth the calculation of the distribution of electrons, $dN(E_i)/dE_i$, set in motion by monoenergetic photons. Using this energy distribution we have then calculated the spectrum of electrons, $d\Phi(E)/dE$, that cross unit area in the irradiated medium. Many of the ideas behind these calculations can be found in a series of earlier publications (B6, C3, C4, J8).

6.17   RESTRICTED STOPPING POWERS AND LINEAR ENERGY TRANSFER (LET)

In the last three sections we have been concerned with the way charged particles, and in particular electrons, lose energy as they are slowed down in a scattering medium. A parameter called stopping power (expressed in MeV cm²/g) was used to characterize the rate at which the electrons lose energy. Another parameter, closely related to the stopping power, is the linear energy transfer (LET) or "restricted" stopping power. This quantity is useful for some purposes in dosimetry (see Chapter 7), radiation biology, and radiotherapy. The focus of attention is now on the way the energy is actually deposited along the track in the medium. For example, it may be that an electron in slowing down suffers such a violent collision with another electron that this latter electron rebounds away with such energy that it forms a track of its own. These tracks are called "delta rays" (see also Fig. 7-1). The energy they carry away is included in the stopping power but is excluded from restricted stopping power or LET. Stopping powers for electrons are calculated using equation 6-26. Restricted stopping powers are calculated by using the following expression:

$$L_\Delta = 2\,\pi r_0^2\,N_e \frac{\mu_0}{\beta^2}\left[\ln \frac{2(E + 2\mu_0)(E - \Delta)\Delta}{\mu_0 I^2} + \frac{E}{E - \Delta} \right.$$

$$\left. + \frac{\Delta^2/2 + \mu_0(2E + \mu_0)\ln\left(\frac{E - \Delta}{E}\right)}{(E + \mu_0)^2} - 1 - \beta^2 - \delta \right] \quad (6\text{-}46)$$

where the symbols have the same meaning as for equation 6-26 except Δ. In the restricted stopping power, only energy exchanges less than Δ are to be counted. Restricted stopping powers for $\Delta = .0001$ to $\Delta = 0.1$, along with unrestricted stopping powers, are given in Table 6-4 for water for the energies given in Table 6-3.

TABLE 6-4
Ionizational Stopping Power, S_{ion}, and Restricted Stopping Power L_Δ for Electrons in Water in MeV/cm

(MeV)	S_{ion}	$L_{.0001}$	$L_{.001}$	$L_{.01}$	$L_{.1}$
.01	22.56	14.64	19.59		
.02	13.17	8.300	10.90	13.16	
.04	7.777	4.781	6.170	7.441	
.08	4.757	2.859	3.633	4.373	
.1	4.115	2.471	3.106	3.735	
.2	2.793	1.632	2.037	2.436	2.793
.4	2.148	1.231	1.517	1.801	2.068
.8	1.886	1.061	1.292	1.523	1.748
1	1.852	1.034	1.256	1.477	1.695
2	1.839	1.002	1.208	1.414	1.619
4	1.896	1.008	1.209	1.410	1.611
8	1.970	1.023	1.223	1.422	1.621
10	1.994	1.028	1.227	1.426	1.625
20	2.063	1.042	1.239	1.437	1.634
40	2.125	1.050	1.246	1.442	1.638
80	2.184	1.053	1.248	1.444	1.639
100	2.204	1.054	1.249	1.445	1.640

From the second column in Table 6-4 we note that a 2 MeV electron loses energy to ionization in water at the rate of 1.839 MeV/cm. If we consider only energy exchanges that are less than $\Delta = 0.0001$ MeV or 100 eV, the (restricted) stopping power is much lower—only 1.002 MeV/cm. As we include larger energy losses the restricted stopping power increases, and in the limit is equal to the (unrestricted) stopping power.

LET is usually expressed as keV per micrometer. There are 10^4 micrometers in 1 cm and so the LET (unrestricted) for 2 MeV electrons is $L_\infty = 0.184$ keV/μm. This is the minimum unrestricted LET since both higher and lower energy electrons (see Table 6-4 or Fig. 6-9) lose energy more rapidly. In any actual irradiation we will have electrons of many initial energies (see Figs. 6-5, 6-7) and each of these in turn will pass through all energies from its initial value down to zero as it slows down. We will thus have a spectrum of LET values. This will be discussed in Chapter 17.

Imagine a 20 MeV electron incident on a water phantom. We wish to determine the rate of energy deposition along this track as the electron slows down. If we assume all interactions are small ones, so the electron track is straight, then we can use the data of Table 6-4 to describe the LET pattern of the track. The result is shown as the curve ABCDEF of Figure 6-16. Since the initial LET of this particle is .206 keV/μm, this locates point A; since the range is 9.24 cm, this locates the end of the track point F where the rate of energy deposit falls to zero. As the electron loses energy the LET first falls slightly from A to B to reach a minimum at C (about 2 MeV), and then the rate of energy loss increases very rapidly as we near the end of the track. This large LET near the end of the track was first observed by Bragg and is called the Bragg peak. To understand how this curve was obtained consider the example.

Example 6-15. Show that when the electron's energy falls to 2 MeV, the electron will be at point C on the track and its LET will be .184 keV/μm.

From Table 6-3 we note that a 2 MeV electron has a range of 0.97 cm. Point C should therefore be 0.97 cm from the end of the track or at a depth of 9.24 − .97 = 8.27 cm. At this point the LET should be the value appropriate to 2 MeV or 0.184 keV/μm (see Table 6-4). C is correctly plotted.

Curve ABCDEF of Figure 6-16 is based on Table 6-4 or equation 6-26. It does *not,* however, take into account the multiple changes in direction that occur as the electron slows down. This completely smears out the Bragg peak so that it is *not observed for electrons.* The relative energy deposited as a function of depth for electrons is also discussed in Chapter 10 (see Fig. 6-10). *There is no increase in energy deposited near the end of the track and the Bragg peak for electrons is never observed.*

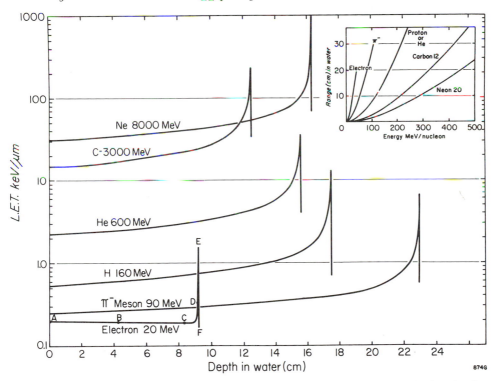

Figure 6-16. Bragg curves for charged particles slowing down in water, calculated using equation 6-26 for electrons and equation 6-25 for the other charged particles. Since the effect of change in direction during the slowing down process is not taken into account, the curve for electrons is quite inadequate but for the heavier particles is a reasonable approximation. The insert shows the range as a function of energy for the charged particles.

BRAGG CURVES FOR HEAVY PARTICLES: For heavy charged particles such as π mesons (mass 273 m_0), protons, and nuclei of helium, carbon, and neon the particles maintain their direction as they pass through water and so a well-defined range, a sharp Bragg peak, and an initial flat or plateau region are observed. These are shown in Figure 6-16 and were calculated using equation 6-25. The initial LET values increase from 0.185 to 31 keV/μm as the mass and energy of the particles is increased. For each particle the LET in the Bragg peak achieves a value of about 4 times the initial value for that particle.

A little thought will convince the reader that the area under any of these curves gives the energy of the particle. For example, the average LET for neon is about 50 keV/μm and the range is about 16 cm (see Fig. 6-16) so the area is:

$$50 \,\frac{\text{keV}}{\mu\text{m}} \times 16 \times 10^4 \,\mu\text{m} = 8 \times 10^6 \,\text{keV} = 8000 \,\text{MeV}$$

The insert of Figure 6-16 shows the range of these particles as a function of energy. It is left as an exercise for the student to prove that protons and helium of the same energy per nucleon should have the same range.

PROBLEMS

The difficult problems are marked with an asterisk.

1. Equation 6-2 defines the classical electron radius, r_0. Show that the expression is dimensionally correct, and that the radius $r_0 = 2.81777 \times 10^{-15}$ m.
2. Show that the classical scattering cross section per unit solid angle at 0° is $r_0^2 = 7.94 \times 10^{-30} \text{m}^2$.
3. Show that the solid angle subtended by the corner of a room is $\pi/2$ steradians.
4. Integrate equation 6-5 and show that the total Thomson classical cross section is given by equation 6-6.
5. Find the number of photons scattered between cones of angle 30° and 35° when a beam of 10^6 low energy photons impinges on a scattering medium containing 10^{23} electrons/cm². Assume classical scattering.
6. Repeat the calculations of problem 5 for a beam of 10 MeV photons.
7. Eliminate v and ϕ from equations 6-8a, 8c, and 8d and derive equations 6-9a, 9b, and 9c.
8. The 1 MeV curve of Figure 6-4 gives the differential cross section per unit solid angle as a function of θ. Multiply this curve by $2\pi \sin\theta \, d\theta$ to give $d\sigma/d\theta$ and plot this as a function of θ. Find the area under this curve graphically and thus obtain σ, the total cross section. Check your answer against Figure 5-7.
9. Multiply $d\sigma/d\theta$ obtained in problem 8 by E/hν of equation 6-9a. Plot this product as a function of θ, find the area under the curve and so determine σ_{tr}, and check your answer against Figure 5-7.
10. A detector of area 2.5 cm² is placed 30 cm from a block of scattering material containing 10^{23} electrons/cm². The block is bombarded by a beam of 10^6 photons with 1 MeV energy. The detector is placed along a line making an angle of 45° with the direction of the photon beam. Find the number of scattered photons that reach the detector (use Fig. 6-4).

11. A beam of 10^6 photons with energy 0.8 MeV bombards a block of scattering material containing 10^{23} electrons/cm^2. Find the number of electrons produced with energies in the range of 0.2 to 0.25 MeV (use Fig. 6-5).

12. Show that the area under one of the curves of Figure 6-5 is equal to the total coefficient plotted in Figure 5-7.

*13. Multiply equation 6-11 by $2\pi \sin \theta \, d\theta$ and integrate over all angles to give the value of σ of equation 6-12.

*14. Multiply equation 6-13a by $2\pi \sin \theta \, d\theta$ and integrate over all angles to give σ_{tr} of equation 6-13.

15. Show that equation 6-17 follows from 6-16 when α is small.

*16. Hubbell gives data for S(q,Z). Evaluate $d\sigma_c/d\theta$ of equation 6-18 for carbon at 20 keV and so obtain a curve similar to those of Figure 6-6. Obtain the area under this curve and so obtain σ_c according to equation 6-19. Compare with the value in the appendix.

*17. Using the atomic form factor F(q,Z) of Hubbell, evaluate $d\sigma_{coh}/d\theta$ of equation 6-17 for carbon at 20 keV. Find the area under this curve and check with the value for σ_{coh} given in the appendix.

*18. Using the data obtained in problem 17, find the angle that includes half the coherent scattered radiation. Compare with the value obtained by Hubbell (see NSRDS-NBS #29, 1969).

19. From Figure 6-7 determine the number of positrons set in motion with energies between 2.0 and 2.5 MeV when a beam of 10^6 photons of energy 20 MeV impinges on a foil of lead of thickness 0.10 g/cm^2.

20. A slab of carbon 2 cm thick (density 2.25 g/cm^3) is bombarded by 10^6 photons, each with an energy of 20 MeV. Use data from Table A-4b to determine the following: number Compton interactions, energy converted to K.E. by Compton interaction, energy scattered by Compton process; number of pair and triplet processes, energy radiated as bremsstrahlung; total energy diverted from beam, total energy converted to K.E., total energy radiated. Make an energy balance. Calculate the energy absorbed using μ_{ab}/ρ. Compare with total energy converted to K.E.

21. A slab of carbon 0.1 g/cm^2 is bombarded by 10^6 photons, each with an energy of 10 keV. Use the data of Table A-4b to calculate the number of Compton collisions, the number of coherent scattering events, and the number of photoelectric processes. Determine the energy converted into K.E. by each process and the energy scattered by each process. Make an energy balance. Calculate the energy absorbed using μ_{ab}/ρ and compare with the energy converted to K.E.

22. In the case history of Table 6-1, involving 76 photons of energy 61 keV at interaction point L, show that on the average 71 Compton electrons with mean energy 6 keV and 5 photoelectrons with 61 keV energy are produced. Show also that the average distance to the next interaction is 4.7 cm.

23. Using the principle of conservation of energy and momentum, show that a photoelectric process cannot take place with a free electron.

*24. Using the principles of conservation of energy and momentum, show that triplet production cannot occur below $4m_0c^2$ (2.04 MeV).

25. Show that the angles ϕ and θ in the Compton process are related by $\cot \phi = -(1 + \alpha) \tan \theta/2$.

*26. A beam of photons of energy 1 MeV and energy fluence 1.00 J/m^2 is allowed to impinge on an aluminum foil 0.5 cm^2 in area and 10 mg/cm^2 thick. Calculate:
   a. The total number of recoil electrons that will emerge from the plate. Assume no self-absorption.
   b. The number of photons scattered through an area 4 cm^2 at a distance of 10 cm in

a direction making 90° with the incident radiation.

c. The energy fluence scattered through the area in b.

d. Suppose a gamma counter were placed as in b. Where would you place a beta counter to observe coincidences? What angular width in the plane of scattering should this counter have? Assume all "particles" originate at a "point" in the aluminum.

e. A counter that is sensitive only to β particles with a circular window of effective radius 1 cm is placed 40 cm from the aluminum foil, making an angle of 30° with the photon beam. Calculate the number of betas counted, assuming 100% efficiency. What energy β particles will be received?

27. Evaluate S_{ion} for electrons in water for E = 400 keV using only the first term inside the square brackets of equation 6-26 and compare with the value in Table 6-3. Determine the important terms in the equation for electrons with energies less than 0.5 MeV.

28. A beam of 1 MeV photons with a fluence of 10^4 photons per cm² interacts with 1 mm layer of water. Use Figure 6-5 to determine the spectrum of electrons set in motion. Now use equation 6-40 to obtain the spectrum of electrons seen at any point in the water. Plot the number per cm² as a function of energy and the number per LET interval.

29. Show that equations 6-43 and 6-44 lead to the same value for $\bar{\bar{S}}$.

30. Perform the numerical integration discussed in section 6.13 leading to the range of a 2 MeV electron in water, and show the range is 0.96 cm.

31. Derive equation 6.29.

32. Show that $\bar{\bar{S}}$ as given by equation 6-41 is the same as equation 6-42.

33. Find the area under the LET curve for carbon given in Figure 6-16 and show that it is equal to the energy of the particle.

34. Show why protons and helium nuclei of the same energy per nucleon will have the same range.

*35. The differential cross section, $d\sigma(E)/d(E)$, gives the number of Compton collisions that lead to electrons with energies in the range E to E + dE. This cross section is related to $d\sigma/d\theta$ by the relation $d\sigma(E)/dE = (d\sigma/d\theta)(d\theta/dE)$. By manipulation of the basic Compton expressions show that

$$\frac{d\sigma(E)}{dE} = \frac{3}{8}\,\sigma_0 \cdot \frac{1}{\alpha h\nu}\left\{1 + \cos^2\theta + \frac{\alpha^2\,(1 - \cos\theta)^2}{1 + \alpha(1 - \cos\theta)}\right\} \tag{a}$$

Now, using the relation between E and θ (eq. 6-9a)

$$E = \frac{h\nu\alpha(1 - \cos\theta)}{1 + \alpha(1 - \cos\theta)} \tag{b}$$

eliminate the angle of scattering θ from (a) and (b) and so obtain the differential cross section, $d\sigma(E)/dE$, in terms of the energy of the electron, E. This substitution should give

$$\frac{d\sigma(E)}{dE} = \frac{3}{8}\frac{\sigma_0}{\alpha h\nu}\left\{2 - \frac{2E}{\alpha(h\nu - E)} + \frac{E^2}{\alpha^2(h\nu - E)^2} + \frac{E^2}{h\nu(h\nu - E)}\right\} \tag{c}$$

This expression was plotted in Figure 6-5. By substituting a few values such as E = 0 and E = E_{max} = hν · 2α/(1 + 2α), check that expression (c) actually is represented by the curves of Figure 6-5.

Chapter 7

MEASUREMENT OF RADIATION: DOSIMETRY

There are two distinctly different considerations in dosimetry: to describe a radiation beam itself and to describe the amount of energy it may deposit in some medium. Both of these topics will be discussed in this chapter. A number of quantities and some units will be defined first and then discussed in detail later.

7.01 QUANTITIES TO DESCRIBE A RADIATION BEAM

FLUENCE: Radiation from an x ray generator or a radioactive source consists of a beam of photons, usually with a variety of energies. If we consider that the beam is monoenergetic, then one way to describe the beam would be to specify the number of these photons, dN, that would cross an area, da, taken at right angles to the beam. The ratio of these would yield what the International Commission on Radiological Units and Measurements (ICRU) (I2) has called fluence, or photon fluence, represented by the capital Greek letter phi, Φ:

$$\text{Fluence or photon fluence; } \Phi = \frac{dN}{da} \left[\frac{\text{number photon}}{\text{area}} \right] \quad (7\text{-}1)$$

ENERGY FLUENCE: An alternative and equally good way to describe a beam would be in terms of the energy flow in it. The amount of energy crossing unit area is called the energy fluence and is represented by the capital Greek letter psi, Ψ:

$$\text{Energy fluence; } \Psi = \frac{dN \cdot h\nu}{da} \left[\frac{\text{energy}}{\text{area}} \right] \quad (7\text{-}2)$$

FLUENCE RATE: At times one may be interested in the number of photons that pass through unit area per unit time. This is called the fluence rate and is represented by the lower case Greek letter phi, ϕ, thus:

$$\text{Fluence rate; } \phi = \frac{d\Phi}{dt} \left[\frac{\text{number photon}}{\text{time} \times \text{area}} \right] \quad (7\text{-}3)$$

ENERGY FLUENCE RATE: The energy carried across unit area per unit time is called the energy fluence rate, or energy flux density or intensity. It is represented by the lower case Greek letter psi thus:

$$\text{Energy fluence rate; } \psi = \frac{d\Psi}{dt} \left[\frac{\text{energy}}{\text{time} \times \text{area}} \right] \quad (7\text{-}4)$$

217

Although these concepts are simple, the actual representation of a radiation beam by any one of them is difficult, because beams almost always contain photons of many different energies. To describe a real beam using these quantities one would need to know the *number* and *energy* of all of the photons in the beam and this information is very difficult to obtain. A distribution giving the number of photons that have given energies is called a spectrum (see Chapters 6 and 8).

EXPOSURE: A beam may be described in terms of exposure measured in roentgens. It is a measure of radiation in terms of its ability to ionize air; it will be discussed in detail in section 7.07.

ABSORBED DOSE: This is a measure of the energy absorbed from a radiation beam per unit mass of material. It will be discussed in the next section.

7.02   ENERGY TRANSFER—A TWO STAGE PROCESS—KERMA AND ABSORBED DOSE

KERMA: In Chapters 5 and 6 it was shown that the transfer of energy from a photon beam to the medium takes place in two stages. The first stage (a) involves the interaction of the photon with an atom, causing an electron or electrons to be set in motion. The second stage (b) involves the transfer of energy from the high energy electron to the medium through excitation and ionization. These are illustrated in Figure 7-1.

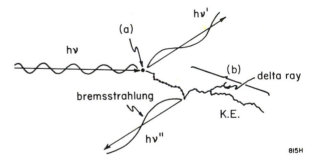

Figure 7-1. Schematic representation of the transfer of energy from a photon (hν) to the medium. The photon interacts at a, transferring some of its energy to an electron giving it K.E. This electron in turn gives up its energy mostly in small collisions along its track b. The transfer of energy at a is called kerma, and along b is called absorbed dose. The photon hν' is scattered from a. The photon hν'' is bremsstrahlung resulting from a collision between the electron and a nucleus. The delta ray is another electron track resulting from a relatively violent electron-electron collision. The absorbed dose equals the kerma less the energy carried away by bremsstrahlung. Kerma occurs at a point, while absorbed dose occurs farther downstream over a range equal to the range of the electron.

A quantity called kerma has been introduced by the ICRU (I2) to describe the initial interaction. Kerma stands for *K*inetic *E*nergy *R*eleased in the *M*edium (the "a" has been added only for phonetic reasons).

$$\text{Kerma; } K = \frac{d\overline{E}_{tr}}{dm} \left[\frac{\text{energy}}{\text{mass}} \right] \qquad (7\text{-}5)$$

where $\overline{dE}_{tr}$ is the kinetic energy transferred from photons to electrons in a volume element whose mass is dm. It is the quantity that most directly connects the description of the radiation beam with its effects. For example, if we have a beam of photons with energy hν and photon fluence Φ, then the kerma is given by:

$$K = \Phi \cdot \left(\frac{\mu}{\rho}\right) \cdot \overline{E}_{tr} \qquad (7\text{-}6)$$

where (μ/ρ) is the mass attenuation coefficient for the medium and $\overline{E}_{tr}$ is the average amount of energy transferred to electrons of the medium at each interaction. The product $\Phi(\mu/\rho)$ gives the number of photon interactions that take place per unit mass of material irradiated by a photon fluence Φ and $\overline{E}_{tr}$ is the average energy that is transferred to electrons by these interactions. The units of kerma are joules per kilogram, the same as those of absorbed dose, but there is no special unit (like the gray) for kerma.

In any actual irradiated medium, there will of course be a spectrum of photon energies. If this spectrum is described by dΦ(hν)/d hν, the kerma will be given by:

$$K = \int_0^{h\nu_{max}} \frac{d\Phi(h\nu)}{d\,h\nu} \cdot \left(\frac{\mu(h\nu)}{\rho}\right) \cdot \overline{E}_{tr}(h\nu) \cdot d\,h\nu \qquad (7\text{-}6a)$$

which is the sum of the kermas from all of the photons in the spectrum.

Example 7-1: Suppose a beam of 10.0 MeV photons with fluence of $10^{14}/m^2$ is incident on a small block of carbon. Calculate the kerma.

(Table A-4b) $\qquad\qquad \left(\dfrac{\mu}{\rho}\right) = 0.00196$ m²/kg

Average energy trans- $\qquad \overline{E}_{tr} = 7.30$ MeV
ferred (Table A-4b)

$$\begin{aligned}\text{Kerma} \\ \text{(eq. 7-6)}\end{aligned} = K = \frac{10^{14}}{m^2} \times .00196\,\frac{m^2}{kg} \times 7.30\text{ MeV} = 1.43 \times 10^{12}\,\frac{\text{MeV}}{kg}$$

$$= 1.43 \times 10^{12}\,\frac{\text{MeV}}{kg} \times 1.602 \times 10^{-13}\,\frac{J}{\text{MeV}} = 0.229\text{ J/kg}$$

Kerma is a useful concept for clarifying the principles of radiation dosimetry. It is easy to calculate, but difficult to measure.

ABSORBED DOSE: The quantity that is of more interest in radiotherapy and radiobiology is absorbed dose. The difference between kerma and absorbed dose can be seen by referring to Figure 7-1. Energy is transferred to an electron at (a) but not all of it is retained in the medium; some of it is radiated away as bremsstrahlung. The absorbed dose is the energy actually retained in the medium and it will be brought about by the ionizations and excitations that take place all along the track indicated by (b). Because the length of the electron tracks may be appreciable, *kerma and absorbed dose do not take place at the same location.* The ICRU (I2) has defined the quantity called absorbed dose to be:

$$\text{Absorbed dose; } D = \frac{d\overline{E}_{ab}}{dm} \left[\frac{\text{energy}}{\text{mass}} \right] \qquad (7\text{-}7)$$

$d\overline{E}$ is the mean energy imparted by the ionizing radiation to a mass, dm, of matter. The increment of mass, dm, should be considered small enough so that absorbed dose is defined at a point. It must not be so small, however, that statistical fluctuations in the energy deposition are significant.

A special unit called the *rad* was introduced for this quantity in 1953 and more recently, in keeping with SI conventions, a new special unit called the *gray* (Gy) has been defined:

$$1 \text{ rad} = 100 \text{ erg/g}$$
$$1 \text{ Gy (gray)} = 1 \text{ J/kg} = 10^7 \text{ erg/}10^3 \text{ g} = 100 \text{ rad} \qquad (7\text{-}7a)$$

In time the rad will cease to be used and will be replaced by the gray. In this chapter we will use both rads and grays with an emphasis on the latter.

The meanings of kerma and absorbed dose may be further clarified by following the history of a (typical) photon of an energy of, say, 10 MeV as it interacts with the carbon of example 7-1. The average energy transferred to such an electron would be 7.30 MeV ($\overline{E}_{tr}$ of Table A-4b). Of this, 7.06 MeV ($\overline{E}_{ab}$ of Table A-4b) will be absorbed along the electron track and the difference, 0.24 MeV, will leave the track as bremsstrahlung. The length of the track of the 7.30 MeV electron will be about 4.2 gm/cm^2 or about 1.9 cm (Table A-6). In traveling along this track the electron will cause some 2×10^5 ionizations.* The energy imparted to the medium in bringing about these ionizations is the important quantity and is the absorbed dose.

One atom of the irradiated material was ionized at the site of the photon interaction but 2×10^5 atoms were disrupted along the electron track.

7.03   **ELECTRONIC EQUILIBRIUM**

In the previous section it was noted that the transfer of energy (kerma) from the photon does not take place at the same location as the absorption of the energy by the medium (absorbed dose). This has very severe

---

*Since on the average 33.85 eV is required to produce an ion pair, a 7.3 MeV electron on dissipating its energy will produce $7.3 \times 10^6/33.85 \approx 200,000$ ions. Although this calculation applies strictly to air, the number for carbon would be similar.

implications for the calculation of absorbed dose. Kerma can be related to fluence very simply by equation 7-6. Absorbed dose on the other hand cannot be calculated in this simple way unless a state of equilibrium exists between the two quantities. The following section illustrates the reason for this.

Figure 7-2 shows, very schematically, the electrons that are set in motion when a clean (electron free) beam of high energy photons bombards a medium. For purposes of illustration, the electrons are shown in motion at a slight angle to the direction of the beam and all the electron tracks are shown traveling (in this same direction) a distance equal to the range R. Two cases will now be presented.

No Attenuation of the Photon Beam

In Figure 7-2a we have assumed that in the distance R there is no attenuation of the photons and the same number of electron tracks (100) are set in motion in each square from A to G. If we now examine square D, we see that it is traversed by 400 tracks, 100 of which started in each of A, B, C, and D. Thus, if one measures the ionization in D, it will be the same as the *total* ionization produced by the track that started in A. The absorbed dose is proportional to the ionization produced in each of the squares, and it is readily seen that this will start at zero and reach its maximum value at depth R. The portion of the medium from the surface to depth R is called the buildup region, and the portion beyond it is loosely called the region of electronic equilibrium where as many electrons stop in any volume as are set in motion in it. The kerma is constant with depth, as shown by the dotted horizontal line in Figure 7-2a. If we also assume that no bremsstrahlung losses occur, the absorbed dose is equal to the kerma beyond the buildup region.

Attenuation of the Photon Beam

In Figure 7-2b is shown a condition in which electronic equilibrium is not attained. Here it has been assumed that the primary radiation is attenuated exponentially with a reduction of 5% in a distance equal to the distance between A and B, B and C, etc., so that the numbers of electrons set in motion in successive squares are 100, 95, 90, 86, 82, 78 respectively. The ionization in square D is composed of 100 tracks of electrons that started in A, 95 from B, etc. Now, the ionization in D is less than the full ionization produced by all the tracks starting in A. The kerma will decrease continually but the absorbed dose will first increase, as it did above, then decrease. Well beyond this "equilibrium thickness" the absorbed dose and kerma both decrease exponentially, but the absorbed dose curve is always above the kerma curve if we neglect bremsstrahlung losses. The student may see that this is the case since the absorbed dose

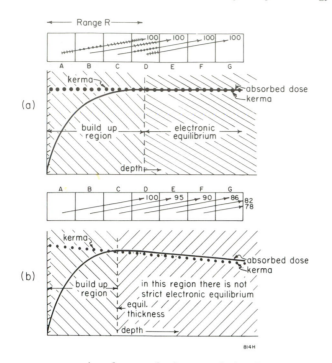

Figure 7-2. (a) Graph showing schematically why the absorbed dose increases with depth and how electronic equilibrium is achieved when there is no attenuation of the primary. (b) Situation similar to that of a when attenuation of the primary occurs. Now electronic equilibrium is not produced even at depths beyond the equilibrium thickness. Kerma and dose have the same units and so the curves can be plotted on the same graph.

at any point beyond the peak is due to the kerma further upstream. Although a peak does occur in the dose curve, which is sometimes called the point of equilibrium, true electronic equilibrium is never established, for at no place in the medium are as many electrons set in motion as are brought to rest in it.

The diagrams of Figure 7-2 are schematic and greatly oversimplified, for as we saw in Chapter 6, a spectrum of electrons of *all* energies from zero to a maximum value is always set in motion; furthermore, these are projected in many different directions. To illustrate these ideas consider Table 7-1. Column 2 shows the maximum energy transferred (calculated from eq. 6-9a) to electrons in water by photons that had energies given in the first column. The third column gives the range of these electrons in water expressed in g/cm² (taken from Table A-6). This range increases continually with increase in energy. The fourth column gives the attenuation coefficient in water expressed in cm²/g. This falls rapidly in the region 0.1 to 1.0 MeV and then falls more slowly and finally becomes nearly constant above 10 MeV. The fifth column gives the percent attenuation of the photons in a distance equal to the electron range of column 3. For even approximate electronic equilibrium to exist, the percent attenuation of the photons in the range R should be very small. This is certainly the case from 0.1 to 0.5 MeV, but at higher energies this attenuation becomes increasingly large and even at 3.0 MeV it exceeds 5%.

We have discussed a very simple special case of the attainment of electronic equilibrium, starting with a "clean" photon beam that included no electrons and produced monoenergetic electrons all in the forward direction. Real situations are never this simple. For example, at a bone–soft tissue interface, electrons set in motion in one material produce part of their tracks in the other. This transition region extends over a distance determined by the range of the electrons in each of the materials. Kerma and absorbed dose are not in equilibrium with each other and the calculation of dose becomes very difficult. This case will be dealt with in section 7.13.

TABLE 7-1
Attenuation of Photons in Distance Equal to Range of Electrons in Water

(1)	(2)	(3)	(4)	(5)	(6)
Photon Energy MeV	Max. Electron Energy MeV	Range R, in Water of Electrons with Energies given in Column 2 g/cm²	Total Attenuation Coeff. in Water cm²/g	Percent Attenuation in Range R	Range in Air of Electrons with Energies given in Column 2 (cm)
0.1	0.1	.014	.1706	.24	13
0.2	0.2	.045	.1370	.62	42
0.5	0.4	.128	.0969	1.2	120
1.0	0.8	.329	.0707	2.3	308
2	1.8	.865	.0494	4.3	970
3	2.8	1.40	.0397	5.7	1500
5	4.76	2.40	.0303	7.3	
10	9.8	4.82	.0222	11.	
20	19.7	9.10	.0182	18.	
50	49.7	19.6	.0167	39.	
100	99.7	32.5	.0172	75.	

In section 7.02 an equation (7-6) was given that allows one to calculate kerma if the photon fluence at a point is known. There is no equation for dose that corresponds to this unless there is an equilibrium between kerma and absorbed dose. In the special case that there is such an equilibrium, absorbed dose is given by:

$$D = \Phi \left(\frac{\mu}{\rho}\right) \overline{E}_{ab} = K (1 - g) \qquad (7\text{-}8)$$

where $\overline{E}_{ab}$ is the part of the average kinetic energy transferred to electrons that contributes to ionization (it excludes energy lost by bremsstrahlung), g is the fraction of the energy that is lost to bremsstrahlung (see section 6-13), and K is the kerma of equation 7-6. The dose calculated from this expression is sometimes called "collision kerma" (A2).

The most common relation between kerma and absorbed dose is that depicted in Figure 7-2b where the kerma and dose curves are parallel to each other but the curve for absorbed dose is slightly above the curve for kerma. In this case the absorbed dose differs from the kerma by a factor, b, slightly greater than 1.00. In practice, b is usually assumed to be 1.0. It is discussed by Roesch (R3).

$$D = \Phi \left(\frac{\mu}{\rho}\right) \overline{E}_{ab}\, b \qquad\qquad (7\text{-}8a)$$

7.04   THE BRAGG-GRAY CAVITY

The only direct method of measuring absorbed dose is by calorimetry (Chapter 9) in which the rise in temperature of an isolated mass of the medium is measured. Although the method has been extensively developed by various users of radiation, unfortunately, it has not yet been fully adopted by standardization laboratories. As a result, most absorbed dose measurements made today are based on a measurement of ionization followed by calculations involving a number of troublesome correction factors. These factors are derived from Bragg-Gray Cavity theory.

Figure 7-3 shows a medium traversed by a beam of photons, which produce electron tracks as shown in the diagram. Suppose now a small gas-filled cavity is placed in the medium (for purposes of illustration this cavity is shown rather large). Ionizations will be produced in the gas in

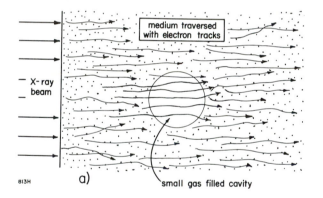

Figure 7-3. A Bragg-Gray cavity in a medium traversed by electron tracks.

the cavity by the electrons (whose tracks are shown in Fig. 7-3), which eject other electrons from atoms and molecules of the gas, giving rise to absorbed energy in the gas. It is possible, by electrical means, to collect and measure the charge thus liberated in the gas. It turns out also that the average energy required to cause one ionization in the gas is constant over widely varying conditions of gas pressure and electron energies (I3). It is represented by W and for air has the value:

$$W = 33.85 \frac{eV}{\text{ion pair}} = 33.85 \frac{\text{joule}}{\text{coulomb}} \text{ *(for air)}$$

The dose absorbed in the gas can therefore be related to the ionization

---

*The student may show that W has numerically the same value in eV/ion pair or joules/coulomb.

produced in the gas by the equation:

$$D_{gas} = \frac{Q}{m_{gas}} W \qquad (7-9)$$

If Q is expressed in coulombs and m_{gas} in kg, then the absorbed dose is in joules/kg or grays. The mass of gas in the cavity can be determined from the volume of the cavity and the density of the gas. The most commonly used gas is air, whose density is:

$$\rho_{air} = 1.293 \text{ kg/m}^3 \text{ at STP } (0° \text{ C, } 101.3 \text{ kPa})†$$

Example 7-2. A cavity with 1 cm³ volume, filled with air at STP, is exposed to a radiation field that liberates 3.336×10^{-10} C in a given time. Determine the dose to the air.

$$m_{gas} = 1 \times 10^{-6} \text{ m}^3 \times 1.293 \text{ kg/m}^3 = 1.293 \times 10^{-6} \text{ kg}$$

$$D_{air} \text{ (eq. 7-8)} = \frac{3.336 \times 10^{-10} \text{ C}}{1.293 \times 10^{-6} \text{ kg}} \times 33.85 \frac{J}{C} = 0.873 \times 10^{-2} \frac{J}{kg}$$

$$= .873 \times 10^{-2} \text{ Gy}$$

In this example the numerical value chosen for Q is the charge that would be liberated by an exposure of 1 roentgen, to be discussed later.

Equation 7-9 gives the energy imparted to the gas, but we require the net energy imparted to unit mass of the wall surrounding the gas and exposed to the same electron fluence. In section 6-15 we showed how the electron fluence spectrum could be determined at a point in a medium for a given spectrum of photon energies. Since the air cavity is assumed to be so small that it does not affect the electron spectrum, the gas in the cavity will "see" the same electron fluence as does the wall. It follows then that:

$$\frac{D_{wall}}{D_{gas}} = \frac{\int_{E_{min}}^{E_{max}} \left(\frac{d\Phi(E)}{dE}\right)_{wall} S_{ion} (E)^{wall} dE}{\int_{E_{min}}^{E_{max}} \left(\frac{d\Phi(E)}{dE}\right)_{wall} S_{ion} (E)^{gas} dE} = \bar{\bar{S}}_{gas}^{wall} \qquad (7-10)$$

The ratio of these two integrals will be referred to by the symbol $\bar{\bar{S}}_{gas}^{wall}$, the superscript and subscript signifying that a ratio is being calculated and the two bars signifying that it is averaged over both the photon spectrum and the spectrum of electrons in the medium. The ratio of these two integrals is frequently called the "average stopping power ratio" although more correctly it is a ratio of averaged stopping powers. It is a rather special ratio because *both* integrals involve the electron fluence

---

†The pascal (Pa) is the fundamental unit of pressure and is expressed in newton/m². The student may show that a column of mercury 760 mm high (i.e. 1 atmosphere) produces a pressure of 101.3 kPa.

spectrum *in the wall*. E_{max} is the maximum electron energy and E_{min} is the energy of an electron which can just cross the cavity. In our calculations we have chosen E_{min} to be 1 keV.

Typical values for $\bar{\bar{S}}$ relative to *air* for wall materials of carbon, Bakelite,® Lucite,® polystyrene, and water are listed in Table 7-2 for the spectrum of electrons set in motion by spectra of photons produced by x ray machines, two isotopes, and by linacs or betatrons. Calculations are included for different filtrations of some beams and illustrate that the stopping power ratio is not very sensitive to the assumed photon spectrum. For example, spectrum 8 is for primary cobalt radiation, while spectrum 9 is for primary plus scattered radiation for a large field in a phantom and the stopping power ratios are within 0.3%. Two spectra for 26 MV photon beams, one for a betatron and the other for a linear accelerator, give data within about 0.8% of each other although the photon spectra are quite different. The values in Table 7-2 are in very close agreement with similar data obtained for $\bar{\bar{S}}_{air}^{water}$ by Nahum (N3).

TABLE 7-2

Ratio of averaged stopping powers, $\bar{\bar{S}}_{air}^{med}$ for a number of materials relative to air for a series of photon spectra. Data was calculated using equation 7-10. For comparison, $\bar{\bar{S}}$ water/$\bar{\bar{S}}$ air, determined using equation 6-45, is entered in the last column.

Spectrum Number*	Description	$\bar{\bar{S}}_{air}^{med}$ for Various Media					$\dfrac{\bar{\bar{S}}_{water}}{\bar{\bar{S}}_{air}}$
		Carbon	Bakelite	Lucite	Poly-styrene	Water	
1	60 kV$_p$, HVL—1.6 mm Al	1.022	1.094	1.125	1.137	1.140	1.141
2	100 kV$_p$, HVL—2.8 mm Al	1.022	1.095	1.126	1.138	1.140	1.141
3	250 kV$_p$, HVL—2.6 mm Cu	1.021	1.090	1.121	1.132	1.139	1.139
4	270 kV$_p$ primary only, 2.7 mm Cu	1.020	1.089	1.120	1.131	1.138	1.138
5	270 kV$_p$ primary plus scatter	1.022	1.094	1.124	1.136	1.139	1.137
6	400 kV$_p$, HVL—4 mm Cu	1.019	1.086	1.116	1.127	1.138	1.137
7	Cs-137	1.015	1.075	1.104	1.112	1.133	1.132
8	Co-60, primary only	1.009	1.071	1.099	1.105	1.129	1.128
9	Co-60, primary plus scatter	1.011	1.073	1.101	1.109	1.131	1.129
10	6 MV, Linac	1.000	1.064	1.092	1.098	1.123	1.120
11	8 MV, Linac	.993	1.058	1.085	1.091	1.117	1.114
12	12 MV, Schiff spect.	.976	1.043	1.069	1.073	1.102	1.100
13	18 MV, Schiff spect.	.965	1.033	1.059	1.063	1.092	1.091
14	26 MV, Betatron	.960	1.028	1.053	1.057	1.086	1.083
15	26 MV, Linac	.968	1.035	1.061	1.065	1.094	1.092
16	35 MV, Schiff spect.	.946	1.015	1.039	1.043	1.073	1.073
17	45 MV, Schiff spect.	.940	1.009	1.034	1.037	1.068	1.068

*Spectra 1 and 2 are taken from Yaffe (Y1); 3 and 6 are from Johns, appendix B, (J9); 4 and 5 are taken from Skarsgard, Table 8-1 (S8); 7 is monoenergetic radiation at 0.662 MeV; 8 has two energies at 1.17 and 1.33 MeV; 9 is taken from Bruce, Fig. 13x (B4); 10 is from Bentley et al., Fig. 3, calculated thick target (B8); 11 is taken from Levy et al., Fig. 5 (L3); 12 and 13 are calculated thin target spectra filtered by 2 cm tungsten and 2 cm water; 14 is from Sherman et al. representing an Allis Chalmers betatron (S9); 15 is from Levy et al., Fig. 6, experimental spectrum for Saggittaire (L4); 16 and 17 are calculated thin target spectra plus 2.2 cm tungsten and 10 cm of water representing high energy betatrons.

Equation 7-10 is not quite correct for the calculation of average stopping powers because it does not take into account the fact that in many collisions a fast moving electron (the δ-rays of Fig. 7-1) is produced. These "secondary" electrons should be added to the "primary" electron spectrum, $d\Phi(E)/dE$, increasing the number of low energy electrons. At the same time, as pointed out by Spencer and Attix (S7), the restricted stopping power (LET) should be used (see also sec. 6.17) and the integration should extend from some low energy limit, Δ, to E_{max} instead of from E_{min}. There is some arbitrariness in the choice of a value for Δ, but it is generally associated with the size of the cavity in the ionization chamber and taken to be the energy possessed by an electron that can just cross the cavity. For practical dosimeters this is about 10 keV. Fortunately, the ratio of the average stopping powers is not very sensitive to the choice of Δ. Nahum (N3, N4) has determined the ratio of averaged restricted stopping powers, $\bar{\bar{L}}_{air}^{water}$, using Monte Carlo techniques, for a selection of photon spectra similar to some of those presented in Table 7-2. His results are presented in Table 7-3 where they are compared with the corresponding Bragg-Gray stopping powers from Table 7-2. The ratios of restricted stopping powers tend to be somewhat higher than the Bragg-Gray stopping powers for water but differ by not more than 0.5%. This difference would be greater and in the opposite direction for materials of higher atomic number.

TABLE 7-3

Ratios of Averaged Restricted Stopping Powers for Water to Air, $\bar{\bar{L}}_{air}^{water}$

$\bar{\bar{L}}_{air}^{water}$ calculated by Nahum (N4) is compared to $\bar{S}_{air}^{water}$ calculated using equation 7-10 and given in Table 7-2.

Photon Spectrum*	$\bar{S}_{air}^{water}$ (eq. 7-10)	$\bar{\bar{L}}_{air}^{water}$ (Nahum) $\Delta = 10$ keV	% Diff.
8 ^{60}Co	1.130		
9 ^{60}Co plus scatter	1.131	1.135	+.4
10 6 MV	1.123	1.129	+.5
12 12 MV	1.102	1.109†	+.6
13 18 MV	1.092	1.101†	+.8
14 26 MV, betatron	1.087	1.092	+.4
15 26 MV, linac	1.094	1.099	+.5
16 35 MV	1.073	1.076†	+.3

*Spectrum 8 has two energies at 1.17 and 1.33 MeV; 9 is taken from Bruce, Fig. 13x (B4); 10 is from Bentley et al., Fig. 3, calculated thick target (B8); 12 and 13 are calculated thin target spectra filtered by 2 cm tungsten and 2 cm water; 14 is from Sherman et al. representing an Allis Chalmers betatron (S9); 15 is from Levy et al., Fig. 6, experimental spectrum for Saggittaire (L4); 16 is a calculated thin target spectrum plus 2.2 cm tungsten and 10 cm of water representing high energy betatron.

†Interpolated or extrapolated from Nahum's data

In view of the fact that these results are so close to each other and that stopping powers are not known to better than 2%, we will use the Bragg-Gray stopping power ratios (eq. 7-10) for calculations in this book.

In Table 7-2 we also show the ratio of $\bar{\bar{S}}_{\text{water}}/\bar{\bar{S}}_{\text{air}}$, i.e. the ratio of the mean stopping powers calculated using equation 6-45. It is seen that this ratio is nearly the same as $\bar{\bar{S}}_{\text{air}}^{\text{water}}$ showing that it does not matter much whether one uses precisely the same spectrum (that pertaining to the medium) for both the numerator and the denominator of this expression. Using the tabulated values for $\bar{\bar{S}}_{\text{air}}^{\text{wall}}$ we can now calculate the dose to the wall material surrounding our air cavity. Combining equations 7-9 and 7-10 we obtain:

$$D_{\text{wall}} = \frac{Q}{m_{\text{gas}}} W \cdot \bar{\bar{S}}_{\text{gas}}^{\text{wall}} \quad \text{or} \quad D_{\text{wall}} = \frac{Q}{m_{\text{gas}}} W \cdot \bar{\bar{L}}_{\text{gas}}^{\text{wall}} \quad (7\text{-}11)$$

which is the important Bragg-Gray formula that relates the ionization in a cavity to the absorbed dose in the wall surrounding the cavity.

Example 7-3. A 1 cm³ air cavity in a block of carbon is exposed to Co-60 gamma rays and a charge of 3×10^{-8} C is produced and collected from the cavity. Find the absorbed dose to the carbon, assuming the air is at STP.

$$m_{\text{gas}} = 10^{-6} \text{ m}^3 \times 1.293 \frac{\text{kg}}{\text{m}^3} = 1.293 \times 10^{-6} \text{ kg}$$

$$\bar{\bar{S}}_{\text{air}}^{\text{carbon}} = 1.009; \text{ see Table 7-2 for Co-60 (spectrum no. 8)}$$

$$D_{\text{carbon}} \text{ (eq. 7-11)} = \frac{3 \times 10^{-8} \text{ C}}{1.293 \times 10^{-6} \text{ kg}} \times 33.85 \frac{\text{J}}{\text{C}} \times 1.009$$

$$= 0.792 \frac{\text{J}}{\text{kg}} = 0.792 \text{ Gy} = 79.2 \text{ rad}$$

The simple relation of equation 7-11 thus allows us to calculate the dose to the medium from a measurement of the ionization produced in an air-filled cavity within the medium. Unfortunately, the medium in which we are usually interested is water and this does not make a very satisfactory wall for an ion chamber! One is, therefore, forced to place a practical ion chamber with its wall in the water phantom and from the reading of the ion chamber determine first the dose to the wall using equation 7-11, and then from the properties of the wall relative to water, calculate the dose to the water. This procedure is described in the next section.

7.05 **DETERMINATION OF ABSORBED DOSE USING AN ABSOLUTE ION CHAMBER**

An ionization chamber made of a known material and having a cavity of a known volume is called an absolute ionization chamber. It may be used to determine absorbed dose in a medium. It is necessary to collect *all* of the charge, Q, liberated in the cavity by the radiation and to measure this charge accurately. One must also know the volume of the cavity so that one can calculate the mass of gas, m. The actual determination of Q and m with precision is not easy, but here we are primarily interested in the principles involved. It is desired to determine the dose to the medium at point P (Fig. 7-4) when the medium is placed in a radiation field. At P we place the Bragg-Gray cavity (see Fig. 7-4b), of outside radius c and inner radius a. *The wall thickness (c − a) must be greater than the range of the electrons in it to ensure that the electrons that cross the cavity arise in the wall and not in the medium.* Suppose after a given irradiation a charge Q is measured. From this measurement we may use equation 7-11 to calculate the dose to the wall of the chamber. We wish to first relate this to the *dose to the medium* and then determine a correction factor to take into account the fact that the insertion of the chamber with its wall and air cavity has perturbed slightly the dose to point P in the homogeneous phantom.

Figure 7-4. Determination of absorbed dose using an absolute ion chamber. (a) Homogeneous phantom: dose is to be determined at point P using the ion chamber illustrated in (b), which is centered at point P' identical in position to P. The chamber has a wall of outer radius c and inner radius a.

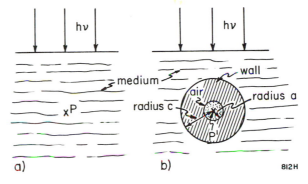

The situation depicted in Figure 7-4 is more complicated than that of Figure 7-3 since now *three* materials are involved—the gas, the wall of the cavity, and the medium in which the ion chamber is placed. The Bragg-Gray formula (eq. 7-11) gives the dose to the walls of the cavity. We want the dose to the medium. Since the amount of wall material introduced into the medium is assumed to be small and in composition not very different from the medium, it is assumed that the photon spectrum is not changed by the introduction of the wall material. The absorbed dose in the wall material may, however, be different from its value in the medium. The ratio of doses in the two materials resulting from the same photon spectrum should be very nearly the ratio of the "collision" part of the kermas in the two materials.

$$\frac{D_{med}}{D_{wall}} = \frac{K_{med}}{K_{wall}} \tag{7-12}$$

$$= \frac{\int_0^{h\nu_{max}} \left(\frac{d\Phi(h\nu)}{d\,h\nu}\right)_{med} \left(\frac{\mu(h\nu)}{\rho}\right)_{med} \overline{E}_{ab}^{med}(h\nu)\,d\,h\nu}{\int_0^{h\nu_{max}} \left(\frac{d\Phi(h\nu)}{d\,h\nu}\right)_{med} \left(\frac{\mu(h\nu)}{\rho}\right)_{wall} \overline{E}_{ab}^{wall}(h\nu)\,d\,h\nu} = \left(\frac{\overline{\mu}_{ab}}{\rho}\right)_{wall}^{med}$$

It must be remembered that this ratio is subject to the same requirements of electronic equilibrium that were discussed in section 7.03.

The quantity $(\bar{\mu}_{ab}/\rho)^{med}_{wall}$ defined in this way arises in many dose calculations and so we use a single symbol for it, the (μ/ρ) signifying its connection with photon interactions and the bar to signify that it is an average. Values of $(\bar{\mu}_{ab}/\rho)^{med}_{wall}$ calculated using equation 7-12 for the photon spectra of Table 7-2, are given in Table 7-4.

TABLE 7-4

Values of $\left(\dfrac{\bar{\mu}_{ab}}{\rho}\right)^{water}_{med}$ for Carbon, Bakelite, Lucite, and Polystyrene and $\left(\dfrac{\bar{\mu}_{ab}}{\rho}\right)^{med}_{air}$ for Water, Muscle, and Fat Determined Using Equation 7-12 for Photon Spectra Listed in Table 7-2.

(1) Photon Spectrum*	$\left(\dfrac{\bar{\mu}_{ab}}{\rho}\right)^{water}_{med}$				$\left(\dfrac{\bar{\mu}_{ab}}{\rho}\right)^{med}_{air}$			
	(2) Carbon	(3) Bakelite	(4) Lucite	(5) Polyst.	(6) Water	(7) Muscle	(8) Fat	(9) Bone
1. 60 kV$_p$	2.399	1.931	1.622	2.518	1.016	1.057	.617	4.873
2. 100 kV$_p$	2.112	1.758	1.519	2.152	1.026	1.062	.670	4.524
3. 250 kV$_p$	1.155	1.086	1.056	1.076	1.103	1.098	1.073	1.427
4. 270 kV$_p$	1.170	1.098	1.065	1.092	1.100	1.097	1.060	1.530
5. 270 kV$_p$	1.372	1.253	1.181	1.303	1.073	1.085	.924	2.668
6. 400 kV$_p$	1.129	1.065	1.040	1.050	1.108	1.101	1.095	1.217
7. ^{137}Cs	1.111	1.051	1.029	1.032	1.112	1.102	1.112	1.064
8. ^{60}Co	1.111	1.051	1.029	1.032	1.112	1.103	1.113	1.061
9. ^{60}Co	1.116	1.055	1.032	1.037	1.111	1.102	1.107	1.105
10. 6 MV	1.112	1.053	1.030	1.035	1.111	1.101	1.109	1.066
11. 8 MV	1.114	1.055	1.032	1.038	1.109	1.098	1.104	1.067
12. 12 MV	1.120	1.062	1.039	1.049	1.101	1.090	1.087	1.078
13. 18 MV	1.125	1.068	1.044	1.059	1.095	1.083	1.073	1.087
14. 26 MV	1.129	1.073	1.049	1.067	1.089	1.078	1.061	1.094
15. 26 MV	1.124	1.068	1.044	1.058	1.095	1.084	1.074	1.085
16. 35 MV	1.135	1.081	1.056	1.080	1.081	1.069	1.043	1.102
17. 45 MV	1.137	1.085	1.059	1.085	1.077	1.065	1.035	1.106

*Spectra 1 and 2 are taken from Yaffe (Y1); 3 and 6 are from Johns, appendix B, (J9); 4 and 5 are taken from Skarsgard, Table 8-1 (S8); 7 is monoenergetic radiation at 0.662 MeV; 8 has two energies at 1.17 and 1.33 MeV; 9 is taken from Bruce, Fig. 13x (B4); 10 is from Bentley et al., Fig. 3, calculated thick target (B8); 11 is taken from Levy et al., Fig. 5 (L3); 12 and 13 are calculated thin target spectra filtered by 2 cm tungsten and 2 cm water; 14 is from Sherman et al. representing an Allis Chalmers betatron (S9); 15 is from Levy et al., Fig. 6, experimental spectrum for Saggittaire (L4); 16 and 17 are calculated thin target spectra plus 2.2 cm tungsten and 10 cm of water representing high energy betatrons.

We are now in a position to calculate the dose to the medium from our determination of the dose to the walls. Combining equation 7-11 with equation 7-12 we obtain:

$$D_{med} = \left(33.85 \ \frac{J}{C}\right) \cdot \frac{Q}{m} \cdot \bar{\bar{S}}^{wall}_{air} \left(\frac{\bar{\mu}_{ab}}{\rho}\right)^{med}_{wall} \qquad (7\text{-}13)$$

This expression allows us to calculate the dose to the medium from a measurement of Q/m in the gas inside the wall material of the chamber. It is correct provided the air cavity (radius a) is small enough to produce negligible perturbation of the radiation field, and provided the shell of wall material has essentially the same atomic number and density as the medium.

Example 7-4. Suppose a carbon ion chamber with a 1 cm³ air cavity is placed in a water phantom and exposed to Co-60 gamma rays, which produce a charge of 3×10^{-8} C. Find the dose to the *water*. Assume the carbon walls are slightly thicker than the range of electrons.

From example 7-3, the dose to the carbon walls is 0.792 Gy

Table 7-4 shows that $\left(\dfrac{\bar{\mu}_{ab}}{\rho}\right)^{water}_{carbon} = 1.111$ (for spectrum no. 8)

Dose to water (eq. 7-13) = 0.792 Gy × 1.111 = 0.890 Gy

CORRECTION FACTORS FOR THE FINITE SIZE OF THE ION CHAMBER: We now attempt to correct for the fact that the introduction of a finite-sized ion chamber (radius c) with a finite air-filled cavity of radius "a" will alter the kerma slightly, and therefore the dose in equilibrium with it. That is, with a measurement made with the geometry of P′ we wish to determine the dose delivered to P. First consider the air cavity. If it were made smaller, the dose to a point at its center would be smaller because of the extra photon attenuation provided by the additional wall material. Hence, the true dose would be calculated from the measured one by multiplying the measured one by an attenuation factor $k(a_{wall})$, which is less than 1.0. If the air cavity were vanishingly small we would have a composite phantom composed of a shell of wall material of radius c instead of medium of radius c. The measured dose should be multiplied by $k(c_{med})$ and divided by $k(c_{wall})$. This will give a correction factor greater than 1.0 if the wall attenuates the beam more than an equivalent thickness of medium. Combining all these factors we obtain a correction factor, k_c, for the perturbing effect of the chamber.

$$k_c = \frac{k(a_{wall}) \cdot k(c_{med})}{k(c_{wall})} \qquad (7\text{-}14)$$

The precise determination of these attenuation factors is not possible, but Cunningham (C5) has determined approximate values theoretically and some of these are given in Figure 7-5. Combining equations 7-13 and 7-14 we obtain

$$D_{med} = \left(33.85 \frac{J}{C}\right) \cdot \frac{Q}{m} \cdot \bar{\bar{S}}^{wall}_{air} \cdot \left(\frac{\bar{\mu}_{ab}}{\rho}\right)^{med}_{wall} \cdot k_c \qquad (7\text{-}15)$$

which allows us to calculate the dose to the medium from a measurement of Q/m for an air-filled cavity in some wall material placed in the medium. $\bar{\bar{S}}$ can be obtained from Table 7-2, (μ_{ab}/ρ) from Table 7-4, and k_c from Figure 7-5.

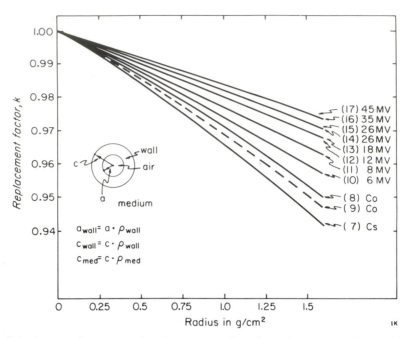

Figure 7-5. Attenuation correction factors as a function of the equivalent radius in cm of water. The insert shows how the three equivalent radii (a_{wall}, c_{wall}, c_{med}) are calculated. The numbers affixed to the graph correspond to the spectra of Table 7-2.

In Figure 7-5, the attenuation factors are plotted as a function of radius, r, for a number of the spectra listed in Table 7-2. To determine the three radii, a_{wall}, c_{med}, c_{wall}, one needs to know the radius of the air cavity, a, the outer radius of the chamber, c, and the densities relative to water of the wall material and the medium. We illustrate the use of Figure 7-5 by an example.

Example 7-5. Suppose the carbon chamber used in example 7-4 had an outer diameter of 1.4 cm and an inner diameter of 0.8 cm. Determine k_c using Figure 7-5 and thus the dose to the water corrected for the various attenuation factors. Density of carbon is 2.25 g/cm³. (Assume spectrum no. 9 for cobalt 60 gamma rays.)

$$
\begin{aligned}
a &= 0.4 \text{ cm} & a_{carbon} &= 0.4 \times 2.25 = .90 \text{ g/cm}^2 & k(a_{wall}) &= .972 \\
c &= 0.7 \text{ cm} & c_{carbon} &= 0.7 \times 2.25 = 1.57 \text{ g/cm}^2 & k(c_{wall}) &= .948 \\
c &= 0.7 \text{ cm} & c_{water} &= 0.7 \times 1.00 = 0.70 \text{ g/cm}^2 & k(c_{med}) &= .980
\end{aligned}
$$

$$
k_c \text{ (eq. 7-14)} = \frac{.972 \times .980}{.948} = 1.007
$$

$$
D_{water} = 0.890 \text{ Gy} \times 1.007 = 0.897 \text{ Gy}
$$

Because carbon has a density considerably greater than water, the shell of the carbon chamber more than compensates for the air cavity.

7.06   EFFECTS OF TEMPERATURE AND PRESSURE ON IONIZATION MEASUREMENTS

In the above discussion it would be necessary to specify the temperature and pressure of the gas, since these determine its density. The mass, $m(t, p)$, of a given volume of air at temperature t and pressure p is related to its mass $m(0, 101.3)$ at $0°$ C and 101.3 kPa (760 mm Hg) pressure by:

$$m(t, p) = m(0, 101.3) \left(\frac{273.2}{273.2 + t} \right) \left(\frac{p}{101.3} \right) \qquad (7\text{-}16)$$

The first bracketed term corrects for the expansion of the gas with increased temperature and the second for changes due to changes in pressure. Since the mass of gas appears in the denominator in equation 7-11, the correction factor k_{tp} that must be applied to the dose determination is:

$$k_{tp} = \left(\frac{273.2 + t}{273.2} \right) \left(\frac{101.3}{p} \right) \qquad (7\text{-}17)$$

The student may readily see that this expression is correct as follows. Suppose in the last example the temperature had been $20°$ C and the pressure 100 kPa. The air would have expanded from the cavity and hence too small an ionization would have been obtained, so the temperature correction would have to be larger than 1.00—in this case 293.2/273.2 = 1.073. Because the pressure is too low, too little air is present, hence the measured ionization is again too small, and the correction factor for it is 101.3/100 = 1.013. The total correction is 1.087. When extreme accuracy is desired, a correction must be made for the water vapor in the air (I3).

Usually instruments are calibrated to read correctly at room temperature ($22°$ C) and 101.3 kPa. When this is the case the correction factor is:

$$k_{tp} = \left(\frac{273 + t}{273.2 + 22} \right) \left(\frac{101.3}{p} \right) \qquad (7\text{-}18)$$

Whenever absolute ionization measurements are made, corrections must be applied to take into account the change in density of the gas with pressure and temperature. Often in what follows this fact will not be specifically mentioned. It should be noted that this correction assumes that the air cavity is not sealed and that there is free passage of air in and out of the chamber, so that the pressure inside the chamber is atmospheric. Whether this is true or not for a chamber can only be determined by experiment.

7.07   **EXPOSURE—THE ROENTGEN**

In the previous sections we discussed the principles involved in making a determination of absorbed dose from a measurement of the ionization within a cavity. Another approach to the problem is to first determine the *exposure* at the point of interest and then calculate the dose from the exposure. We now define *exposure* and the unit in which it is measured, the *roentgen*.

The quantity exposure was defined by the International Commission on Radiological Units and Measurements (ICRU) about a half century ago in an attempt to quantify radiation beams. The roentgen was a practical unit, and in the early days, its definition was based largely on the technique employed for its measurement, namely the standard air chamber as described below. The roentgen is only defined for photons and may not be used for particles such as electrons, protons, and neutrons, which have come into radiological practice. Furthermore its definition makes it difficult to apply it to photon beams of energy greater than about 3 MeV. For these reasons exposure is of limited value in radiotherapy today but is still useful in diagnostic radiology. Exposure is now defined by the ICRU as:

$$X = \frac{dQ}{dm} \qquad (7\text{-}19)$$

where dQ is the absolute value of the total charge of the ions of one sign produced in air when all of the *electrons liberated by photons** in a volume element of air having a mass dm are completely stopped in air. *Exposure is thus a measure of the ability of the radiation to ionize air.* Exposure is measured in coulombs per kg, and its special unit is the roentgen, defined as:

$$1 \text{ R} \equiv 2.58 \times 10^{-4} \text{ C/kg of air (exactly)}\dagger$$
$$\text{or} \quad 1 \text{ C/kg} = 3876 \text{ R} \qquad (7\text{-}20)$$

The roentgen could equally well have been defined in terms of the ionization produced per cm^3. Since air at STP has a density of 0.001293 g/cm^3, 1 kg of air has a volume of $10^3/.001293 = 7.734 \times 10^5$ cm^3 and 1 roentgen is equivalent to:

$$\frac{2.58 \times 10^{-4} \text{ C kg}^{-1}}{7.734 \times 10^5 \text{ cm}^3 \text{ kg}^{-1}} = 3.335 \times 10^{-10} \text{ C/cm}^3 \text{ of air} \quad (7\text{-}21a)$$

---

*Exposure is connected to the photon interactions and is thus more closely allied to kerma than to absorbed dose. Exposure in C/kg multiplied by W in J/C gives the part of kerma that is associated with ionization (bremsstrahlung excluded) and can also be called "collision kerma."

†The student may wonder why such a curious sized unit was defined. The roentgen was originally defined as the radiation that produced 1 esu of charge in 1 cm^3 of air at STP. Since 1 esu = 3.335 × 10^{-10} C, equation 7-20a shows that the numerical size of the roentgen has not been altered although its definition has been changed.

From section 7.04 we know that to produce 1 coulomb of charge by the ionization of air requires an energy absorption of 33.85 joules. Hence, an exposure of 1 R is equivalent to an energy absorption in air of:

$$2.58 \times 10^{-4} \frac{C}{kg} \times 33.85 \frac{J}{C} = 0.00873 \text{ J/kg of air} \quad (7\text{-}21b)$$

1 roentgen is defined as: 2.58×10^{-4} C/kg of air (7-21c)
is equivalent to: 3.335×10^{-10} C/cm³ of air
and to: 0.00873 J/kg of air

Strictly speaking, exposure can only be measured directly, by one instrument, the "Standard Air Chamber." This device is used by standardization laboratories and provides (exposure) calibrations for ionization chambers for radiology and radiobiology. Although the roentgen has been used extensively in radiological practice for many years, the ICRU now recommends that it be phased out and that exposures be expressed in C/kg.

7.08   STANDARD AIR CHAMBER

A standard ionization chamber is represented schematically in Figure 7-6 (A3, W4, G5). X rays from the focal spot of an x ray tube are limited by the circular diaphragm, D, of area, A, and enter the ionization chamber. Electrons will be set into motion everywhere within the cone, FQR, but will not be confined to this cone. Some of the electrons will be projected forward from their point of origin, and some at right angles to the beam. Thus, ions will be produced in a much larger volume than that represented by the cone, FQR. This region will extend from the volume FQR a distance x in all directions, where x is the maximum range of the electrons that travel at right angles to the beam. Typical electron tracks are shown in the insert to Figure 7-6.

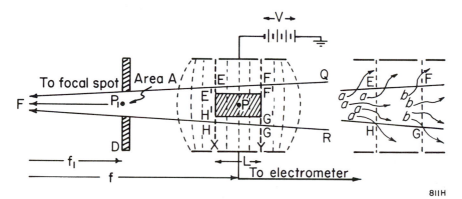

811H

Figure 7-6. Schematic diagram of the standard ionization chamber.

The ions are collected by two metal plates placed parallel to the x-ray beam and at a distance greater than x from the cone FQR. The lower plate is made up of three sections with the outer two grounded and the middle one connected to a charge measuring electrometer. The upper plate is raised to a negative potential V. The upper plate will attract positive charges, and negative charges will be driven onto the lower plates including the sensitive central electrode. The directions in which the ions will move is represented by the dotted electric lines of force. In the central region the lines of force are straight so that all the negative ions produced between the planes X and Y will be collected by the electrometer.

However, not all the ions produced between X and Y will arise from electrons originating in the volume EFGH. Some electrons originating in front of X (tracks a) will produce ions between X and Y, and similarly tracks b, originating between X and Y, will produce some of their ions beyond plane Y. In general, the number of ions lost through tracks b will equal the number gained through tracks a. Because of this equilibrium, we can consider that all the ions collected between the planes X and Y actually were produced by electrons originating in the volume EFGH. We can thus segregate a known mass of air and measure the ionization produced by electrons set into motion within it and so determine exposure according to equation 7-19. We wish to calculate the exposure at P, a point on the axis and midway between planes X and Y. We note that ions are collected from the volume EFGH, which is $A_f L$, where L is the length of the collecting plate and A_f is the cross-sectional area of the beam in the plane of P, at distance f from the source. If ΔQ is the charge collected and ρ is the density of air then:

$$\text{Exposure at P} = \frac{\Delta Q}{\rho \cdot A_f \cdot L} \qquad (7\text{-}22)$$

In practice it is more convenient to determine the exposure at a point outside the collecting volume such as P_1, which is situated on the axis at the position of the limiting diaphragm. Neglecting attenuation of the beam by the air path $P_1 P$, the exposure at P_1 will be larger than that at P by the inverse square factor $(f/f_1)^2$ (see page 313). Hence:

$$\text{Exposure at } P_1 = \left(\frac{f}{f_1}\right)^2 \cdot \frac{\Delta Q}{\rho A_f L} \qquad (7\text{-}23)$$

The area A of the limiting diaphragm and A_f are also related by the inverse square factor: $A = A_f \cdot (f_1/f)^2$ so equation 7-23 becomes:

$$\text{Exposure at } P_1 = \frac{\Delta Q}{\rho A L} \qquad (7\text{-}24)$$

The volume AL is shown schematically in Figure 7-6 as the shaded rectangle E′F′G′H′.

Example 7-6. In a standard air chamber the limiting diaphragm has an area of 0.500 cm² and the length of the sensitive electrode is 8.00 cm. In an irradiation a charge of 1.12×10^{-7} coulombs is collected. Air is at STP (density 1.293 kg m⁻³). Determine the exposure X at point P.

$$X \text{ (eq. 7-22)} = \frac{1.12 \times 10^{-7} \text{ C}}{.5 \times 10^{-4} \text{ m}^2 \times 8.0 \times 10^{-2} \text{ m} \times 1.293 \text{ kg m}^{-3}}$$

$$= .02166 \frac{\text{C}}{\text{kg}}$$

Exposure in R (eq. 7-20) = $.02166 \times 3876$ R = 83.9 R

The accurate realization of the roentgen requires considerable care and the correction for a number of effects. If the plates of the chamber are closer to the volume EFGH of Figure 7-6 than the maximum range of the electrons, an electron could strike the plate before it had expended all its energy and produced its full quota of ions. Under these circumstances the charge collected would be too small. By the same argument the sensitive volume EFGH must be placed so that P_1P is at least equal to the range, R, of electrons in the forward direction. If this condition is not satisfied, more ions will be lost through tracks b than are gained through tracks a. Also, electrons released from the collimator at P_1 might reach the collecting volume EFGH. As these would not be balanced by an equal number leaving the volume, the equilibrium condition described above would not exist.

To get some idea of the difficulty of meeting this requirement, the maximum ranges, R of electrons set in motion by monoenergetic photons are given in the last column of Table 7-1. We see, for example, that 3 MeV photons produce electron tracks 1.5 m long, giving some idea of the size of the standard air chamber that could be required to measure the exposure from such radiation. This thickness of air will attenuate this photon beam by 5.4% and so large corrections are required to correct for the attenuation by the thickness of air between the diaphragm and the sensitive volume. For these reasons the standard air chamber cannot be used for energies greater than about 3 MeV. Since most radiotherapy today is carried out with energies above 3 MeV, the concept of exposure and the roentgen are of limited value to radiotherapy.

7.09 PRACTICAL ION CHAMBERS—THE THIMBLE CHAMBER

The large standard chamber lacks mobility and could not be used for calibration purposes except in special circumstances or in a standardization laboratory. This has led to the development of practical ion chambers that, although convenient, must be standardized at intervals against a standard chamber. Suppose we consider a unit volume of air, completely surrounded by air, and bathe the air with x irradiation (Fig. 7-7a).

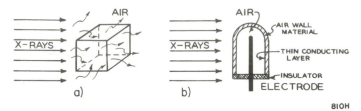

Figure 7-7. Diagram illustrating the nature of air "air wall" chamber.

There will be some electrons entering this volume from outside and some leaving it. In general the number of ions produced outside the volume by electrons from inside it will be equal to the number of ions produced inside the volume by electrons originating outside. We may then consider that all the ions produced inside the volume were produced by electrons originating there and that they expended all their energy inside the volume. This would, of course, be true only if the air around the volume extended to a distance equal to or greater than the maximum range of the electrons. If now all this "air" were condensed into a solid air wall, we would not alter the state of affairs and we would have a thimble chamber, as represented in Figure 7-7b. The inside of this chamber is now covered with a conducting layer and an electrode is inserted. If the electrode is charged, the ions produced can be collected. We have thus isolated a given mass of air and collected the charge liberated by the radiation and have so fulfilled the spirit of the definition of exposure. The basis of the practical chamber depends on an "air wall," and this may be difficult to achieve in practice, since air is not available as a conducting solid. In practice, ion chambers are usually made of plastic (for example Bakelite with composition $C_{43}H_{38}O_7$ and coated on the inside with carbon ($Z = 6$) and with an inner electrode made of aluminum ($Z = 13$). By properly adjusting the size of the aluminum electrode and the amount of carbon, it is possible to produce a chamber whose response varies with photon energy in nearly the same way as the standard air chamber.

To calibrate a practical ion chamber against a standard chamber, they are arranged in such a way that they may be alternatively moved into the same x ray beam so that the practical chamber can occupy the same point in space as the diaphragm of the standard air chamber. This procedure will yield an exposure calibration factor, which we will represent by $N_X(h\nu)$, the X indicating exposure and $h\nu$ the fact that the calibration factor is a function of photon energy. If after a given irradiation the exposure meter reads M, then the exposure X is given by:

$$X = M \cdot N_X \tag{7-25}$$

Usually N_X is very close to 1.00 but if it is quite different the manufacturer of the chamber may decide to alter the response in the following way. Suppose a chamber is found to be correct at 200 kV but gives too high a reading at 100 kV. Its response at the latter radiation quality may be reduced by decreasing the effective Z (see next section) of the chamber. One way to do this would be to shorten the aluminum electrode, thus reducing the amount of material of Z greater than 7.7 in the chamber. If the response at both qualities is too high, then the volume of the chamber may be reduced. Kemp (K5) has shown that very small amounts of impurities in the colloidal graphite, which is placed on the inside of the chamber, can produce a large effect on the chamber performance. Once the best compromise in the response at low and high energies has been achieved, the chamber should not be tampered with further. The calibration factors for this chamber at a number of photon energies should be obtained by the standardization laboratory and used by the user.

Typical exposure calibration factors for two chambers are given in Figure 7-8 as a function of the equivalent photon energy, with an auxiliary scale giving the half-value layer (see Chapter 8). Curve A is for an ionization chamber designed for general use. For low energies its response is too low because its walls are too thick and hence absorb a large fraction of the low energy x rays. At high energies its walls are too thin to give equilibrium, but this situation can be rectified by adding a "cobalt cap," which fits snugly over the ion chamber when cobalt measurements are being made. The dashed curve is for a chamber designed primarily for low energy x rays. Over the range HVL 4.0 mm Cu to 2 mm Al, the calibration factor is very nearly 1.00. At very low energies its response is too low because of attenuation in the wall.

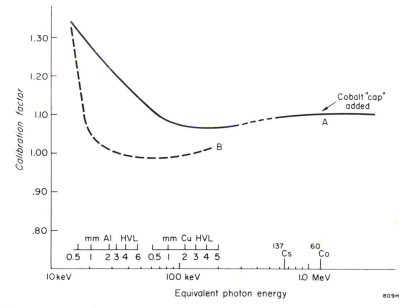

Figure 7-8. Exposure calibration factors for 2 types of ion chambers. (a) Farmer exposure meter. (b) Low energy 100 R Victoreen chamber. These are typical curves and should *not* be used in a calibration procedure.

When charge is collected, the instrument measures exposure. If, instead, the rate of charge liberation, or ion current, is determined the instrument measures exposure rate. Ion chambers, together with their electrometers (the charge measuring device) have in the past been loosely called dosimeters. To be consistent with current terminology it would be more accurate to use the terms exposure meters and exposure rate meters.

WALL THICKNESS IN PRACTICAL ION CHAMBER: In the standard ionization chamber it was necessary to provide a thickness of air on all sides of the sensitive volume equal to or greater than the range of the electrons. In a practical chamber, in an exactly analogous way, the "air wall" material must be thicker than the maximum range of electrons, otherwise too small a reading will be obtained. The response of a Farmer type chamber exposed to cobalt 60 gamma rays as a function of wall thickness is shown in Figure 7-9. It is seen that as the chamber wall is increased, the response rises to a maximum when the "equilibrium" wall is attained, and then falls slowly. The reduction in response for a thick walled chamber is due to the attenuation in the wall in exactly the same way as in the standard chamber when appreciable attenuation occurred between the limiting diaphragm and the sensitive volume. The chamber wall thickness should be close to the value that gives the maximum reading. To extend the useful energy range over which a given chamber may be used, an extra cap is often provided with a wall thickness of 2 to 3 mm. The chamber is used without this cap over the equivalent photon energy range up to about 400 keV and with the cap added for measurements of Cs-137 or Co-60 gamma rays (see Fig. 7-8). The chamber should be calibrated by the standardization laboratory with the cap for high energy radiation and without it for low energy radiation.

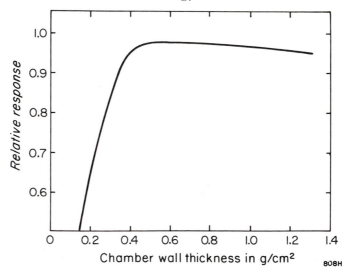

Figure 7-9. Response of a Farmer type ion chamber as a function of wall thickness, for Co-60 radiation.

7.10 **EFFECTIVE ATOMIC NUMBER**

In dealing with a compound or a mixture of molecules, for example, air, it is sometimes convenient to describe the mixture by an effective atomic number ($\overline{Z}$). The concept is useful in dealing with ion chambers since one often wishes to design a chamber with walls that absorb x rays in the same way as does the air in the chamber. Now air contains nitrogen (Z = 7), oxygen (Z = 8), and argon (Z = 18). The question is can one assign a single atomic number to the mixture that will correctly predict its absorption properties for x rays for a range of photon energies?

In the energy range where Compton absorption is important, the absorption is independent of Z so all one needs to know is the number of electrons per gram in the mixture, and the effective atomic number is unnecessary. The energy region of interest in discussing the effective atomic number is then from about 30 keV to 80 keV, where the photoelectric process is dominant over the Compton process. In section 5.07 it was pointed out that the photoelectric coefficient per electron depends upon Z^m where m is about 3 for high Z materials and about 3.8 for low Z materials. It was also noted that m varies with photon energy.

To investigate this problem, we have plotted the energy absorption coefficient per electron versus Z using data derived from Plechaty et al. (P5). These were obtained from their data by dividing their cross sections in cm^2 per atom by Z and multiplying by $\overline{E}_{ab}/h\nu$. The curves shown in Figure 7-10 are smooth functions of Z. It should be noted that if one plots (μ/ρ) or (μ_{ab}/ρ) versus Z the curves are not smooth because the number of electrons per gram ($N_e = N_0 Z/A$) fluctuates with atomic number. For example, oxygen (Z = 8) has 3.01×10^{23} el/g, fluorine (Z = 9) has 2.85×10^{23}, and neon (Z = 10) has 2.98×10^{23}.

In the appendix the elemental compositions of a variety of materials such as air, water, fat, muscle, and bone are given. Using these and the tables of Plechaty et al., one can calculate the energy absorption coefficient of a gram of the mixture and divide this by the number of electrons per gm to give the energy absorption coefficient in cm^2 per electron for the mixture (see section 5.11). These are located by the horizontal lines in Figure 7-10. At 30 keV, for example, air has an energy absorption coefficient of 0.464×10^{-24} cm^2 per electron. This locates point P and shows that air at 30 keV has an effective atomic number of 7.75. Similarly at 40 keV, the location of P' yields an effective atomic number for air of 7.80. For bone the effective atomic numbers at these two energies are 12.11 and 12.22. By this procedure one can evaluate $\overline{Z}$ for any material at any photon energy. The procedure is, however, only useful if it yields the same or nearly the same $\overline{Z}$ for any energy or any of the various absorption coefficients that could be plotted. We have chosen to use the energy absorption coefficients in Figure 7-10 because it is the most useful one in dealing with dosimetry problems. When this process is carried out one

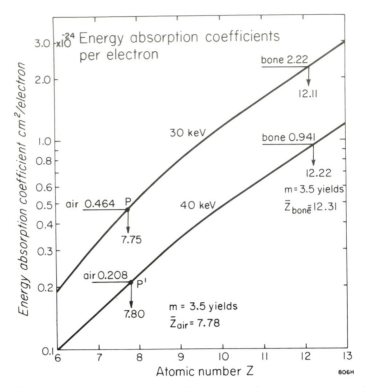

Figure 7-10. Plot of energy absorption coefficient in cm² per electron as a function of atomic number using data from Plechaty (P5) for 30 and 40 keV photons. The coefficients for air and bone are also shown, allowing one to determine an effective atomic number for air and bone.

finds that $\overline{Z}$ is nearly independent of $h\nu$ and the coefficient used and so is a meaningful concept.

The determination of $\overline{Z}$ by the above procedure, however, involves considerable effort and the question arises, can one calculate it? We know that the photoelectric cross section per *electron* varies at Z^m where m is in the range 3-4. The effective atomic number, $\overline{Z}$, of a mixture may be defined by:

$$\overline{Z} = \sqrt[m]{a_1 Z_1^m + a_2 Z_2^m + \ldots a_n Z_n^m \ldots} \tag{7-26}$$

where a_1 to a_n are the fractional numbers of electrons per gram belonging to materials of atomic number Z_1 to Z_n. To illustrate the use of this formula we calculate $\overline{Z}$ for air using m = 3.5. The calculations are laid out in tabular form below. The fourth column gives w, the fractional content, by weight for the components of air taken from Table A-3 (p. 720). The fifth column gives $N_0 Z w / A$ where N_0 is Avogadro's number and A the atomic weight. The total of this column gives the total number of electrons per gram in air. Dividing each of the entries of column 5 by 3.0061×10^{23}, we obtain the fractional number of electrons belonging to each element and the total of these yields 1.000, as it should. In the last column aZ^m is evaluated and totaled. $\overline{Z}$ is then determined from equation 7-26 and yields $\overline{Z} = 7.78$ for air, which agrees reasonably well with Figure 7-10.

(1) material	(2) Z	(3) A	(4) w	(5) N_0Zw/A	(6) Calc. of a's	(7) $aZ^{3.5}$
N_2	7	14.007	.755	2.2722×10^{23}	$a_1 = .75586$	685.9
O_2	8	16.000	.232	$.6986 \times 10^{23}$	$a_2 = .23329$	337.8
A	18	39.948	.013	$.0353 \times 10^{23}$	$a_3 = .01175$	290.7
				3.0061×10^{23}	1.00000	1314.4

$$\overline{Z}_{air} \text{ (eq. 7-26)} = \sqrt[3.5]{1314.4} = 7.78$$

A similar calculation for bone yields 12.31, in fair agreement with the interpolated values of 12.11 and 12.22. This procedure was carried out for air, water, fat, muscle, bone, polystyrene, Lucite, LiF, and ferrous sulphate for photon energies from 30 to 80 keV. The value of m that gave the best fit ranged from 3.4 to 3.8, with most of the best fit values ranging around 3.5. For this reason all values of $\overline{Z}$ given in this text (for example in Appendix A-3) were determined using $m = 3.5$. The fact that no single value for m will fit all the data should convince the reader that there is little point in specifying the effective atomic number to more than 2 significant figures.

The effective atomic number was first introduced by Mayneord (M6) who recommended an exponent $m = 2.94$. Since that time many equations similar to equation 7-25 have appeared in the literature with quite different values of m (M7, S10, W5, W6). The effective atomic number might be used as follows. Suppose one wished to determine $\overline{E}_{tr}$ for air at 30 keV. Table A-4 shows $\overline{E}_{tr} = 9.93$ keV for nitrogen and 13.0 keV for oxygen. Interpolating between these one obtains for $\overline{Z} = 7.8$ the value 12.4 keV. An evaluation by determining the contribution from each component of air separately is much more work and yields 12.3.

7.11 DETERMINATION OF ABSORBED DOSE IN "FREE SPACE"

A concept that has been of some use in practical dosimetry is the absorbed dose in "free space." It is useful for two reasons: with it one may characterize the "output" of a radiation unit and it may also serve as a reference for tumor dose calculations that involve tissue-air ratios and backscatter factors. (These quantities are discussed in Chapter 10.) The concept is also useful in providing a discussion of some of the physics that is relevant to photon dosimetry and because of this will now be discussed in some detail.

The meaning of "dose in free space" may be clarified by referring to Figure 7-11. Part a of this diagram depicts a beam of photons irradiating nothing but air. Let us assume that we know the exposure (or exposure rate) at point P. It could have been determined, for example, from a measurement made with an ionization chamber for which we have an exposure calibration factor, N_X, and equation 7-25. Let the exposure determined in this way be denoted by X. It is the exposure at point P in the absence of dosimeter and is dependent on the dosimeter that was used to determine it only through its calibration factor.

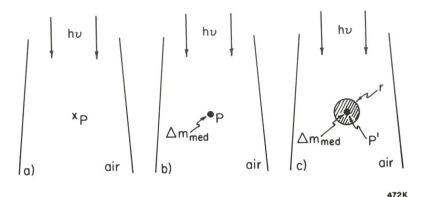

472K

Figure 7-11. Diagram illustrating the meaning of "dose in free space." (a) An exposure, X, is measured at P. (b) A small mass of phantom material is introduced at P and kerma is calculated. (c) More material is added until there is electronic equilibrium and finally absorbed dose may be calculated.

It was pointed out in section 7.07 that exposure is directly related to the part of kerma associated with the production of ionization. This is called "collision kerma" and is given by:

$$K_{air} = X \left(0.00873 \, \frac{J}{kg \, R} \right) \qquad (7\text{-}27a)$$

from equation 7-21c.

Next imagine that at point P we introduce a very small mass, Δm, of phantom-like material, as depicted in Figure 7-11b. Δm is just large enough to avoid statistical fluctuations due to the photon interactions taking place in it. We could not calculate the dose in it but we could determine the collision kerma. It would be:

$$K_{\Delta m} = K_{air} \, (\overline{\mu}_{ab}/\rho)_{air}^{\Delta m} \qquad (7\text{-}27b)$$

where $(\overline{\mu}_{ab}/\rho)_{air}^{\Delta m}$ is the ratio of averaged mass energy absorption coefficients for the material of Δm to air as defined by equation 7-12.

We require absorbed dose rather than kerma and to obtain it we must add material around Δm so that electronic equilibrium will be established in it. This situation is indicated in Figure 7-11c where point P, now labelled P', is surrounded by phantom-like material of radius r. The kerma to mass Δm will now be slightly smaller:

$$K'_{\Delta m} = K_{\Delta m} \, k(r_{med}) \qquad (7\text{-}27c)$$

where $k(r_{med})$ is the attenuation factor discussed in section 7.05 and given in Figure 7-5.

We can now determine the absorbed dose at point P′ but first we must decide how large the radius, r, should be and this is not easy. A minimum would be the maximum range of the electrons set into motion; for example, for ^{60}Co radiation this would be about 0.44 g/cm² (see Table A-6 for 1 MeV electrons in water). A value for the attenuation correction factor for material of this radius can be obtained from Figure 7-5 and would be about 0.985. In the past the attenuation correction factor for such a minimal mass of phantom-like material has been given the symbol A_{eq} and the value 0.985. It is probable, in view of the shape of the kerma and dose curves shown in Figure 7-2b, that r should be somewhat larger, more like 0.8 cm. This would imply an attenuation correction of $k(r_{wat}) = k(0.8) = 0.978$. Such a size also has the advantage of being about equal to the outside diameter of practical ion chambers used for cobalt radiation.

We may finally determine the absorbed dose at point P′:

$$D_{\Delta m} = K'_{\Delta m} \cdot b \qquad (7\text{-}27d)$$

where b is the factor appearing in equation 7-8a. It is the ratio of absorbed dose to kerma at point P. In all practical dosimetry situations this factor is assumed to be equal to 1.00. It is discussed by Roesch (R3) who gives a maximum value of 1.0045 for b, for cobalt radiation. In this book it will be assumed to be 1.00.

Finally, all steps can be combined so that the absorbed dose in "free space" at a point in air where exposure is known can be determined from:

$$D_{fs} = X \left(0.00873 \, \frac{J}{kg \, R}\right) \left(\frac{\overline{\mu}_{ab}}{\rho}\right)^{med}_{air} k(r_{med}) \qquad (7\text{-}28)$$

Dose "in free space" is of limited use for energies much above 1 MeV because it tends to be coupled directly to exposure as just described and the use of exposure is limited to a few MeV. The dose in free space could be determined for high energies using methods discussed in section 7.12, but this is not done for the very practical reason that the buildup cap that would be required for the ion chamber would be so large as to be inconvenient. It might also preclude the use of small radiation beams because the cap might not be covered by the beam. Treatment machine calibrations can also be carried out by making measurements directly in phantoms and this can be done at any energy. The physics of this procedure will be discussed next.

7.12   DETERMINATION OF ABSORBED DOSE IN A PHANTOM USING AN EXPOSURE CALIBRATED ION CHAMBER

Figure 7-12 shows an absorbing medium (for example, water) being irradiated. We wish to determine the dose at point P by placing the center of our calibrated dosimeter at P′ (as illustrated in Fig. 7-12b). Suppose after a given irradiation a reading, M, is obtained. When this is multiplied by the exposure calibration factor, N_X, and corrected for temperature and pressure and if necessary for loss of ionization by recombination (see Chap. 9), one obtains the exposure, X, at the point. The exposure, X, is for the situation depicted in Figure 7-12c, i.e., for a point at the center of an air-filled sphere (or cylinder) of radius c in the phantom. *Our task is then to calculate the dose at P from the exposure measured at P″*. Such an exposure would correspond to the (collision) kerma to the air that would occupy the cavity depicted in Figure 7-12c and this kerma would be given by:

$$K_{air} = X \left(0.00873 \ \frac{J}{kg \ R} \right) \tag{7-29a}$$

This equation is exactly the same as 7-27a. We now proceed just as for the previous section and imagine a small mass, Δm, of phantom material placed at point P″, at the center of the air cavity. The (collision) kerma to Δm would be:

$$K_{\Delta m} = K_{air} \ (\mu_{ab}/\rho)_{air}^{med} \tag{7-29b}$$

The next step is to fill in the cavity, of radius c, with phantom material. This would alter the kerma to the small mass, Δm, by the attenuation factor, $k(c_{med})$, and the kerma to mass Δm would now be:

$$K'_{\Delta m} = K_{\Delta m} \ k(c_{med}) \tag{7-29c}$$

Again, $k(c_{med})$ is discussed in section 7.05 and values for it may be obtained from Figure 7-5.

Finally, the absorbed dose at point P in the homogeneous phantom may be obtained from:

$$D_{med} = M \cdot N_X \cdot \left(0.00873 \ \frac{J}{kg \ R} \right) \cdot \left(\frac{\bar{\mu}_{ab}}{\rho} \right)_{air}^{med} \cdot k(c_{med}) \cdot b$$

$$\tag{7-30}$$

This is exactly the same as equation 7-28 except that the radius c, the outer radius of the chamber, takes the place of r, the radius of the phantom-like material. Again in using this relation we will assume that b, the ratio of dose to kerma, is 1.00.

It should be noted that neither equation 7-30 nor 7-28 depend directly on the nature of the dosimeter. It is, of course, necessary that it have a

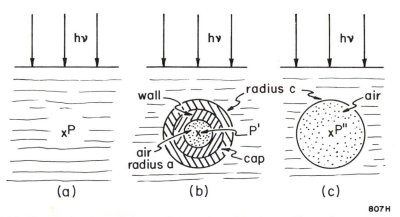

807H

Figure 7-12. Determination of dose using an ion chamber calibrated to measure exposure. (a) Homogeneous phantom showing point P where the dose is to be determined. (b) Phantom showing the exposure meter with its air cavity, wall, and buildup cap of radius c situated at P', the same depth. (c) The exposure meter determines the exposure at P'' at the center of an air-filled cavity of radius c.

rather flat response to the radiation, that is, respond as an air-like detector, since it is measuring exposure. It is not necessary for us to know what materials make up the walls of the ion chamber nor the size of the air cavity in it. In fact it is not necessary that it be an ion chamber; it could be any device that would respond to radiation in an "air-like" manner and that has an exposure calibration factor. The attenuation factor k depends on the size of the chamber (through radius c) but not on its composition. It relates to the material of the phantom that is replaced by dosimeter; because of this it is sometimes also called the replacement factor.

It is possible to have a dosimeter calibrated in terms of absorbed dose instead of exposure. If this is done and the dosimeter used to measure dose in a phantom irradiated by a beam of the same energy as the one for which the dose calibration was determined, the absorbed dose at a point such as P of Figure 7-12a would be given by:

$$D_{med} = M \cdot N_D \qquad (7\text{-}31)$$

The relation between dose calibration factor and exposure calibration could be determined by equating equation 7-31 to equation 7-30. An example will now illustrate the use of an exposure-calibrated dosimeter for the determination of absorbed dose.

Example 7-7. A Farmer type ionization chamber is used to make a determination of absorbed dose in a water phantom irradiated by Co-60 gamma rays. It is protected against the water by thin rubber tubing and is held with its center at a point such as P of Figure 7-12. After a given irradiation the electrometer connected to it gives a scale reading of 74.0. The exposure calibration factor N_X for the chamber with this electrometer is 1.06 for Co-60 radiation. Determine the absorbed dose in the phantom. The outer radius of the chamber with its cap is 0.8 cm. Determine also the dose calibration factor:

$$X = 74.0 \times 1.06 = 78.4 \text{ R}$$

Since phantom is water $c_{med} = c = .8 \text{ g/cm}^2$ and $k(c_{med}) = .977$ (Fig. 7-5)

Table 7-4 (spectrum 9) $\left(\dfrac{\bar{\mu}_{ab}}{\rho}\right)^{water}_{air} = 1.111$ for Co-60

$$\therefore D_{water} = .00873 \, (1.111) \, (78.4) \, (.977) = 0.743$$

$$N_D = 0.743/74.0 = 0.0104 \text{ Gy per meter reading}$$

Equation 7-30 is very useful since it enables us to calculate the dose from a measurement of exposure in the phantom. Its use, however, requires a knowledge of the exposure factor N_X for the dosimeter. Unfortunately, therefore, the method cannot be used above 3 MeV.

7.13   DETERMINATION OF ABSORBED DOSE
AT ENERGIES ABOVE 3 MeV

The precise determination of dose for energies above 3 MeV is important since much radiotherapy is carried out at such energies. The only truly satisfactory way to do this is to calibrate an ion chamber or some type of transfer instrument to read in grays using a calorimeter to make the basic energy absorption measurement. Although several standardization laboratories have calorimeters, this calibration service is not yet generally available. In the meantime we look at a number of approximate methods. It is hoped that soon absorbed dose calibrations over a range of energies will become available, making many of the sections of this chapter obsolete. We now discuss the two methods that are currently available.

Absolute Dosimetry

The dose at some convenient reference point in the medium can be determined using equation 7-15. Experimentally, we need to accurately measure the charge, Q, liberated by a given irradiation. This can be achieved by methods described in Chapter 9. We also need to determine the mass of gas, m, in the chamber. This can be calculated if we know the volume; although the physical volume can be determined precisely, there may be regions in the cavity where the electric field does *not* collect the ions, and this portion of the volume should not be included. Even with great care the determination of m to 2% accuracy is very difficult.

Next we must determine $\bar{\bar{S}}^{wall}_{air}$ and $(\bar{\mu}_{ab}/\rho)^{med}_{wall}$. This is not easy since the composition of the walls is often not well known, and furthermore, their radiological properties are often adjusted by adding impurities to the conducting layer on the inside of the wall. In addition, usually neither the photon spectrum nor the electron spectrum are known. The product of these two factors can therefore seldom be known to within 2%.

Finally, we have the troublesome attenuation factors. Although Cunningham (C5) has attempted to determine these with precision, their calculation (Fig. 7-5) is complex. Furthermore, many radiation physicists do not even accept the idea that some factor k_c is required. It is easy, therefore, to introduce from this cause also an error of 2%. Combining all the possible errors an accuracy of better than about 5% by this method would seem to be difficult to achieve. We conclude then that absolute dosimetry is not the method of choice.

Use of Exposure Meter with Calibration Factor at Cobalt 60 to Determine Absorbed Dose at Energies above 3 MeV

An exposure calibrated dosimeter may be used to determine absorbed dose using equation 7-30. This equation is useful up to energies of about 3 MeV, and the question arises whether its range could be extended to higher energies, that is, could one make a measurement in a high energy beam (say 26 MV) using a dosimeter given an exposure calibration with Co-60 and apply suitable corrections to allow determination of absorbed dose at the higher energies. This can, in fact, be done and is a procedure that has found favor and that we now describe in detail, but the reader should bear in mind that it, too, is an approximate procedure.

It was shown above that the dose at a point in a medium can be determined using equation 7-15 but that the mass of air in the chamber must be known and this, for reasons also discussed, is difficult. It can, however, be determined indirectly from the exposure calibration procedure as follows.

Consider a radiation beam, say ^{60}Co, for which an exposure calibration factor, N_X, has been obtained. The dose in a medium at a point such as P in Figure 7-12 can be determined from both equations 7-15 and 7-30. Since the same dose is being calculated by both equations we can equate them and solve for $(Q/m)(1/M)$, the charge per unit mass of air per meter reading, M:

$$\frac{Q}{m}\frac{1}{M} = N_X \left(2.58 \times 10^{-4} \frac{C}{kg\,R}\right) \left[\frac{(\bar{\mu}_{ab}/\rho)_{air}^{wall}}{\bar{\bar{S}}_{air}^{wall}}\right] \left[\frac{k(c_{wall})}{k(a_{wall})}\right] \qquad (7\text{-}32)$$

To get this result we have also used equation 7-14 and the fact that $(\bar{\mu}_{ab}/\rho)_{air}^{wall} = (\bar{\mu}_{ab}/\rho)_{air}^{med}/(\bar{\mu}_{ab}/\rho)_{wall}^{med}$. The quantity calculated in equation 7-32 is a constant of proportionality and would be unique for each dosimeter. It connects the charge released and the meter reading. Its dimensions are coulombs per kg of gas per roentgen. The charge released can

be determined accurately by electrical means and this procedure therefore effectively determines the mass of air in the chamber. Because we
are more concerned with absorbed dose than exposure, it is convenient
to multiply equation 7-32 by W and form a quantity referred to (L5,
D5) as the "cavity-gas calibration factor," N_{gas}, which is an expression of
the absorbed dose to the gas per unit signal of the dosimeter.

$$N_{gas} = \frac{Q}{m}\frac{W}{M} = N_X \left(0.00873 \frac{J}{kg\ R}\right)\left[\frac{(\bar{\mu}_{ab}/\rho)_{air}^{wall}}{\bar{\bar{S}}_{air}^{wall}}\right]_{Co}\left[\frac{k(c_{wall})}{k(a_{wall})}\right]_{Co} \quad (7\text{-}33)$$

The variables in N_{gas} depend on the gas in the cavity (air) and the material making up the walls that surround it but not on the medium. Although in this case the variables are to be evaluated for ^{60}Co radiation,
the same value would be obtained for N_{gas} for any beam for which an exposure calibration, N_X, was available. N_{gas} can also be obtained from an
absorbed dose calibration as will be discussed later.

The following examples will illustrate the determination of N_{gas}.

Example 7-8. A cylindrical ionization chamber with walls made of
Bakelite has an outside radius of 0.8 cm and an inside radius of 0.3 cm.
Determine the cavity-gas calibration factor, N_{gas}. Assume ^{60}Co radiation
(spectrum 8, Table 7-2).

$(\bar{\mu}_{ab}/\rho)_{air}^{bak} = (\bar{\mu}_{ab}/\rho)_{air}^{wat}/(\bar{\mu}_{ab}/\rho)_{bak}^{wat} = 1.112/1.051 = 1.058$ (Table 7-4)

$\bar{\bar{S}}_{air}^{bak} = 1.071$ (Table 7-2)

$c_{bak} = 0.8 \times 1.4 = 1.12$ g/cm^2 and   k(1.12) = 0.967 (Fig. 7-5)

$a_{bak} = 0.3 \times 1.4 = 0.42$ g/cm^2 and   k(0.42) = 0.988 (Fig. 7-5)

$N_{gas} = N_X \left(0.00873 \frac{J}{kg\ R}\right) \times \frac{1.058}{1.071} \times \frac{0.967}{0.988}$

$= 0.00844\ N_X$ J/kg per unit signal

Example 7-9. Determine N_{gas} for an ionization chamber made of
Lucite with the same dimensions as the Bakelite chamber of example
7-8. Again assume spectrum 8.

$(\bar{\mu}_{ab}/\rho)_{air}^{luc} = 1.112/1.029 = 1.081$ and $\bar{\bar{S}}_{air}^{luc} = 1.099$

$c_{luc} = 0.8 \times 1.2 = .96$ g/cm^2 and   k(.96) = 0.972 (Fig. 7-5)

$a_{luc} = 0.3 \times 1.2 = .36$ g/cm^2 and   k(.36) = 0.990 (Fig. 7-5)

$N_{gas} = N_X \left(0.00873 \frac{J}{kg\ R}\right)\frac{1.081}{1.099} \times \frac{0.972}{0.990} = 0.00843\ N_X$ J/kg

Note that almost the same result (within 0.2%) was obtained for the two
chambers.

Once N_{gas} is known, the absorbed dose for a beam of any energy may be obtained from the equation:

$$D_{med} = M \cdot N_{gas} \left[(\bar{\mu}_{ab}/\rho)_{wall}^{med} \ \bar{\bar{S}}_{air}^{wall} \right]' \ k'_c \qquad (7\text{-}34)$$

where k'_c is given by equation 7-14. The primed quantities are to be evaluated at the beam energy for which D_{med} is desired. An application of this expression will now be given.

Example 7-10. Assume the ion chamber of example 7-8 has an exposure calibration described by curve A of Figure 7-8, giving, for cobalt: $N_X = 1.11$ R per unit signal. This dosimeter is placed in a water phantom and irradiated by a beam from a 26 MV linac (use spectrum 15 of Table 7-2) until the dosimeter reads 87.0. Determine the absorbed dose.

$N_{gas} = 0.00844 \times 1.11 = 0.00937$ J/kg (from ex. 7-8)

$(\bar{\mu}_{ab}/\rho)_{bak}^{wat} = 1.068$ (Table 7-4)   and $\bar{\bar{S}}_{air}^{bak} = 1.035$ (Table 7-2)

$c_{wat} = 0.8 \times 1.0 = 0.8$ g/cm²   and $k'(0.8) = 0.986$ (Fig. 7-5)

$c_{bak} = 0.8 \times 1.4 = 1.12$ g/cm²   and $k'(1.12) = 0.981$ (Fig. 7-5)

$a_{bak} = 0.3 \times 1.4 = 0.42$ g/cm²   and $k'(0.42) = 0.993$ (Fig. 7-5)

$k'_c = 0.993 \times 0.986/0.981 = 0.998$ (eq. 7-14)

$$D_{water} = 87.0 \times 0.00937 \ \frac{J}{kg} \times 1.068 \times 1.035 \times 0.998 = 0.899 \text{ Gy}$$

In calculating the dose in this example it was assumed that all of the electrons causing ionization in the cavity arose from the Bakelite walls. At such a high energy, where some of the electrons have ranges of several cm, this will certainly not be the case. In fact, a very appreciable part of the ionization will be due to electrons coming from the water beyond the Bakelite walls. If all the electrons came from the water, the absorbed dose would be given by the relation:

$$D_{med} = M \cdot N_{gas} \left[\bar{\bar{S}}_{air}^{med} \right]' \ k' \ (a_{wat}) \qquad (7\text{-}35)$$

The difficulty is to know the proportion of each. The range of uncertainty caused by this is not great, however, as may be judged from the following example.

Example 7-11. Repeat the calculation of absorbed dose for the conditions described in example 7-10 but assume that the chamber acts as an "electron detector," that is, that all of the electrons "seen" come from the medium (water) beyond the ion chamber walls.

$\bar{\bar{S}}_{air}^{wat} = 1.094$ (Table 7-2)

$a_{wat} = 0.3 \times 1.0 = 0.3$ g/cm²   and $k'(0.3) = 0.995$

$$D_{water} = 87.0 \times 0.00937 \ \frac{J}{kg} \times 1.094 \times 0.995 = 0.887 \text{ Gy}$$

The two results are within 1.4% of each other, suggesting that fairly precise dosimetry can be achieved even with incomplete knowledge about the relative contributions from the walls and the medium.

Sometimes, also, the actual composition of the walls is not well known. To illustrate the effect that this might have, consider the following example.

Example 7-12. Repeat the calculations of example 7-10, assuming the chamber walls are made of Lucite instead of Bakelite.

$$N_{gas} = 0.00843 \ \frac{J}{kg} \times 1.11 = 0.00936 \ J/kg \ \text{(ex. 7-9)}$$

$$(\bar{\mu}/\rho)^{\prime \, wat}_{luc} = 1.044 \ \text{(Table 7-4)}$$

$$\bar{\bar{S}}^{\prime \, luc}_{air} = 1.061 \ \text{(Table 7-2)}$$

$$c_{wat} = 0.8 \times 1.0 = 0.8 \ g/cm^2 \quad \text{and} \quad k'(0.8) = 0.986$$

$$c_{luc} = 0.8 \times 1.2 = 0.96 \ g/cm^2 \quad \text{and} \quad k'(0.96) = 0.983$$

$$a_{luc} = 0.3 \times 1.2 = 0.36 \ g/cm^2 \quad \text{and} \quad k'(0.36) = 0.994$$

$$k'_c = 0.994 \times 0.986/0.983 = 0.997$$

$$D_{water} = 87.0 \times 0.00936 \ \frac{J}{kg} \times 1.061 \times 1.044 \times 0.997 = 0.902 \ Gy$$

This answer is almost exactly the same as that given in example 7-10. Such close agreement could not always be expected, but it does suggest that a detailed knowledge of the composition of the walls is also not critical. Of course, if some material, say aluminum, quite different from water were used, the results would not be so close (see problem 14).

In the above examples, the cavity-gas calibration factor was determined from an exposure calibration. It can just as easily be determined from an absorbed dose calibration. To do this we replace equation 7-30 by the much simpler equation 7-31.

$$D_{med} = M \cdot N_D \tag{7-31}$$

where N_D is the absorbed dose (to the medium) per unit signal of the dosimeter; N_D is the absorbed dose calibration factor.

To determine N_{gas} we solve for $N_{gas} = WQ/mM$ from equations 7-15 and 7-31 to yield:

$$N_{gas} = N_D \left[\frac{(\bar{\mu}_{ab}/\rho)^{wall}_{air}}{\bar{\bar{S}}^{wall}_{air}} \right]_{Co} \left[\frac{k(c_{wall})}{k(a_{wall})} \right]_{Co} \left[\frac{(\bar{\mu}_{ab}/\rho)^{air}_{med}}{k(c_{med})} \right]_{Co} \tag{7-33a}$$

Absorbed dose calibrations are available for certain reference energies, such as ^{60}Co radiation, at a number of standardization laboratories throughout the world. It is still up to the user of radiation, however, to be able to determine the absorbed dose at any other energy by evaluating equation 7-34 or 7-35.

Agreed-on Dose Calculation Factors for High Energy Photons

Although we have developed a theoretical framework for the calculation of absorbed dose for high energy photon beams, the difficulties that have been mentioned are such that we do not seriously recommend direct evaluation of these equations for any given ionization chamber. They are presented here rather to increase the radiation user's understanding of the principles of radiation dosimetry.

For purposes of dose determination at high energies, the ICRU (I1) has published numerical values for a quantity that has come to known as C_λ, which is to be used in the following equation:

$$D_{med} = M \, N_X \, C_\lambda \qquad (7\text{-}36)$$

The ICRU values for C_λ are based partly on calculations and partly on measurements. Their values for a number of photon beams are given in column 2 of Table 7-5 along with a number of values calculated using the methods outlined in examples 7-8 through 7-12. The photon spectra listed in column 1 are taken from Table 7-2. A Farmer type chamber as described in example 7-8 is assumed and for column 3 it is taken to be made of Bakelite. Stopping power ratios are taken from Table 7-2. For columns 4 and 5 the chamber (and its buildup cap) was assumed to be made of Lucite and polystyrene respectively. For the calculations so far mentioned it is assumed that the dosimeter acts as a photon detector. That is, it is assumed that the photons interact with the walls of the chamber and that the ionization detected results from the electrons produced by these interactions. Equation 7-34 has been used.

In high energy beams some of the electrons will have ranges of several cm (see Table A-6) and will exceed the thickness of the walls, and the ionization will be caused in part by electrons that are set in motion in the medium. The limit of this would be when all of the electrons detected come from the medium and the dosimeter acts as an electron detector. In this case equation 7-35 would apply and the values in column 6 have been calculated this way. This latter assumption is also equivalent to assuming the ion chamber is made of truly water-equivalent material. In the lower energy part of the table, the ion chamber undoubtedly acts mainly as a photon detector, while for high energies it acts more and more like an electron detector. For energies in between these limits the ion chamber will act as a combination of the two, and this could be taken into account by combining equations 7-34 and 7-35 as follows (A4):

$$D_{med} = M \cdot N_{gas} \left\{ f \left(\frac{\overline{\mu}_{ab}}{\rho} \right)_{wall}^{med} \overline{\overline{S}}_{air}^{wall} \, k_c + (1 - f) \, \overline{\overline{S}}_{air}^{med} \, k(a) \right\} \qquad (7\text{-}37)$$

In this expression f is the fraction of the dosimeter signal that results from photon interactions which take place in the walls. $(1 - f)$ is the fraction that results from photon interactions in the medium that produce electrons which penetrate the walls and give rise to ionization in the chamber. All quantities within the braces must be evaluated for the radiation beam that is being measured, but it must be noted that the electron spectra will be different for each of the two stopping power ratios. The first term, for example, will be more concerned with high energy electrons while the second term would involve electrons that have penetrated the walls and have expended much of their energy. The fraction f is not generally known but can be estimated from the results of buildup measurements such as that depicted in Figure 7-9. Fortunately, as shown by the previous examples and the results given in Table 7-5, it is seldom necessary to make dose calculations so complicated.

TABLE 7-5

Values for C_λ

This table contains values for the factor C_λ, which may be used to convert the reading, M, of an exposure meter to absorbed dose in grays in water. $D_{water} = M \cdot N_x \cdot C_\lambda$ where N_x is the exposure calibration factor for cobalt 60 radiation. It is assumed the ionization chamber is of the Farmer type and has, with its buildup cap, an external radius c = 0.8 cm and an internal radius a = 0.3 cm. The photon spectra used are taken from Table 7-2. Values recommended by the ICRU (I2) are given in col. 2. The remainder of the table contains calculated data. For col. 3 it is assumed the chamber and its cap are made of Bakelite, for col. 4 Lucite and for col. 5 polystyrene. For col. 6 it was assumed that the walls were of negligible thickness and that it acted as an electron detector. Stopping power ratios from Table 7-2 were used for all calculations.

Spectrum (1)	Recommended by ICRU (2)	Calculated (for C_λ in Gy per Roentgen Divide by 100)			
		(3)	(4)	(5)	(6) no wall
		Bakelite	Lucite	Polyst.	
8. ^{60}Co, prim.	.95	.948	.948	.958	—
9. ^{60}Co, prim. + scat.	.95	.958	.952	.957	—
10. 6 MV	.94	.944	.943	.947	.940
11. 8 MV	.93	.940	.939	.944	.936
12. 12 MV	.92	.933	.933	.939	.920
13. 18 MV	.91	.929	.929	.929	.909
14. 26 MV	.90	.928	.927	.941	.904
15. 26 MV	.90	.930	.930	.940	.913
16. 35 MV	.88	.924	.922	.940	.889
17. 45 MV		.922	.920	.940	.883

Although our simple calculations are in fairly good agreement with each other and with the ICRU values, we recommend that the ICRU values be used until absorbed dose calibrations are supplied for individual chambers at a wide range of energies by standardization laboratories (G4). An example will illustrate the use of C_λ.

Example 7-13. A linear accelerator operating at 26 MeV is to be calibrated for therapy. A Farmer type dosimeter placed at a depth of 5 cm in a water phantom (or equivalent) gives a reading of M = 80.0 in 1.20 min. Temperature is 26° C; pressure is 100.6 kPa. The calibration factor as supplied by the standardization laboratory for cobalt 60 for this chamber is 1.04 and C_λ = .0090 (see Table 7-5). Determine the dose rate in water.

$$\text{Dose rate (uncor.)} = M \cdot N_X \cdot C_\lambda = \frac{80(1.04)(.0090)}{1.20} = .624 \text{ Gy/min}$$

$$\text{Dose rate} = \frac{(273.2 + 26)}{(273.2 + 22)} \times \frac{101.3}{100.6} \times .624 \frac{\text{Gy}}{\text{min}} = .637 \text{ Gy/min}$$

Dosimetry for Electron Beams

High energy electrons produced in linacs and betatrons are used in radiotherapy. The dosimetry of these particles is quite different from that of photons for the following reasons. When a photon beam interacts with a scattering medium, the spectrum of electrons at all points in the phantom is essentially the same, although there will be some slight change with depth (see Chapter 8). On the other hand, with high energy electrons the energy of the electrons in the beam continuously decreases with depth. For example, a 20 MeV electron beam will contain only 20 MeV electrons on the surface, 10 MeV electrons at a depth of about 5 cm, and 1–2 MeV electrons near the end of the electron range.

There is another important difference—with high energy photons a buildup region is required to develop electronic equilibrium, while for electrons no buildup cap is required and in fact it would be an advantage if one could measure an electron beam with a chamber having a very thin wall and shallow air cavity (as illustrated in Fig. 9-11). With such a chamber, which is an electron detector, the energy deposited in the medium (water) at the depth at which the electrons of initial energy E_0 have energy E can be determined from the Bragg-Gray relation (eq. 7-11), which we now write as:

$$D_{\text{water}} = \frac{Q}{m} \left(33.85 \frac{J}{C} \right) \bar{S}_{\text{air}}^{\text{water}} \qquad (7\text{-}38)$$

where $\bar{S}_{\text{air}}^{\text{water}}$ is the ratio of the ionizational stopping powers evaluated over the energy spectrum of the electrons that exists at the location of the chamber. Although equation 7-38 for electron beams is simpler than the corresponding equation for photon beams, it is more difficult to apply because, as mentioned above, the spectrum continually changes with depth.

Since many radiological laboratories are not equipped with facilities for absolute dosimetry, it is frequently necessary to use an instrument, such as a Farmer type dosimeter, which has been calibrated for exposure (with its buildup cap) at Co-60 energies in a standardization laboratory. If such a device is placed in a phantom irradiated by an electron beam, the dose may be determined from equation 7-38. As before we avoid the need to determine Q/m in absolute terms by using the cavity-gas calibration factor, N_{gas}, as given by equation 7-34. Thus:

$$D_{med} = M \cdot N_{gas} \cdot \overline{S}_{air}^{med} \cdot k_E \qquad (7\text{-}39)$$

$\overline{S}_{air}^{med}$ is again the ratio of ionizational stopping powers averaged over the spectrum of electrons "seen" at the point of measurement and k_E is a correction factor not unlike the attenuation correction factor, k_c, introduced in section 7.05 for photon dosimetry. k_E will depend on the shape and size of the dosimeter and is required for two reasons: (1) the introduction of the air cavity surrounded by walls of non–phantom-like material perturbs the electron flux slightly and (2) because the electrons came from one direction only, the point of measurement of the absorbed dose will be displaced from the center of the chamber towards the source of the electron beam. This correction is called a perturbation correction factor and is discussed in some detail in ICRU Report 21 (I5). For a cylindrical chamber the point of measurement can be shown to be at a point 2/3 to 3/4 of the cavity radius in front of the center of the chamber, provided it is irradiated from a direction perpendicular to the chamber axis. The perturbation and displacement correction is not required for the thin flat ionization chamber of Figure 9-11.

Normally, the electrons in an electron beam are all of the same energy, and as the beam penetrates the phantom the electron energy gradually decreases. This is only approximately so, however, because it has been shown (I5) that at any depth in a high energy electron beam the electron spectrum does contain an appreciable number of low energy electrons. Nevertheless, a useful approximation to the mean energy at depth d is given by $\overline{E} = E_0 (1 - d/R_0)$ where E_0 is the incident electron beam energy and R_0 is the practical range of electrons with energy E_0 (for a discussion of range, see sec. 6-13). The use of this relation and stopping power data for monoenergetic electrons (Table A-6) will be illustrated by an example.

Example 7-14. The Farmer type ionization chamber of example 7-8 is used to determine the absorbed dose in a water phantom irradiated by a 20 MeV beam of electrons. It is placed at a depth of 3 cm and gives a reading of 112 (corrected for temperature and pressure) for 10 units on the beam monitor. Determine the absorbed dose per monitor reading. The exposure calibration factor for this chamber is $N_X = 1.11$. Assume the perturbation correction factor is 1.00.

$\overline{E} = 20 (1 - 3/9.2) = 13.5$ MeV (use Table A-6 for range)
$\overline{S}_{air}^{water} \approx S(13.5)_{water}/S(13.5)_{air}$ (Table A-5)
$\qquad = 2.019/2.031 = 0.994$
$N_{gas} = 0.00844 \; N_X$
$D = 112 \times 1.11 \times 0.00844 \times 0.994 = 1.04$ Gy
$D = 0.104$ Gy per monitor unit.

For purposes of practical dosimetry a quantity known as C_E has been adapted for electron beam dosimetry in a way that is completely analogous to the use of C_λ for photon beams (eq. 7-36). The corresponding relation is:

$$D_{med} = M \cdot N_X \cdot C_E \qquad \text{(7-36a)}$$

where M is the dosimeter reading and N_X is the exposure calibration factor for a reference photon beam such as that from ^{60}Co.

Agreed on Dose Calibration Factors for Electrons

The ICRU (I5) has published values for C_E that are based on both theoretical and experimental data and that have become more or less accepted. They are given in Table 7-6 for a few energies and depths. The use of this factor will be illustrated by an example.

Example 7-15. Using data from Table 7-6, and considering the 20 MeV electron beam and irradiation conditions of example 7-14, determine the absorbed dose at depth of 3 cm for a dosimeter reading of 112. Again assume the exposure calibration factor, N_X, is 1.11.

$C_E = 0.00848$ (Table 7-6)
$D_{med} = 112 \times 1.11 \times 0.00848 = 1.05$ Gy

The answer in example 7-14 was 1% lower than this. In both examples the perturbation factor, k_E, was ignored. As a first step in taking account of it, the measurement could be thought of as being made not at a depth of 3 cm but at $3 - 0.3 \times (2/3) = 2.7$ cm.

Electron beam dosimetry is still at a relatively early stage in its development. For more "in depth" treatments, the student should consult ICRU Report 21 (I5) and literature referred to in that document.

Discussion of C_E and C_λ

The factors C_E and C_λ both decrease with increase in energy. The main factor bringing about this decrease is the stopping-power term. At high energies both $\overline{S}_{air}^{water}$ and $\overline{L}_{air}^{water}$ are a good deal less than 1.00 because of the polarization effect discussed in section 6.12. In the condensed medium (the water), this effect reduces the stopping power of the water

TABLE 7-6

Values for C_E

Recommended values for C_E, the factor to convert the reading, M, of an exposure meter to absorbed dose in water irradiated by an electron beam. $D_{water} = M \cdot N_x \cdot C_E$, where N_x is the exposure calibration factor for ^{60}Co radiation

| | C_E (for Gy per Roentgen Divide by 100) | | | | | | | | | |
| | Initial Electron Energy, E_0 | | | | | | | | | |
Depth d	5	10	15	20	25	30	35	40	45	50
1	0.922	.877	.843	.823	.808	.795	.784	.775	.768	.762
2		.893	.858	.835	.819	.806	.795	.786	.778	.771
3		.915	.871	.848	.830	.816	.804	.794	.786	.778
4		.947	.886	.859	.840	.824	.812	.801	.792	.785
5		.963	.901	.871	.847	.831	.819	.809	.799	.791
6			.933	.885	.856	.839	.825	.815	.806	.798
7			.965	.902	.867	.846	.832	.821	.812	.803
8				.941	.882	.854	.839	.827	.816	.808
9				.959	.898	.865	.847	.832	.820	.814
10				.926	.917	.878	.856	.840	.827	.819
12					.939	.906	.879	.857	.841	.829
14						.959	.907	.877	.857	.842
16							.954	.903	.876	.857
18								.940	.900	.874
20									.935	.895
22									.921	.924
24										.918

Data from ICRU, Report 21 (I5)

relative to the same material in the gaseous phase (steam). Thus, less energy is given to the water than one would expect on the basis of the ionization in the air.

The factors for C_E given in Table 7-6 are less than the corresponding values of C_λ given in Table 7-5 for at least two reasons. Consider the entry for 35 MV. The photon beam that is produced when 35 MeV electrons bombard a target contains all photons from 0 to 35 MeV and the average photon energy will be about 35/3 = 12 MeV. The average energy of the electrons that are set into motion by these photons will be still less, again by almost a factor of 1/3, or 4–5 MeV. The entry in Table 7-5 for 35 MV is 0.88 and the entry in Table 7-6 for 5 MeV electrons at a depth of 1 cm is 0.922. The value for a 5 MeV electron at the surface of a phantom would be somewhat less, likely not very different from 0.88. This calculation can only be a rough approximation but illustrates why we would expect the value for C_E to always be less than C_λ for any stated energy.

7.14   ABSORBED DOSE IN THE NEIGHBORHOOD OF AN INTERFACE BETWEEN DIFFERENT MATERIALS

In section 7.03 we discussed the problem of electronic equilibrium. When this condition is met, absorbed dose can be calculated from the photon fluence, Φ, thus:

$$D = \Phi \left(\frac{\mu}{\rho}\right) \overline{E}_{ab} = \psi \left(\frac{\mu_{ab}}{\rho}\right) \qquad (7\text{-}40)$$

where (μ/ρ) is the mass attenuation coefficient, $\overline{E}_{ab}$ is the average energy absorbed per interaction, ψ is the energy fluence, and (μ_{ab}/ρ) is the mass energy absorption coefficient. A closely related quantity is the kerma, K, given by:

$$K = \Phi \left(\frac{\mu}{\rho}\right) \overline{E}_{tr} = \psi \left(\frac{\mu_{tr}}{\rho}\right) \qquad (7\text{-}41)$$

where $\overline{E}_{tr}$ is the average energy transferred to electronic motion per interaction, $\overline{E}_{ab}$ is less than $\overline{E}_{tr}$ by the energy radiated from the system as bremsstrahlung, and (μ_{tr}/ρ) is the mass energy transfer coefficient.

In section 7.03 we saw that electronic equilibrium is not present at an air–phantom interface. Neither is it present at any interface between two different materials. Such a situation is illustrated in Figure 7-13 where we show a phantom consisting of 1 cm of muscle next to 1 cm bone. We wish to calculate kerma and dose for such a phantom irradiated by Co-60 representing high energy radiation, and 50 keV radiation representing soft radiation.

Imagine beams of these radiations incident from the left on composite phantoms. If the area of the beam is large, scattered radiation becomes important, making the problem very difficult. Here we will assume the beam is of small area so that the complications of scattered radiation are avoided. To solve this problem we need the basic data shown in Table 7-7 which were collected from the appendix. $\overline{E}_{tr}$ is assumed to be equal to $\overline{E}_{ab}$ for the energies and materials considered.

For a spectrum of photon energies, these two simple equations must be replaced by integrals as indicated by equation 7-6a.

Low Energy X Rays

Consider first the situation on the right side of Figure 7-13. We imagine a kerma of 100 J/kg on the incident side of the phantom locating point A on the curve. Point B is for a depth of 1 cm of muscle, which reduces the surface value of kerma by the factor $e^{-.224} = .799$, yielding point B at 79.9 J/kg. For point B the beam enters bone where the mass energy absorption coefficient is nearly 4 times that of muscle. The kerma therefore jumps by the factor $.1590/.0409 = 3.89$ to yield C with a value of 311. In the bone the beam is attenuated by the factor $e^{-(.3471)(1.65)} = .563$ to yield point D at 175 J/kg. At D we enter muscle so the kerma is now reduced by the factor 3.89 to yield point E at 45.0 J/kg. Point F is located at $45.0\,(.799) = 36.0$ J/kg.

The kerma in the phantom is thus composed of three exponentials AB, CD, and EF with "jumps" between them.

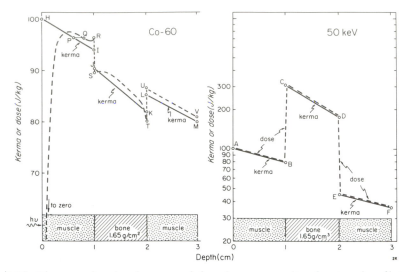

Figure 7-13. Diagram showing kerma and dose in a composite phantom irradiated from the left by cobalt 60 radiation and 50 keV radiation.

We now sketch the absorbed dose curve arising from this kerma. Table 7-7 shows that the range of electrons in muscle and bone produced by 50 keV photons is about 0.04 and 0.03 mm respectively. This means that, for all practical purposes, the energy is deposited at the point where the energy transfer occurred, and thus the energy absorption curve is identical to the kerma curve. The dose curve is shown by the dashed lines.

TABLE 7-7
Absorption Data for Co-60 and 50 keV Radiation

	Material	(μ/ρ) cm²/g	$\overline{E}_{tr} = \overline{E}_{ab}$	(μ_{ab}/ρ) cm²/g	S_{ion} MeV cm² g⁻¹	Range* mm	Table for Data
⁶⁰Co	muscle	.0626	.588 MeV	.0294	2.55	5	A-3c
	bone	.0604	.588 MeV	.0283	2.37	3	A-3d
50 keV	muscle	.2240	9.13 keV	.0409	15.3	.04	A-3c
	bone	.3471	22.9 keV	.1590	11.3	.03	A-3d

*Ranges taken from Table A-6 for the electron of maximum energy.

High Energy Radiation

The left side of Figure 7-13 shows the results of similar calculations using cobalt 60 radiation for a kerma at the surface of 100 J/kg. The kerma curve now consists of three exponentials, HI, JK, and LM, but now JK is below the others—in contrast to the situation depicted for 50 keV radiation. It is left as an exercise for the student to show that the kerma is given by these lines and to explain why J is below I. From these kerma curves we now attempt to sketch in the dose curve. For this radiation the highest energy electrons have a range of about 5 mm in muscle, so the dose curve must reach its maximum at a depth of 5 mm. If the beam is uncontaminated with electrons, then the surface dose is zero. Beyond the peak, the dose will decrease along a line parallel to kerma but above it. Since the dose at a point such as P is due to kerma "upstream" from it, the distance QP should be some *average* range or about 2 mm. As we approach the interface, the situation is confused but probably the dose rises slightly to R due to electrons scattered back from the layer of bone.

Now consider the situation at the interface. A point just to the left of the interface will "see" the same electron fluence as does a point just to the right of the interface. At the interface the mass stopping power changes from 2.55 in muscle to 2.37 in bone (see Table 7-7) so the absorbed dose must suddenly decrease by the factor 2.37/2.55 = 0.93, which locates point S. Once inside the bone the dose rises above kerma and runs parallel to it until the next interface is approached when it probably falls below kerma due to loss of backscattered electrons. At the interface, the dose suddenly increases by the factor 1.08 (2.55/2.37) to yield point U.

From this discussion it is evident that the accurate analysis of this problem is very complex, and careful measurements of the dose near interfaces is required. This problem will be returned to again in Chapter 11. This complex problem has been dealt with in the literature. Spiers (S10) has examined the problem in cavities in bone and Dutreix et al. (D3) have dealt with the dose near interfaces between various metals and carbon. Epp et al. (E3) and Nilsson et al. (N5) have studied dose buildup beyond small air cavities such as the larynx. The effects of buildup can extend over great distances for very high energy x rays (L6).

**7.15   RELATION BETWEEN ENERGY FLUENCE
                        AND EXPOSURE**

In some calculations involving integral dose (sec. 11.08) and protection (Chapter 15) and in dealing with exposure from radioactive sources, it is convenient to have a relation between energy fluence and exposure in roentgens. Consider an x ray beam incident on unit area. We want the relation between the energy fluence, Ψ, through this area, and the exposure X at the point P in the center of the area. Imagine a small mass of air at P. The energy absorbed by it from the beam is simply $\Psi\,(\mu_{ab}/\rho)_{air}$. Since 1 roentgen corresponds to an energy absorption in air of .00873 J/kg, an alternative expression for the same energy absorption is (.00873 J/kg R) X. Equating these and rearranging we have:

$$\text{energy fluence per roentgen:} \quad \frac{\Psi}{X} = \frac{.00873 \text{ J}}{(\mu_{ab}/\rho)_{air} \text{ kg R}} \quad (7\text{-}42)$$

If (μ_{ab}/ρ) is expressed in m²/kg, the energy fluence per roentgen is in joules per m² per R. Values of energy fluence per roentgen for a range of photon energies are given in Appendix A-2b and are plotted in Figure 7-14. At low energies the mass energy absorption coefficient is large and the energy fluence per roentgen is small; at high energies the reverse is the case. There is a rapid rise from 10 keV but relatively little change beyond 100 keV.

The rather complicated curve of Figure 7-14 results from the complicated variation of the energy absorption coefficient of air with photon energy. The energy absorption coefficient shows a minimum at 0.1 MeV and a maximum at 0.5 MeV. It follows that the energy fluence per R will show a maximum at 0.1 and a minimum at 0.5 MeV as indicated in Figure 7-14. The auxiliary scale of Figure 7-14, relating the photon energy to half-value layer, is the same as for Figure 7-8.

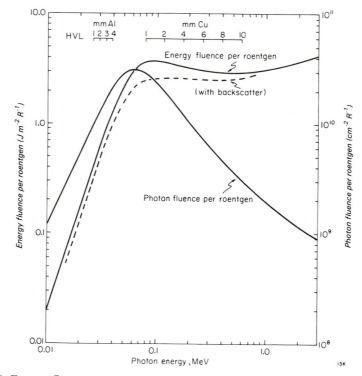

Figure 7-14. Energy fluence per roentgen and photon fluence per roentgen as a function of photon energy. The upper scale shows the HVL in mm Al and in mm Cu. (HVL is discussed in Chapter 8).

In Figure 7-14 the unit area was imagined to be in free air, so that there was no scattering to it from surrounding objects. If, however, the unit area is imagined to lie on a scattering surface, then it will be traversed by scattered radiation as well as primary. The exposure for the same primary radiation will be increased by the backscatter factor (see Chapter

10) and the energy fluence per R is thus reduced by this factor. The dotted curve of Figure 7-14 is calculated assuming a backscatter factor for an area of 400 cm².

Photon Fluence per Roentgen

In some circumstances one may be interested in relating photon fluence to exposure. The relation between energy fluence, Ψ, and photon fluence, Φ, is simply $\Psi = \Phi \cdot h\nu$ and hence from equation 7-42 the photon fluence per roentgen is:

$$\text{photon fluence per roentgen;} \quad \frac{\Phi}{X} = \frac{0.00873 \text{ J}}{h\nu(\mu_{ab}/\rho)_{air} \text{ kg R}} \quad (7\text{-}43)$$

We illustrate these ideas by an example.

Example 7-16. Calculate the energy fluence and photon fluence per R for $h\nu = 1$ MeV. Check your calculations with data in Table A-2b and plotted in Figure 7-14.

For 1 MeV photons $(\mu_{ab}/\rho)_{air} = .0279 \dfrac{\text{cm}^2}{\text{g}} = .00279 \dfrac{\text{m}^2}{\text{kg}}$
(Table A-3a)

$$\frac{\Psi}{X} = \frac{.00873 \text{ J kg}^{-1} \text{ R}^{-1}}{.00279 \text{ m}^2\text{kg}^{-1}} = 3.13 \frac{\text{J}}{\text{m}^2\text{R}} \quad (\text{eq. 7-42})$$

Substituting $h\nu = 1.0$ MeV $= 1.602 \times 10^{-13}$ J (see Table A-1) yields

$$\frac{\Phi}{X} = \frac{0.00873 \text{ J kg}^{-1} \text{ R}^{-1}}{1.602 \times 10^{-13} \text{ J} \times 0.00279 \text{ m}^2 \text{ kg}^{-1}}$$

$$= 1.95 \times 10^{13} \text{ photons m}^{-2} \text{ R}^{-1} \text{ (eq. 7-43)}$$

These check with the values in Table A-6 and Figure 7-14. These calculations tell us that we require an energy fluence of 3.13 J/m² of 1 MeV photons or a photon fluence of 1.95×10^{13} photons/m² to register an exposure of 1 R.

Exposure Rate from Gamma Emitters (Exposure Rate Constant)

In dealing with the dosimetry of isotopes, we require a relation between the activity of the source in becquerels (or curies) and the exposure rate at some reference point in air near this source. The exposure rate constant, Γ (Greek capital letter gamma), is defined as the exposure rate in R/hr at a point 1 meter from a 1 Ci source. From the inverse square law the exposure rate, X/t, at any point P, distance d, from a source of activity A is then simply:

$$\frac{X}{t} = \frac{\Gamma \cdot A}{d^2} \quad (7\text{-}44)$$

Γ has dimensions R m² hr⁻¹ Ci⁻¹. We illustrate this idea with a simple example.

Example 7-17. A therapy center purchases an 8000 Ci source of cobalt 60. Determine the expected exposure rate at 80 cm from this source. Γ for cobalt 60 is 1.29 R m² hr⁻¹ Ci⁻¹.

$$\text{exposure rate } \frac{X}{t} = \frac{1.29 \text{ R m}^2 \text{ hr}^{-1} \text{ Ci}^{-1} \times 8000 \text{ Ci}}{(.8 \text{ m})^2} = 16100 \frac{R}{hr}$$
(eq. 7-42)

The actual output of the source would be somewhat less than this because some of the radiation would be attenuated and absorbed in the source. The strengths of sources are often described in terms of Rhm, which stands for the exposure rate in roentgens per hr at 1 meter. The above source would be referred to as having an Rhm value of 8000 × 1.29 = 10,320. For smaller sources Γ is sometimes expressed in R cm² hr⁻¹ mCi⁻¹. The student can easily show that with this definition Γ is then numerically 10 times as large. For example for ⁶⁰Co: Γ = 12.9 R cm² hr⁻¹ mCi⁻¹.

Determination of Γ for an Isotope that Emits 1 Photon of Energy hν per Disintegration

If the disintegration scheme for an isotope is known, then Γ can be calculated using the ideas of energy fluence per roentgen. First, assume each disintegration of the isotope gives rise to *one photon of energy hν*.

Since 1 Ci undergoes 3.7 × 10¹⁰ dis/s (see sec. 3.03) and since the area of a sphere of radius 1 m is 4π m² and since 1 hr = 3600 s it follows that:

$$\frac{\text{photon fluence in 1 hr}}{\text{1 m from a 1 Ci source}} = \frac{3.7 \times 10^{10} \times 3600}{4\pi} = 1.060 \times 10^{13} \frac{\text{photons}}{\text{m}^2}$$

Substituting this photon fluence in equation 7-42 and solving for the exposure X we obtain:

$$\frac{\text{exposure in 1 hr}}{\text{1 m from a 1 Ci source}} = \frac{h\nu(\mu_{ab}/\rho)_{air}}{.00873} \frac{\text{kg R}}{J} \times 1.060 \times 10^{13} \frac{\text{photons}}{\text{m}^2}$$

If we agree to express the absorption coefficient in m²/kg and the photon energy in MeV (1 MeV = 1.602 × 10⁻¹³ J) then the right side simplifies and becomes:

$$h\nu(\mu_{ab}/\rho)(194.5) \text{ R}$$

This has dimensions of exposure as it should. The quantity on the left is *numerically* equal to Γ so the relation we seek is:

$$\Gamma = 194.5 \; h\nu(\mu_{ab}/\rho)_{air} \text{ R m}^2 \text{ hr}^{-1} \text{ Ci}^{-1} \qquad (7-44)$$

which is the relation between the exposure rate constant and the energy, hν, of the photon emitted. To use this relation, hν must be expressed in MeV and the energy absorption coefficient for air in m²/kg. Γ as given by equation 7-44 is tabulated in Table A-2b and plotted in Figure 7-15. As the photon energy is increased from 0.01 MeV, Γ falls rapidly because of the rapid decrease in the energy absorption coefficient, reaching a minimum at about 60 keV. Beyond this minimum it increases, because (μ_{ab}/ρ) is essentially constant and the dependence is then mainly on the photon's energy.

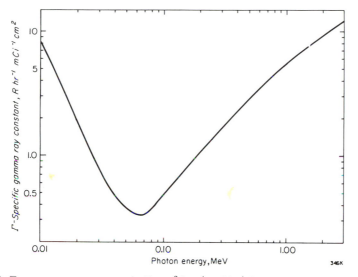

Figure 7-15. Exposure rate constant in R cm^2 hr^{-1} mCi^{-1} for a point source emitting 1 photon per disintegration of energy, hν. It also gives the exposure rate in R/hr 1 meter from a point source of 1 curie emitting 1 photon per disintegration of energy hν.

Example 7-18. Evaluate Γ for an isotope that emits 1 photon of 1 MeV per disintegration.

For 1 MeV photon: $(\mu_{ab}/\rho)_{air} = .00279$ m^2/kg   (Table A-3a)

$\Gamma = 194.5 \ (1.00) \ (.00279) \ = .543$ R m^2 hr^{-1} Ci^{-1} (eq. 7-44)

This checks with Figure 7-14 and Table A-2b.

Calculation of Γ (Exposure Rate Constant) for a Radionuclide

In the last section we showed how one could calculate Γ for an isotope that emitted 1 photon per disintegration. Here we are concerned with a real isotope, which may have a complex decay scheme emitting many gammas, each with different probability. Suppose the isotope emits photons hν_1, hν_2 . . . hν_n and the number of these per disintegration is N_1, N_2 . . . N_n. The total exposure rate constant is:

$$\Gamma = N_1\Gamma \ (h\nu_1) + N_2\Gamma(h\nu_2) \ . \ . \ . \ N_n\Gamma(h\nu_N)$$

To illustrate this type of calculation, we determine Γ for cobalt 60 whose decay scheme is given in Figure 3-7. Using the data from this diagram we construct the following chart:

hν (MeV)	N (Fig. 3-7)	Γ (Fig. 7-15 or Table A-2b)	N · Γ
1.173	.998	.617	.616
1.332	1.000	.681	.681

Total Γ (Rm² hr⁻¹ Ci⁻¹) = 1.297

For cobalt 60 the two gammas are nearly the same energy with an average value of 1.25 MeV and are emitted in almost equal numbers of 1 per disintegration, so it would be accurate enough to take Γ as twice the value of hν = 1.25 MeV.

The type of calculation shown above was used to determine Γ for the commonly used isotopes. See Tables 13-2 and 14-1. The student should note that this calculation gives the exposure due to gamma rays, which could be converted to dose using the f factors of Table A-7. It does not include the dose due to the beta particles that may be emitted in the disintegration of the isotope. The contribution from the beta particles to the dose is important when the isotope is ingested. This will be discussed in Chapter 15.

7.16 SUMMARY OF METHODS TO DETERMINE ABSORBED DOSE

(1)
$$D_{med} = \frac{Q}{m_{air}} \left[33.85 \frac{J}{C} \right] \bar{\bar{S}}^{med}_{air} \qquad (7\text{-}11)$$

This is the Bragg-Gray relation and relates the absorbed dose at a point in a medium to Q, the charge liberated in an air cavity centered at the point. m_{air} is the mass of the gas and $\bar{\bar{S}}^{med}_{air}$ is the ratio of averaged mass stopping powers discussed in section 7.04. This relation forms the basis of all dosimetry using ion chambers.

(2)
$$D_{med} = \frac{Q}{m_{air}} \left[33.85 \frac{J}{C} \right] \bar{\bar{S}}^{wall}_{air} \left(\frac{\bar{\mu}_{ab}}{\rho} \right)^{med}_{wall} k_c \qquad (7\text{-}15)$$

This equation extends the Bragg-Gray relation to a practical ion chamber whose walls are made of some known material. Q is the charge liberated in a cavity containing a known mass, m, of air; $\bar{\bar{S}}^{wall}_{air}$ is the ratio of averaged stopping powers and can be obtained from Table 7-2; $(\bar{\mu}_{ab}/\rho)^{med}_{air}$ is the ratio of averaged mass energy absorption coefficients, obtainable from Table 7-4; k_c is the attenuation or replacement factor discussed in section 7.05. This equation is used for absolute dosimetry and is valid for all photon energies.

(3)
$$D_{fs} = M \cdot N_X \left[0.00873 \frac{J}{kg\ R} \right] \left(\frac{\bar{\mu}_{ab}}{\rho} \right)^{med}_{air} k(r_{med}) \qquad (7\text{-}28)$$

This is the "dose in free space" and is the dose to a small mass of phantom-like material, of radius r, placed at a point in a beam. M is the dosimeter reading; N_X is its exposure calibration factor; $(\bar{\mu}_{ab}/\rho)$ is the ratio of averaged mass energy absorption coefficients; and $k(r_{med})$ is the attenuation correction for the material of radius r. All quantities must be evaluated for the energy of the beam being measured. This method is useful in providing a reference dose for tissue-air ratios and backscatter factors. It may also be used to calibrate the output of a treatment unit. It is limited to radiation energies for which an exposure calibration factor is available.

(4)
$$D_{med} = M \cdot N_X \left[0.00873 \frac{J}{kg\ R} \right] \left(\frac{\bar{\mu}_{ab}}{\rho} \right)_{air}^{med} k(c_{med}) \qquad (7\text{-}30)$$

This is the dose at a point in a phantom. All quantities are the same as described for the dose in free space except that c is the outer radius of the dosimeter as it was configured (with buildup cap) for the exposure calibration N_X. This method can be used to determine a reference dose for tissue-phantom ratios and also for calibrating the output of a treatment unit. Like the dose in free space, it is used for the same beam energies for which the exposure calibration applies.

(5)
$$D_{med} = M \cdot N_D \qquad (7\text{-}31)$$

This again determines the absorbed dose at a point in a phantom. N_D is an absorbed dose calibration factor. The dose being measured must again be in a beam of the quality to which the calibration factor applies.

(6)
$$D_{med} = M \cdot N_{gas} \cdot \left[\left(\frac{\bar{\mu}_{ab}}{\rho} \right)_{wall}^{med} \cdot \bar{\bar{S}}_{air}^{wall} \right] \cdot [k_c] \qquad (7\text{-}34)$$

This method can be used for determining absorbed dose in a beam of any energy provided the dosimeter is acting as a "photon detector." N_{gas} is the "gas calibration factor" and is a constant of the dosimeter, which may be determined at a calibration energy from either an exposure calibration or an absorbed dose calibration. The terms in square brackets must be evaluated for the energy of the beam being measured and can be obtained from Tables 7-2 and 7-4, equation 7-14, and Figure 7-5.

(7)
$$D_{med} = M \cdot N_{gas} \cdot \left[\bar{\bar{S}}_{air}^{med} \right] \cdot \left[k(a_{med}) \right] \qquad (7\text{-}35)$$

This equation holds if the ion chamber is an "electron detector." The bracketed terms must apply to the beam energy being measured and can be obtained from Table 7-2 and Figure 7-5. This equation can also be used for electron beams.

(8)
$$D_{med} = M \cdot N_X \cdot C_\lambda \qquad (7\text{-}36)$$

This equation can be used for dose calculations in high energy photon beams where C_λ is a practical dose calculation factor and can be obtained from Table 7-5, column 7.

(9)
$$D_{med} = M \cdot N_X \cdot C_E \tag{7-36a}$$

This equation can be used for high energy electron beams. C_E can be obtained from Table 7-6.

PROBLEMS

1. The principal gamma ray lines from radium, in equilibrium with its daughter products, are given in Table 13-1. Determine the following: (a) the photon fluence rate at a distance of 1 cm from a "point source" of 1 mg of radium (3.7×10^7 Bq), (b) the energy fluence rate at the same point, (c) the average photon energy, (d) the single photon energy, which has an attenuation coefficient in water equal to the apparent attenuation coefficient of the spectrum given.

2. For the gamma ray spectrum given in problem 1, calculate the kerma rate to a small mass of water placed at 1 cm from the source. Calculate also the dose rate to the water, assuming equilibrium between kerma and dose.

3. Starting with the spectrum given in problem 1, assume the radiation to have passed through 10.0 cm of water. Again find the equivalent energy as in problem 1d.

4. Radiation has an HVL of 1.5 mm Cu. Find the equivalent kilovoltage, V_e. Assuming the mean photon energy is equal to V_e, calculate the mean energy of the recoil electrons. For simplicity consider that only Compton electrons are set in motion.

5. A small cavity of volume 0.4 cm³ placed in a block of tissue records an ionization of 6.67×10^{-10} C when irradiated with the radiation of Problem 4. Find the absorbed dose in soft tissue. Assume a mean stopping power ratio of 1.18.

6. Using the data for the energy absorption coefficient of the Table A-3d, calculate the f factor for bone for a photon energy of 0.10 MeV. Check your result with the f value given in Table A-7 or in Figure 8-10.

7. A very small, correctly calibrated, dosimeter records an exposure of 200 R when imbedded in solid bone and irradiated with HVL 2.0 mm Cu. Calculate the absorbed dose in the bone.

8. A small carbon chamber with volume of 0.1 cm³ is placed in muscle and a charge of 6.67×10^{-9} coulomb is liberated by radiation with HVL 1.5 mm Cu. Find the absorbed dose in the muscle. Assume mean stopping power of carbon relative to air is 1.02.

9. Explain why electronic equilibrium can never be achieved by very high energy radiation.

10. Find the mean energy of electrons set in motion by 4.0 MeV photons. What is the range of such electrons in water, in air (density 0.001293 gm/cm³), and in bone (density 1.65 gm/cm³)?

11. The exposure rate from a cobalt unit as measured with a correctly calibrated Victoreen® dosimeter is 80 R/min. This measurement was made under conditions of backscatter and with a chamber of the proper wall thickness. Calculate the absorbed dose rate in muscle at the peak of the buildup curve.

12. A carbon chamber of volume 1.5 cm³ is placed in a carbon block and centered in a 24 MV betatron beam. The block is adjusted in thickness to give the maximum ionization. An ionization of 3.0×10^{-8} coulomb is collected in 30 seconds. The temperature is 25°C, the pressure is 75.5 cm of Hg. Find the absorbed dose rate in water at the peak of the buildup curve. Assume mean stopping power of carbon relative to air is 0.95.

13. The energy absorption coefficients for air are tabulated in Table A-3. For photon energies of 0.10, 0.50, and 2.0 MeV, calculate the energy fluence/R and the photon fluence/R. Check your values with the answers given in Table A-2.

14. An ionization chamber has walls made of aluminum and is used to measure absorbed dose in a water phantom from a beam from a 10 MV linear accelerator. A cobalt exposure calibration factor is obtained and has a value 1.07. The ion chamber has an inner radius of 1.5 mm and a wall thickness of 2 mm. For one unit on the linac monitor, the dosimeter gives a reading of 1.43. Following example 7-10, determine the absorbed dose and discuss the assumptions that are required in order to obtain its value. Estimate the accuracy of the value you have obtained.

Chapter 8

THE QUALITY OF X RAYS
(HALF-VALUE LAYER)

8.01 QUALITY

In the last chapter methods for measuring an amount of radiation were described. In this chapter, methods for describing the *kind* of radiation in the beam will be presented. Since in radiology one is interested in the penetration of the beam into or through the patient, it is logical to describe the nature of the beam in terms of its ability to penetrate some material of known composition. Quality is expressed in terms of the half-value layer. *The half-value layer (HVL) is the thickness of some standard material required to reduce a beam to half its original value as measured by a device calibrated to read exposure in roentgens.* Over the range 120 to 400 kV, half-value layers are usually given in mm of copper, while below 120 kV aluminum is used.

The specification of the quality of a beam in terms of HVL is really a very crude specification, since it tells very little concerning the number and energy of the photons present in the beam. A complete specification of the quality requires a knowledge of the amount of energy present in each energy interval as indicated in Figure 2-13. For most purposes, such a complete specification is not necessary because the biological effects of x rays are not very sensitive to the energy of the radiation. For this reason, the specification of the quality in terms of HVL is usually sufficient.

8.02 **EFFECTS OF FILTERS ON AN X RAY BEAM**

When monoenergetic electrons bombard a *thick target* the spectral distribution of the *unfiltered* beam is the straight dashed line A of Figure 8-1 described by equation 2-5. This distribution would not be suitable for deep therapy because the low energy photons would not penetrate to the tumor and would merely increase the dose to the superficial layers of the body; neither would it be useful in diagnostic radiology since none of the low energy photons would penetrate through the patient to reach the imaging device but they would contribute to the dose. The unwanted low energy radiation may be removed from the beam by the use of appropriate filters.

Curve B results when beam A is filtered by 1 mm aluminum. Curve C results when beam B is filtered by an additional 0.25 mm tin. It will be seen that this reduces the energy fluence practically to zero in the region

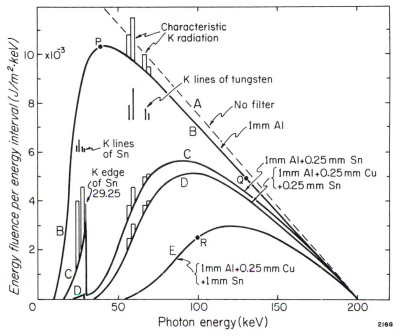

Figure 8-1. Graph showing how the spectral distribution of radiation generated by 200 keV electrons bombarding a thick W target changes with filtration. Dashed line A, unfiltered beam. Curves B, C, D, and E are obtained from A by calculating the attenuation produced by the indicated layers of Al, Cu, and Sn.

from 30 to 40 keV but allows a band of radiation to pass through the filter just below the K absorption edge of tin at 29.2 keV. Above 29.2 keV the tin absorbs strongly by the photoelectric process but just below this energy the photons have insufficient energy to eject the K electrons, so the photoelectric absorption is small. (For details of the attenuation coefficient in the region of an absorption edge see Figure 5-5). In addition, the photons that strongly interact with the tin by a photoelectric process above 29.2 keV will produce tin atoms with holes in the K shell and when these holes are filled, the characteristic radiation of tin at energies from 25 to 29 keV will be produced. This characteristic radiation will add to curve C as indicated by the spikes on the curve below the absorption edge.

The radiation below 29.2 keV may be filtered out by placing a thin layer of copper between the tin filter and the patient as shown by curve D. The copper absorbs strongly in the region below 29.2 keV and so removes most of the spike in curve C. In addition, the copper strongly absorbs the characteristic radiation of tin. It is usual to place a thin layer of aluminum next to the copper to absorb the characteristic radiation from the copper. Composite filters of this kind are called *Thoraeus filters* (T2, T3). It is important that they be arranged in the proper order with the highest atomic number material nearest the x ray tube; otherwise, the characteristic radiation will not be stopped. A more penetrating beam E can be obtained by further filtration of D.

8.03　　　THE MEASUREMENT OF HALF-VALUE LAYER

The half-value layer of an x ray beam can be obtained by measuring the exposure rate of an x ray machine for a series of different attenuators placed in the beam. The components should be arranged as indicated in Figure 8-2. The sensitive volume of the exposure meter should be positioned with a clamp at point C on the axis of the beam. The detector should be at least 50 cm from the end of the treatment cone or beam-defining system of the unit so that radiation scattered from B is avoided. In addition, the x ray beam should be directed in such a way in the room that detector C is at least 50 cm from any scattering objects such as the floor or the walls.

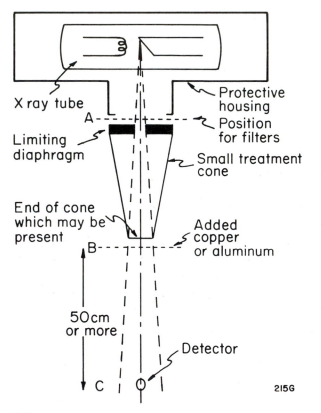

Figure 8-2. Ideal arrangement for accurate measurement of half-value layer.

The beam from the machine should be reduced in size until it is about 5 by 5 cm at the detector. Care should be taken to ensure that the detector is in the center of this 5 by 5 cm field. When the x ray machine is provided with a light localizer and continuously adjustable diaphragms, centering of the detector is easily carried out. One way to check the alignment is to mount a fluorescent screen just beyond the detector and momentarily turn on the x ray machine. Standing well to the side of the unit one can quickly observe whether or not the shadow of the detector is centered in the field. Too small an x ray field should not be used to avoid the possibility of part of the detector being outside the field.

The x ray unit is provided with a slot at A into which filters may be positioned. A clamp should be arranged on a retort stand to hold additional attenuators of aluminum or copper at position B. A series of such attenuators about 5 by 5 cm in area should be assembled. Care should be taken to insure that the aluminum or copper attenuators are of uniform thickness and do not contain impurities as do many alloys that may "look like" copper or aluminum.

The exposure rate in R/min should be determined for a series of attenuators placed at B, while the kV and mA of the tube are held as constant as possible. Results of a typical experiment are given in Figure 8-3. In Chapter 5, it was noted that an exponential attenuation curve should appear as a straight line when plotted on semilog paper. The curve of Figure 8-3 is not linear because the beam of radiation from the x ray machine is not monoenergetic. Each layer of attenuating material acts very much like the filters described in section 8.02 and progressively changes the quality of the beam. However, under heavy filtration, the softer components are almost completely removed and the radiation transmitted is more nearly monochromatic and the attenuation curve approaches a straight line.

Examination of Figure 8-3 shows that the HVL of the unfiltered beam is 0.35 mm Cu (0.35 mm Cu reduces the exposure rate from 68 R/min to 34 R/min). If 1.0 mm of copper is used as the filter, then an extra 1.3 mm is required to reduce the exposure rate by one-half (20 R/min to 10 R/min) so the HVL has been increased to 1.3 mm Cu. By further filtration the HVL may be increased still more to yield an HVL of 2.7 mm Cu for 4 mm Cu filtration. A few of the possible filter and HVL combinations are shown in the insert to Figure 8-3. For each filtration, the exposure rate relative to that obtained with 1.0 mm Cu filtration is given. It should be noted that by operating the machine with HVL 2.7 mm Cu, the exposure rate is only 27% of the value that may be obtained with HVL 1.3 mm Cu.

After obtaining the data of Figure 8-3 the user would decide on the filter to be used in the routine operation of the machine and the appropriate filter or filters would be locked into place in the filter slot. The beam from the machine with the filter at A (Fig. 8-2) might now be slightly different from the beam with the filter at B because of the influence of scattered radiation from the cone or material on the end of the cone.

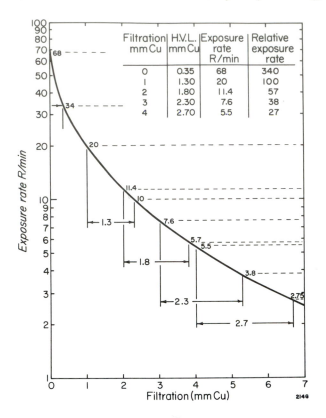

Filtration mm Cu	H.V.L. mm Cu	Exposure rate R/min	Relative exposure rate
0	0.35	68	340
1	1.30	20	100
2	1.80	11.4	57
3	2.30	7.6	38
4	2.70	5.5	27

Figure 8-3. Experimentally determined attenuation curve for 200 kV radiation, showing how the HVL may be determined for a number of filtrations.

To check this possibility, three measurements should be made: first with no added filter at B, the second and third with thicknesses just less and just more than the expected HVL allowing one to determine the HVL by interpolation.

Effect of Scatter on HVL Measurements

If scattered radiation is not avoided, very erroneous values for the HVL may be obtained. To illustrate this, an experiment was performed on a 250 kV unit and the results are summarized in Figure 8-4. A detector was placed on the axis of the beam at a point P, 100 cm from the source. Measurements were first made using a small field at the detector (about 5 by 5 cm) with the attenuator first at position A and then with it against the detector at position B. In the first case, curve A_1 is obtained; in the second, B_1. These curves are very different, the beam in B_1 being apparently much more penetrating than in A_1 since more radiation is transmitted through any given thickness. This discrepancy arises from the effects of scattered radiation. With the attenuation at A, a negligible fraction of the scattered radiation from the attenuator reaches the detector, while at B, because of its close proximity to the detector, a large fraction of the scattered radiation reaches P. These two conditions are referred to as attenuation experiments in "good geometry" and in "bad geometry."

The geometry may be changed again by altering the field size as illustrated in the lower part of the insert of Figure 8-4. With a field size of 30 by 30 cm at P curves, A_2 and B_2 were obtained. B_2 gives what appears to be an even more penetrating beam than B_1 because now the detector sees even more scattered radiation from the attenuator.

The half-value layers that may be read off Figure 8-4 range from 2.0 to 2.8 mm of copper (see numbers affixed to graph at the 50% level). The correct half-value layer is the minimum value, 2.0, obtained in the experiment in which the scattered radiation from the attenuator was avoided.

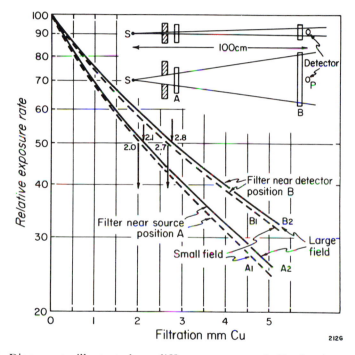

Figure 8-4. Diagram to illustrate how different apparent half-value layers may be obtained for the same beam by using different arrangements of field size and attenuator position in making the measurements.

Effect of Detector on HVL Measurement

The measurement of HVL requires the availability of an exposure meter calibrated to read in roentgens, that is an ion chamber with walls equivalent to air (see Chapter 7). A perfect exposure meter would for example give the same reading for 1 roentgen of radiation regardless of whether it were produced by 10 or 1000 keV photons or any energy between these. If the measuring device does not have such a "flat" response for the spectrum of radiations in the beam, the HVL measurement will be in error, since the spectrum and hence the response will be dependent on the amount of attenuator added during the HVL determination. An extreme example of this situation is illustrated in Figure 8-5 where an attenuation experiment was performed on a 130 kV x ray beam used in CT scanning (see Chapter 16). Two sets of measurements were carried out. One set—using a correctly calibrated air wall detector—gave an HVL of 5.7 mm Al; the second set—obtained using a high pressure xenon chamber as the detector—gave an incorrect HVL of 8.6 mm Al. The air wall detector gives a reading proportional to the energy absorbed in air while the xenon detector gives a reading essentially proportional to the energy fluence of the beam. The difference between the two curves is a striking illustration of the effects of "detector response" on the measured HVL.

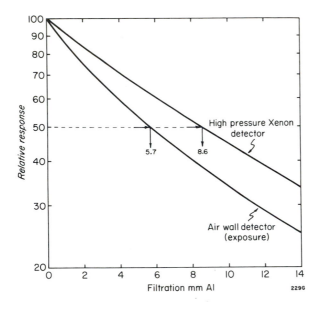

Figure 8-5. Graph showing that the measured attenuation of a beam from a 130 kV x ray machine depends upon the type of detector used in the experiment. The HVL of the beam is 5.7 not 8.6 mm of Al.

HVL and Filters for Therapy

When 200 to 400 kV machines were used in radiotherapy, the precise determination of the HVL was essential because the HVL determined the depth dose distribution achieved. Today HVL determinations for this range of energies are less important. In the 100 to 140 kV range, an HVL determination is still necessary. These beams are usually filtered with Al and are operated at an HVL of 2.0 to 3.0 mm Al. They are used to treat superficial tumors.

Cobalt 60 and cesium 137 emit essentially monoenergetic radiation so filters are not required. Although the specification of the HVL of a cobalt beam as 1.1 cm of Pb is true, it is not a useful statement; it is much more relevant to specify the average energy of the emitted radiation as 1.25 MeV.

Linacs in the energy range 4 to 20 MeV and betatrons at 20 to 30 MeV produce continuous distributions of radiation from about 1 MeV to their peak energy. Examination of Figure 5-11 will convince the reader that for this energy range there is no *good* filter material. The attenuation coefficient for lead passes through a minimum value at 3 MeV. A lead filter will therefore discriminate against both the low and the high energy radiation from a linac and will transmit radiation at 3 MeV. A filter made with high Z material therefore will make the beam less useful. A medium Z material such as Cu has an attenuation coefficient essentially constant with energy, so filters of such materials will have no preferential filtering effect and will only reduce the intensity of the beam. A low atomic number filter of carbon or aluminum will reduce the low energy radiation slightly more than the high energy radiation; hence, if a filter is to be used it should be of such material. There is a difficulty, however, since these have small density and thick layers would be required. Such machines are therefore usually used without a filter.

The specification of the quality of these high energy beams is not easy. Certainly the specification of the HVL in copper or lead is useless since a beam that contains the useful high energy photons, which can penetrate into water, would be more easily stopped in lead than lower energy less useful photons. High energy beams from linear accelerators and betatrons should be specified in terms of the penetration of the beam in water. Unfortunately, however, no consensus has emerged as to how the quality of such beams should be described.

High energy beams from betatrons and linacs are sharply "peaked" along the axis (see Fig. 2-16) so flattening filters are required. They should be made of low atomic number material (Chapter 4) so that the desirable high energy photons will not be removed.

HVL and Filters in Diagnostic Radiology

Unless care is taken, a diagnostic x ray examination may involve enough radiation to be a real hazard to the patient. Often the judicious use of filters can reduce the dose to the patient without any deleterious effect on the diagnostic value of the radiograph. In general, enough filters should be used to remove low energy photons, which cannot reach the imaging device and which only serve to increase the dose to tissues where the beam enters the patient. All diagnostic x ray machines used in routine examinations should be equipped with a total filtration (inherent plus added) of 3 mm Al permanently locked into place. These will have an HVL of 1 to 3 mm Al dependent on kV. For xeroradiography at 45 to 50 kV, the total filter should be 1.5 mm Al, while for special mammography studies using 30 kV with film as the detector, the total filter should be 0.5 mm Al. These beams usually have HVL values less than 1 mm Al.

It is obvious that photons with insufficient energy to pass through the patient can serve no useful purpose and should be removed from the beam. It is not so obvious that high energy photons should also be removed. This will be dealt with in section 8.05.

8.04   EQUIVALENT PHOTON ENERGY

In certain investigations, it is convenient to express the quality of an x ray beam in terms of the equivalent photon energy $\overline{h\nu}$ derived from a knowledge of the half-value layer. The type of x ray beam used in radiology is always heterogeneous, consisting of many different energies; however, we can refer to it as having an equivalent photon energy $\overline{h\nu}$ if monoenergetic radiation of this energy has the same HVL as the radiation in question. The relationship between $\overline{h\nu}$ and HVL is shown in Figure 8-6. It was obtained from the total mass attenuation coefficients given in the appendix. For example, from Table A-4g we note that Cu (density 8.96 g/cm³) has a $\mu/\rho = 0.455$ cm²/g at 100 keV. Hence

$$\mu = 8.96 \, \frac{g}{cm^3} \times 0.455 \, \frac{cm^2}{g} = 4.08 \, cm^{-1}$$

$$HVL = 0.693/4.08 \, cm^{-1} = 1.70 \, mm \, Cu \quad (eq. \, 5\text{-}3)$$

Thus a heterogeneous beam with HVL 1.70 mm Cu has an equivalent photon energy $h\overline{\nu} = 100$ keV. This point is marked P in Figure 8-6.

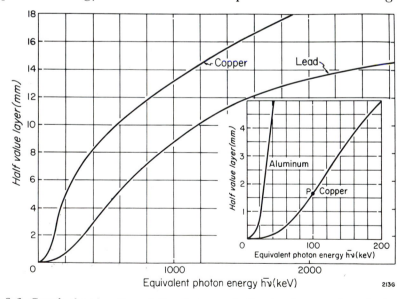

Figure 8-6. Graph showing the relation between half-value layer and equivalent photon energy, calculated from the total attenuation coefficients given in the appendix.

8.05   MEASURED SPECTRAL DISTRIBUTIONS

For many years, experimentally determined spectral distributions were not available, and it was necessary to rely on empirical formula such as equation 2-6, which was used to plot Figure 8-1. In the 1940s Greening (G6, G7), using an air wall ion chamber, carefully measured the transmission through known thicknesses of copper and aluminum and by appropriate mathematical manipulation determined the spectral distribution. A more direct approach was made possible with the development of the NaI scintillation spectrometer and more recently with the germanium lithium drifted, Ge(Li), spectrometer described in detail in Chapter 9. In these devices individual photons are detected, and the voltage output pulse is proportional to the energy of the detected photon. The voltage pulses are sorted for size in a pulse height analyzer and recorded in 400 or more different channels, each channel corresponding to a particular photon energy. The number of counts in a channel gives a measure of the number of photons with a particular energy.

The Ge(Li) detector yields remarkable resolution, allowing one to see the two $K\alpha$ and two $K\beta$ lines from tungsten (see curve D of Fig. 8-7). The resolution achievable with it is much better than with NaI (see Fig. 14-5) but there is one practical difficulty. Ge(Li) crystals cannot be made large and deep enough to fully absorb photons with more than about 150 keV. In contrast, NaI crystals can be grown to some 30 cm in diameter and up to 10 cm thick. The one-to-one correspondence between photon energy and output depends upon the *total* absorption of the photons incident on the device. For this reason Ge(Li) crystals are ideal for investigating diagnostic x rays but less useful in studying the more energetic radiations from therapy installations.

Since these spectrometers detect every photon emitted and since a second photon cannot be analyzed as to energy until the previous one has been processed, there is a finite counting rate of about 2000 c/s that cannot be exceeded. To reduce the counting rate to a small enough value, the spectrum must be observed through a very small pinhole (0.5 mm) at a distance of some 10 meters. The small pinhole can itself introduce artifacts unless great care is taken, and the large distance of 10 meters is awkward, to say the least, and will require appreciable air attenuation corrections. One way to overcome the counting rate problem is to first scatter the beam to be studied by a foil and then measure the scattered beam in the spectrometer. This was the technique used by Yaffe (Y1) to obtain the data of Figure 2-13. Although this scattering technique overcomes the counting rate problem, it degrades the resolution. The individual kα lines are well resolved in Figure 8-7 but are combined into a single peak in Figure 2-13. Although in principle the measurement of an x ray spectrum is easy, there are a number of rather complex corrections that must be applied to the measured spectrum to obtain the true incident spectrum (S11).

Special Filters of High Atomic Number for Diagnostic Radiology

The germanium detector is an ideal device to help in the design of an optimum beam for certain special techniques in diagnostic radiology. A band of radiation whose energy is matched to the imaging device is required. Each imaging device, whether a film screen-combination or an image amplifier, has a maximum response to a particular band of radiation, usually in the range 30 to 70 keV. Photons with energies above 70 to 80 keV penetrate the patient but are not efficiently absorbed in the detector and so reduce the contrast in the image. These should be removed. The way this may be done is illustrated by the spectra of Figure 8-7, obtained with a germanium detector in our laboratory (D4).

Distribution A is obtained with the tube excited at 70 kV constant potential with an inherent filtration of about 1 mm Al. The kilovoltage is close to the K edge, so essentially no K lines appear. By adding a filter of holmium—a rare earth—a band of radiation just below its K edge (56 keV) is isolated, as illustrated by curves B and C. This band of radiation is heavily absorbed by contrast agents such as iodine (K edge 33 keV) and barium (K edge 37 keV) making the beam useful in angio contrast studies or in intravenous pyelograms.

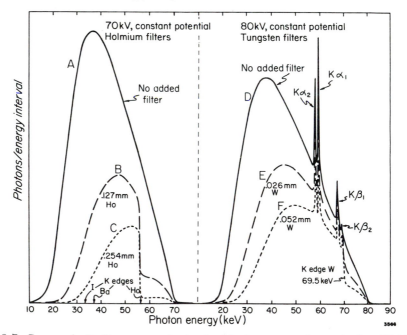

Figure 8-7. Curves A, B, C: spectra obtained with the x ray tube excited at 70 kV constant potential using no added filter, 0.127 mm, and 0.254 mm holmium respectively. Curves D, E, F: spectra generated at 80 kV constant potential with no added filter, 0.026 mm, and 0.052 mm of tungsten respectively.

Curves D, E, and F show how a tungsten filter used with a tube excited at 80 kV can produce a useful band of radiation in the 30 to 70 keV range. Experiments by Villagran (V2) show that with such filters matched to the proper kilovoltage, patient dose can be reduced to half with no loss in diagnostic information. More studies of this kind are required to select the right combinations of kV, filter thickness, and filter material for each type of image receptor. This will be discussed further in Chapter 16.

8.06   TYPES OF SPECTRAL DISTRIBUTIONS

The curves of Figure 8-7 illustrate one way to present data concerning a beam. There are, however, several other ways in which spectral distributions may be presented, which are useful in certain situations. A few of these will be dealt with here.

Photon Fluence per Energy Interval

Curve A in Figure 8-8 gives the number of photons per unit area per energy interval at 1 meter from the focal spot. The actual measurements were carried out at a distance of 10 m from the focal spot and the counting rate was observed through a pinhole of diameter 0.51 mm. Point P curve A shows that there were 3.5×10^{13} photons per m² in the energy interval 39.5 to 40.5 keV. The photon fluence is represented by Φ (phi), and since it is a function of hν we represent it by $\Phi(h\nu)$. Since the ordinate is the portion of the photon fluence between hν and hν + dhν, we represent this by the derivative $d\Phi(h\nu)/dh\nu$. The total area under the curve of Figure 8-8 is the total number of photons given by

$$\Phi = \int \frac{d\Phi(h\nu)}{dh\nu} \cdot dh\nu \qquad (8\text{-}1)$$

Numerical integration shows that the area under this curve is 1.57×10^{15} photons/m². The student may show that this is reasonable by noting that a rectangle of height 2×10^{13} photons/keV · m² and width 80 keV encloses about the same area.

Energy Fluence per Energy Interval

The data of Figure 8-8 can be presented in a different form. If we multiply the ordinate at each value of hν by hν, the energy of the photon, we obtain the differential energy fluence represented by Ψ (psi). Thus,

$$\frac{d\Psi(h\nu)}{dh\nu} = h\nu \cdot \frac{d\Phi(h\nu)}{dh\nu}$$

This is plotted as curve B. It has the same general shape as curve A but the multiplication of each ordinate by hν shifts the distribution towards

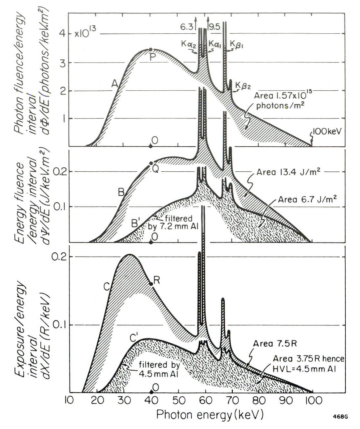

Figure 8-8. Curve A: Photon fluence per energy interval at 1 meter from a 100 kV constant potential x ray source. Measurements were made with a Ge(Li) detector placed 10 meters from the source behind a 0.51 mm pinhole in lead. The $K\alpha_1$ and $K\alpha_2$ at 59.321 and 57.984 keV are off scale. The $K\beta_1$ is really a mixture of $K\beta_3$ and $K\beta_1$ at 67.143 keV, while the $K\beta_2$ is a mixture of several lines with an average of 69.192 keV. Curve B: Same basic data converted to energy fluence per keV interval. Curve B′ is obtained from B by attenuation with 7.2 mm Al. Curve C: Same basic data as curve A but presented as an exposure distribution in roentgens per keV interval. Curve C′ contains half the area of curve C showing that the HVL = 4.5 mm Al.

the high energy end of the spectrum. The area under this curve is

$$\Psi = \int \frac{d\Psi(h\nu)}{dh\nu} \cdot dh\nu = \int h\nu \cdot \frac{d\Phi(h\nu)}{dh\nu} \cdot dh\nu \qquad (8\text{-}2)$$

and gives the total energy fluence in the beam. For our example this area is 13.4 J/m². The reader may show that this is about right by noting that a rectangle of height 0.2 J/keV m² and width 70 keV encloses the same area.

Exposure per Energy Interval

In order to relate these spectra to an HVL measured with an exposure meter, we need to determine the differential exposure, $dX(h\nu)/$

dhν, corresponding to the differential photon fluence, dΦ(hν)/dhν. It will be remembered from Chapter 7 that the roentgen corresponds to an energy absorption of 87.3 $\times$ 10^{-4} J/kg in air. To obtain the energy absorbed by air from a photon fluence, we multiply the energy fluence by the energy absorption coefficient for air to yield:

$$\text{Energy absorbed} = \frac{d\Phi(h\nu)}{dh\nu} \cdot h\nu \cdot \left(\frac{\mu_{ab}}{\rho}\right)_{air}$$

Now, dividing by the factor 87.3 $\times$ 10^{-4} J/kg we obtain

$$\frac{dX(h\nu)}{dh\nu} = \frac{d\Phi(h\nu)}{dh\nu} \cdot h\nu \cdot \left(\frac{\mu_{ab}}{\rho}\right)_{air} \cdot \frac{1}{87.3 \times 10^{-4} \text{ J/kg}} \text{ R} \quad (8\text{-}3)$$

which gives us the required relation between dX(hν)/dhν and dΦ(hν)/dhν. Taking each ordinate in turn of curve B (Fig. 8-8), we thus calculate dX/dhν, which is plotted as curve C. For this calculation the required energy absorption coefficients for air are given in Table A-3a of the appendix. Since μ_{ab}/ρ decreases rapidly with energy from 20 to 100 keV, distribution C is shifted to the left relative to B. The total area under the curve is the exposure in roentgens arising from the spectral distribution. The area under this curve is 7.5 R.

To clarify some of these ideas we will calculate the ordinate on each of curves B and C from curve A of Figure 8-8.

The ordinate OP = 3.5 $\times$ 10^{13} $\dfrac{\text{photons}}{\text{keV m}^2}$ at 40 keV

40 keV = 4 $\times$ 10^4 eV = 4 $\times$ 10^4 $\times$ 1.602 $\times$ 10^{-19} J = 6.41 $\times$ 10^{-15} J

$\therefore$ OQ = 3.5 $\times$ 10^{13} $\times$ 6.41 $\times$ 10^{-15} $\dfrac{\text{J}}{\text{keV m}^2}$ = .224 $\dfrac{\text{J}}{\text{keV m}^2}$

From Table A-3a, μ_{ab}/ρ for air at 40 keV = 0.00625 m^2 kg^{-1}

Now using equation 8-3 we obtain

$$\text{OR} = \frac{.224 \text{ J}}{\text{keV m}^2} \times .00625 \frac{\text{m}^2}{\text{kg}} \times \frac{1}{87.3 \times 10^{-4} \text{ J kg}^{-1} \text{ R}^{-1}}$$

$$= 0.160 \frac{\text{R}}{\text{keV}}$$

Note that the units cancel, leaving the answer in R/keV. The value 0.160 R/keV appears as point R on curve C.

Half-Value Layer

We are now in a position to calculate the HVL from the spectral distribution. To do this we imagine curve C attenuated in turn by increasing thicknesses of aluminum and find the thickness that reduces the area from 7.5 R to half this value, or 3.75 R. This was easily done with a computer, which showed that the required thickness was 4.5 mm Al. That this is reasonable can be seen from curve C^1, which was obtained from curve C by calculating at each energy the attenuation produced by 4.5 mm Al using the total attenuation coefficients for Al given in Table A-4e in the appendix. By inspection it is clear that the area under curve C^1 is about half that of curve C.

In Figure 8-5 the effects of using a non–air wall detector on the measured HVL were illustrated. This can now be understood. If, for example, the detector gave a response proportional to the energy fluence, the measured HVL would be obtained by finding the thickness of aluminum that reduced the area under curve B to half its value. Using a computer to calculate the attenuation by increasing thicknesses of aluminum, it can be shown that curve B^1 obtained with a filter of 7.2 mm Al encloses half the area of curve B. Using a detector with a response proportional to energy fluence one would obtain an incorrect HVL of 7.2 mm Al, a value much larger than the correct one of 4.5 mm Al, illustrating again the importance of using a detector with the correct response.

8.07   SPECTRAL DISTRIBUTIONS OF SCATTERED RADIATION

A number of people have investigated the quality of the radiation within a scattering medium (E3, H10, M8, S8, S12). This is done by using the arrangement shown in Figure 8-9. A crystal photomultiplier, or Ge(Li) detector, is placed in a well-shielded enclosure connected to a hollow tube whose closed end is placed at the point of interest in the water phantom. Scattered radiation traveling in the direction of the tube is thus conducted down it without attenuation to the detector. By keeping the end of the tube at a fixed point in the phantom and setting the assembly at different angles, it is possible to determine the spectrum of the scattered radiation in each direction. By summing over all angles, one may then determine the total scattered radiation at the point. By moving the end of the hollow tube to other points within the water phantom, the scattered radiation at other points may be determined.

A few of the results obtained in this way (S8) are given in Figure 8-9 and Table 8-1. The figure shows the spectrum of scattered radiation at depths of 0, 2.5, and 10 cm for primary radiation with HVL 2.0 mm Cu. As the depth is increased, the amount of scattered radiation increases initially and then decreases but the general shape of the scattered spectra does not change much with depth. On the same graph is plotted the spectral distribution of the primary. The K lines of tungsten are not resolved but give a broad peak at about 65 keV. The primary spectra contain many more energetic and fewer low energy photons than the scattered spectra. The total spectral distribution is found by adding the scattered radiation to the primary.

Table 8-1 gives the spectral distributions of primary scattered and total

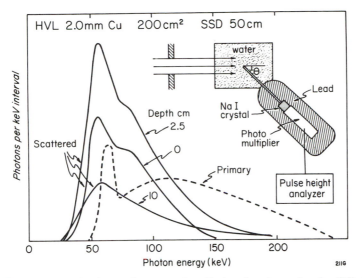

Figure 8-9. Spectral distributions of scattered radiation for three depths (S8). The insert shows the arrangement of the apparatus for making these measurements.

radiation for 6 field sizes at a depth of 10 cm (S8). The photon energy intervals are given in the first column. The second column gives the number of primary photons in each of the energy intervals of column 1. The numbers are normalized to an exposure of 100 roentgens in air at the surface of the phantom. The next two columns, for a field size of 25 cm², give the scattered spectrum (S) and the total spectrum (T), consisting of primary plus scattered radiation. For example, between 40 and 60 keV, there are 197×10^8 primary photons/cm² and 955×10^8 sec-

TABLE 8-1

Spectral Distributions

Photon fluence per energy interval for primary scattered and total radiation as a function of field size at 10 cm depth for HVL 2.2 mm Cu. Multiply table values by 10^8 to give the number of photons/cm² in the photon intervals of column (1) for 100 R in air.

(1) Area (cm²) Energy (keV)	(2) 0 P	(3) 25 S	T	(4) 50 S	T	(5) 100 S	T	(6) 200 S	T	(7) 400 S	T
20-40	3	222	226	393	397	641	645	946	950	1270	1274
40-60	197	955	1152	1488	1685	2149	2346	2988	3185	3725	3922
60-80	323	802	1125	1191	1514	1615	1938	2151	2474	2623	2946
80-100	287	652	849	801	1088	1052	1339	1330	1617	1611	1898
100-120	310	402	712	559	869	720	1030	884	1194	1055	1365
120-140	299	265	564	369	668	442	741	554	853	645	944
140-160	263	173	436	235	498	282	545	325	588	392	655
160-180	216	116	332	150	366	168	384	179	395	234	450
180-200	166	66	232	85	251	92	258	98	264	118	284
200-220	117	34	151	43	160	41	158	48	165	54	171
220-240	71	9	80	12	83	13	84	11	82	11	82
240-260	30	0	30	2	32	1	31	0	30	2	32

From Skarsgard and Johns (S8)

ondary photons, yielding a total of 1152×10^8 photons/cm^2 in the 25 cm^2 field. The rest of the table gives the number of scattered photons (S) and the total number (T) for field areas of 50, 100, 200, and 400 cm^2. The original publications give a detailed description of the spectrum at points on the axis for various qualities of radiation, various depths and a selection of areas.

Summary of Scattered Radiation

Detailed investigations of the spectral distributions within a scattering material such as water lead us to the following conclusions.

a. The softer components in the primary beam are gradually filtered out by the water so the HVL of the primary increases with depth.

b. At the surface the scattered radiation is all backscattered and very soft compared with the primary. With a large field the total radiation is soft compared with the primary.

c. The amount of scattered radiation increases with depth to a broad maximum and then slowly decreases. The quality of the scattered radiation becomes slightly broader with increase in depth, reaches a maximum value, and then slowly decreases. The *total* radiation becomes softer with increase in depth, the amount of softening increasing with field size.

d. At the edges of the field there is less scattered radiation than on the axis, so for a given depth the beam becomes slightly harder with increase in distance from the axis.

e. The variations in quality within a radiation field are maximum for beams with HVL in the Cu range of 0.15 to 1.5 mm Cu. The effects are less important for radiation in the 1 to 25 MeV range.

f. Detailed knowledge of the variation of quality in the field may be of value in certain detailed radiobiological investigations.

8.08   CONVERSION FROM EXPOSURE TO ABSORBED DOSE

It is important in principle to know the quality of the radiation at points within the scattering medium because the conversion from exposure to absorbed dose, discussed in the last chapter, depends on photon energy and hence on the spectral distribution of the beam. Because we very frequently wish to relate absorbed dose to the exposure at a point, it is convenient to establish a simple relation between the two quantities. This problem was discussed in Chapter 7 and a simple relation was given by equation 7-30. We now rewrite this equation as $D_{med} = X \cdot f_{med}$ where f_{med} is given by:

$$f_{med} = \left(0.00873 \; \frac{Gy}{R}\right) \left(\frac{\mu_{ab}}{\rho}\right)_{med} \bigg/ \left(\frac{\mu_{ab}}{\rho}\right)_{air} \qquad (8\text{-}4)$$

This relation would hold for radiation consisting only of a single photon energy. Values of f_{med} using this relation are plotted in Figure 8-10 for

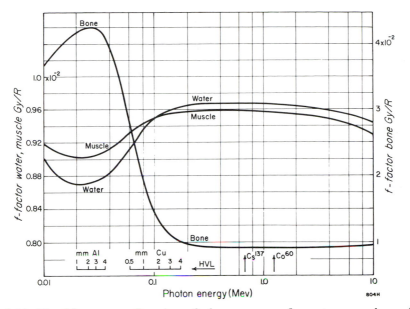

Figure 8-10. The f-factor as a function of photon energy for water, muscle, and bone taken from data in Table A-7. The auxiliary scale relates the HVL in Al and Cu to the energy scale.

water, muscle, and bone and are given in Table A-7 for a number of materials.

For a spectrum it would be necessary to find the average, or effective, value for this quantity by integrating it over the entire spectrum of photon energies present at the point. Thus:

$$\bar{f}_{med} = \left(0.00873 \ \frac{Gy}{R}\right) \frac{\int \left(\frac{\mu_{ab}(h\nu)}{\rho}\right)_{med} \cdot \left(\frac{d\Phi(h\nu)}{dh\nu}\right) \cdot dh\nu}{\int \left(\frac{\mu_{ab}(h\nu)}{\rho}\right)_{air} \left(\frac{d\Phi(h\nu)}{dh\nu}\right) \cdot dh\nu} \quad (8\text{-}4a)$$

where $d\Phi(h\nu)/dh\nu$ is the photon fluence per photon energy interval.

A few values of $\bar{f}_{med}$ were obtained in this way for water and bone using data from Table 8-1 and the results are given in Table 8-2. For water the variation of $\bar{f}$ with area and depth is only a few percent. With increase in area the beam becomes slightly softer and $\bar{f}$ decreases slightly (see Fig. 7-12). Water and air absorb radiation in a very similar manner, hence the variation of $\bar{f}$ from point to point in the phantom is very small.

The second part of Table 8-2 gives data for bone. Now the variation is quite important. With increase in field size and depth the beam becomes softer and photoelectric absorption more important so that $\bar{f}_{bone}$ increases considerably. For example, a 1 gram sample of bone at the surface of the phantom exposed to a small field would absorb 1.756 times as much energy as 1 gram of air. If the bone were placed on the axis of a

400 cm² field at depth 15 cm it would absorb 2.592 times as much energy as air placed at this point. The relative energy absorbed by bone is nearly 50% greater when it is placed in a part of the beam where scattering is important.

TABLE 8-2
Values of f̄ for Water and Bone
Calculated from tables similar to Table 8-1 for HVL = 2.2 mm Cu (Values are in rad/R)

Depth (cm)	0 cm²	25 cm²	50 cm²	100 cm²	200 cm²	400 cm²
Water						
0	.946	.942	.941	.940	.939	.938
5	.949	.940	.938	.934	.932	.931
10	.950	.945	.942	.940	.938	.937
15	.952	.937	.934	.931	.928	.925
Bone						
0	1.756	1.920	1.961	1.999	2.038	2.068
5	1.643	1.989	2.083	2.238	2.312	2.361
10	1.590	1.803	1.903	2.005	2.093	2.142
15	1.505	2.114	2.244	2.368	2.482	2.592

PROBLEMS

1. In an experiment to determine the HVL of a beam from a therapy unit, the following exposure rates were measured with the corresponding added filtration: 0 mm Cu—90 R/min; 1 mm Cu—42 R/min; 2 mm Cu—25.5 R/min; 3 mm Cu—17.7 R/min; 4 mm Cu—13.3 R/min; 5 mm Cu—10.5 R/min; 6 mm Cu—8.7 R/min; 7 mm Cu—7.7 R/min. Plot this data and determine the approximate half-value layer when an added filter of 3 mm Cu is used.

2. Discuss the precautions to be used in making a precise determination of an HVL.

3. Using the attenuation coefficients in the appendix, calculate a few points on curve E from curve A of Figure 8-1.

4. From data in the appendix find the HVL in Cu and Pb for an equivalent photon energy of 200 keV. Check with Figure 8-6.

5. To determine the spectral distribution from a diagnostic x ray tube, a pinhole in Pb (diameter 0.50 mm) was placed 10 meters from the source and tube operated at 2 mA for 800 seconds yielding 60,000 counts in the 30 keV channel. Calculate, neglecting air attenuation, the photon fluence rate (photons/cm²s) to be expected at 50 cm with the tube operating in a more normal manner at a current of 100 mA. Calculate the exposure rate.

6. For problem 5, estimate the air attenuation correction factor for air at 98.6 kPa and 22°C for 30 keV photons (ρ = .001293 g/cm³ at 101.3 kPa and 0°C).

7. Take one point on curve A of Figure 8-8 and calculate the corresponding points on curves B and C. Estimate the areas under curves A, B, and C of Figure 8-8 and discuss the meaning of these areas.

8. The energy and intensities of the K lines of tungsten are given by Storm and Israel

(S1) and are reproduced here with the number in parentheses representing the relative intensities.

K-L$_2$	57.984	(57.6)	K-M$_4$	67.654	(.233)	K-N$_4$	69.269	(.063)
K-L$_3$	59.321	(100)	K-M$_5$	67.716	(.293)	K-N$_5$	68.283	(.063)
K-M$_2$	66.950	(10.8)	K-N$_2$	69.033	(2.45)	K-O$_2$	69.478	(.53)
K-M$_3$	67.244	(20.8)	K-N$_3$	69.100	(4.77)	K-O$_3$	69.489	(.53)

What lines, and with what intensity, would you expect to see resolved with a Ge(Li) detector? (Assume the full width at half maximum response is 1% of the photon energy.)

9. The last column of Table 8-1 gives the photon fluence of primary plus scattered radiation at 10 cm depth in a 400 cm^2 field. Find the half-value layer of this spectral distribution. Could this HVL be determined experimentally? Discuss.

10. Equation 8-4 shows how one could calculate $\bar{f}$. Suggest other relations that would be just as logical.

11. A 1 gram sample of air-like material placed at point P absorbs 174×10^{-7} J from an x ray beam. Determine the exposure at the point P. If the point P were on the axis of a 200 cm^2 field at depth 10 cm and the beam had an HVL of 2.2 mm Cu, what energy absorption would be produced in 1 g of water, and in 1 g of bone?

3   17.7

8.85

Chapter **9**

MEASUREMENT OF RADIATION
(Instrumentation and Techniques)

In Chapter 7 the concepts of exposure and absorbed dose were discussed. It was shown that measurements of charge produced by ionization enable one to calculate exposure, or under certain circumstances determine the absorbed dose. In this chapter we are concerned with the instrumentation and the techniques to measure radiation and from these measurements determine either dose or exposure, and in some cases both.

9.01 **SATURATION IN ION CHAMBERS**

In Chapter 7 it was tacitly assumed that all the ions produced in the chamber were in fact collected. Whether this is true or not will depend upon the design and dimensions of the chamber, the polarizing voltage, and whether the source produces pulsed or continuous radiation. In this and the following two sections we will discuss this problem in detail.

This problem is important, as may be demonstrated by placing two aluminum plates 1 cm apart in an x ray beam and measuring the current as the voltage between the plates is varied from 0 to 300 V. Typical results are illustrated in Figure 9-1 for three different exposure rates. For an exposure rate of 50 R/min it is seen that practically all the ions are collected when 300 volts is applied between the plates. Under these circumstances we say that the saturation current is collected. When the exposure rate is increased to 200 R/min, there will be 4 times as many ions produced per minute, hence a greater concentration of ions and a greater chance for their recombination. For this concentration of ions, saturation is not attained with 300 volts across the chamber. To predict the fraction of ions collected we must first investigate the basic mechanism involved in their motion in an ion chamber.

Mobility

In an ion chamber, positive ions move towards the negative electrode and negative ions in the opposite direction, with velocities proportional to the electric field thus:

$$v_+ = k_+ \epsilon \quad \text{and} \quad v_- = k_- \epsilon \tag{9-1}$$

290

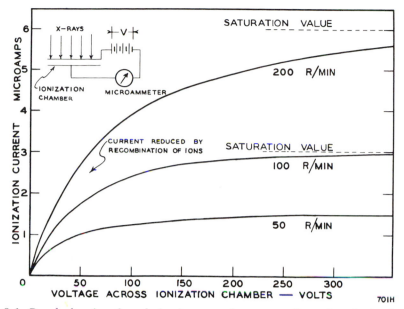

Figure 9-1. Graph showing the relation between the current through an ionization chamber and the voltage across it for three different exposure rates.

where v_+ and v_- are the velocities of the positive and negative ions, ϵ is the electric field in volts/cm, and k_+ and k_- are the mobilities of these ions. In inert gases the negative ions are the electrons and they have mobilities many times that of the positive ions. In gases such as air, however, the electrons produced by the ionization quickly attach themselves to molecules of air so that both positive and negative ions have nearly the same mobility. Thus

$$k_+ \approx k_- \approx 1.8 \,\frac{\text{cm}}{\text{s}} \cdot \frac{\text{cm}}{\text{V}} \text{ (for air)} \qquad (9\text{-}2)$$

In a parallel plate ion chamber with 300 volts applied between plates 2 cm apart, the electric field is 150 V/cm and the velocity of the ions about $(150 \text{ V/cm})(1.8 \text{ cm}^2/\text{sV}) = 270$ cm/s. The time for an ion to cross the chamber is 2 cm/(270 cm/s) = 7.41 ms. In this time the ions have a finite chance of bumping into an ion of the opposite sign to become neutral. Once neutral they can no longer be collected and so are lost to the measuring circuit. The number lost is determined by the recombination coefficient.

Recombination Coefficient

The chance of an ion recombining with an oppositely charged one is proportional to the product of the two ion concentrations and the time, t, and the constant of proportionality is called the recombination coefficient (α). Thus

$$\frac{\text{number of recombinations}}{\text{per unit volume in time, t}} = \alpha\, C_+\, C_-\, t \qquad (9\text{-}3a)$$

where C_+ and C_- are the concentrations of the positive and negative ions respectively. For air α is about 1.6×10^{-6} cm^3 s^{-1}. For ion chamber calculations it is more useful to deal with the *charge* lost to recombination and to calculate this in terms of the *charge* concentrations Q_+ and Q_- in the chamber. Since the ions are usually singly charged, Q and C are related by $Q = eC$ where e is the charge on the electron (1.60×10^{-19} C). With this notation equation 9-3a becomes

$$\frac{\text{charge lost to recombination}}{\text{per unit volume in time, t}} = \frac{\alpha}{e} Q_+ Q_- t \qquad (9\text{-}3b)$$

Example 9-1. In an air ion chamber there are present initially 10 pC of positive ions and an equal number of negative ions in each cm^3. Determine the charge lost to recombination in the first ms.

$$Q_+ = Q_- = 10 \text{ pC/cm}^3 = 10^{-11} \text{ C/cm}^3$$

$$\begin{array}{l}\text{charge lost} \\ \text{(eq. 9-3b)}\end{array} = \frac{1.6 \times 10^{-6} \text{ cm}^3 \text{ s}^{-1}}{1.60 \times 10^{-19} \text{ C}} \times 10^{-22}\, \frac{\text{C}^2}{\text{cm}^6} \times 10^{-3}\text{s} = 10^{-12}\, \frac{\text{C}}{\text{cm}^3}$$

This calculation shows that 10% of the charge is lost to recombination in the first ms.

In using equation 9-3b, we have tacitly assumed that the ion concentration remains constant with time—this is almost true over 1 ms but would certainly not be true over longer times. If we wish to solve the problem accurately, we must replace equation 9-3b by the differential equation, which for equal concentrations of positive and negative ions become

$$dQ = -\frac{\alpha}{e} Q^2 \, dt \qquad (9\text{-}4)$$

The student may easily integrate this to yield

$$Q = \frac{Q_0}{1 + \left(\dfrac{\alpha}{e}\right) Q_0\, t} \qquad (9\text{-}5)$$

where Q is the charge concentration at time t, and Q_0 is the initial concentration. The student should note that this is an example of a decay that is *not* exponential. It is a common reaction in chemistry referred to as second order kinetics because it depends on the square of the concentration.

Example 9-2. Repeat the calculation of example 9-1 using the accurate expression that takes into account the reduction of the concentration with time.

$$\frac{\alpha}{e} Q_0 t = \frac{1.6 \times 10^{-6} \text{ cm}^3 \text{ s}^{-1}}{1.60 \times 10^{-19} \text{ C}} \times 10^{-11} \frac{\text{C}}{\text{cm}^3} \times 10^{-3} \text{ s} = 0.100$$

Hence, charge conc. after 1 ms. (eq. 9-5) $= \dfrac{10}{1 + 0.100} \dfrac{\text{pC}}{\text{cm}^3} = 9.09 \dfrac{\text{pC}}{\text{cm}^3}$

Thus, the charge concentration lost to recombination is $10 - 9.09 = .91$ pC/cm^3, a little less than the value of 1.0 pC/cm^3 obtained in example 9-1, showing that the depletion of ions during the ms is not quite negligible.

9.02   **CALCULATION OF EFFICIENCY OF ION COLLECTION—PULSED RADIATION**

The exact calculation of the charge lost to recombination in an ion chamber is complicated. Here we will discuss the principles involved and give approximate expressions that may be used to estimate it. This discussion is based on a detailed analysis by Boag (B9) and Greening (G8).

Pulsed Radiation

Imagine pulsed radiation producing a concentration Q_0 of positive and negative ions uniformly in the space between the plates P and N of a parallel plate chamber (Fig. 9-2). Assume the plates to be a distance d apart and held at a potential difference V. The diagram shows the charge pattern at time t after the pulse. The positive ions will occupy the space to the right as they are pulled to plate N, while the negative ions will occupy the space to the left as they are attracted to plate P. The boundary of negative charges will move to the left with velocity $v_- = k_- V/d$ and after time t will be distance $x_- = k_- t V/d$ from plate P, while the boundary of positive ions will be x_+ from plate P. The overlap region where both positive and negative ions are present has width x, given by

$$x = d - (x_+ + x_-) = d - t(k_+ + k_-) V/d \qquad (9\text{-}6)$$

By placing $x = 0$ and solving for t we obtain the time t_r, during which there is an overlap of positive and negative charges so that recombination can take place.

$$t_r = \frac{d^2}{V(k_+ + k_-)} \qquad (9\text{-}7)$$

In this overlap region the charge concentration will decay according to equation 9-5. To obtain the total charge lost to recombination we must

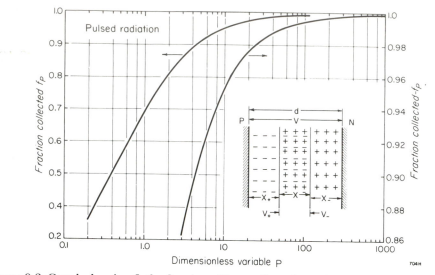

Figure 9-2. Graph showing f_p the fraction of ions collected as a function of the dimensionless variable p given by equation 9-12. The insert shows a parallel plate chamber in which a pulse of radiation has produced a uniform distribution of positive and negative ions, which are shown being collected.

take into account the decreasing volume of the overlap region as collection takes place. The amount of charge lost to recombination in time dt will be given by dQ × available volume, ie. $dQ \cdot A \cdot x$. Using equations 9-4, 9-5 and 9-6, the total charge lost to recombination in time t_r will be:

$$R = A \int_0^{t_r} \frac{\alpha}{e} \left[\frac{Q_0}{1 + \dfrac{\alpha}{e} Q_0 t} \right]^2 \cdot \left\{ d - \frac{V}{d} (k_+ + k_-) t \right\} dt \qquad (9\text{-}8)$$

With a little effort the student may show that this integral is

$$R = Q_0 d A \left[1 - p \ln \left(1 + \frac{1}{p} \right) \right] \qquad (9\text{-}9)$$

where

$$p = \frac{e}{\alpha} (k_+ + k_-) \frac{V}{Q_0 d^2} = \mu' \frac{V}{Q_0 d^2} \qquad (9\text{-}10)$$

and

$$\mu' = \frac{e}{\alpha} (k_+ + k_-)$$

Now the charge per pulse produced in the ion chamber is QdA and the fraction of this charge that is collected is

$$f_p = 1 - \frac{R}{Q_0 d A} = p \ln \left(1 + \frac{1}{p} \right) \qquad (9\text{-}11)$$

To evaluate f for a given condition we must determine μ' of equation 9-10, which involves the properties of the gas in which the ionization is

taking place. Using the value of μ' suggested by Boag* for air, the dimensionless variable p becomes:

$$p = 0.306 \times 10^{-12} \frac{V}{d^2 \, Q_0} \qquad (9\text{-}12)$$

V is in volts, d in cm, Q_0 in coulombs per cm^3 per pulse in air.

The fraction of the charge collected, f_p, given by equation 9-11 is plotted in Figure 9-2 against the dimensionless variable p. Since p is proportional to V, the curve of Figure 9-2 is like a saturation curve, but it is more than a saturation curve since p involves all the variables on which collection depends. If, for example, d is doubled, then for the same Q_0, V would have to be increased by a factor of 4 to allow collection of the same fraction of ions. That the dimensionless variable should involve d^2 can be seen as follows. Doubling d increases the distance the ions have to travel by a factor of 2 and also reduces the ion velocity by a factor of 2, so that the collection time is increased by a factor of 4. These ideas are illustrated by an example.

Example 9-3. Find the fraction of the ions collected in a parallel plate ion chamber exposed to radiation that liberates 10 pC per cm^3 per pulse when the plate separation is 1.5 cm and 300 volts is applied to the chamber. What voltage would be required to collect 99.5% of the ions?

We first determine the dimensionless quantity p using equation 9-12.

V = 300 volt; d = 1.5 cm; and Q_0 = 10 pC = 10^{-11}C

$$p = .306 \times 10^{-12} \times \frac{300}{2.25 \times 10^{-11}} = 4.08$$

For p = 4.08 the fraction collected (Fig. 9-2) is 0.893.

To collect 99.5% of the ions requires p $\approx$ 100 (see Fig. 9-2). This means the potential would have to be increased by a factor of 25 to about 7500 V, which might well cause breakdown of the insulation. A better way to insure 99.5% collection would be to reduce d by a factor of about 2 and increase the potential by a factor of about 6, yielding a p of about 100, which would insure the collection of 99.5% of the ions. (Methods for handling the problem of pulsed radiation when the chamber is cylindrical or spherical rather than a parallel plate will be dealt with at the end of the next section.)

9.03   **CALCULATION OF EFFICIENCY OF ION
COLLECTION—CONTINUOUS RADIATION**

Imagine a parallel plate ion chamber (insert to Fig. 9-3) exposed to a continuous radiation field that produces a charge Q_c of positive ions and

---

*In reference (B9) Boag uses the dimensionless variable $\mu = 1/p$ where $\mu = (1090$ volt cm/esu) (d^2Q_0/V). This leads to our value of p when electrostatic units are converted to coulombs.

an equal charge of negative ions in each unit volume of the chamber per second. The subscript c is used to indicate continuous radiation and to distinguish this case from pulsed radiation dealt with above. The student should note that Q_c is a charge per unit volume per second while Q_0 was a charge per unit volume per pulse. We wish to determine f, the fraction of charges collected. If no recombination occurs, the charge collected per second, i.e. the current, is:

$$I = Q_c \, d \, A \qquad\qquad (9\text{-}13)$$

Now in the collection process the positive ions will move to the right with velocity $k_+ V/d$ and the negative ones to the left with velocity $k_- V/d$. Consider first the positive ions. Since they are produced uniformly everywhere in the chamber and since they all move with constant velocity to the right, their concentration will start at zero at plate P and increase linearly to a maximum value just next to the negative plate. Let $Q_+(x)$ represent the concentration of positive ions at distance x from plate P. Right next to plate N the charge concentration will be $Q_+(d)$ and since this layer of charges has velocity $k_+ V/d$ the charge collected per second is

$$Q_+(d) \cdot \frac{k_+ V}{d} A = I$$

This is an alternative expression for equation 9-13 so we may equate the two and solve for $Q_+(d)$ to yield

$$Q_+(d) = \frac{Q_c \, d^2}{k_+ V} \qquad\qquad (9\text{-}14)$$

Hence, the concentration of positive charges at distance x from plate P is

$$Q_+ = \frac{Q_c \, d}{k_+ V} x \qquad\qquad (9\text{-}15)$$

This concentration is shown graphically in the insert to Figure 9-3 as the line OR. It rises linearly from zero at plate P to its maximum value at plate N. In an analogous way the concentration of negative ions is given by:

$$Q_-(x) = \frac{Q_c \, d}{k_- V} (d - x) \qquad\qquad (9\text{-}16)$$

It falls from its maximum value at plate P to zero at plate N. In deriving these two expressions we have so far taken no account of the fact that some charges are lost to recombination.

Equations 9-15 and 9-16 give the concentration of positive and negative ions at all points in the chamber, allowing us to calculate the charge

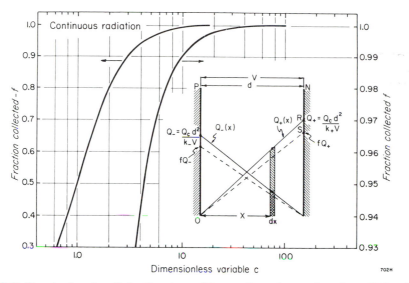

Figure 9-3. Graph showing f the fraction of ions collected as a function of the dimensionless variable c given in equation 9-22. The insert shows a parallel plate chamber in which charges are generated continuously and uniformly through the volume. The concentration of the positive and negative charges are shown as a function of the distance x.

lost to recombination using equation 9-3b. Consider the region of area A and width dx:

$$\text{Charge lost to recomb. per second in width dx} = \frac{\alpha}{e}(Q_-)(Q_+)A\,dx = A\frac{\alpha}{e}\frac{Q_c^2\,d^2\,x(d-x)dx}{k_+\,k_-\,V^2}$$

To obtain the total charge lost to recombination per second we integrate this expression from x = 0 to x = d to yield

$$A\frac{\alpha}{e\,k_+\,k_-}\frac{Q_c^2\,d^2}{V^2}\int_0^d x(d-x)dx = A\frac{\alpha}{e\,k_+\,k_-}\frac{Q_c^2\,d^2}{V^2}\left(\frac{d^3}{6}\right) \qquad (9\text{-}17a)$$

If we divide this by $Q_c\,d\,A$ we obtain f_r', the fraction that recombines:

$$f_r' = \frac{1}{6}\frac{\alpha}{e\,k_+\,k_-}\frac{Q_c\,d^4}{V^2} \qquad (9\text{-}17b)$$

It is convenient to introduce a dimensionless variable c that includes all the parameters in this equation and depends upon the voltage V to the first power, thus:

$$c = \sqrt{\frac{6e\,k_+\,k_-}{\alpha}}\frac{V}{d^2\,\sqrt{Q_c}} \qquad (9\text{-}18)$$

With this notation, equation 9-17b, giving the fraction that recombine, becomes

$$f_r' = 1/c^2 \qquad (9\text{-}19a)$$

This expression is correct, provided recombination removes a negligible fraction of the ions. If, however, recombination is not negligible it will *overestimate* the recombination loss since it assumes *too high* a concentration of ions at every point in the chamber. At the negative plate the charge density is not really $Q_c d^2/k_+V$ as represented by point R but rather a smaller value $f\, Q_c d^2/k_+V$ as shown by point S (f is the fraction collected). If we assume the distribution shown by the dotted line OS applies *throughout* the chamber, the student may carry through the calculation and show that equation 9-19a becomes

$$f_r'' = f^2/c^2 \qquad\qquad (9\text{-}19b)$$

This expression will *underestimate* the recombination loss. The correct answer f_r will lie between f_r' and f_r''. The problem is difficult to solve accurately since the ions in the space between the plates will affect the electric field. Greening (G8) and Boag (B9) suggest that a good compromise solution is found by taking the geometric mean of the two estimates to give

$$f_r = f/c^2 \qquad\qquad (9\text{-}20)$$

Now since f (the fraction collected) $= 1 - f_r$ we write $f = 1 - f/c^2$, which we solve for f to give

$$f = \frac{1}{1 + 1/c^2} \qquad\qquad (9\text{-}21)$$

which allows us to calculate the fraction collected in terms of the dimensionless variable c. Our expression for c involves the properties of the gas in the chamber. Using values for air suggested by Boag* our expression becomes

$$c = 1.219 \times 10^{-6} \frac{V}{d^2 \sqrt{Q_c}} \qquad\qquad (9\text{-}22)$$

V is in volts, d is in cm, and Q_c is in coulombs per sec per cm^3 of air.

To aid in calculations, the fraction f of ions collected is plotted in Figure 9-3 using equation 9-21. These ideas are now illustrated with an example.

Example 9-4. A parallel plate ion chamber with 1.20 cm gap is placed in a continuous radiation field, which produces 10.0 nC of charge/cm^3s. The potential across the chamber is 150 volts. Estimate the fraction of ions collected. What conditions would allow for collection of 99.9% of the ions?

---

*In reference (B9) Boag uses a dimensionless variable that is the reciprocal of ours. Our value was obtained from his by taking this into account and making the appropriate conversions from esu to coulombs. In our expression the quantity 1.219×10^{-6} has dimensions

$$\sqrt{\frac{cm\ C}{V^2\ s}}$$

We first express Q_c, V, and d in the correct units.

$Q_c = 10.0$ nC $= 10^{-8}$C; V $= 150$ volt; d $= 1.20$ cm

$$c \text{ (eq. 9-22)} = 1.219 \times 10^{-6} \times 150 \times \frac{1}{1.44 \times 10^{-4}} = 1.27$$

f (eq. 9-21 or Fig. 9-3) $= .617$; i.e. 62% are collected.

To collect .999 of the ions, Figure 9-3 shows that c should be about 30, that is, increased from 1.27 by a factor of about 24. For the same charge production we could decrease d by a factor of 4 (d^2 by 16) and increase V by a factor of 3/2. This would ensure collection of 99.9% of the ions.

Cylindrical and Spherical Chambers

Most practical ionization chambers are either cylindrical or spherical in form. In these chambers the electrical field varies with the distance from the central electrode and the calculations are more complicated than for a parallel plate ionization chamber. Boag (B9) has shown that this problem can be dealt with by imagining that the real gap is replaced by a larger equivalent gap in a parallel plate chamber and then calculating the fraction collected by the methods described above. In a cylindrical chamber the quantity of importance is the ratio of the radius of the shell *a* to the radius of the inner electrode *b*. The equivalent gap length is $K_{cyl}(a - b)$, where K_{cyl} is plotted in Figure 9-4. For a spherical chamber with a spherical central electrode, the equivalent gap length is $K_{sph}(a - b)$. K_{sphere} is also shown in Figure 9-4.

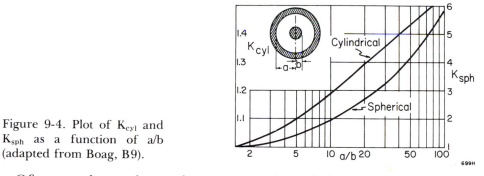

Figure 9-4. Plot of K_{cyl} and K_{sph} as a function of a/b (adapted from Boag, B9).

Often we do not know the concentration of charges produced in an ion chamber but do know the exposure rate. These are related by equation 7-20 thus:

$$1 \text{ roentgen} = 3.335 \times 10^{-10} \text{ C/cm}^3 \text{ for air at NTP} \quad (9\text{-}23)$$

We now illustrate these ideas with a few examples.

Example 9-5. A cylindrical air wall chamber of radius 0.5 cm with a central electrode of radius 0.05 cm is used to measure continuous radiation from a cobalt unit with an exposure rate of 240 R/min with a collection voltage of 150 volts. Find the efficiency of ion collection.

ratio $a/b = 0.5/.05 = 10$

K_{cyl} (Fig. 9-4) $= 1.19$

equivalent gap length $= 1.19(0.5 - 0.05) = 0.535$

exposure rate $= 240$ R/min $= 4$ R/s

Q_c (eq. 9-23) $= 4 \times 3.335 \times 10^{-10} \dfrac{C}{cm^3 s} = 13.34 \times 10^{-10} \dfrac{C}{cm^3 s}$

$\sqrt{Q_c} = 3.65 \times 10^{-5}$; $V = 150$ volt; $d = .535$ cm

c (eq. 9-22) $= \dfrac{1.219 \times 10^{-6} \times 150}{(.535)^2 \times 3.65 \times 10^{-5}} = 17.5$

f (eq. 9-21 or Fig. 9-3) $= .997$

We should collect 99.7% of the ions.

Example 9-6. Suppose the measurements described in the last example were performed on a pulsed machine giving 100 pulses per second using the same average exposure rate. Determine the collection efficiency.

Q_0 (charge per pulse per cm^3) $= 13.34 \times 10^{-12} \dfrac{C}{cm^3 s}$

$p = .306 \times 10^{-12} \dfrac{150}{(.535)^2\, 13.34 \times 10^{-12}} = 12.02$

f_p (eq. 9-11 or Fig. 9-2) $= .960$

For continuous radiation a given chamber design allows 99.7% collection, while with pulsed radiation only 96.0% is collected. With high energy linacs of high output, the pulsed radiation may create collection problems unless care is taken in the design of the ion chamber.

Sometimes the situation is neither pulsed nor continuous, as when radiation is produced by a half-wave rectified x ray generator. The duration of each burst of x rays is about 1/120 s, which is long compared with the collection time so the radiation may not be considered pulsed. The situation could be dealt with in an approximate way by considering the radiation as continuous with an effective average intensity about 2 times the actual average value.

9.04   **OPERATIONAL AMPLIFIERS**

In general the currents produced in ion chambers are small and cannot be readily measured with a microammeter but require either special, very sensitive electrometers or some type of electronic amplifier. In the last decade very small and inexpensive solid state operational amplifiers with gains of 10^5 or more have become available. These have greatly simplified many problems relating to the measurement of small ionization currents. Since they are now used so universally a brief discussion of them is in order.

An operational amplifier is represented by a triangular structure as indicated in Figure 9-5, with open loop gain G. The device has two input points, P and Q, and one output terminal, O. The input terminal P is marked (−) and is called the inverting terminal since a small *negative* voltage applied to it will give a *positive* output voltage G times as large. In contrast, a positive voltage applied to Q will give a positive output voltage G times as large. The operational amplifiers are always used with a feedback connection of some kind between the output point O and the inverting input P. In the circuit of Figure 9-5 this feedback connection is the resistor R_f. We wish to determine the output voltage V_o, when an input voltage V_i is applied to the circuit, i.e. the gain of the circuit (closed loop gain). *This gain should not be confused with the open loop gain G.*

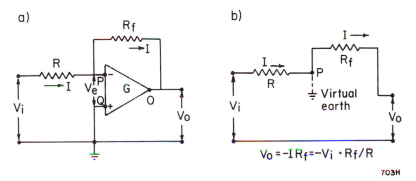

Figure 9-5. (a) Operational amplifier used as a voltage amplifier. (b) Simplified circuit equivalent to a, using the idea that P is a virtual ground.

Assume as a result of an input signal V_i that a current I flows into R. Since these amplifiers have a very large input impedance, essentially no current will flow into the amplifier, so I must also flow through R_f. From Ohm's law, it follows that

$$V_o = V_i - (R + R_f) \, I \qquad (9\text{-}24)$$

The potential of P will change by $V_i - IR$ and since Q is at ground potential the error voltage V_e appearing between P and Q is

$$V_e = V_i - R \, I \qquad (9\text{-}25)$$

Since for a signal applied to P, the amplifier has a gain of $-G$

$$V_o = -G \, V_e = -G(V_i - R \, I) \qquad (9\text{-}26)$$

Eliminating I from 9-25 and 9-26 and rearranging we obtain

$$V_o = -V_i \frac{R_f}{\dfrac{R(G+1)}{G} + \dfrac{R_f}{G}}$$

Now in these amplifiers G is usually about 10^5 so $(G+1)/G \approx 1$ and R_f/G becomes negligible in comparison with R. Hence

$$V_o = -V_i(R_f/R) \qquad (9\text{-}27)$$

We now estimate how much error voltage appears across the input terminals of the amplifier. Substituting equation 9-27 into equation 9-26 we obtain

$$V_e = -\frac{V_o}{G} = \frac{V_i}{G}\left(\frac{R_f}{R}\right) \qquad (9\text{-}28)$$

This circuit has a number of very attractive features. From equation 9-27 we see that the gain of the circuit is simply R_f/R and *does not depend on the open loop gain G of the operational amplifier.* This leads to exceedingly stable operation. In addition, the gain of the circuit can be altered easily. For example, if $R_f = R$ the circuit gain is 1.0; if $R_f = 10\,R$ the gain is 10 so the gain may be altered in a precise way by merely altering R_f. Because the amplifier has a very high gain the input terminal P effectively does not budge from its initial value regardless of input signal. This means P can be considered as a "virtual ground," which we will see simplifies calculations immensely. The one serious limitation these amplifiers have is that voltages in excess of 10 to 15 volts may not be applied to any of the input or output terminals. We now clarify these ideas by a simple example.

Example 9-7. Suppose the amplifier of Figure 9-5 has an open loop gain of 10^5 and an input voltage of 1.0 volts is applied to the circuit. Let $R = 1.0$ MΩ, and $R_f = 10.0$ MΩ. Calculate the output voltage and the error voltage.

Output voltage (eq. 9-28) $V_o = -1.0\,\dfrac{10.0}{1.0} = -10.0$ V

Error voltage (eq. 9-29) $V_e = -V_o/G = 10/10^5 = 0.1$ mV

Thus, when 1 volt is applied to the input, the potential of P increases very slightly (0.1 mV), and point O drops by 10 volts. Because point P remains very nearly at ground potential it is called a virtual ground, and the circuit can essentially be replaced by Figure 9-5b. By Ohm's law $V_i = I\,R$ and $V_o = -I\,R_f$ which leads immediately to $V_o = V_i(R_f/R)$ in agreement with equation 9-28.

Some idea of the size of one of these devices can be obtained from Figure 9-6a, which shows one such amplifier. It includes some dozen transistors and sells for about 1 dollar. There are hundreds of operational amplifiers on the market today, and some care should be exercised in the proper choice of one for radiation measurements. For such measurements an amplifier with very high input impedance, that is one with very small leakage current, should be chosen. By combining some dozen operational amplifiers in a sophisticated circuit, manufacturers have created electrometer operational amplifiers with leakage currents less than 10^{-15}A. Such an amplifier is shown in Figure 9-6B. These sell for about 100 dollars.

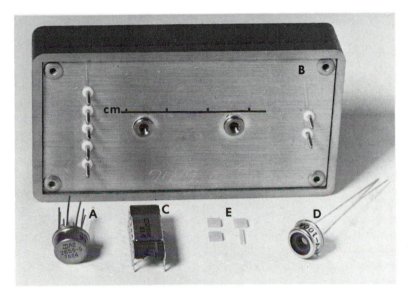

Figure 9-6. (A) Photograph of an operational amplifier, including some dozen transistors. (B) Combination of many amplifiers, in one case creating an electrometer amplifier with very high input impedance. (C) Assembly of 4 FET high impedance switches. (D) Light and x ray sensitive diode detector—EG&G-PV-100. (E) Thermoluminescent dosimeter chips of LiF.

9.05   TYPICAL CIRCUITS USING OPERATIONAL AMPLIFIERS

Most operational amplifiers require positive and negative power supplies at 15 volts as illustrated in Figure 9-7a with a current drain of about 5 mA from each power supply. They also often include an offset adjustment that can be used to zero the output when the input voltage is zero. They sometimes require a frequency compensator on the feedback loop as illustrated in Figure 9-7a. Because operational amplifiers are so inexpensive and small they can easily be combined to form circuits with special properties. We will consider a few of these.

Current to Voltage Converter

If in Figure 9-5 we remove the voltage source V_i and make $R = 0$, then our device becomes a current-to-voltage converter with input current I and output voltage V_o. Since the amplifier may be considered as having an infinite impedance, the ion current I flows through R_f to the output terminal, and since P may be considered a virtual earth we obtain immediately

$$V_o = -I\ R_f \qquad\qquad (9\text{-}29)$$

Example 9-8. A circuit similar to Figure 9-5 with the voltage source V_i removed and $R = 0$ is to be used to measure a current of 10^{-9}A. Determine the output voltage when $R_f = 10^9 \Omega$.

$$V_o(\text{eq. 9-29}) = -10^{-9}\ A \times 10^9 \Omega = -1\ \text{volt.}$$

The output may be measured using a simple voltmeter or recorded on a chart recorder. To measure a relatively large current of 10^{-9}A or more a simple operational amplifier is satisfactory, but if one desires to measure a much smaller current, say 10^{-12}A, then one would require a feedback resistance $R_f \approx 10^{11} \Omega$ and the use of a high input impedance electrometer amplifier of the type illustrated in Figure 9-6B.

Current Integrator

If we wish to integrate a small ion current over some period of time t we merely replace the feedback resistor R_f by a capacitor C as illustrated in Figure 9-7b. Again, since the input impedance to the amplifier is very large the current I must flow into the capacitor C and since the input terminal is a virtual ground, the charge collected is $Q = \int I dt$ and the output voltage V_o is simply

$$V_o = -\frac{Q}{C} = -\frac{1}{C} \int I dt \qquad\qquad (9\text{-}30)$$

Example 9-9. A current of 10^{-8} A is to be integrated for 50 ms on a capacitor, $C = .01\ \mu F$. Determine the output voltage.

$$Q = 10^{-8} A \cdot dt = 10^{-8}\ A \times 5 \times 10^{-2} s = 5 \times 10^{-10} C$$

$$V_o\ (\text{eq. 9-30}) = \frac{-5 \times 10^{-10} C}{10^{-8}\ F} = -0.05\,V$$

At the end of the integration period the capacitor would be discharged by closing the switch S in preparation for the next integration cycle. The switch could be a solid state device with no moving parts. They take many different forms and are turned on or off in a fraction of a microsecond by a 5 volt logic pulse. The voltage pulse effectively squeezes

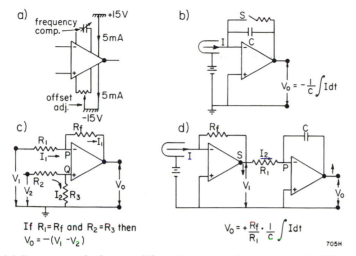

Figure 9-7. (a) Power supply for amplifier, (b) current integrator, (c) differential voltage amplifier, (d) current-to-voltage converter followed by a current integrator.

charge carriers out of the region between the source and drain of the transistor to increase the resistance between these terminals to more than 10^{12} ohms and thus to effectively open the circuit. Such a switch is shown in Figure 9-6C. This component actually contains 4 separate switches.

Differential Amplifier

In the circuits we have dealt with so far, the terminal Q of the amplifier has been connected to the ground. If this point were connected instead to a second signal as illustrated in Figure 9-7c, we can obtain an output voltage proportional to the difference between the two input signals. That this is so can be seen as follows. Because of the properties of the operational amplifier, P and Q are held at the *same* potential although in this case *not* at ground potential. If $R_2 = R_3$ then $V_Q = V_2/2$ and the current $I_1 = (V_1 - V_p)/R_1 = (V_1 - V_2/2)/R_1$. If $R_f = R_1$ the reader can easily show that

$$V_o = -(V_1 - V_2) \qquad (9\text{-}31)$$

Thus, the circuit enables one to determine an output signal equal to the difference between two input signals. If $R_1 \neq R_f$ and $R_2 \neq R_3$ the arithmetic is more complicated and we now obtain an output signal equal to the difference between one signal and a weighted value of the other (see problem 13).

Several Amplifiers in Series

Because the amplifiers are so small and relatively inexpensive, several of them can be used in series as illustrated in Figure 9-7d. Here the first stage is a current-to-voltage converter, yielding $V_1 = -I\,R_f$, causing the potential of S to drop. This voltage generates a current ($I_2 = V_1/R_1 = -I\,R_f/R_1$) into point P, which is integrated in the last stage. The student may show that the output voltage is

$$V_o = +\frac{1}{C} \cdot \frac{R_f}{R_1} \int I\,dt \qquad (9\text{-}32)$$

9.06   PRACTICAL DEVICES FOR MEASURING RADIATION

The simplest way to measure radiation is to connect a well-designed ion chamber on the end of shielded cable to a suitable commercially available electrometer as illustrated in Figure 9-8. In the system shown, the outer shell of the ion chamber is connected via the outer shield of the cable through R to the polarizing voltage. The outer shield of the cable is usually covered with rubber insulation to prevent accidental grounds and the resistance $R \approx 10\ \Omega$ gives further protection against possible damage arising from the inadvertent grounding of the outer wall of the ion chamber. The wall of the ion chamber is usually made of a conducting plastic with "air wall" (see section 7.09) characteristics. The electrometers often have digital readout and feature automatic ranging so that the device automatically selects the proper range on which to make the measurement. The electrometer contains a grounding switch S and a zero adjustment. We will now describe in detail the steps required to use such a device to measure exposure from a cobalt unit. We will assume that the ion chamber has been calibrated with its buildup cap in the standardization laboratory and that its sensitivity N_X is known in roentgens/coulomb or roentgens/scale reading.

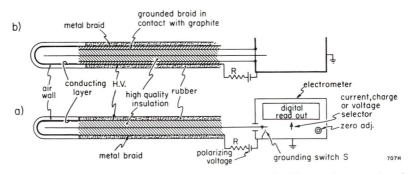

Figure 9-8. (a) Ion chamber connected to electrometer. (b) Alternative ion chamber configuration with guarded construction to minimize leakage.

1. Position the center of the ion chamber with its buildup cap at the point where one wishes to determine the exposure rate.

2. Set the electrometer to measure current.
3. Ground the sensitive lead of the electrometer with switch S and use the zero adjustment to null the reading. Open S and observe the leakage current, I_L.
4. Open S and turn on the unit. A steady current reading should appear on the electrometer. Observe it for a few seconds and record its average value I. If I is large compared with I_L the calibration is complete. If it is not, an attempt should be made to reduce the leakage current by carefully cleaning the insulation at the end of the cable.
5. The exposure rate is $N_X(I - I_L)$. For example, suppose $N_X = .211 \times 10^{10}$ roentgen/coulomb and $I - I_L = 5.12 \times 10^{-10}$ C/s. Then the exposure rate is

$$0.211 \times 10^{10} \frac{R}{C} \times 5.12 \times 10^{-10} \frac{C}{s} = 1.08 \text{ R/s}$$

6. This should now be corrected for temperature and pressure (section 7.06). The user should evaluate the dimensionless variable p or c (sections 9.02 and 9.03) to assure that essentially 100% of the ions are being collected. If they are not, a correction can be made or the polarizing voltage may be increased.

A calibration can equally well be performed using the electrometer as a charge measuring device and the same answer should be obtained. One would proceed as follows:

1. Set the electrometer to measure charge.
2. Ground S and null the device, open S.
3. Turn on the unit for 10 s and measure the charge Q_1.
4. Ground the electrometer and readjust the zero, open S.
5. Turn on the unit for 70 s and measure a charge Q_2.
6. The charge produced in the ion chamber in 1 min is $Q_2 - Q_1$.
7. Measure the leakage Q_L in 1 min with the machine off. It should be negligible compared to $Q_2 - Q_1$. If it is not, clean the insulator. For the experiment described above $(Q_2 - Q_1) - Q_L = 307.1 \times 10^{-10}$ C. Hence exposure in 1 min is

$$S_x(Q_2 - Q_1 - Q_L) = .211 \times 10^{10} \frac{R}{C} \times 307.1 \times 10^{-10} \text{C} = 64.8 \text{R}$$

Exposure rate = 64.8 R/60s = 1.08 R/s as above.

Note that two exposures (10 s and 70 s) are required because of the finite and unknown time required for the cobalt unit to come "on." For measuring a cobalt calibration, current or charge are equally effective. If, however, the output of the radiation source fluctuates with time, greater precision can usually be achieved by measuring the charge produced in a measured time than trying to record the average current.

Guarded Construction

If the ion chamber has a large air volume (several cm³) and is being used to measure a large exposure rate (50 R/min or more), leakage is usually not a problem. If, however, the ion chamber is small, the cable of inferior quality and very long, and the signal small, leakage may be a problem. Sometimes, the problem can be overcome using the guarded construction of Figure 9-8b. The cable now has three conductors; the central one, as before, is imbedded in a good insulator. This insulator is covered with a thin layer of graphite and surrounded by a metal braid. This is covered by a sheath of insulation and another metal braid, which is finally covered by a rubber sheath. The inner braid making contact with the graphite layer is grounded and the high voltage is carried to the chamber on the outer shield. With this arrangement the sensitive central electrode is surrounded by ground at *all* places except in the ion chamber where it "looks" at the high voltage across the air gap. Leakage from the high voltage to ground can take place but this cannot affect the measured signal. The graphite layer reduces the noise in the cable and makes the system less sensitive to spurious signals that may arise when the cable is flexed.

Condenser Chambers

In some applications the long cable of the device described in Figure 9-8 is a disadvantage. It may be dispensed with in a condenser ion chamber illustrated in Figure 9-9. The central electrode of the ion chamber on the right is permanently connected to the capacitor on the left. The plates of the capacitor consist of the conducting layer of carbon on the inside of the hollow insulator, and the outer metal shield that is connected to the conducting layer of carbon on the inside wall of the ion chamber. To use the device, the central electrode is charged to potential V_1 (some 300 volts) and the left hand end then covered with a protective cap to prevent touching the central electrode, causing charge leakage. The device is positioned in the radiation field with the ion chamber centered at the point of interest and exposed. During the exposure, ionization causes charge to leak off the central electrode so that at the end of the exposure the potential has dropped to V_2. If C is the capacity of the condenser ion chamber system, then the charge liberated by the radiation is

$$Q = C(V_1 - V_2) \tag{9-33}$$

To measure Q, we first connect the device to a battery and measure V_1 on a good electrometer, then expose the device and remeasure the potential V_2 on the same electrometer. The charge is then determined from equation 9-33 using the known capacity C of the chamber; the exposure is proportional to $V_1 - V_2$; the constant of proportionality de-

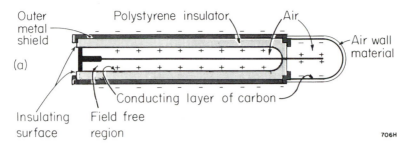

Outer metal shield
Polystyrene insulator
Air
Air wall material
(a)
Insulating surface
Field free region
Conducting layer of carbon

706H

Figure 9-9. Schematic diagram of condenser ion chamber. Ions are produced in the two compartments containing air, but since there is no electric field in the region on the left, no ions are collected here and the sensitive region is confined to the thimble chamber on the right.

pends on C and the volume of air in the ion chamber. Rather than obtaining these separately, it is more convenient to expose the device to a known radiation field and determine the calibration factor N_X in roentgen/volt; the exposure then is simply

$$X = N_X(V_1 - V_2)$$

Condenser chambers of the type illustrated in Figure 9-9 were widely used for calibration of x-ray generators for many years. One of the most popular was the Victoreen R-meter, which is shown with its protective electrode cover in Figure 9-11C. The voltages were measured on a *string* electrometer (a glorified gold leaf electroscope). Condenser chambers are still used, especially as dosimeters for personnel protection (see Figs. 9-11D and E). They are charged to a known voltage, carried by the person for a day or a week and then remeasured. Some types include a built-in string electrometer so that the drop in voltage with exposure can be seen by the wearer. This is an advantage when one wishes to determine the part of a procedure that contributes the most radiation to the wearer. It should be noted that the polarizing voltage in a condenser chamber decreases as the exposure continues. The exposure should be terminated before the voltage drops below the level required for good ion collection.

Townsend Balance

An integrating dosimeter that involves a slightly different principle is illustrated in Figure 9-10. It uses an ion chamber with guarded construction and an electrometer device that detects zero voltage between R and G. The potentiometer contact point P is placed at O, the central electrode of the ion chamber is grounded by closing S, and the electrometer is adjusted to read zero. Now S is opened and the radiation turned on. Negative charges will flow onto RR′ and the upper plate of C and the electrometer will indicate a negative reading. After exposing for a time t, the radiation is turned off and the contact point P of the potentiometer moved slowly upward until the electrometer returns to its initial null reading. When this happens the charges on RR′ will be as they were initially, and the *total charge liberated* by the radiation will appear on the standard capacitor C. The charge produced in time t is simply Q = CV. Since the measurement involves a capacity C, which can be determined with great precision, and a voltage V, which can also be measured precisely, this technique is often favored in standardization laboratories. Of course, to measure exposure or dose in absolute terms requires that we also know the volume and properties of the ion chamber. The Farmer dosimeter (F3) based on these ideas is widely used.

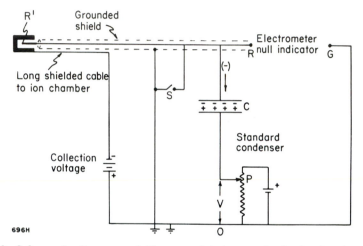

Figure 9-10. Schematic diagram of Townsend balance, the basic circuit used in the Farmer dosimeter.

9.07					**TYPES OF ION CHAMBERS**

To answer many of the practical questions that may arise in a radiology department, one requires a selection of ion chambers that have been developed for particular purposes. A few of them will be discussed. A selection of typical ion chambers are shown in Figure 9-11.

ABSOLUTE DOSIMETRY: For this application one requires a stable ion chamber with a precisely known calibration factor. A Farmer type dosimeter is shown in Figure 9-11A together with its Co-60 buildup cap. For such a chamber to be useful as a standard it should be kept locked up and only used by one or two people to calibrate a secondary dosimeter that then may be used by many others. An absolute dosimeter that has been used frequently is no longer a standard and should be returned to the standardization laboratory for recalibration. The charge liberated can be measured precisely by a good solid state electrometer such as a Keithley or a Townsend balance.

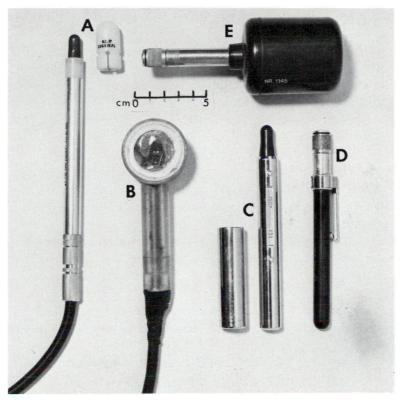

Figure 9-11. (a) Farmer ion chamber with Co-60 cap. (b) Thin walled chamber. (c) Victoreen condenser chamber with electrode cover. (d) Pencil ion chamber for personnel protection. (e) Large volume sensitive chamber for measurement of low levels of radiation.

BUILDUP MEASUREMENTS: In section 7.09 we discussed buildup. Often in a clinical situation one needs to know the dose to the surface of the skin. To measure this requires an ion chamber with a very thin front window or wall. They are usually made by constructing a "pill box" type of structure about 1.5 cm in diameter and 1 mm deep. The front window is made from thin carbon coated Mylar® stretched over the cavity. Such an ion chamber is shown in Figure 9-11B. To measure the buildup region this device is placed in the beam; the response is measured as increasing layers of Mylar or paper, whose thicknesses can be measured in g/cm², are placed over the front window.

BEAM PROFILE MEASUREMENTS: Often one requires a device to explore the edges of a beam where the radiation intensity varies rapidly. For such applications one requires a cylindrical ion chamber of small diameter (6 mm or less) that may be moved slowly across the beam in a direction perpendicular to its axis. To get the required sensitivity, the chamber can be made relatively long (3 cm), since in this direction the dose does not change rapidly. A chamber suitable for this type of work is shown in Figure 9-11A.

DOSE TO PERSONNEL: Dosimeters for this purpose are usually of the condenser type (see Fig. 9-11D). To yield the required sensitivity they should have a relatively large volume, 10 to 20 cm^3. They need not give high precision but they should be reliable and show negligible leakage. Often it is convenient to wear two chambers simultaneously. The lower reading is likely the correct one.

STRAY RADIATION MEASUREMENTS: To measure stray radiation outside a radiation room or near a cobalt unit with the source off, a chamber with high sensitivity and hence a very large volume is required. These may be condenser types (Fig. 9-11E) or connected to an electrometer. The latter is more convenient to use.

LEAKAGE: Leakage of current is always present and the possibility of it being important should be considered. Often the experiment can be done in such a way to eliminate its effects. If leakage is severe look for a conducting fiber or hair across the insulator. If such is not found, carefully wipe the insulator with a brush dipped in absolute alcohol.

STEM IONIZATION: By making an ion chamber small enough, one can approximate the dose at a "point." This may, however, create an unexpected problem for it may be that the measured ionization is not arising solely in the small air cavity of the chamber but also in the stem leading to the air volume. To test this the air volume can be shielded from radiation and the stem exposed. In a good chamber this should give a negligible reading relative to that arising from the air volume.

ISOTROPIC RESPONSE: To explore the dose in a scattering medium one needs to be assured that the detector used does not perturb the radiation being measured. An ion chamber with a heavy and large stem will cut off scattered radiation directed towards the cavity from the direction of the stem and so give too small a reading.

MONITORS: If an x ray machine is stable, then the dose delivered by the device is controlled by the kilovoltage and the tube current in milliamps. If these are held constant, then the dose may be set by the timer. Most therapy machines are fitted with two such timers so that if one fails the second one will terminate the exposure.

Cobalt units are exceedingly stable from hour to hour or day to day so for them a simple timer is all that is required. Again, these are often used in pairs to avoid possible malfunction and overdose. Cobalt units should have lights to indicate when the source is "on." The "on" light should also indicate that the source is *completely* "on" otherwise the patient may be underexposed.

Linear accelerators and betatrons are not stable in output so their beams must be continually monitored. These monitors terminate the dose and also often control the beam by continuously adjusting the bending magnets so that the electron beam is continually centered on the target. A typical monitor for a linac is shown in Figure 9-12. It consists of four separate quadrant collecting electrodes, Q_1, Q_2, Q_3, and Q_4. The signals from these electrodes are used to control the current in the various bending magnets so that the beam is centered on P. When the beam is centered, $Q_1 + Q_2 = Q_3 + Q_4$ and in addition $Q_3 + Q_2 = Q_1 + Q_4$. The chamber has in addition two circular electrodes, M_1 and M_2, covering the area of the beam. These plates are maintained between circular high voltage plates marked HV. The plates are connected to integrating circuits and counters that deliver a pulse after a dose of about 0.1 rad. The operator sets the machine to deliver a certain dose, i.e. a certain number of pulses, and the machine shuts off when this dose is reached. M_1 and M_2 are connected to completely separate electronic systems so that the chance of both of them malfunctioning at the same time is remote. The monitors must, of course, be checked frequently with an accurately calibrated chamber. Many centers perform such a calibration every morning before treatment starts. Because linacs are pulsed and have very high outputs, care must be taken in the design of the monitor to ensure that close to 100 percent of the ions are collected. To ensure efficient ion collection, the plate separations are usually about 1 mm and several hundred volts are used on the HV plates.

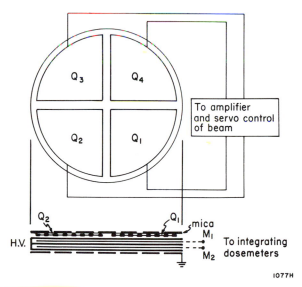

Figure 9-12. Schematic diagram of a monitor ion chamber used in a linac.

1077H

CORRECTION FOR INVERSE SQUARE LAW: Often the ion chamber cannot be placed exactly at the place where one wishes to measure exposure or dose. This situation could arise, for example, at the end of a treatment cone as illustrated in Figure 9-13b. We cannot measure the exposure at

Q but are forced to put the measuring device with its center at P a distance f + r from the radiation source. The dose at Q will be larger than that at P by the inverse square law factor, $(f + r)^2/f^2$. That this is so can be seen from Figure 9-13a. All the radiation that passes through A will pass through B if there is negligible absorption of the radiation between A and B. If f_2 is exactly twice f_1, then b will be 2a and the area of B will be 4 times A. Hence the photon fluence (number of photons per unit area) at B will be 1/4 the value of A. In general it follows that:

$$\Phi_A = \Phi_B \frac{f_2^2}{f_1^2}$$

This is a simple statement of the inverse square law.

Inverse square law corrections are large when f is small and r is large. Imagine using an ion chamber with r = 0.8 cm to measure the exposure from a superficial therapy x ray machine at a focal skin distance of 15 cm. The correction factor is $(15 + .8)^2/15^2 = 1.11$ or 11 percent. Suppose the same chamber were used to measure at a point 80 cm from a cobalt unit. Now, the correction is only 2% $[(80 + .8)^2/80^2 = 1.02]$.

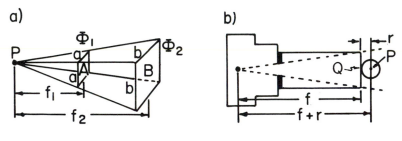

1076H

Figure 9-13. (a) Diagram to illustrate the *inverse square law.* (b) Diagram to illustrate the method for correcting the measured exposure at P to the exposure at the end of the treatment applicator.

9.08   SOLID STATE DETECTORS—THE DIODE

So far in this chapter we have been concerned with the detection of radiation by the ionization produced in a gas and, in particular, in air. Under certain conditions the ionization produced in *solids* can be exploited to allow the detection of radiation. The devices using this principle are called solid state detectors. These have many useful applications and are under rapid development at the time of this writing.

In section 2.03 the p-n silicon rectifier was described. It was designed to conduct large currents (up to amperes) in the forward direction, i.e. with p positive, and to withstand voltages up to 470 volts without much conduction in reverse bias, with p negative. The device was used as a rectifier. By altering the doping of the device it can be made into a detector of light or x rays. Figure 9-14a shows how the device is fabricated. The main part of the detector is a slab of silicon 1 mm thick lightly doped with n type carriers. Into this base a thin layer about one μm thick of p type carriers is diffused. This layer is thin enough to be essentially transparent to light so that light is transmitted into the depletion region where the p and n type carriers are in contact. The depletion region is about 2 μm thick. Electrical connection is made to the p type region by a metalized deposit around the edge of the window. Connection is made to the n type carrier through a layer of heavily doped n type carrier in contact with the lightly doped region. By careful design the leakage current (dark current) can be made very small (10^{-13}A). Some idea of the size of the device can be seen from Figure 9-6D.

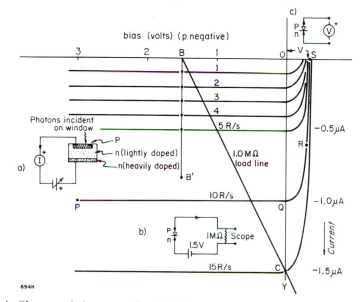

Figure 9-14. Characteristic curves for EG&G UV-100 diode used as a detector of x rays generated at 100 kV. (a) Schematic representation of diode used in the bias mode with p negative. (b) Diode used with a 1 MΩ load resistor giving operation along line BC. (c) Diode used on open circuit along line OS.

Figure 9-14 shows the current as a function of bias voltage for a typical diode for exposure rates from 1 to 15 R/s. Consider the curve marked PQRS corresponding to 10 R/s. With 3 volts bias the current is 1.01 μA (point P). This current decreases slightly to 1.0 μA (point Q) as the bias is reduced to zero. At point Q there is no voltage across the device but there is a current produced by the radiation. For this reason the device at Q is referred to as being operated in the *photo-voltaic* mode. If now the voltage on the device is reversed and P made increasingly positive by a few mV, the current is reduced rapidly to zero along QRS and then increases very rapidly in the opposite direction when P is made more positive. Great care should be exercised in operating the device in this quadrant as the inadvertent application of more than about 300 mV would cause it to conduct heavily in the forward direction, and destroy it.

The most useful region in which the device may be used is with P negative. The characteristic curves were obtained by measuring the current with a zero impedance device as a function of bias voltage for a series of exposure rates. A plot of current as a function of exposure rate at fixed bias (along line BB^1) shows that the device is linear for exposure rates from 1 mR/s up to at least 15 R/s. The sensitivity is about 0.1 μA per R/s using 100 kV$_p$ radiation. This sensitivity increases by about 10% as the bias is increased from 0 to about 15 volts. This increased sensitivity is not, however, useful since the dark current also increases. A bias voltage of more than about 15 volts should *not* be used because the device will start to conduct, as shown by the curves of Figure 2-4. Operating along the line BB^1 requires a current measuring device, I, with small resistance or a current amplifier such as shown in Figure 9-5. In some situations it is simpler to use the circuit of Figure 9-14b, where the signal is observed with an oscilloscope with 1 MΩ impedance. Now the bias decreases with increase in current due to the voltage drop across the 1 MΩ, and we operate along line BC. The sensitivity is now about 0.1 V per R/s. The system is linear, provided the point C is not to the right of the Y axis. Figure 9-14 shows that the system would not be linear for an exposure rate greater than 15 R/s. For higher dose rates the system can be made linear again by either using a larger bias or a smaller load resistance or both.

LOGARITHMIC RESPONSE: The diode may be used on open circuit along the line OS of Figure 9-14. In this situation the voltage generated must be measured by a voltmeter of infinite impedance (as illustrated in Fig. 9-14c). Under these circumstances, theory shows and observations substantiate that the open circuit voltage is proportional to the logarithm of the exposure rate, thus

$$V = k \log (X/t)$$

This mode may be useful when one wishes to evaluate the ratio of two exposure rates.

PROPERTIES AND USES OF THE DIODE DETECTOR: The diode detector has properties that make it a powerful tool in determining the performance of a diagnostic x ray generator. Its use in this way will be dealt with in detail in Chapter 16. Here we summarize its properties and how it may be used.

Study of Wave Form

Air chambers have a slow response because of the time taken to collect the ions (see section 9.2, 9.3). In contrast, in the diode, collection time is very short and it is possible, using the oscilloscope connection of Figure 9-14b, to study the yield of x rays as a function of time in periods as short as 0.1 ms. A diode connected to an oscilloscope provides one with a powerful diagnostic tool to study the wave forms from a diagnostic x ray unit. One can, for example, measure exposure times, study the switching transients, observe damage in the rotor, and see whether the phases exciting the x ray tube are balanced, etc.

MEASURE DOSE: The diode detector may be used to measure exposure or dose for applications where great precision is not required. Since the device is made of silicon ($Z = 14$), it shows a large energy dependence relative to an air ion chamber. This follows from the ratio of the energy absorption coefficient of Si relative to air, which decreases by a factor of 4.6 as the photon energy is increased from 60 keV to Co-60. Therefore, the device is not useful in measuring beams containing photons of many different energies, but it is ideal in measuring dose from diagnostic x ray machines where 10% accuracy is all that is required. Because silicon has a density of about 2000 times that of air, and because W for silicon is about 3.5 eV/ion pair relative to 35 eV/ion pair air, the diode is some 20,000 times as sensitive as an air wall chamber of the same volume. Further, if one is measuring soft radiation in the range 60 to 100 keV where photoelectric absorption is important, there is another five fold sensitivity increase over an air chamber, giving an overall factor of about 10^5.

Diodes have an enormous dynamic range allowing exposure rates from 20 R/s to 0.1 mR/s to be measured. Thus, the output from powerful (1000 mA diagnostic units) x ray machines down to exposure rates used in fluoroscopy and the even smaller ones incident on the input phosphor of an image amplifier can be measured. Since the diode is also sensitive to light, the device may be used to measure the light output from an image amplifier and thus study its performance. For further details on such uses of diodes, see Yaffe (Y2), Thomas (T4), and Chapter 16.

9.09   THERMOLUMINESCENT DOSIMETRY (TLD)

Certain crystalline materials, when heated, emit light proportional to the amount of radiation damage previously inflicted on them. The emission of light by the application of heat is called thermoluminescence. By measuring the light emitted one can determine the radiation dose previously received. This technique is called thermoluminescent dosimetry, or TLD. This technique can also be used by geologists: by making a few assumptions they can estimate the age of rocks or how long ago they were last heated. TLD has been rapidly developed during the 1970s and now provides the radiation physicist with a powerful technique for measuring dose to personnel, calibrating high energy machines, and determining the dose in small inaccessible places in the body. Lithium fluoride

(LiF) is the most popular material for TLD. It has a regular crystalline structure, but when impurities are included imperfections arise in the lattice. The energy levels of such a material are illustrated in Figure 16-10. This diagram shows energy traps that arise from these imperfections. When the material is irradiated the energy is absorbed from the radiation beam; some of the electrons of the crystals of LiF are raised to higher energy levels. Most of the electrons immediately return to the ground state, but a few remain trapped in the impurity levels. Upon subsequent heating of the LiF, these trapped electrons are elevated to still higher electron levels from which they *can* return to the ground state with the emission of light. The total amount of light emitted will be proportional to the number of electrons that were trapped; this in turn is proportional to the amount of energy absorbed from the radiation.

When a previously irradiated sample of LiF is heated at a constant rate, the light output as a function of time follows the pattern shown in Figure 9-15a and is called a "glow curve." The different peaks in this diagram correspond to different "trapped" energy levels. The area under the whole glow curve can be used to measure dose. The arrangement for measuring the light output is shown schematically in Figure 9-15b. The irradiated sample is inserted into a heater and a photomultiplier tube converts the small amount of light emitted into an electrical current so that it may be amplified and measured.

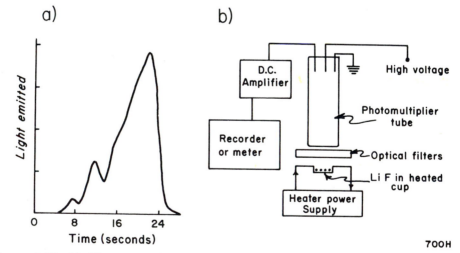

Figure 9-15. (a) Glow curve for LiF showing relative light output as a function of heating time. (b) Schematic diagram showing apparatus for measuring light output from a thermoluminescent material.

TLD material may take a number of different forms. It may be a chip of material, a small cylindrical rod, or powder, and in fact can have almost any desired shape. Figure 9-6E shows several pieces of material used for TLD. For quantitative measurement, care must be exercised to heat the sample and measure the light output in a reproducible way. Many types of automatic commercial equipment are available for this purpose.

PRECISION OF TLD AND DOSE RANGE: LiF may be used to measure dose over a very wide range, from 10^{-5} Gy to 10^3 Gy. Over very wide dose ranges, the sensitivity is not absolutely constant so when precision is required the TLD samples should be calibrated against dose over the range of interest. If the rods and chips are individually calibrated, they give slightly better precision than does powder. These can be reused after careful annealing. With great care a reproducibility of about 2% is possible using chips or rods.

MATERIALS FOR TLD: LiF has an effective atomic number of 8.31, a value close to tissue, and so is the most useful material for medical work. Materials of higher atomic number such as CaF_2 and $CaSO_4$ with various added impurities are useful for the dosimetry of cobalt 60 because they are 10 to 100 times as sensitive as LiF. Because of their high Z, however, they show a rapid variation in response between 30 keV and Co-60.

USES OF TLD—CLINICAL DOSIMETRY: Because TLD material may be fused into chips or rods of very small dimensions, it may be placed in body cavities to explore dose patterns produced by radiation. TLD is particularly useful to explore the dose in regions where the dose varies rapidly, for example around radium needles, or in the buildup region of a high energy beam or where interface effects, such as described in Chapter 7, make dose calculations nearly impossible. Every radiotherapy department should have TLD capabilities so that dose calculations for complex situations can be checked experimentally.

PERSONNEL MONITORING: TLD has found an important place in radiation monitoring and is rapidly replacing the use of film. It offers greater precision than film and is more easily automated, a distinct advantage when thousands of samples are involved, as in a government-organized service.

DOSE CALIBRATION SERVICES: In the earlier sections of this chapter we discussed some of the problems of correctly calibrating a high energy therapy unit. TLD may be used to compare these procedures from one center to another. TLD samples can be mailed to a group of centers and the user in each requested to expose the samples to a specified dose, of perhaps 5.00 Gy. The exposure is carried out by the user for each of his machines and the exposed TLD samples mailed back to the coordinating center for measurement. This is an ideal way to compare the absolute dosimetry of the various centers at minimum cost. Precision of about 2% can be achieved with TLD. For further details on TLD see books by Cameron (C6) and Attix (A5), and for a recent paper on its clinical use see Van Dyk and Leung (V3).

9.10   **CHEMICAL DOSIMETRY**

The energy absorbed from radiation may produce a chemical change in the absorbing medium, and the amount of this may be used to measure dose. One of the most useful chemical radiation dosimeters is the Fricke dosimeter, which depends upon the oxidation of an acidic aqueous solution of ferrous sulphate to ferric sulphate. The amount of ferric ion produced can be readily measured by absorption spectrometry, since ultraviolet light at 304 nm is strongly absorbed by the ferric ion.

G VALUE: The radiation chemical yield is expressed as the number of molecules of product produced per 100 eV of absorbed energy. This number is known as the G value. Consider a sample of ferrous sulphate of density ρ in kg/m^3 is given a dose D and in the process a concentration ΔM (moles/liter) or ferric ions are produced. Since the energy absorbed is $D\rho$ we may write G as

$$G = \Delta M/D\rho \tag{9-34}$$

Since ΔM may be measured by spectrometry and G may be determined from other experiments we may solve for the dose D:

$$D = \frac{\Delta M}{G\rho} \tag{9-35}$$

We want D in grays so we must convert moles to number of molecules, m^3 to liters and eV to joules. The student may show that

$$D = \frac{\Delta M}{G\rho} \times 9.65 \times 10^9 \text{ Gy} \tag{9-36}$$

DETERMINATION OF AMOUNT OF FERRIC ION PRODUCED: The quantity of ferric ion produced by the radiation may be determined by measuring the "optical density" of an irradiated solution and comparing it with that of an unirradiated solution. The absorbance A or optical density of a solution is defined by the equation

$$A = \log \frac{I_0}{I_t} \tag{9-37}$$

where I_0 is intensity of the incident light impinging on a quartz cell containing the solution and I_t that of the transmitted light. If only 1/10 of the incident light is transmitted, the optical density is 1.0 ($\log 10 = 1$). The absorbance, as defined by this equation, is directly proportional to the amount of the absorbing species present. For example, if twice the amount of material were present, this would be equivalent to twice the thickness of solution and the transmitted intensity would be $1/10 \times 1/10 = 1/100$, then the optical density would be 2 ($\log 100 = 2$). Spectrophotometers are devices that enable one to determine precisely the absorbance, A_λ, of a solution at any suitable wavelength, λ, from the ultraviolet (200 nm) up to the infrared (1000 nm).

Since optical density is proportional to the amount of material in a solution, it may be expressed thus

$$A_\lambda = \epsilon_\lambda \cdot l \cdot M \tag{9-38}$$

where l is the path length of the cell in cm, M is the concentration of the absorbing species in the solution in moles/liter, and ϵ_λ is the constant of proportionality called the molar extinction coefficient. Since A_λ is dimensionless, ϵ_λ has dimension liter moles^{-1} cm^{-1} = 1000 cm^2 moles^{-1}. Thus, it has dimensions of area/mole and is really an attenuation coefficient similar to those defined in Chapter 6 (see problem 22). If ϵ_λ is known, the concentration may be determined from a measurement of A_λ using equation 9-38. Solving equation 9-38 for M and substituting it in equation 9-36, we obtain for the absorbed dose

$$D = \frac{\Delta A_\lambda}{\epsilon_\lambda l \rho G} (9.65 \times 10^9) \text{ grays} \tag{9-39}$$

where ΔA_λ is the change in absorbance at λ following a dose D to the ferrous sulphate; ϵ_λ is the molar extinction coefficient of the ferrous ion (which has been precisely determined to be 2196 ± 5 liter moles^{-1} cm^{-1} at 304 nm); ρ is the density of the solution in kg/m^3; and G is the yield in number per 100 eV. The precise value for G is not easily arrived at since it varies with the energy of the radiation. Recommended values for G taken from ICRU (I6) are given in Table 9-1.

TABLE 9-1

Recommended G Values for the Production of Ferric Ion Fe^{+++} in 0.4 Mole/Liter H_2SO_4 as a Function of Photon Energy

Radiation	G Value (no. per 100 eV)
^{137}Cs	15.3 ± 0.3
2 MV	15.4 ± 0.3
^{60}Co	15.5 ± 0.2
4 MV	15.5 ± 0.3
5–10 MV	15.6 ± 0.4
11–30 MV	15.7 ± 0.6

From ICRU #14 and 21 (I6, I5)

TECHNICAL ASPECTS OF THE USE OF FERROUS SULPHATE: In principle the use of ferrous sulphate as a dosimeter is simple, but for accuracy considerable care must be taken (see I5, I6). It is necessary to create an environment for the ferrous ion in which it is stable, so that its concentration may be measured accurately some time after the irradiation. To provide this stability, it is usual to prepare a stock solution of 1 millimole per liter $FeSO_4$, 1 millimole per liter NaCl in aerated 0.4 mol/liter H_2SO_4 in clean glassware. Such a solution, often called a Fricke solution, has a density of 1024 kg/m^3. The presence of the sulphur in the solution (mainly from the H_2SO_4) causes a slight increase in absorption over water for soft radiation but has negligible effect at the energies listed in Table 9-1, f-values for water and Fricke solution are listed in Table A-7. At 10 keV the Fricke solution absorbs about 10% more energy than water due to the extra photoelectric absorption in the sulphur and a true correction for this extra absorption would require a knowledge of the spectral distribution. Since soft radiation can be measured easily with ion chambers, the Fricke dosimeter is not generally used for such radiations. The Fricke dosimeter is of particular value in dealing with high energy x ray and electron beams. Now, the main problem is a precise knowledge of the G value (see Table 9-1). This problem cannot be solved until better measurements of the G value have been made using calorimeters.

The Fricke dosimeter is very useful in determining the average dose to an irradiated volume of complex shape. A container the shape of the region of interest is fabricated and filled with the Fricke solution and then irradiated. The solution is agitated to mix the ferric ion uniformly throughout the volume, and then its average concentration is measured. The system is linear up to about 350 Gy. It is not useful for measuring doses of less than about 10 Gy because of the difficulty in measuring precisely the small change in absorbance of the solution due to the presence of the ferric ion. For accuracy, one should try to irradiate the volume of interest to an average dose of at least 50 Gy.

Example 9-10. It is required to determine the average dose to a sample of water in a complexly shaped radiation container near a cobalt source. This is most easily done using the Fricke dosimeter. The container is filled with Fricke solution and exposed. A sample of the well-mixed irradiated solution is then placed in a quartz cuvette of 2 cm path length and its absorbance measured against the stock solution at 304 nm. Suppose the measured absorbance is 0.360. Calculate the dose.

$$\frac{D(\text{eq. 9-39})}{\text{to Fricke sol.}} = \frac{0.360 \times 9.65 \times 10^9}{2196 \times 2.0 \times 1024 \times 15.5} = 49.8 \text{ Gy}$$

Because of the presence of sulphur in the Fricke solution, 1 gram of it will absorb slightly more than 1 gram of water. The correction can be made approximately by taking the ratio of the mass energy absorption coefficients for Fricke solution and water using Table A-3, yielding

$$D(\text{water}) = 49.8 \times \frac{0.0297}{0.0296} = 49.9 \text{ Gy}$$

A more correct value would be obtained by averaging the coefficients over the photon spectrum using equation 7-12. This would make little difference in this case.

9.11 FILM AS A DOSIMETER

X rays have the property of affecting a film in much the same way as light. The film contains very small crystals of silver bromide. When radiant energy strikes these crystals, they become more susceptible to chemical change and form what is referred to as a *latent image*. When the film is developed, the crystals that have been altered by the radiation are reduced to small grains of metallic silver. The film is then *fixed;* this dissolves the unaffected silver bromide, leaving a clear film, but does not affect the metallic silver. Thus areas that have been exposed to x rays appear dark and a negative film results.

The concentration of metallic silver grains is measured by determining the optical density or absorbance of the film, using a densitometer illustrated in the insert to Figure 9-16. Light from the source, S, is passed through a diffusing screen and is incident on a small aperture just below the film under test. The light transmitted through the film (I_t) is measured by a photocell placed above the film. This light detector is arranged to collect essentially all the light that comes through the aperture regardless of its direction. This light reading is compared with the value obtained with no film in place (I_0) and the optical density is calculated from $\log (I_0/I_t)$ using equation 9-37. In most densitometers the optical density can be read directly on a linear scale without the necessity of any calculation. This simplification is achieved by zeroing the instrument so that with no film in place the density reads zero. Densitometers usually have a series of apertures so that the area of the film whose density is sampled can be varied at will. Apertures with openings down to 0.5 mm diameter can often be used, allowing one to essentially measure at a "point."

Figure 9-16 shows the optical density of two films as a function of x ray exposure. Graph B is for a relatively fast film giving an optical density of 2.8 for an exposure of 100 mR. In contrast, graph C is for a very slow film yielding a density of 1.2 for an exposure of over 100 R. For zero exposure both films have a density of about 0.2; this is called the background or fog, which is always present. With increase in exposure the optical density increases rather linearly and then gradually saturates as the exposure is increased. Saturation starts to set in when the unexposed silver bromide starts to be used up. The curves of Figure 9-16 should not be confused with the characteristic curves of Figure 16-12 where density is plotted against the *log* of the exposure.

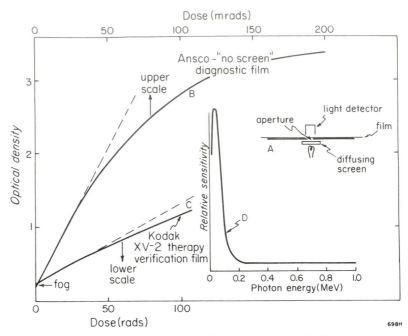

Figure 9-16. (a) Schematic representation of a densitometer. Calibration curves for (b) fast and (c) slow films showing optical density as a function of exposure. (d) Sensitivity as a function of photon energy, due to Ehrlich (E5).

The optical density of a film depends on the exposure, but it also depends very critically on the development procedure. To be useful as a dosimeter the development of the film must be carefully controlled using the correct chemicals, time, temperature, and agitation. For consistent results automatic processors should be used as discussed in Chapter 16. Furthermore, a careful calibration of density versus exposure over the range of interest must be made for each batch of film used and each development protocol. The need for a calibration over the exposure range of interest is obvious from Figure 9-16, which shows that film is *not* a linear system except for very small exposures.

ENERGY RESPONSE. The blackening of a film by radiation depends primarily on the absorption of the radiation by the silver salts. Silver (Z = 47) absorbs radiation below 150 keV very strongly by the photoelectric process, so in the range from 0 to 150 keV the response is very dependent on energy. This is illustrated by curve D in Figure 9-16, which shows that the speed or sensitivity of the film is some 25 times as great for photons at energy near 25 keV (K edge of silver is 25.5 keV) as it is for photons above 200 keV. From this graph it is clear that film *may not* be used for precise dosimetry if a wide band of radiation is present with energies in the range 10 keV to 1 MeV. However, above 200 keV the response is "flat" with energy, and films now make good dosimeters. For investigations involving high energy beams from cobalt units and linear accelerators, films provide a useful tool for dosimetry. Film also makes a good *practical* dosimeter for the diagnostic range excited by 50 to 150 kV_p as discussed in section 16.07.

Uses of Film in Dosimetry. For high energy radiations, films are useful in obtaining a quick quantitative pattern of a radiation distribution. For example, a single exposure of a film in a water phantom can be used to determine the complete isodose pattern (see Chapter 10). Densitometers are available that mechanically seek out and plot constant density lines, which can be related to isodose lines once a dose calibration curve has been obtained. They are also useful for checking the alignment of diaphragms in treatment cones, the size and shape of a radiation field, the accuracy of a light localizer, the size of the penumbra around a field, leakage radiation around collimators, and the positioning of special radiation shields. They may also be used to measure in the buildup region of a beam. To do this a sheet of film in its light-tight paper envelope would be placed on the surface of the phantom and covered with a step wedge made of increasing thicknesses of low atomic number material. The film, covered with the step wedge, is given one exposure and developed, and the density pattern is measured with a densitometer. This technique should give results similar to LiF powder.

Protection: Films have been used for many years as personnel monitors. They are very sensitive and so can measure small doses. By covering the film with various types of filters one can determine the type of radiation causing the exposure, as well as the amount. The lack of great accuracy for this application is not a serious drawback.

Films may be used to locate radiation leaks by simply placing them at the suspected spot and leaving them there for a suitable time. They may also be used to measure the integrated dose over a week or month at points of interest around a therapy or diagnostic installation. For the latter, care must be taken to calibrate the film using radiation of the same quality as that being investigated.

9.12   **DIRECT MEASUREMENT OF ABSORBED DOSE—THE CALORIMETER**

When a medium is bombarded by radiation, most of the energy absorbed will give rise to heat while a small amount may appear in the form of chemical change. Neglecting for the moment the latter, we can calculate the rise in temperature produced by the absorption of 1 Gy in water as follows:

$$1 \text{ Gy} = 1 \frac{\text{J}}{\text{kg}} = \frac{1}{4.18} \frac{\text{calories}}{\text{kg}} \qquad (9\text{-}40)$$

Since the specific heat of water is 10^3 cal/kg °C the rise in temperature produced by 1 Gy is

$$\Delta T = \frac{1}{4.18} \frac{cal}{kg} \times \frac{1}{10^3} \frac{kg}{cal} °C = 2.39 \times 10^{-4} °C$$

This small change in temperature can be measured using a thermistor. These are semiconductors that exhibit a large change in resistance (about 5%) for a 1 degree change in temperature. Useful thermistors for this work are about the size of a pinhead and have resistances in the range 10^3 to 10^5 ohms. In the above example, the change in resistance of a $10^5\Omega$ resistor produced by one Gy in water will be

$$\Delta R = \frac{5}{100} \times 10^5\Omega \times 2.39 \times 10^{-4} = 1.2\Omega$$

By using a carefully designed Wheatstone bridge, this change in resistance may be measured precisely. Calorimeters may be designed to measure energy fluence or to measure energy locally absorbed. Each of these types will be described.

ENERGY FLUENCE. If the beam of radiation is directed into a thermally insulated block of lead, the beam can be totally absorbed and the rise in temperature measured (G9). The energy fluence of the beam in J/m^2 can thus be determined. This basic energy measurement can be compared to the exposure in roentgens, and may thus be used to check the calculation of energy flux per roentgen dealt with in section 7.15. The measurement of energy fluence is of considerable interest in basic physics but of less importance in radiology and so will not be dealt with further here.

ENERGY LOCALLY ABSORBED. A calorimeter designed to measure energy locally absorbed is illustrated in Figure 9-17a. The absorber or core of the device is placed inside a jacket and a shield, which is in turn placed in a large thermally controlled mass of buffer. The core, jacket, shield, and buffer are made of the same material and are thermally insulated from each other by maintaining a vacuum between all of the components, which minimizes heat losses by conduction and convection. Radiation losses are minimized by covering the components with a very thin layer of aluminum. The components are fitted with thermistors and small electrical heaters so the temperature of each can be measured and controlled. The "nested" components are designed to simulate a phantom. Calorimeters may be made of graphite or tissue-equivalent plastic. Each of these has advantages and disadvantages, which will be dealt with later.

Suppose the core, jacket, shield, and buffer are brought to the same temperature, and then the radiation beam is turned on. As radiation is absorbed, the core will rise in temperature as will the jacket and shield. Since the core and jacket "see" essentially the same radiation and since

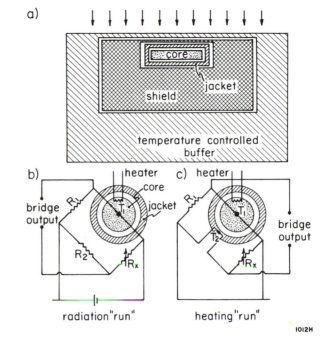

Figure 9-17. (a) Schematic diagram of calorimeter designed to measure energy locally absorbed. (b) Arrangement of components in a Wheatstone bridge to measure the rise in temperature of the core when the calorimeter is exposed to radiation. (c) Arrangement of components to measure the rise in temperature of the core when heat is injected electrically. With this configuration most of the heat lost from the core to the jacket is automatically corrected for. (Adapted from Domen, D6, 7.)

they are made of the same material, they will show the same temperature rise; heat transfer from core to jacket during an experiment will be minimized. The rise in temperature is measured by a Wheatstone bridge as illustrated in Figure 9-17b. The change in temperature, ΔT_r, is measured by connecting the bridge output to an amplifier recorder system. If the mass and specific heat of each component of the core were accurately known, one could determine the energy input from the measured rise in temperature, ΔT_r. In practice, it is simpler to dissipate a known amount of electrical energy, E_h, in the core and measure the rise in temperature, ΔT_h, produced. The energy absorbed from the radiation beam is then

$$E_{ab} = E_h \frac{\Delta T_r}{\Delta T_h} \qquad (9\text{-}41)$$

By carefully measuring these quantities and correcting for heat losses the energy locally absorbed can be measured to an accuracy of about 0.1%.

The determination of E_{ab} from equation 9-41 tacitly implies that the heat losses from the core for the radiation experiment are the same as for the electrical heating experiment. A little thought will convince the reader that this is not true. In the heating "run," the core increases in temperature but the jacket does not, leading to an increase in the heat loss from the core to jacket. Domen (D6,7) at NBS has introduced a convenient way to overcome this heat loss by placing T_2 (a thermistor in the jacket) in the opposite arm of the Wheatstone bridge, as illustrated in Figure 9-17c. In this configuration the student may easily show that the output of the bridge is now proportional to the sum of the temperature rises of core and jacket. If now the jacket is adjusted to have the *same* thermal capacity as the core, then the output voltage is proportional to the heat deposited in the core added to the heat lost from the core to the jacket. Of course, as the jacket warms up from energy that has reached it from the core, it in turn will start to lose energy to the shield. The amount of energy escaping this way is very small and can easily be corrected for. The efficacy of this mode of operation is illustrated in Figure 9-18a. The temperature of the core during and after a 100 s heating period is the curve OAB. The temperature rise of the jacket is given by OC, while the temperature change of the core plus jacket is OA′B′. This is measured directly with the configuration of Figure 9-17c. The line A′B′ is very nearly parallel to the axis and the true temperature rise of the core after a heating run is PA′.

MATERIALS FOR CALORIMETERS. One of the most troublesome problems with calorimetry is the long-term drifts that take place after injection of energy into any part of the system. These drifts arise because of thermal gradients in the material and the fact that thermal isolation cannot be made perfect. For example, after a pulse of heat is injected into one part of the core, it will take several seconds for all points of the core to reach one temperature; during this period the heat loss from the core to jacket cannot be calculated. The parameter that is important in determining the time for thermal gradients to disappear is $k/\rho c$, where k is the thermal conductivity, ρ the density, and c the specific heat. This parameter is called the temperature diffusivity; the larger its value the more rapidly temperature gradients will disappear. A calorimeter should be made of material with large thermal conductivity, k, and small ρc. Typical values for these parameters are given in Table 9-2, where we see that carbon (graphite) is slightly better than copper and 1000 times as large as water or tissue equivalent plastic (TEP) A-150. From this point of view, carbon makes the best calorimeter.

TABLE 9-2
Temperature Diffusivity

Material	ρ-Density g/cm^3	c-Specific Heat Jg^{-1}°C^{-1}	k-Thermal Conductivity Jcm^{-1}s^{-1}°C^{-1}	Temperature Diffusivity $k/\rho c$ [cm^2/s]
Carbon	2.25	.71	2	1.25*
Copper	8.96	.38	4.0	1.16
Water	1.00	4.2	6.1×10^{-3}	1.4×10^{-3}
A-150 (TEP)	1.13	1.7	1.3×10^{-3}	$.68 \times 10^{-3}$*

*Courtesy Domen (NBS)

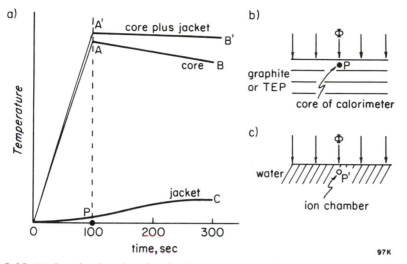

Figure 9-18. (a) Graphs showing the rise in temperature of the core, jacket, and core plus jacket of a graphite calorimeter during and following a 100 s heating period (adapted from Domen, D6). (b) Calorimeter in radiation field Φ. (c) Transfer ion chamber at point P, in the same radiation field.

HEAT DEFECTS. The whole basis of calorimetry rests on the idea that the energy input will appear as heat, giving rise to a change in temperature. For many materials this is not the case. Bewley (B 10) and McDonald (M9,10) have shown that when tissue-equivalent plastic is irradiated, the rise in temperature may be too large or too small. Apparently oxygen is trapped in the plastic when it is made and on irradiation a chemical reaction takes place yielding a temperature rise as much as 15% too high. After doses of some 10^3 gray this effect disappears, presumably due to the depletion of the trapped oxygen. The effect can also be removed by expelling the oxygen by an annealing and degassification program. Now the plastic shows the opposite effect, in which about 3% of the input energy produces some unknown chemical effect and does not appear as heat. Many careful experiments on TEP will have to be carried out before precise absolute dosimetry with TEP is feasible. To date there is no evidence for either thermal excess or defect in graphite, making it the material of choice from this point of view.

DETERMINATION OF DOSE IN WATER. Imagine a calorimeter placed in a radiation field Φ as illustrated in Figure 9-18b. For a given irradiation the calorimeter yields the absorbed dose, D_0, in the material of the calorimeter, which may be TEP or graphite. We then slide the calorimeter out of the beam and in its place put a water phantom with a high quality ion chamber connected to its electrometer at P_1 (Fig. 9-18c). We expose this chamber to the *same* irradiation, giving a meter reading M_0. This process calibrates our ion chamber as a "gray meter" for any beam with properties similar to Φ. For example, suppose the chamber in the water phantom yields a reading M when placed in a similar beam; then the dose D is

$$D = \frac{M}{M_0} \cdot D_0 \cdot K = M \cdot N_D \qquad (9\text{-}42)$$

$$\text{where } K = \frac{\text{Energy absorbed by sample water at } P_1}{\text{Energy absorbed by calorimeter material at } P} \qquad (9\text{-}43)$$

and N_D is the absorbed dose calibration factor of equation 7-31.

If the calorimeter material is TEP, which is very similar to water, and if P_1 and P are at the same depth, then K = 1 and our calibration is complete. The precision of this calibration depends upon the precision of the TEP calorimeter and our knowledge of the heat defects present. Careful investigations of these heat defects are necessary. Perhaps a better approach would be to use some type of water calorimeter as described many years ago by Bernier (B11).

The other approach is to use a carbon calorimeter as described by Domen (D6); such a device can yield the absorbed dose in carbon to a precision of about 0.1%. Now our uncertainty will arise in calculating the absorbed dose to water at point P' from the absorbed dose in carbon at point P. One could add a layer of graphite to the water phantom to make the primary dose at P and P_1 identical. If this were done then K would to a first approximation be given by

$$K = \frac{(\mu_{ab}/\rho)_{water}}{(\mu_{ab}/\rho)_{graphite}} \qquad (9\text{-}44)$$

The validity of determining K in this way would have to be established by careful experiments. If it could be established, we would avoid the many troublesome cap corrections, displacement corrections, stopping power ratios, etc. dealt with in Chapter 7. Clearly the optimum path to absorbed dose calibration has yet to be established and more research is required. (For a review of this field, see N6.)

9.13   SUMMARY OF CALIBRATION PROCEDURES

In this section we discuss some practical considerations concerned with determining the output of diagnostic x ray machines and radiotherapy treatment units. For machines producing radiation with photon energies less than about 3 MeV, this can conveniently be done by measuring exposure rate in air. We are ultimately, however, more concerned with absorbed dose rate in a phantom, and this can be calculated from the exposure rate by using appropriate multiplying factors, some of which have been discussed in Chapter 7 and some of which will be discussed in Chapter 10. For photon energies above 3 MeV and for other modalities of radiation (such as beams of neutrons or charged particles), it is necessary to determine the absorbed dose rate directly in a phantom under some specified reference conditions without the intermediate step of first measuring exposure in air.

Exposure Rate Determinations

Exposure rates for diagnostic x ray machines and x and γ ray therapy machines of energies up to 3 MeV are determined as follows.

a. Select a suitable treatment applicator or reference field size (for example 10 by 10 cm) and direct the beam in such a way as to avoid scattering from nearby objects.

b. Select filter, tube current (mA), and voltage (kV) and determine the half-value layer (see section 8.03) for these settings of the machine.

c. Select a suitable practical dosimeter that has an exposure calibration factor traceable to a standardization laboratory (see section 7.09) for the half-value layer of the radiation beam to be measured. The ionization chamber should be one that has been designed specifically for the energy of radiation being measured. Such chambers and the relevant considerations are discussed in sections 7.09, 7.10, and 9.07. It may be necessary to interpolate between two calibration factors to obtain the required one.

d. Fasten the dosimeter in a clamp so that its position is accurately known and can be reproduced for repeated readings. The center of the sensitive volume of the ion chamber should be at the center of the field and even with the end of the treatment cone if there is one, or else at the reference distance chosen for the calibration. Sometimes this is not possible, in which case an inverse square correction will have to be made (section 9.07).

e. Set the timer to an appropriate value, turn on the machine, and bring it to the operating point selected in b. Open the shutter, or in the case of a cobalt unit simply turn the beam on. If the ion chamber is operated as an exposure rate measuring instrument, its reading can now be taken directly. If it is to be operated as an exposure meter, timer, settings should be chosen so that a set of readings are obtained at both relatively high scale readings (say about 3/4 scale) and relatively low scale readings. The exposure rate may then be obtained by taking differences of sets of readings to determine the slope of the "reading versus time" curve. That is:

$$\frac{\Delta M}{\Delta t} = \frac{M_2 - M_1}{t_2 - t_1}$$

where M_2 and M_1 are high and low meter readings for times t_2 and t_1. Several sets of readings should be averaged to give $\Delta M/\Delta t$, the "reading per unit time." Alternatively, since many computers and calculators are equipped with "least squares routines," it is convenient to take a series of readings M_i at times t extending across the range of the dosimeter and determine the slope, $\Delta M/\Delta t$, of the M versus t line. This latter procedure gives information about the precision of determining this slope; it can also give information about the shutter timing error.

f. During the exposure, for an x ray machine it may be necessary to adjust either the kV or mA. If this is not possible the average tube current and voltage over the time of the exposure should be recorded.

It will be helpful to construct a small table with the headings time, reading, mA, kV, and corrected reading. The corrected reading will be the actual reading multiplied by correction factors for mA and kV as follows. Output is directly proportional to mA, for small variations at least; if the actual tube current were 19.6 mA on the average when the selected current was 20.0 mA, the reading should be corrected by the factor 20.0/19.6 = 1.020, or 2%. The correction for kV is more difficult. To obtain it properly an experiment should be performed in which the exposure is measured for a series of kV settings, keeping the tube current constant. Such an experiment might show that a 1% change in kV produced a 2.5% change in exposure. If this is not done, one may assume that the exposure depends on the square of the kV so that a 1% change in kV produces a 2% change in exposure. The correction factor for such a change would be 1.02 if the kV were 1% low.

g. Measure temperature and pressure. The exposure calibration factor as issued by the standardization laboratory is valid only for the temperature and pressure stated by them. It is usually 22°C and 101.3 kPa but this should be confirmed.

h. The corrected exposure rate is:

$$\frac{\Delta M}{\Delta t} \left(\frac{f + x}{f}\right)^2 \left(\frac{101.3}{P} \times \frac{273 + T}{273 + T_x}\right) N_x$$

where $\Delta M/\Delta t$ is the average uncorrected exposure rate as obtained in paragraph e, f is the SSD, x is the distance from the SSD to the center of the chamber, P and T are the pressure and temperature of the gas in the ion chamber when the measurement is made, and T_x is the temperature for which the calibration factor, N_x, applies.

i. A number of other small corrections may be required. Efficiency of ion collection is discussed in sections 9.02 and 9.03. The problems of leakage stem ionization are discussed in section 9.07. A dosimeter should also be checked for constancy of sensitivity, and if it has changed since the calibration was performed, allowance must be made. Some instruments are equipped with a device containing a long-lived radioactive isotope for this purpose. Alternatively, careful measurements of a cobalt unit can be used.

j. These procedures, carefully carried out, should allow an output calibration for the conditions measured, to an accuracy of better than ±2.5% (17).

Determination of Absorbed Dose Rate in Free Space

Proceed as in paragraphs c, d, e, f, g, h, and i above. The dose rate in free space can then be calculated using equation 7-28, using data from Table 7-4 and Figure 7-5.

Determination of Absorbed Dose Data in a Phantom

a. An appropriate phantom must be chosen. Ideally, the phantom should be composed of water but since they are somewhat inconvenient to handle, phantoms made of plastics such as polystyrene are frequently used. The dimensions must be such that a margin of at least 5 cm is provided around all sides of the largest field being measured. The phantom should also extend to a depth at least 10 cm deeper than the point of measurement, to provide complete backscatter.

b. If a water phantom is used, the ion chamber must be provided with a watertight sleeve and clamped securely in the phantom at a known position. If a solid phantom is used it must have a hole drilled in it to allow the ion chamber to be inserted to a well-known position. The ion chamber should fit the hole so that no appreciable air spaces surround it, particularly the sensitive part of the chamber. The distance from the surface of the phantom to the center of the ion chamber should be known with a precision of at least ±1 mm.

c. The phantom should be clamped to the treatment unit or located in such a way that its position can be reproduced for repeated measurements and the distances from the source to the ion chamber should be known with a precision of at least ±2 mm.

d. All steps from b through i of the exposure calibrations will also apply.

e. The absorbed dose in the phantom is calculated using expressions and factors given in sections 7.12 and 7.13.

f. These procedures, carefully carried out, should yield an absorbed dose determination in the phantom to an accuracy of approximately ±2.5%.

PROBLEMS

1. A pulse of radiation produces equal concentrations of positive and negative ions in air for which $\alpha = 1.6 \times 10^{-6}$ cm^3 s^{-1}. If the initial charge concentration $Q_0 = 20$ pC/cm^3, plot the charge concentration as a function of time. What times are required for Q_0 to drop to 1/2 the original value; 1/4 the original value? Is this exponential decay?

2. The plates of an ion chamber are 5.0 cm apart and 600 volts is applied between them. A pulse of radiation produces an instantaneous uniform charge distribution

in the air between the plates. Determine the time during which recombination can take place.

3. Find the fraction of ions collected in a parallel plate ion chamber exposed to radiation, which liberates 18.0 pC/cm^3 per pulse. The plates are 1.8 cm apart and 360 volts is applied between them.

4. A parallel plate chamber with plates 1.5 cm apart and 300 volts between them is exposed to continuous radiation, which liberates 8 μC/cm^{3}s in the air between the plates. Find the fraction of ions collected.

5. A cylindrical air-filled ion chamber of radius 0.6 cm with a central electrode of radius 0.1 cm is exposed to a cobalt 60 beam at an exposure rate of 200 R/min. If the collecting voltage is 180 volts, determine the fraction of ions collected.

6. The chamber of problem 5 is exposed to a pulsed beam with an exposure of 2.05 R per pulse. Find the fraction of ions collected.

7. Perform the integration of equation 9-8 and show that the integral is given by equation 9-9.

8. Perform the integration of equation 9-17a to yield equation 9-17b.

9. Perform the calculation involved in proceeding from equation 9-19a to equation 9-19b.

10. The chamber described in problem 5 is used to measure the radiation from a full wave diagnostic x ray unit, which yields an average exposure rate of 100 R/min. Determine the fraction of ions lost to recombination assuming first a uniform exposure rate and then square pulses each lasting 1/120 sec.

11. A high power high energy linac gives an average dose rate of 10 Gy/min at 1 meter. This is equivalent to about 3.33 × 10^5 pC/cm^3 min in an air-walled cavity. A cylindrical chamber with a radius of 0.5 cm and an inner electrode 0.05 cm radius is used to measure this radiation. With 400 volts across the chamber and the linac producing 100 pulses/s, estimate the fraction of ions collected.

    The same linac has a parallel plate monitor chamber 40 cm from the target. If the plates are 1 mm apart and a potential of 200 volts is applied between them, estimate the fraction of the charge lost to recombination.

12. Derive equation 9-27 from equations 9-24, 9-25 and 9-26.

13. Show that for the circuit of Figure 9-7c, $V_0 = V_2 \ R_1/(R_1 + R_2) - V_1 \ R_f/R_3$. What resistor values would you choose to make $V_0 = 10V_2 - V_1$?

14. An ion chamber with outer diameter 1.00 cm is used to measure the output of an x ray machine that has a treatment cone designed to treat at a distance of 50.0 cm. The chamber is placed in contact with this treatment cone with its center 50.5 from the target. The chamber has a calibration factor of 0.315 × 10^{10} roentgens per coulomb at a temperature of 20°C and a pressure of 101.3 kPa for the radiation being measured. It is connected to a good solid state electrometer and exposed for 60.0 seconds, yielding a charge of 3.05 × 10^{-8}C. The temperature and pressure at the time of the measurement was 25°C and 99.2 kPa. Determine the exposure rate at the *end* of the treatment cone.

15. A cobalt 60 unit is to be calibrated with an exposure meter that has a calibration factor of 1.032 roentgens per meter reading at 20°C and 101.3 k Pa. The ion chamber with its buildup cap has a diameter of 1.80 cm. It is exposed for 5 seconds, yielding a reading of 6.1, and then for 65 seconds giving a reading of 91.1. The temperature is 18°C and the pressure 100.1 kPa. Determine the exposure rate.

16. A Farmer ion chamber is connected in a Townsend balance as in Figure 9-10. It was found that the point P had to be raised in potential by 10.0 V to maintain balance during the exposure of an ion chamber in the radiation field. The condenser C had

a capacity of 501 pF and the air wall chamber a volume of .506 cm^3. Calculate the exposure.

17. Figure 9-14 shows the characteristic curves for a diode. Such a device is biased at 3 volts and used in configuration of Figure 9-14b with a 1 MΩ load resistor. Draw the load line and estimate the exposure rate at which it will become nonlinear.

18. Determine the buildup of dose with depth for either a cobalt unit or a linac using TLD powder. Repeat, using film.

19. Calculate the amount of ferric sulphate that is produced in a ferrous sulphate solution after a dose of 1.00 Gy. Determine the change in optical density of the solution as measured in a 1 cm cell. Can you see why the ferrous sulphate dosimeter is not useful in measuring small doses?

20. After a given exposure to Co-60 radiation, the change in absorbance at 304 nm of a ferrous sulphate solution as measured in a 1 cm cell is 0.482. Find the dose in grays.

21. Derive equation 9-36 from equations 9-34 and 9-35.

22. We showed that the molar extinction coefficient, ϵ_λ, had the dimension of area/mole. Show that the cross section σ in cm^2/molecule is related to ϵ_λ by

$$\sigma = \frac{2.303 \; \epsilon_\lambda \times 1000}{N_0}$$

where N_0 is Avogadro's number. Determine σ for the ferric ion at 304 nm. Note that it is some million times as large as most of the cross sections for x ray absorption given in the appendix. Discuss.

23. A sample of ferrous sulphate solution is exposed to radiation from a 10 MeV linac. The change in absorbance produced by the radiation was 0.415 as measured in a 5 cm cell. Determine the dose in grays to the solution. Calculate the dose to a sample of water placed at the same place in the radiation field.

24. Figure 9-17c shows a configuration involving two thermistors—one in the core, and one in the jacket. Show that the output of the bridge is proportional to the sum of the temperature rises of core and jacket.

25. A nearly infinite slab of material is brought to one temperature, T_0, and at time zero one face of the slab is placed in contact with a heat source at temperature T. Write down the differential equation for the temperature T of any point in the material at time t. Show that the important parameter in determining the rate at which the temperature diffuses through the block is $k/\rho c$, where k is the thermal conductivity, ρ the density, and c the specific heat.

26. A cobalt 60 beam of area 1.0 cm^2 gives an exposure rate of 100 R/min at a point in space. Determine the energy fluence rate and the photon fluence rate. Design a total absorption calorimeter of Pb to measure the energy fluence rate. Determine the rise in temperature in 1 min assuming no heat loss, density of lead 11.3 g/cm^3, specific heat 0.038 cal g^{-1} $^\circ$K^{-1}.

Chapter 10

THE INTERACTION OF SINGLE BEAMS OF X AND GAMMA RAYS WITH A SCATTERING MEDIUM

10.01   INTRODUCTION

In radiotherapy, one is concerned with the *absorbed dose* received by tissues in the irradiated volume. Since it is seldom possible to measure this directly, it must be calculated. Because this calculation must be done on a routine basis, it is further necessary that the calculations be simple and reliable. In this and following chapters we will be concerned with defining and illustrating various concepts that are useful in this dose determination.

In Chapter 7 we described in detail methods for determining the absorbed dose in a phantom. These procedures gave us the dose at a reference point. Functions have been developed to enable us to calculate the dose at any other point once the dose at this reference point is known. These functions have been developed as a result of a long series of careful systematic measurements made by many workers over many years. For greater clarity the order of presentation we will follow differs from the historical development. Furthermore, although we recognize the importance of beams of electrons, our discussions are strongly oriented toward the use of photons. Much of the formalism applies equally well to both.

10.02   PHANTOMS

When a patient is placed in a photon beam of known quality and quantity, the photons will be absorbed and scattered and both the quality and quantity of the beam will be changed. The changes in quality were dealt with in Chapter 8. In this chapter, the changes in quantity will be discussed. To study these changes, experiments have been performed using phantoms to replace the patient. The phantom should be of a material that will absorb and scatter photons in the same way as tissue. Spiers (S13) long ago showed that the phantom material should have the same density as tissue and contain the same number of electrons per gram. Water and wet tissues absorb photons in almost the same way, and for this reason water has been used in many investigations. Since ionization chambers show troublesome leakage effects when damp, water phantoms introduce some difficulties; to avoid these, dry phantoms have been developed. White has made by far the most extensive study of phantom materials and his papers (W7, H11) should be referred to. For most purposes, nonetheless, water remains the most practical phantom material.

10.03   FUNCTIONS USED IN DOSE CALCULATIONS

The right side of Figure 10-1 shows a beam of radiation incident on a phantom and the left side shows the same beam with the phantom removed. The size of the beam is usually characterized by stating the dimensions of the rectangular or square field at some specified distance from the source. In Figure 10-1 the field has a width W_0 at distance F, or width W_m at distance $(F + d_m)$, or width W_d at distance $(F + d)$. Consider two points on the beam axis: point Y at depth d_m is the point where the dose is maximum, while point X is a point at any depth d. For radiations having a half-value layer less than a few mm of Cu (for example radiation generated up to 250 kV$_p$) point Y is on the surface of the phantom while for energies above a few hundred keV the maximum dose is below the surface. For cobalt 60 radiation, which is nearly monoenergetic with an energy of 1.25 MeV, $d_m = 0.5$ cm. The depth of maximum dose increases with energy, reaching a value of about 5 cm for a continuous spectrum with peak energy 25 MeV. The points Y′ and X′ shown in the left side of Figure 10-1 are at the same positions in space as Y and X but are "in air," that is, with no phantom present. To make a statement about dose in air the points in air must be considered to be surrounded by enough phantom-like material to establish electronic equilibrium (sec. 7.11). After a given irradiation the doses delivered to a small mass of phantom material at these points will be referred to as $D_{Y′}$ (dose at Y′); $D_{X′}$ (dose at X′), while D_X and D_Y are the corresponding doses in the phantom. Four functions—the *tissue-air ratio*, the *backscatter factor*, the *percentage depth dose*, and the *inverse square law*—may be used to interrelate the doses at these four points. An additional function, *tissue-phantom ratio*, is specially useful for high energy radiation.

The tissue-air ratio (T_a) is the ratio of the dose at X to the dose at X′ and is represented by:

$$T_a(d,W_d,h\nu) = D_X/D_{X′} \qquad (10\text{-}1)$$

It depends on the depth d below the surface of the phantom, the size W_d of the beam measured at depth d, and on the quality of the radiation, represented here by $h\nu$. The dependence on these variables is indicated by including them within parentheses after the symbol T_a. At times we are interested in the *area* of the field at depth d and could then refer to the tissue-air ratio as $T_a(d,A_d,h\nu)$.

The backscatter factor (B) is the tissue-air ratio for the special case when the depth d is equal to the depth of maximum dose, that is d_m. We represent it by:

$$B(W_m,h\nu) = T_a(d_m,W_m,h\nu) = D_Y/D_{Y'} \qquad (10\text{-}2)$$

The backscatter function gives the factor by which the radiation dose is increased by radiation scattered back from the phantom. The concept was first developed for low energy radiation, where the depth, d_m, was for all practical purposes equal to zero, so the maximum dose was on the surface. The term has been carried over to high energy radiation even though the point, Y, is no longer on the surface. Since the backscatter factor is a function of field size and quality, we represent it by $B(W_m,h\nu)$.

The percentage depth dose (P) is the ratio of the dose at X to the dose at Y, both points being within the phantom. It is expressed as a percentage thus:

$$P(d,W_m,F,h\nu) = 100\ D_X/D_Y \qquad (10\text{-}3)$$

The percentage depth dose depends on the depth d, the width of the beam W_m, the distance F from the source to the surface of the phantom, and on the quality of the radiation $h\nu$.

Usually the field size is specified at the depth of the reference point, although frequently the surface is also used and W_m in equation 10-3 becomes W_o. Since a number of different conventions are used, it is essential that the user be aware of the convention that applies to a specific set of data before it is used, otherwise errors in dose calculations will be made.

At times it is convenient to relate doses in the phantom to a reference point other than Y—for example Y_r, which might be at a depth of 10.0 cm. When this is done, percentage depth doses can exceed 100 and are often referred to as "relative depth doses."

The Inverse Square Law (I): Points X' and Y' are in air and if there is no attenuating or scattering material between them or near to them, the dose at one point will be related to the dose at the other inversely as the square of their distances from the source (see also section 9.07). That is:

$$I(F,d,d_m) = \frac{D_{X'}}{D_{Y'}} = \left(\frac{F + d_m}{F + d}\right)^2 \qquad (10\text{-}4)$$

The inverse square relationship is valid provided the dimensions of the source of radiation are small compared to the distance F. This function is independent of beam quality.

RELATIONSHIP BETWEEN THE FUNCTIONS: The square insert between the two halves of Figure 10-1 illustrate how the doses are related. For example the dose at Y can be obtained from the dose at Y' by multiply-

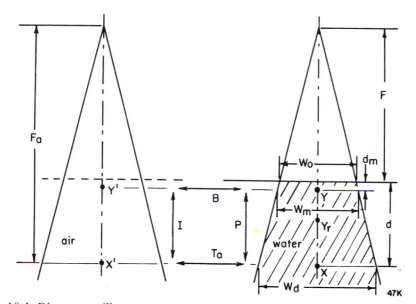

Figure 10-1. Diagram to illustrate the meaning of functions that facilitate the calculation of absorbed dose in a patient or in a phantom.

ing by the backscatter factor B along the arrow B. The dose at X can be obtained from that at Y by multiplying by P along the arrow P. In a similar way the dose at X′ is related to that at Y′ through the inverse square factor I (vertical arrow I). Finally the dose at X is related to that at X′ by the tissue-air ratio, T_a.

By going clockwise around the rectangle we may relate D_X to $D_{Y'}$ thus:

$$D_X = D_{Y'} \cdot B \cdot P$$

and by going counterclockwise we obtain:

$$D_X = D_{Y'} \cdot I \cdot T_a$$

Dividing the second equation by the first we obtain the relation between B, P, T_a, and I for a given radiation quality thus:

$$P(d, W_m, F) = \frac{100\ T_a\ I}{B} = 100\ \frac{T_a(d, W_d)}{B(W_m)} \left(\frac{F + d_m}{F + d} \right)^2 \quad (10\text{-}5)$$

This is an important relation between the four functions. Before discussing the properties of each of these functions in detail, we will introduce the tissue-phantom ratio.

Tissue-Phantom Ratio (T_p). For high energy radiation, measurements in air such as at point X′ are not practical and tissue-air ratios are not used. This is chiefly because it would be necessary to supply the dosimeter with such a large buildup cap that it would not be fully irradiated by small area beams. As an alternative, the arrangement shown in Figure 10-2 is used. The right side of this diagram is the same as the right side of Figure 10-1 but only point X is shown. The left side shows a phantom arranged so that point X″, which is the same distance from the source, is at a depth d_r below the surface. The tissue-phantom ratio is the ratio of the dose at X to the dose at X″ thus:

$$T_p(d, d_r, W_d, h\nu) = D_X / D_{X''} \tag{10-6}$$

This quantity, like T_a, depends on the depth d, the field size W_d, and on the radiation quality $h\nu$. Like tissue-air ratio it does not depend on distance from the source. We have also included d_r, the reference depth, within the parentheses because the ratio would also depend on this quantity. The field size, W_d, is designated at the position of the point and is the same for the two configurations of Figure 10-2.

Tissue-phantom ratios may be related to tissue-air ratios through the dose in air, $D_{X'}$.

$$D_X = D_{X'} \cdot T_a(d, W_d, h\nu)$$

$$D_{X''} = D_{X'} \cdot T_a(d_r, W_d, h\nu)$$

and hence: $$T_p = \frac{T_a(d, W_d, h\nu)}{T_a(d_r, W_d, h\nu)} \tag{10-7}$$

This relation can be seen to be like equation 10-5 for percent depth dose, but without the inverse square term.

Tissue-phantom ratio can be thought of either as an extension of tissue-air ratio where the reference dose in air, $D_{X'}$, is replaced by one at a reference depth in a phantom, $D_{X''}$, or as an extension of percent depth

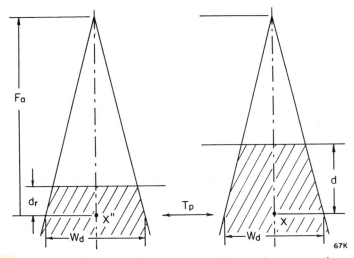

67K

Figure 10-2. Diagram to illustrate the meaning of tissue phantom ratio, useful for the calculation of absorbed dose in a patient or a phantom.

doses where the distance to the source is infinite and the inverse square term of equation 10-5 becomes unity.

10.04 **TISSUE-AIR RATIO**

Tissue-air ratio was originally introduced by Johns (J10) in 1953 as "tumour-air ratio." It was at that time specifically intended to simplify calculations for rotation therapy. In this type of treatment, the patient is located so that the tumor is on the axis of rotation of the machine and the source moves in a circle about this point. The source-to-axis distance is a constant quantity in such motion and so is the size of the beam at the axis. Attention is thereby focused on this point for calculations. Since the time of its introduction it has become more and more widely used, especially in dosimetry involving isocentric units. Because it is perhaps the simplest of all the functions used in radiotherapy calculations, it is introduced first.

Tissue-air ratio was defined by equation 10-1. Its meaning, as applied to a patient, is illustrated in Figure 10-3. The left side of this diagram shows a circular beam of radiation having cross-sectional area A_d at a distance F_a from the source. The beam is in air, and F_a is the distance from source to axis. After a given irradiation let the dose to a small mass of tissue on the axis be $D_{X'}$.

The solid line contour in Figure 10-3b represents a patient in place being irradiated by the same beam. The depth of tissue overlying the axis is d and the dose at this point, $D_{X'}$, may be calculated directly by the relation:

$$D_X = D_{X'}\, T_a(d, W_a, h\nu) \qquad (10\text{-}1a)$$

Tables of tissue-air ratios for rectangular beams are given in Appendix

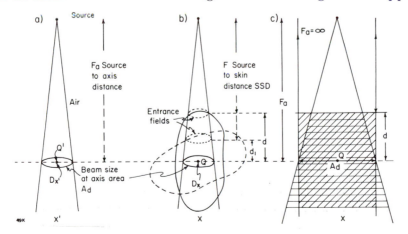

Figure 10-3. (a and b) Schematic diagram to illustrate the use of tissue-air ratio in dose calculations. (c) The scattering to point X from the cylindrical block of phantom material is the same as from the conical-shaped section when the two beams have the same area at depth d and receive the same primary radiation at X.

B-5d. We illustrate their use by an example.

Example 10-1. An isocentric cobalt 60 unit delivers a dose of 1.00 Gy in one minute to a small mass of tissue in air on the axis of the machine at point X'. A patient is introduced into the beam with the center of the tumor at the point X'. The tumor is 10 cm below the skin and the field size at the point X' is 10 × 10 cm. Determine the dose to the tumor.

From Table B-5d, the tissue-air ratio = 0.709 for a 100 cm² field at depth 10 cm

Hence D_X (eq. 10-1a) = 1.00 Gy × .709 = .709 Gy

This calculation makes no mention of rotation therapy, but it is clear how the concept can be used in this context. Suppose at a later instant the position of the patient is as indicated by the dotted contour of Figure 10-3b, so that the overlying tissue is 6.0 cm thick. Table B-5d shows that now $T_a = 0.867$ so that for the same irradiation time the dose delivered to the center of the tumor is .867 Gy. For rotation therapy one would merely average all such dose values. A more usual approach today is to direct the beam to the tumor for a few discrete directions and then add up the doses. It should also be noted that in these calculations no mention is made of the source-to-axis distance; this will be discussed in the next section.

When tissue-air ratio was first introduced, it was defined in terms of a ratio of exposures: the exposure in the phantom divided by the exposure at the same point in the absence of the phantom. This is certainly a valid procedure but has the disadvantage that it could not be used for high energy radiation since for these the use of exposure is not recommended. The use of absorbed dose also makes tissue-air ratios conveniently consistent with other functions used for dose calculation, such as percent depth dose. It is also in line with recommendations of the ICRU (I7).

Effect of Distance from the Source on the Tissue-Air Ratio

Experimentally it has been shown that tissue-air ratios are independent of the distance from the source (F_a of Figs. 10-1 and 10-3) at least for distances of 50 cm or more. Figure 10-3c shows two beams, one parallel and the other diverging, which have the *same* cross-sectional area, A_d, at depth d below the surface of the phantom. They will both deliver the same primary dose since both will be attenuated by the same amount of tissue. If, in addition, the scattered doses to X were the same in both cases, the tissue-air ratio would be the same for both configurations. To test this Johns et al. (J11), using the Klein-Nishina formula, compared the once scattered radiation to point X by the cylindrical block of tissue from the parallel beam to that from the cone-shaped block of tissue from the diverging beam. The once scattered radiation proved to be the same to within about 2% for radiations from 100 keV to 1.25 MeV. Since higher orders of scattered radiation would be expected to depend directly on first scattered radiation, the total dose at point X should be very nearly independent of the distance F_a. *Thus a single table of tissue-air ratios can be used for all source distances.*

Variation of Tissue-Air Ratio with Field Size and Depth

Typical tissue-air ratio data for cobalt 60 are shown in Figure 10-4 as a function of depth for a selection of field sizes. It should be emphasized that the field sizes are specified at the depth in question. For example, point G (Fig. 10-4) is for a field size of 400 cm² at 10 cm depth while point H is for a field of 400 cm² at a depth of 20 cm. The curves are nearly straight lines when plotted on a log scale, showing the variation with depth is essentially exponential.

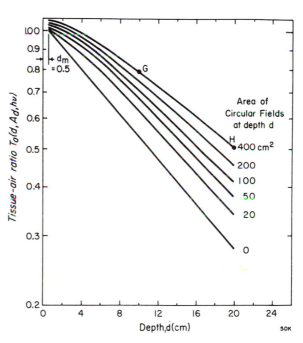

Figure 10-4. Tissue-air ratios for ⁶⁰Co as a function of depth for a selection of circular fields. The areas of these fields are measured at the depth d.

The steepest curve of Figure 10-4 is for zero area. For this case the dose received at a depth d below the surface is due entirely to primary radiation, since the volume that can scatter radiation is zero. If the radiation were monoenergetic, or nearly so, like that from cobalt 60, the dependence on depth of the tissue-air ratio would be the simple exponential $e^{-\mu(d-d_m)}$ where μ is the linear attenuation coefficient for the radiation and the phantom material, and $(d - d_m)$ is the thickness of material in the path of the beam in the phantom that is in addition to that in its path in free space.* The curve thus starts at depth d_m, which for cobalt 60 is 0.5 cm and is a straight line (see Fig. 10-4). As the area of the beam is increased, scatter increases, the tissue-air ratio increases, and the curves are no longer straight.

The dependence of the tissue-air ratio on field size for a constant depth is shown in Figure 10-5 for ^{60}Co. The curves show that the tissue-air ratio increases continuously with field size at all depths. The increase is relatively rapid at first and gradually levels off for very large field sizes. The form of this variation is similar for beams of other qualities.

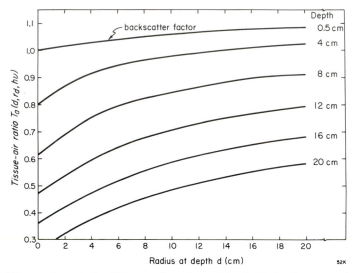

Figure 10-5. Tissue-air ratio for ^{60}Co as a function of the field size for a number of depths.

The effect of scattered radiation may be demonstrated by calculating the ratio of the total dose at a point to the primary dose. For a cobalt 60 beam and a depth of 20 cm $T_a = 0.278$ for a zero area field and $T_a = 0.503$ for a 20 × 20 cm field (Table B-5c). For this field the primary dose is 0.278 and the total dose is 0.503 so the ratio of total to primary increases from 1.0 to $0.503/0.278 = 1.8$ as the field size is increased. In contrast, for radiation with HVL 1.0 mm Cu, scattering is much more important and the student may show using Table B-5a that the ratio for the same conditions is now over 9.0.

Tissue-Air Ratios for Rectangular or Irregular Fields

Tables of tissue-air ratios for a wide range of beam sizes and shapes can be prepared from relatively few measurements by using data for circular beams. Such data can be measured directly as was done by Johns

---

*In determining the dose in free space at point X′ (Fig. 10-1) we require a mass of tissue that has a radius d_m to give maximum electron buildup, hence the extra tissue thickness in the beam in the phantom is $(d - d_m)$. (See sec. 7.11.)

(J10) or may be obtained from measurements made in square beams as discussed in section 10.08. Tissue-air ratios for rectangular beams can then be obtained from data for circular beams by the sector integration procedure first introduced by Clarkson (C7). The method will be illustrated by determining the tissue-air ratio for a 4×15 cm field of cobalt radiation at a depth of 10 cm. Figure 10-6 shows tissue-air ratios for a depth of 10 cm (Table B-5c) plotted as a function of beam radius. The insert shows the 4×15 cm field, and radii have been drawn from its center at angles of 5°, 15°, 25°, to 85° so that the rectangular field may be replaced by a series of sectors of circular fields as indicated. The angles, radii, and corresponding tissue-air ratios, read from the graph in Figure 10-6, are shown in Table 10-1. The tissue-air ratio for the rectangular field is 0.660. The area of the rectangular field is $4 \times 15 = 60$ cm^2. A circular field with this area has a radius of 4.36 cm and gives a tissue-air ratio of 0.681 for 10 cm depth whereas that for the rectangular field is only 0.660. The rectangular field contributes less scatter to its center than would a circular field of equal area because some of its scatter, coming from points near the ends of the rectangle, must travel further than from points near the edge of the circle. The scatter coming from farther away will be attenuated more.

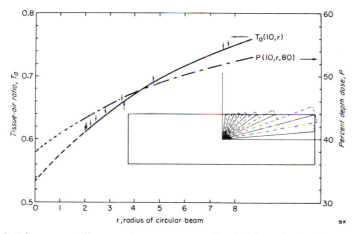

Figure 10-6. Diagram to illustrate how a rectangular field can be broken up into a number of sectors allowing one to calculate the tissue-air ratio, T$_a$, or the percentage depth dose, P, for a rectangular field from the corresponding data from circular fields.

TABLE 10-1
Calculation of Tissue-Air Ratio for a 4×15 Field at Depth 10 cm for ^{60}Co Radiation

Angles	5	15	25	35	45	55	65	75	85	
Radius, r_i	2.01	2.07	2.21	2.44	2.83	3.49	4.73	7.73	7.53	
$T_a(10,r_i)$	.612	.613	.618	.626	.638	.658	.690	.745	.742	total = 5.942

Tissue-air ratio for 4×15 cm field = $5.942 \times 4/36 = 0.660$

A rectangular field, and in fact even a field having an irregular out-line, can be resolved into sectors of circular beams. The tissue-air ratio for a rectangular or irregular beam having a field area A at depth d can be calculated from the equation:

$$T_a(d,A) = \frac{1}{n} \sum_{i=1}^{n} T_a(d,r_i) \qquad (10\text{-}8)$$

where n is the number of sectors in 360°, r_i are the radii from the center to the edge of the field at the center of each sector, and $T_a(d,r_i)$ are the tissue-air ratios for circular fields of radius r_i at depth d. In Table 10-1 the sectors have an angular width of 10°. Although there are 36 such sectors in 360° only 9 of them need be considered in this example be-cause of symmetry. The accuracy of the calculation is improved by using more sectors with smaller angular widths, but little gain is achieved by going below 10°.

Measurement of Tissue-Air Ratios

To obtain a tissue-air ratio it is necessary to determine the dose at pairs of points such as X′ and X of Figure 10-1. Both points must be the same distance from the source and be irradiated with beams having the same field size (G10). The most reliable way to make such measurements is by using ionization chambers. Considerations that need to be taken for such measurements are discussed in sections 7.16 and 9.13. It is convenient to clamp the ion chamber in air on the axis of the radiation beam and with the source of radiation turned on for a fixed time note the reading of the instrument. Let it be $M_{X'}$. For the second reading the dosimeter, still at the same point in space, is surrounded by water so that the depth of water above the chamber is d. A new reading, M_X, is taken for the same exposure time. The tissue-air for that depth and field size is as-sumed to be $M_X/M_{X'}$. This is not quite correct since strictly speaking both the numerator and denominator should be multiplied by factors dis-cussed in sections 7.11 and 7.12. It is usually assumed, however, that these factors cancel, so the ratio of the two readings is considered to be the tissue-air ratio. Readings, M_X, for other depths can be taken by changing the level of the water surface. For a new field size the reading in air must be taken again, since M_X varies in an unpredictable way with field size.

Some additional special precautions must be taken with respect to the reading in air. It is necessary that there be no material in the beam that might contribute scattered radiation to the dosimeter. For some situa-tions, particularly for large field sizes, it is necessary to be surprisingly far from walls or floors that might scatter radiation back to the dosim-eter (V6).

Although the above method of measuring tissue-air ratios is direct, they can also be obtained from measured percent depth doses and backscatter factors using the relations between these quantities given in equation 10-5. All of the early "tumour-air ratios" (J10) were in fact derived in this manner.

10.05   BACKSCATTER FACTOR

When the depth, d, of Figure 10-1 is made equal to the depth of maximum dose, the tissue-air ratio reduces to the backscatter factor and is defined by equation 10-2. The top curve of Figure 10-5 (depth $d_m = 0.5$ cm in a beam of cobalt radiation) is also the backscatter factor. Our attention is now focused upon a special reference point within the phantom, and some detailed discussion about this point is in order. The depth at which electronic equilibrium occurs increases from a fraction of a millimeter for 200 kV radiation to about 5 mm for ^{60}Co radiation and to about 5 cm for 25 MV radiation. The depth, d_m, is frequently also thought of as the depth at which electronic equilibrium (see sec. 7.03) occurs. In some situations this is not true. For example, in the 200 kV range the path lengths of electrons set into motion are so small that d_m must be thought of as zero and we can consider the reference point to be on the surface of the phantom (or the skin of the patient). At these energies, however, because of the great amount of scattered radiation (photons rather than electrons) the maximum dose may actually occur about 1 cm below the surface for a large field. This is because the increase in scattered radiation may, for a short distance, more than compensate for the attenuation of the primary component of the beam. An analogous but very different situation may occur for very high energy radiation. For example, for a 25 MV beam, for a small field size, the maximum dose may be found experimentally to be at a depth of 4–5 cm while for a large field it may be closer to the surface, perhaps 3 cm. This occurs because for large fields a large component of low energy photons and high energy electrons may be scattered from the inner surfaces of the collimator and cause a dose buildup near the surface. This same behavior can also be observed in ^{60}Co beams (L2). The depth of *electronic equilibrium* cannot, therefore, easily be determined experimentally.

The above discussion illustrates that the reference depth, d_m, for high energy radiation has a somewhat arbitrary character. When used, therefore, its magnitude should be stated clearly.

The term "backscatter factor" is applied to the tissue-air ratio for depth, d_m, largely for historical reasons. Backscatter factor was proposed and measured for radiations in the so-called orthovoltage range long before tissue-air ratios were thought of. For these beams, since $d_m = 0.0$, the scatter to the surface is truly backscatter. At high energies, where

$d_m > 0$, not all photons reaching the reference point are scattered back but the term still continues to be used.

Backscatter and Beam Quality

The variation of backscatter with half-value layer is illustrated in Figure 10-7. With soft radiation the backscatter is small; it rises rapidly to a maximum at a half-value layer of about 1.0 mm Cu and then falls slowly to nearly zero for cobalt 60 (HVL 14.8 mm Cu). Figure 10-7 shows the variation of backscatter with quality for five field sizes ranging from a small field (20 cm²) to a large one (400 cm²). The quality at which the maximum backscatter occurs depends on area. For a large field the maximum is shifted slightly towards harder radiation.

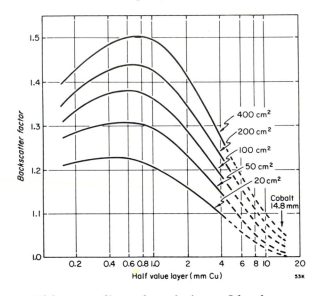

Figure 10-7. Variation of backscatter factor with the quality of the radiation for a number of circular field sizes.

This complicated variation of backscatter with quality can be understood by reference to Chapter 6 and the Klein-Nishina formula. At low energies as many photons are scattered forward as backward and exactly half as many at right angles. This type of scattering is called classical scattering. For soft radiation, the region that can effectively scatter radiation to a point on the surface is very small because this radiation is quickly absorbed in the medium. The backscatter from low energy x rays is thus small. At medium and high energies the same amount is scattered forward as in the classical case but less and less is scattered at right angles or backwards as the energy is increased. At medium energies, although the amount scattered back is small, the region that can effectively scatter to the point is large because of the greater penetrating power of the scattered radiation, and maximum backscatter is obtained. At high energies, the amount scattered backwards is negligible but the reference depth for "backscatter" is no longer zero and some of the foreward scattered photons can contribute to it. The net scatter is, however, relatively small.

10.06 **PERCENTAGE DEPTH DOSE**

Percentage depth dose interrelates doses at points within a phantom. For example, in equation 10-3 the dose at points such as X (of Fig. 10-1) are related to the dose at the reference point Y. Point Y is often at the depth of maximum dose but can in fact be any chosen point. This function can be applied equally well to high or low energy radiations.

$$P(d, W_m, F, h\nu) = 100 \cdot \frac{\text{dose at depth d}}{\text{dose at d}_m} = 100 \cdot \frac{D_X}{D_Y} \quad (10\text{-}3)$$

Example 10-2. A patient is irradiated with a 200 kV (HVL 2.0 mm Cu) beam at a source-to-skin distance of 50 cm using a circular 400 cm^2 field. If the patient's skin is given a dose of 2.00 Gy, determine the doses at depths of 10 cm and 1.0 cm.

P (depth 10, area 400, 50, HVL 2.0) = 46.7   (Table B-2c)

P (depth 1, area 400, 50, HVL 2.0) = 102.4

$$D_{10} \text{ (eq. 10-3)} = \frac{P \cdot D_Y}{100} = \frac{46.7 \times 2.00}{100} = .934 \text{ Gy}$$

$$D_1 \text{ (eq. 10-3)} = \frac{102.4 \times 2.00}{100} = 2.05 \text{ Gy}$$

It should be noted that for this particular quality scattering is severe and the dose at 1 cm depth is slightly larger than the surface dose.

Dependence of Depth Dose on Depth and Photon Energy

Figures 10-8 and 10-9 show the variation of depth dose with depth for a variety of radiations. Figure 10-8 shows the variation for depths up to 16 mm, while Figure 10-9 shows it for depths up to 25 cm. We will first examine the depth dose near the surface. With low energy radiation, as shown by curve A of Figure 10-8 (140 kV), the depth dose decreases with depth from the surface reaching about 80% at 6 mm. The dose from slightly harder radiation (curve B, 200 kV) is almost constant over the depth range shown. More energetic radiation, in the megavoltage range as exemplified by curve C for ^{60}Co, exhibits a rise in depth dose for the first few mm and then reaches a broad maximum that extends over several mm. As the energy is increased still further the surface dose becomes smaller and the maximum occurs at greater and greater depths. With 22 MV betatron radiation (curve E) the surface dose is less than 20% and the maximum occurs some 4 to 6 cm below the surface. The reason for this general behavior was explained in terms of electronic "buildup" discussed in detail in Chapter 7. With high energy radiation the electrons set in motion by the photon interactions are projected primarily in the forward direction; hence, the number of electron tracks will increase with depth until a depth equal to the electron range is reached. From this point on, the dose decreases with depth due to the attenuation of the photon radiation. The result is that the dose first increases and then decreases. With low energy radiation the range of the electrons is so small that this effect is not observed and the dose falls continually with increase in depth.

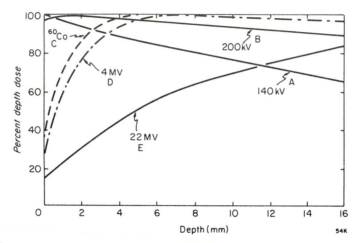

Figure 10-8. Percentage depth dose plotted against depth for the region near the surface for a range of photon beam energies.

The dosage buildup with cobalt 60 occurs in the first few mm and may be lost partially or completely if electron contamination is present. It might be argued that since all the effect occurs in 1 to 2 mm, it cannot be of importance clinically. However, there is clinical evidence that a real skin sparing effect is achieved if care is taken to preserve this buildup (B12). The whole effect will obviously be lost if the patient's skin is covered by bolus, a cast, or the end of a treatment cone.

Figure 10-9 shows the percentage depth dose that may be obtained for low, medium, high, and very high energy photon radiation plotted on a semilogarithmic scale. For all radiation qualities shown, the curves are nearly straight lines for points well beyond the position of maximum dose, indicating that primary attenuation, buildup of scatter, and fall off with inverse square law combine to give essentially exponential attenuation. A useful quantity to use as an index of the penetration of the radiation is the depth at which the dose falls to 50% of its peak value. For 22 MV betatron radiation (curve A), this depth is over 22 cm. This curve and this large half-value depth is representative of very high energy radiation. Curve B, for 8 MV radiation, is considerably less penetrating reaching 50% at a depth of 17 cm. Curves C and D, for 4 MV and ^{60}Co radiation respectively, have a half-value depth of from 12 to 14 cm. Curve E is typical of the depth doses that may be obtained from a 200 to 250 kV x ray machine and yields a depth dose of 50% at a depth of some 7 to 8 cm. Curve F is typical of the depth dose from a 100 to 140 kV x ray machine giving 50% at a depth of only 1 or 2 cm.

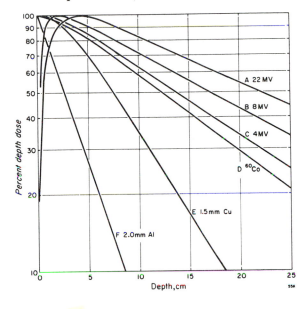

Figure 10-9. Graph showing the variation of depth dose with depth: (a) 22 MeV radiation with copper compensating filter, 10 × 10 cm field, SSD 70 cm; (b) 8 MV radiation from a linear accelerator, 10 × 10 cm field, SSD 100 cm; (c) 4 MV radiation from a linear accelerator, 10 × 10 cm field, SSD 100 cm; (d) cobalt 60, 10 × 10 cm; (e) 200 kV, 10 × 10 cm field, HVL 1.5 mm Cu, SSD 50 cm; (f) 120 kV, HVL 2.0 mm Al. Area 100 cm², SSD 15 cm.

Depth Dose Dependence on Field Area

When the area of the field is very small the dose D_X (of Fig. 10-1) received at a point below the surface is due entirely to primary radiation, since the volume that can scatter radiation is small. As the area of the field is increased, both D_X, and D_Y, at the reference point Y, will increase due to scattered radiation but the increase will be greater at greater depths. Percentage depth dose, therefore, increases with area, at first rapidly and then much more slowly as the area is further increased.

The variation of percentage depth dose with area depends upon the quality of radiation. This is illustrated in Figure 10-10 where the 10 cm depth dose is plotted against the radius of the field for qualities typical of low, medium, and high energy radiation.

The depth dose for zero area is due to primary radiation alone. With large areas the depth dose is due to primary plus scattered radiation. In the case of 25 MV radiation, scatter is very small and the depth dose is very nearly 83% for all field sizes. With cobalt 60, scatter increases the zero area depth dose from 42 to 60% as the field size is increased. With HVL 2.0 mm Cu, the dependence on area is considerable, the depth dose rising from 12 to 46% over the range of field sizes shown. From Figure 10-10, it is evident that high energy radiation offers a big advantage over lower energy radiation especially with small fields.

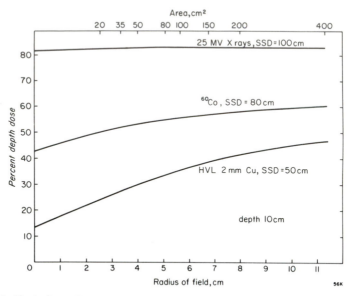

Figure 10-10. Variation of percentage depth dose with area and radius of field for three types of radiation. Depth 10 cm.

Percentage Depth Dose for Rectangular Fields

Percent depth doses for rectangular fields can be obtained from percent depth doses for circular fields by the same sector integration procedure described in section 10.04 for tissue-air ratios. The percentage depth dose for a rectangular field of area A can be obtained from:

$$P(d,A,F) = \frac{1}{n} \sum_{i=1}^{n} P(d,r_i,F) \qquad (10\text{-}9)$$

where F is the source-surface distance, $P(d,r_i,F)$ is the percent depth dose for a circular field of radius r_i, and n is the number of sectors in a complete circle. Percent depth dose for circular beams of cobalt 60 radiation, for a depth of 10 cm at an SSD of 80 cm, were plotted in Figure 10-10 against radius. It is left as an exercise for the student to show that the percent depth dose for a 4 × 15 cm field using the percent depth doses for circular fields given in Table B-2d and the radii given in Table 10-1 is 52.2%. This value appears in Table B-2e (in the appendix).

Percent depth doses are dependent on source-to-surface distance and beam quality and a separate table is required for each of the distances and qualities that are to be used. The method described by equation

10-9 was used for the preparation of the depth dose tables for rectangular fields given in appendix B-2e and for much of the data tabled in Supplement 11 of the *British Journal of Radiology* (B13).

Percent Depth Dose for Isocentric Machines

Most modern linear accelerators and cobalt units have isocentric mounts and the patient is positioned with the tumor on the axis of rotation of the machine. Beams are directed at the tumor from different directions and the source-surface distance and field size at the surface may be different for each beam. The percentage depth dose data discussed above is not convenient for making dose calculations in such beams. The problem is illustrated by the following example.

Example 10-3. A beam from an isocentric cobalt unit is used to irradiate a patient as shown in Figure 10-11. Point Y is on the axis of rotation and is a distance of 80.0 cm from the source. The field size at the axis is 10 × 10 cm and this point is at a depth of 12 cm below the surface. During a course of treatment point Y receives a dose of 2.5 Gy. Determine the dose at point X that is at a depth of 4 cm.

T_a for point Y = 0.636 (Table B-5d)

dose in air at isocenter = 2.5/0.636 = 3.93 Gy

dose in air at point X = 3.93 $(80.0/72.0)^2$ = 4.85 Gy

Field size at point X = 10.0 (72.0/80.0) = 9.0 cm

$T_a(4, 9 \times 9)$, at point X = 0.932 (Table B-5d by interpolation)

Dose at point X = 4.85 × 0.932 = 4.52 Gy

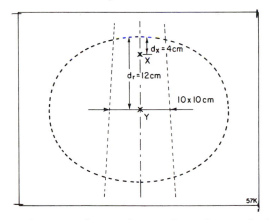

Figure 10-11. Diagram showing two points in a patient irradiated by a 10 × 10 cm beam from an isocentric treatment unit.

In solving this problem we made use of two tissue-air ratios and the inverse square law and combined them in the manner described in section 10.03. Although this is an accurate and useful way to solve this problem, it is not really practical for routine radiation treatment planning purposes where a more direct method is desirable. A direct method using percentage depth doses as discussed earlier in this section requires tables of depth doses for every field size and source-surface distance that might be encountered. This, clearly, is not practical. We can obtain approximate answers using relative depth doses as illustrated in Figure 10-12 where percentage depth doses for 10×10 cm fields at a source-axis distance of 80 cm have been computed by the method of example 10-3 for three different source-surface distances. Curve A is for an SSD of 75 cm and the reference point Y is at a depth of 5 cm and thus coincides with the axis of rotation. The abscissa in this diagram is distance along the axis of the beam measured from the axis of the treatment unit. Thus the surface for curve A is 5 cm above the axis of rotation, for curve B it is 10 cm above, and so on.

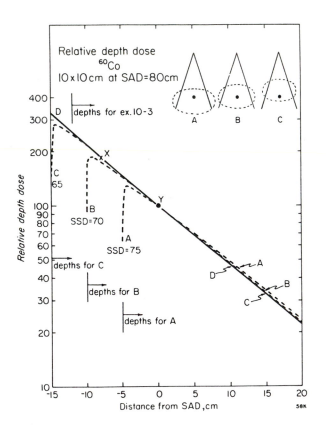

Figure 10-12. Graph of relative depth doses for an isocentric cobalt unit. Field size is 10×10 cm, source axis distance is 80.0 cm. Curve A is for SSD = 75 cm, B is for SSD = 70 cm, C is for SSD = 65 cm, D is for SSD = 60 cm.

We can approximate these curves by a single curve, labelled D, which is within 2% of the accurate curve except for points very near to the surface. Their use can be illustrated by again solving the problem of example 10-3.

Example 10-4. Use the relative depth dose data of Figure 10-12 to solve the problem of example 10-3.

Distance from isocenter to point X = 8 cm

Relative depth dose = 184%   (Fig. 10-12)

Dose at point X = 2.5 × 184/100 = 4.60 Gy

The answer given in example 10-4 is 1.8% higher than the more accurate value given in example 10-3. Relative depth dose data represented by Figure 10-12 are very useful for answering questions like that of example 10-3 in practical situations. The data are accurate for points 4 to 5 cm below the surface but are less so for points near it. Where there is disagreement, the dose is always overestimated for points nearer to the surface than the reference point and slightly underestimated for points below it.

Relative depth dose data for cobalt, SAD = 80 cm, and 25 MV data, SAD = 100 cm, are given in Appendix B-3.

Measurement of Depth Dose

Percentage depth dose may be measured in a number of different ways. One way is to move a probe detector along the axis of the beam and record the reading at a number of depths. These readings are then compared with the reading taken at the reference point to yield the percentage depth dose. This is a straightforward method but is inaccurate because in most treatment units (other than cobalt) there are random fluctuations of dose rate with time. Under these circumstances, the dose at the depth and the dose at the reference point will be measured at different times and the ratio may be inaccurate. This inaccuracy may be avoided if some comparison chamber or monitor is placed at a fixed position in the beam and simultaneous readings are taken on it and on the probe detector. The probe detector readings are first corrected to constant monitor readings, and a comparison is then made between the dose at the depth and the dose at the reference point.

A number of automatic methods have been developed to correct for random fluctuations in dose rate. In one such method, the outputs from the probe detector and the monitor are connected to a ratio circuit and the ratio is recorded directly.

The depth dose measurements from different workers often do not agree too well. This is partly due to fluctuations in output, differences in response of detectors, the use of different phantom materials, and a number of factors difficult to control. The tables presented in this book are those obtained by the authors and collaborators and taken from the excellent summary of depth dose measurements, found in Supplement No. 11 of the *British Journal of Radiology* (B13).

10.07   **TISSUE-PHANTOM RATIOS**

Tissue-phantom ratios were introduced in section 10.03 with the aid of Figure 10-2 as a replacement for tissue-air ratios for high energy radiation. The main reason tissue-air ratios do not lend themselves to use with high energy radiation has to do with the determination of the (reference) absorbed dose in air. The electrons that are set into motion by very high energy photons may travel distances of several cm; in order to make the dose determination in air, a very large buildup cap must be added to the dosimeter. The cap may in fact be so large that not all of it will be irradiated by small field sizes. This has led Karzmark (K6), among others, to suggest that the reference dose in air should be replaced by a dose determined in a phantom at a specified depth. A tissue-phantom ratio is therefore the ratio of the dose determined in a phantom for a chosen depth and field size to the dose determined in the same phantom and same field size but at some reference depth. Like tissue-air ratio, the dosimeter should be at the same distance from the source for both these measurements and the field size should be specified at that same distance.

There is no universal agreement on the reference depth to be used but it is reasonable to use the values recommended by the ICRU (I7) for absorbed dose calibrations. These are given in Table 10-2.

TABLE 10-2
Depths Recommended for Tissue-Phantom Ratios and Absorbed Dose Calibrations

Type of Radiation	Depth in cm
150 kV to 10 MV x rays	5
^{137}Cs and ^{60}Co γ rays	5
11 MV to 25 MV x rays	7
Above 25 MV x rays	10

From ICRU Report 24 (I7)

10.08   **EQUIVALENT SQUARES AND CIRCLES FOR RECTANGULAR AND IRREGULAR FIELDS**

In section 10.06 a precise method for obtaining the depth dose for a rectangular field was given. The same method was applied to tissue-air ratios in section 10.04. We have seen that a rectangular field gives a smaller depth dose and tissue-air ratio than does a circular or square field of the same area. Day et al. (B13), however, have shown that it is possible to choose a circular field that has the same depth dose as a given rectangular field. Such a field is called an equivalent circular field. Radii for equivalent circular fields are given in Table 10-3. It has been taken from Supplement 11 of the *British Journal of Radiology* (B13).

In a more formal way, one could state that the circular field equivalent to a rectangular field would be the one that satisfied the following equation:

$$T_a(d,\hat{r},h\nu) = \frac{1}{n} \sum_{i=1}^{n} T_a(d,r_i,h\nu) \qquad (10\text{-}10)$$

where $\hat{r}$ is the radius of the equivalent circular field.

The data given in Table 10-3 were derived from backscatter factors for x rays in the energy region of 200 to 250 kV_p. More recent studies (V7) have indicated that this table is satisfactory for clinical purposes for all depths and other beam qualities.

In a similar way equivalent squares for rectangular fields have been determined and are presented in Table 10-4. We will now illustrate the usefulness of this data.

Example 10-5. Obtain the 10 cm depth dose for a 4×20 cm field for ^{60}Co by finding the equivalent square and using appendix B-2e. Compare the answer with the percentage depth dose given for this rectangular field in the same table.

    Equivalent square field = 6.7 cm   (Table 10-4)

    Percent depth dose for 6×6 field = 52.0   (Table B-2e)

    Percent depth dose for 8×8 field = 54.0   (Table B-2e)

    Percent depth dose for 6.7×6.7 field = 52.7 by interpolation

    Percent depth dose for 4×20 field = 52.5   (Table B-2e)

The data for rectangular fields in Table B-2e were obtained from careful measurements made using both square and circular fields (B13) and an application of equation 10-9. The percent depth dose (52.7) found by using the equivalent square method is within 0.4% of the value listed in the table for this field. This is representative of the precision that may be expected from this procedure and also illustrates how data for a small number of square fields may be used to produce useful data for any rectangular field chosen for treatment.

A simple rule of thumb method for finding the equivalent square of a rectangular field has been suggested by Sterling (S14). Square fields and rectangular fields are equivalent if the ratios formed by dividing area by perimeter are the same. For the beam of example 10-5, the area is $4 \times 20 = 80$, the perimeter is $2 \times (4 + 20) = 48$. The ratio is $80/48 = 1.67$. The student may show that the square field giving this ratio is 6.67, in very good agreement with the value 6.7 found in Table 10-4.

TABLE 10-3

Radii of Circular Fields Equivalent to Rectangular Fields

Long Axis (cm)	Short Axis (cm)														
	2	4	6	8	10	12	14	16	18	20	22	24	26	28	30
2	1.13														
4	1.50	2.26													
6	1.75	2.70	3.35												
8	1.90	3.0	3.85	4.45											
10	2.00	3.25	4.20	4.95	5.60										
12	2.10	3.40	4.45	5.35	6.10	6.70									
14	2.15	3.55	4.65	5.65	6.50	7.20	7.80								
16	2.20	3.65	4.85	5.90	6.80	7.60	8.30	8.90							
18	2.20	3.70	4.95	6.05	7.05	7.95	8.70	9.40	10.0						
20	2.25	3.75	5.05	6.20	7.25	8.20	9.05	9.85	10.5	11.3					
22	2.25	3.80	5.10	6.30	7.40	8.40	9.35	10.2	11.0	11.6	12.2				
24	2.25	3.80	5.15	6.40	7.50	8.60	9.55	10.5	11.3	12.1	12.7	13.3			
26	2.25	3.85	5.20	6.45	7.60	8.70	9.70	10.7	11.6	12.4	13.1	13.8	14.4		
28	2.30	3.85	5.25	6.50	7.70	8.80	9.85	10.9	11.8	12.7	13.5	14.2	14.9	15.8	
30	2.30	3.85	5.25	6.55	7.75	8.90	10.0	11.0	12.0	12.9	13.8	14.6	15.3	15.9	16.9

From British Journal of Radiology, Supplement 11 (B13).

TABLE 10-4

Side Lengths of Square Fields Equivalent to Rectangular Fields

Long Axis (cm)	Short Axis (cm)														
	2	4	6	8	10	12	14	16	18	20	22	24	26	28	30
2	2.0														
4	2.7	4.0													
6	3.1	4.8	6.0												
8	3.4	5.4	6.9	8.0											
10	3.6	5.8	7.5	8.9	10.0										
12	3.7	6.1	8.0	9.6	10.9	12.0									
14	3.8	6.3	8.4	10.1	11.6	12.9	14.0								
16	3.9	6.5	8.6	10.5	12.2	13.7	14.9	16.0							
18	4.0	6.6	8.9	10.8	12.7	14.3	15.7	16.9	18.0						
20	4.0	6.7	9.0	11.1	13.0	14.7	16.3	17.7	18.9	20.0					
22	4.0	6.8	9.1	11.3	13.3	15.1	16.8	18.3	19.7	20.9	22.0				
24	4.1	6.8	9.2	11.5	13.5	15.4	17.2	18.8	20.3	21.7	22.9	24.0			
26	4.1	6.9	9.3	11.6	13.7	15.7	17.5	19.2	20.9	22.4	23.7	24.9	26.0		
28	4.1	6.9	9.4	11.7	13.8	15.9	17.8	19.6	21.3	22.9	24.4	25.7	27.0	28.0	
30	4.1	6.9	9.4	11.7	13.9	16.0	18.0	19.9	21.7	23.3	24.9	26.4	27.7	29.0	30.0

From British Journal of Radiology, Supplement 11 (B13).

10.09   PATIENT DOSE CALCULATIONS

The functions defined in section 10.03 and described in subsequent sections were all introduced for the purpose of calculating relative doses. In this section we show how they can be combined with machine calibrations so that the dose given to any point in a patient may be known.

The use of tissue-phantom ratios and calibration in a phantom is the most straightforward and will be discussed first.

Tissue Phantom Ratios

The reference dose for the use of tissue-phantom ratios is $D_{X''}$ of Figure 10-2. Procedures for determining absorbed dose in a phantom are discussed in Chapter 7. The depth, d_r, should be chosen according to the beam energy and the phantom should be set up so that the dosimeter is located on the isocenter of the machine at a depth recommended in Table 10-2. The dose should then be determined as a function either of time or of machine monitor units for field sizes covering the range that will be used for treatment. The measurements must include square and rectangular fields as the output from the machine may be strongly dependent on collimator opening. It cannot be assumed that the equivalent squares discussed in the previous section apply. An example set of output data for a high energy linear accelerator is shown in Figure 10-13. Field sizes vary from 4×4 cm to 25×25 cm. As can be seen, the radiation output of such a machine may be strongly dependent on the collimator opening. In this case it is 30% greater for a large field than for a small field. The reasons for this large variation are not clear. Radiation scattered within the phantom can only be a small part of it and therefore the greater part must be due to radiation scattered from the collimator or other structures. The importance of the collimator jaws is illustrated by the dashed lines and the solid line near to it. Both are for the same field sizes. The difference is due to the fact that for one line the short side of the field is defined by the lower set of collimator jaws and for the other line it is defined by the upper jaws.

The data shown in Figure 10-13 is plotted as relative dose. The actual dose would be given by the relation:

$$D_{X''} = M \cdot N_X \cdot C_\lambda \qquad (10\text{-}11)$$

where M is the dosimeter reading, N_X is its exposure calibration factor for cobalt 60 radiation, and C_λ is the factor discussed in section 7.16.

The dose in a patient, calculated using tissue-phantom ratios, is then given by:

$$D = D_{X''} \cdot T_p(d, W_d, h\nu) \cdot (\overline{\mu}_{ab}/\rho)_{\text{wat}}^{\text{tis}} \qquad (10\text{-}12)$$

where d is the depth from the surface of the patient to the isocenter and W_d is the (equivalent) field size. $(\overline{\mu}_{ab}/\rho)_{\text{wat}}^{\text{tis}}$ has been introduced in order to convert the absorbed dose from water to its value for tissue. This quantity is the ratio of mass energy absorption coefficients for tissue to water averaged over the photon spectrum as discussed in section 7.05. Numerical values for this factor can be taken from columns 6 and 7 of Table 7-4.

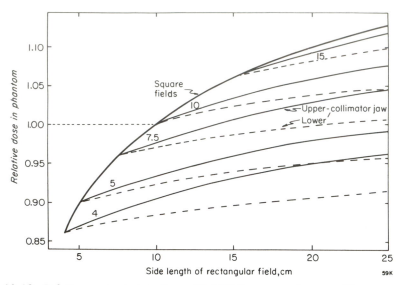

Figure 10-13. Relative output data for a 25 MV linear accelerator. The outputs were measured at a depth of 7 cm in a water phantom and are expressed as fractions of the output for a 10 × 10 cm field.

The factor is very nearly unity (0.99 for beam energies commonly used in radiotherapy) and is frequently neglected.

The reference dose, $D_{X''}$, includes a number of factors that are discussed in sections 7.12 and 7.13. These include an exposure calibration factor for the dosimeter, ratios of averaged stopping powers, ratios of averaged absorption coefficients, and displacement factors. Calibration procedures are discussed in section 9.13. The tissue-phantom ratio is by definition a ratio of two absorbed doses, and it too must include these factors. They will appear, however, both in its numerator and denominator; it is reasonable to assume that cancellation will take place so that the tissue-phantom ratio is taken as the ratio of two dosimeter readings. This is an approximation.

The dose at other depths in the patient may be calculated from D_d by using percent depth doses or relative depth doses.

Percent depth doses

The reference dose, D_Y, of Figure 10-1 may be measured directly in a phantom. The phantom in this case is set up with its surface at the specified source-surface distance. As discussed above, measurements should be made as a function of time or monitor units for a selection of field sizes. Again it cannot be assumed that equivalent squares can be used for these calibrations. The dose in a patient at the reference depth, d_Y, is given by:

$$D = D_Y \cdot (\overline{\mu}_{ab}/\rho)^{\text{tiss}}_{\text{wat}} \qquad (10\text{-}13)$$

where $(\bar{\mu}_{ab}/\rho)^{tiss}_{wat}$ is as discussed above for tissue-phantom ratios. The dose at another depth in the patient is then given by multiplying D by the appropriate percentage depth dose.

Tissue-Air Ratios

The reference dose to be used with tissue-air ratios is $D_{X'}$ of Figure 10-1 and is the dose "in space" to a small mass of phantom-like material located at the appropriate point in air. The principles for determining this dose from a dosimeter reading are the same as those for determining dose in a phantom and are discussed in section 7.11.

In calibrating a treatment machine for use with tissue-air ratios, measurements should be made at the isocenter for a selection of fields. A set of such data for a cobalt unit is shown in Figure 10-14 where the response, M, of the dosimeter is plotted against the length of one side of the field for a range of values of the other side. The data have been normalized to 1.00 for a 10 × 10 cm beam, and this diagram illustrates the way the output in air may change with field size and shape. This may be due to a variety of reasons, including alteration in the amount of scattered radiation from the inside surfaces of the collimator and other structures.

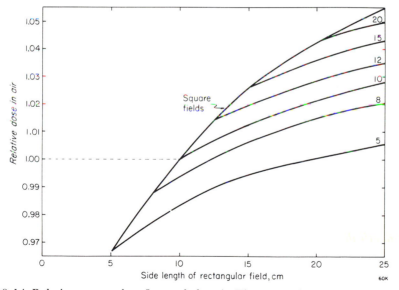

Figure 10-14. Relative output data for a cobalt unit. The output is measured in air and expressed relative to the value for a 10 × 10 field.

The dose in the patient, calculated using tissue-air ratios, is then given by:

$$D_d = D_{X'} \cdot T_a(d, W_d, h\nu) \, (\mu_{ab}/\rho)^{tis}_{wat} \qquad (10\text{-}14)$$

where, as for equation 10-12, d is the depth in the patient and W_d is the field size. $(\overline{\mu}_{ab}/\rho)^{tis}_{wat}$ converts the dose from water to tissue.

Tissue-air ratios, like tissue-phantom ratios and depth doses, are defined as the ratio of two doses. They are usually determined experimentally by making measurements with ion chambers. To convert the readings into doses, both numerator and denominator must by implication contain factors like those appearing in equation 7-30. It has generally been assumed that all factors except the instrument readings will cancel. This is usually a good approximation.

10.10   TABULAR DATA IN THE APPENDIX

Because extensive tables of tissue-air ratios, percentage depth doses, etc. are available elsewhere, we have restricted the tabular material in the appendix of this book to data that is representative of the field. It will enable the student to solve problems that cover the expected range of experience. It is not, however, intended to serve as source material for the practice of radiation therapy. We feel this is particularly important, since for the high energy equipment that is now in such common use the data is specific to the machine. Each user must therefore either measure or acquire the proper data.

For low energy radiations we have supplied percentage depth doses and backscatter factors for circular, square and rectangular fields for typical source surface distances. They are given in Tables B-1 to B-2. We have included more extensive tables for cobalt radiation, since this type of radiation is so widely available and is so convenient for experimental work because of its freedom from random variations in time. Tables B-2 to B-5 for cobalt radiation includes percentage depth doses and tissue-air ratios for circular, square, and rectangular fields. We have included data for three high energy radiations, 6, 10, and 26 MV, for square and circular fields in the form of tissue-phantom ratios and percentage depth doses for source-axis distance of 1 meter. The latter data are given in Tables B-2 to B-4. They are examples only and should not be assumed to apply to any particular machine without thorough testing.

10.11   ISODOSE CURVES

In the preceding sections of this chapter we have confined our attention to the dose at points on the axis of the beam. In any actual treatment we are interested in knowing the dose at many other points in the patient. These may be compared with the dose received at the reference point. When points that have the same dose are joined together, an isodose curve is obtained. A set of isodose curves, for a range of dose values, can be combined to form an isodose chart or isodose distribution. Such a distribution gives a map of the dose pattern in one plane in a radiation beam.

Three typical isodose distributions are shown in Figure 10-15 for low energy, high energy, and very high energy radiation. The 200 kV distribution is typical of the isodose curves obtained in the HVL range from 0.5 to 3.0 mm Cu for a source-to-skin distance of 50 cm. The cobalt 60 curve is typical of the distributions obtainable with cobalt and low energy linear accelerators used at source-to-skin distances from 80 to 120 cm. The 25 MV distribution is typical of super-voltage machines in the range 15 to 50 MV. Study of these three distributions may emphasize some previous observations. Consider first the depth dose along the axis. With 200 kV, the dose falls continuously, reaching about 25% at 10 cm depth. With cobalt 60, the dose rises rapidly to the maximum of 100 at a depth of about 5 mm and then falls slowly to reach some 52% at 10 cm depth. With 25 MV the buildup region that extends to about 4 cm is evident, after which the dose falls to some 83% at 10 cm depth.

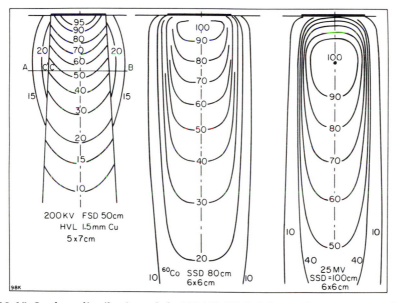

Figure 10-15. Isodose distributions: left, 200 kV, HVL 1.5 mm Cu, SSD 50 cm, field size 5 × 7 cm; middle, ^{60}Co, SSD 80 cm, field size 6 × 6 cm; right, 25 MV, SSD 100 cm, 6 × 6 cm.

The three sets of curves of Figure 10-15 are quite different near the edge of the beam. For the low energy radiation a sharp discontinuity can be seen. This discontinuity may be easily demonstrated by moving a small probe dosimeter across the beam along a path such as shown by the line AB in the diagram. Such an experiment yields the dose profile; the properties of such profiles are discussed in detail in section

10.13. The sharp edge of such a beam may also be demonstrated with photographic film. If the focal spot of the x ray tube were large and the limiting diaphragm some distance from the surface of the phantom, the discontinuity would disappear.

The cobalt 60 isodose curves do not show a sharp discontinuity because of the penumbra effects due to the finite size of the source. The 26 MV radiation shows a somewhat sharper demarcation between the region of high dose and low dose but no discontinuity as with 200 kV radiation. At cobalt 60 and 26 MV energies, no single diaphragm can completely absorb the beam of radiation because of its penetrating power and some radiation always passes through the edge of the diaphragm. The sharpness of the beam is further degraded by the flattening filter.

The three sets of curves of Figure 10-15 are quite different in the region outside the beam. With 200 kV, there is a large amount of side scatter, while with the other two, side scatter is low.

The 26 MV distribution was obtained using a carefully designed and precisely placed beam flattening filter. Without this filter to reduce the beam intensity along the axis, the isodose curves are quite pointed in the forward direction and useless for most radiotherapy. To give the flat isodose curves, the filter must be carefully aligned in the beam.

Isodose Curves with Other Reference Points

Figure 10-16 shows two isodose charts drawn with the reference point at different locations. Both are for 6 × 6 cm beams of cobalt 60 radiation. The chart on the left is for fixed source-surface distance (SSD = 80 cm) use and the reference point is at the position of maximum electronic buildup (see the discussion of depth dose in section 10.06). For this chart the field size is defined at the surface and 100% appears just below it at a depth of 0.5 cm. Percent depth doses are tabulations of the doses along the axis of the beam, and data for this beam are given in Table B-2e and plotted in Figures 10-8 and 10-9. The chart on the right in Figure 10-16 is for use with an isocentric (or rotational) mounted machine. The reference point is chosen to coincide with the axis of rotation (isocenter) and for this chart is located at a depth of 15 cm below the surface (SAD = 80 cm). The field size is defined at the isocenter and 100% appears at this location. All other doses in the beam are expressed as a percentage of the dose at this point.

Percent depth dose data for this beam are plotted as curve C of Figure 10-12. In normal use with an isocentric machine the patient would be placed so the center of the tumor was at the isocenter; using the isodose distribution one can easily compare the dose at other points to the dose at the tumor.

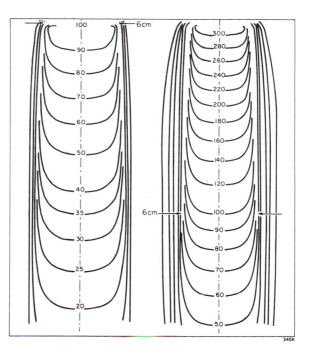

Figure 10-16. Left; Isodose pattern for fixed SSD with percentages referred to the point of maximum electronic buildup. Right; Isodose patterns for isocentric use with percentages and field sizes referred to the axis of rotation. Both beams are for ^{60}Co radiation and are 6 cm square.

Isodose Surfaces—Isodose Curves in Three Dimensions

The isodose curves shown in Figures 10-15 and 10-16 give the distribution of radiation in a plane containing the axis of the beam. This plane is known as the principal plane. It is important to remember, however, that the isodose distribution is three-dimensional in nature and one should think of isodose surfaces rather than isodose curves. It is very difficult to display isodose surfaces, and it is customary to show the distribution in two principal planes at right angles to one another. These principal planes also contain the central ray of the beam. This is illustrated in Figure 10-17, where two distributions for a 15 × 10 cobalt 60 field are shown in perspective at right angles to one another. The isodose curves in the two planes give the intersection of the isodose surfaces with these planes. The three-dimensional nature of the isodose pattern is further illustrated in Figure 10-18 where isodose curves for four different planes are shown for a 6 × 15 beam of cobalt radiation. Figures 10-18a and b are for the principal planes and c is for a plane that is parallel to the plane of b but is 3 cm away from it. Diagram d is for a cross section of the beam taken at a depth of 10 cm. The positions of the intersections of the planes are indicated by the dashed lines in the diagram. The production of these isodose curves requires a computer. The diagrams of Figure 10-18 were produced by methods discussed later in this chapter.

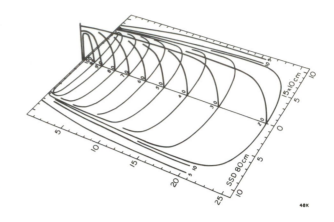

Figure 10-17. Isodose distributions for the two principal planes of a 15 × 10 cm cobalt 60 field at SSD 80 cm drawn in perspective.

From these diagrams one can visualize the isodose surfaces as three-dimensional surfaces. The 95% isodose surface, for example, is shaped somewhat like a rectangular pancake about 13 cm long, 4 cm wide, and 1 cm thick. The 50% isodose surface is like a rectangular block about 15 × 6 × 11 cm with all corners rounded off.

A knowledge of the three-dimensional nature of the isodose surfaces is very important for treatment planning and will be discussed again in Chapter 12.

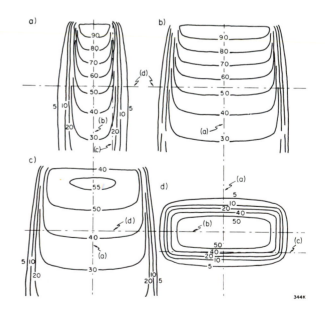

Figure 10-18. Isodose distributions in 4 planes for a 6 × 15 cm beam from a cobalt unit. (a) and (b) are in principal planes. (c) is parallel to b but 3 cm from it. (d) is a cross section at a depth of 10 cm.

With the advent of many new types of therapy machines, it is instructive to compare the isodose curves that may be obtained from them. This will be done in the following section.

10.12   COMPARISON OF ISODOSE CURVES

Side Scatter

In Figure 10-19 are shown two distributions for cobalt 60 and two for HVL 1.0 mm Cu. In the case of cobalt 60, there is very little side scatter for either the 6 × 6 or the 6 × 15 cm curves. To conserve space, only half of each has been drawn; the other half is symmetrical with the part shown. For the softer radiation, side scatter is very evident, especially along the short axis of the 6 × 20 cm field. Along this axis, scattering is received from all parts of the long 20 × 6 strip field. In the case of the 6 × 6 cm field, scattering outside the beam is less because the region that may scatter to points in this plane is smaller. The distributions shown for HVL 1.0 mm Cu are typical of x ray machines operating with half-value layers from 1.0 to 3.0 mm Cu. As the energy is increased, side scatter decreases slowly to yield distributions similar to those of cobalt 60, which are similar to those in the 1 to 4 MeV range. Side scatter is an unfortunate property of low energy beams, as such radiation cannot contribute to the tumor dose but merely raises the dose to healthy tissue surrounding the tumor. Such radiations have been used in the past because no other radiation was available.

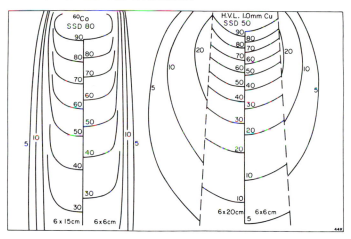

Figure 10-19. Isodose curves demonstrating side scatter. Left, cobalt 60, SSD 80 cm, field size 6 × 15 and 6 × 6. Right, HVL 1.0 mm Cu, SSD 50 cm, field size 6 × 20 and 6 × 6.

Effect of SSD and Source Size on Cobalt 60 Distributions

Figure 10-20 shows four distributions for different types of cobalt 60 units showing the effects of penumbra resulting from different combinations of source-to-skin distance, skin-to-diaphragm distance, and source size. The penumbra has been calculated at the skin surface using the simple concept of geometrical penumbra discussed in section 10.13 and is given for each set of isodose curves. The left-hand diagram compares the type of distribution from a large SSD unit with a short SSD unit. The 10 cm depth dose is reduced by some 12% (from 56 to 50%) and the curving of the isodose curves near the edge of the beam is accentuated. Short SSD units cannot produce as ideal a distribution as can those with a long SSD.

On the right, the isodose curves of a well-designed cobalt unit are compared with one in which no effort has been made to control the penumbra. In the beam with the large penumbra, the fall-off of dose laterally is severe and the beam has lost its incisive character. Many of the inherent advantages of penetrating cobalt 60 beam are lost when used in this way.

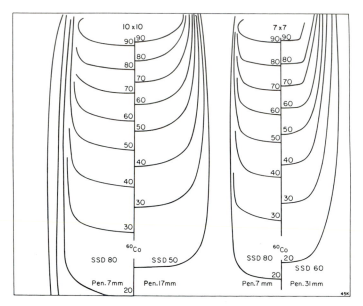

Figure 10-20. Isodose curves for cobalt 60 with different penumbra. Left, 10 × 10 cm field; SSD 80 with penumbra 7 mm compared with SSD 50 and penumbra 17 mm. Right, 7 × 7 cm field; SSD 80 with penumbra 7 mm compared with SSD 60 and penumbra 31 mm.

Comparison of Cobalt 60 with 2 to 4 MV Radiation

Figure 10-21 shows a comparison between cobalt 60 and radiation in the 2 to 4 MV range. On the left, cobalt 60 at SSD 80 cm is compared with radiation from a 2 MeV generator operating at SSD 100. From the point of view of penumbra, the two distributions are identical. This particular 2 MV distribution is highly filtered and gives a slightly higher depth dose at 10 cm depth than the cobalt 60.

The comparison between cobalt 60 and 4 MeV linear accelerators shows that the beams are essentially identical from a penumbra point of view. These linear accelerators give a higher depth dose because of the greater mean energy and the slightly greater SSD. Both give about the same dose rate. The advantage of a slightly greater depth dose from these low energy linear accelerators must be balanced against the absolute reliability and simplicity of a cobalt unit that, when once calibrated, can be expected to deliver radiation in a precise, predictable way for a number of years without need of technical personnel.

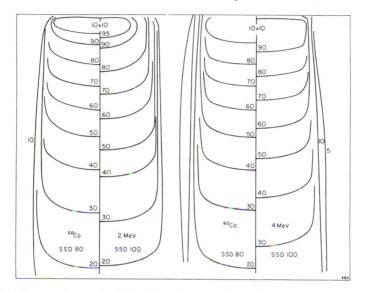

Figure 10-21. Comparison of cobalt 60 and supervoltage 2-4 MV radiation for 10 × 10 fields. Left, cobalt 60 at SSD 80 cm versus heavily filtered 2 MV beam at SSD 100 cm. Right, cobalt 60 at SSD 80 cm versus 4 MV linear accelerator, SSD 100 cm.

10.13 CALCULATION OF DOSE AT ANY POINT

In section 10.03 a set of functions were introduced that can be used to calculate dose at points along the beam axis. In section 10.11 isodose charts were introduced so that doses could be determined in planes. These isodose charts, however, are in general restricted to principal planes, that is, planes that include the beam axis. Frequently one wishes also to determine doses at points that are not included in the principal planes. One may wish to calculate doses at various points in fields that have irregular shapes and so cannot have individual isodose charts. Such calculations are rather complicated, and it is convenient to perform them by considering the primary and scatter components of the beam separately. In what follows, the primary will be discussed first and this will be followed by a discussion of the scatter component.

Description of the Primary Beam

Figure 10-22a shows a radiation beam incident on a point X′ in air. The conditions are the same as for the left side of Figure 10-1, that is no phantom is present. A small dosimeter is moved along the line AF, and its reading is indicated by the solid line in Figure 10-22b. At point A it is shielded by the collimator and at point X' (point X' also of Fig. 10-1) it is in the beam in full view of the source; the dose will be at the maximum value for this line. At point C, the dosimeter is still in full view of the source but it is slightly further away than it was at X' and the dose will be slightly lower. The expected reading is indicated at point C on the dashed line in Figure 10-22b. At point D the collimator blocks off the view of half of the source, and the reading of the dosimeter will be very nearly half of its value at X'. At point E the dosimeter just loses sight of the source, and its reading should drop to zero, as indicated at point E of Figure 10-22b. The distance between points C and E, along the line AB, is called the geometric penumbra. It is dependent on the diameter of the source, S, the distance from the source to the end of the collimator, f_c, and the distance $(f - f_c)$ from the collimator to the line AB. It is given by considering similar triangles and is:

$$p = s(f - f_c)/f_c \qquad\qquad (10\text{-}15)$$

The actual or experimental dose profile is indicated by the solid line of Figure 10-22b. It differs from the theoretical or geometrical dose profile (the dashed curve in Figure 10-22b) in a number of ways: it has no sharp corners, the dose at point C is less than theoretically expected, and the dose at E is greater. These effects arise because the source does not really behave as if it were a sharply defined disk. There will be absorption and scattering within it and scattering from all other structures close to it including the collimators. Although this description directly applies to a cobalt source, the behavior is entirely similar for the "focal spot" in any x ray machine. In a high energy x ray machine such as a linear accelerator or betatron, the "source" is made diffuse also by the flattening filter (for example see section 4.05).

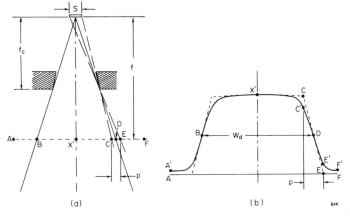

Figure 10-22. Diagrams illustrating properties of the primary component of a radiation beam. (a) The geometrical factors that lead to beam penumbra. (b) A dose profile as measured in air along the line A-F of a.

The dose profile shown in Figure 10-22 is for a cobalt unit. A dose profile for a linear accelerator or other x ray machine will be similar but may be more complicated because of the presence of a beam flattening filter. It may also change from day to day or hour to hour because of drifts in electronic components. In what follows it will be assumed that the beam is from a cobalt source, but all the arguments can in principle be applied to other radiation beams.

In order to calculate the dose at any point in a beam it is convenient to represent the dose profile by a mathematical function. Since the scattering that occurs from the collimator and other structures is too complicated to describe easily, it is more practical to seek an empirical function. A search for a function that would adequately fit experimental data and yet involve few arbitrary constants has suggested the following:

$$f(x) = 1. - 0.5\, e^{(-\alpha_1/p)[(W_d/2)\, -\, |x|]} \text{ for } |x| \le w_d/2$$
$$f(x) = t + (0.5 - t)\, e^{(-\alpha_2/p)[|x|\, -\, (W_d/2)]} \text{ for } |x| > w_d/2 \qquad (10\text{-}16)$$

where $|x|$ is the absolute value of the distance, x, along the line AF from the central ray; $W_d/2$ is half the width of the beam at depth d; p is the geometric penumbra given by equation 10-15; α_1 and α_2 are empirical constants that describe the way in which the actual penumbral region differs from the geometric penumbral region; and t is interpreted as an effective transmission through the collimator. The constants α_1, α_2, and t must be determined by experiment for each treatment machine as required. An example of this procedure is shown in Figure 10-23. An experimental dose profile for a Theratron® 780 cobalt unit is shown as a dashed line along with curves calculated from equation 10-16 and almost coincides with the curve drawn for $\alpha_1 = 5$, $\alpha_2 = 2.5$, and t = 0.02. It can be seen that the choices of numerical values are not very critical.

Primary Dose in a Phantom

If the beam of Figure 10-22a is incident on a phantom and the line AF is at a depth d below the surface of this phantom, then the dose, due

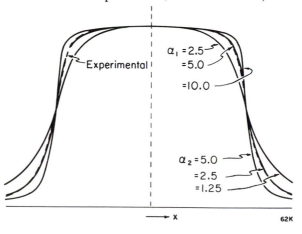

Figure 10-23. Calculated dose profiles showing the effect of changing the constants α_1 and α_2 over a rather wide range.

to primary only, at a point on this line will be given by:

$$D_{Prim} = D_{X'} \cdot f(x) \cdot T_a(d,0) \qquad (10\text{-}17)$$

where $D_{X'}$ is the dose in air at point X' on the beam axis, x is the distance from the axis to the point, $f(x)$ is the function given in equation 10-16, and $T_a(d,0)$ is the tissue-air ratio for depth d but zero field size. It describes the attenuation of the primary beam by the phantom along a line from the source to the point.

Description of Radiation Scattered in the Phantom—Scatter-Air Ratios

The tissue-air ratio (section 10.04) is an expression of the attenuation of primary radiation and buildup of scatter. For calculation of doses in complicated beam shapes, it is useful to have a knowledge of each of these components separately. A procedure for separating out these components can be explained by reference to Figure 10-5. This diagram shows tissue-air ratios for a number of depths plotted against field size. The field size is expressed as the side of a square. As the field size is increased, the tissue-air ratio increases. This increase is due to a change in the scatter component. A field size of zero area would be a "narrow beam" and would contain no scattered radiation. The difference between the tissue-air ratio for a field of finite area and that for a zero-area would be a measure of the contribution from scattered radiation. A tissue-air ratio can therefore be thought of as having two components:

$$T_a(d,r_d,h\nu) = T_a(d,0,h\nu) + S(d,r_d,h\nu) \qquad (10\text{-}18)$$

The first term is the zero-area tissue-air ratio and the second has been called the scatter-air ratio (G10, C8).

The zero-area tissue-air ratio is a mathematical abstraction. It cannot be measured directly. It can only be obtained by extrapolation. This extrapolation is not precise but it is helped by the fact that $T_a(d,0,h\nu)$, as a function of the depth d, has the same shape as a narrow beam attenuation curve, which can be measured.

Derivation of Scatter-Air Ratio Data

The most direct way to compile a table of scatter-air ratios is to first obtain tissue-air ratios and use equation 10-18.

$$S(d,r_d,h\nu) = T_a(d,r_d,h\nu) - T_a(d,0,h\nu) \qquad (10\text{-}18a)$$

The data given in Tables C-1a to c were obtained in this way for HVL 2 mm Al through cobalt radiation. Gupta and Cunningham (G10) also measured scattered radiation directly for cobalt radiation by shielding the dosimeter from primary radiation with a lead block. The scatter-air ratios so obtained, however, were less precise than those derived from tissue-air ratios.

For high energy radiation the situation is not as straightforward, because tissue-air ratio data is not normally available. Tissue-air ratios can be derived from tissue phantom ratios by using equation 10-7, which for circular fields would be:

$$T_a(d,r_d,h\nu) = T_p(d,d_r,r_d,h\nu) \cdot T_a(d_r,r_d,h\nu) \qquad (10\text{-}7a)$$

The first term in the product can be evaluated from measured tissue-phantom ratio data. If data for square fields only is available, conversion to circular fields may be made by assuming that the equivalent circular field has the same areas as the corresponding square. The second term of equation 10-7a is the tissue-air ratio for the reference depth, d_r (see sec. 10.07), and must be determined indirectly. Van Dyk (V7), working with 10 MV radiation, assumed it to be always 1.0. Because of the small amount of scattered radiation at high energies, this is a fairly good approximation. Somewhat better values may, however, be determined as follows:

(a) With the dosimeter at the reference depth, d_r, in a phantom determine dose as a function of field size. This experiment yields both phantom scatter and change in collimator scatter with collimator opening. The readings can be plotted and extrapolated to zero field size (see Fig. 10-13).

(b) With the dosimeter at the same location as for a, but without the phantom, again determine dose as a function of field size. The dosimeter must be equipped with a buildup cap appropriate to the energy of the radiation. This experiment is an attempt at measuring the alteration in machine output as the collimator opening is varied. These data too can be plotted and extrapolated to zero field size. Because of the size of the cap required in this experiment, it may be that measurements cannot be made at small field sizes and this makes the extrapolation more uncertain. The shape of the curve for small field sizes can be examined by using a buildup cap of high density material, and although this procedure certainly introduces more unknowns, the quantity being measured is sufficiently insensitive to them that it is a useful practical procedure.

(c) The data from a and b are renormalized to their values for zero area field and a is divided by b to produce an estimate of the tissue-air ratios for the reference depth.

The data given in Table C-1e for 25 MV radiation was produced in this manner. The values obtained in step c can be inferred from the data for depth 5 cm in Table C-1e. The tissue-air ratios for this depth vary from 1.0 to just over 1.1 for field sizes ranging from 0 to 30 × 30 cm.

Sector Integration of Scattered Radiation

One of the most useful applications of scatter-air ratios is the calculation of relative dose in rectangular or irregularly shaped beams. The sector integration technique was discussed in sections 10.04 and 10.06 but will be described in more detail here. Figure 10-24a shows a cross section of a rectangular beam 5 × 15 cm. The dose is to be calculated at point P, which is at the center of the field and at a depth 5 cm below the surface of a phantom. Six radial lines, spaced at equal angular intervals ($\Delta\theta = 15°$), have been drawn from P to the edge of the field. One of them, r_4, is used as the radius to draw a complete circle about point P. Scatter-air ratio values, for a depth of 5 cm, are plotted against radii (Fig. 10-24). The radius r_4 is 4.11 cm and the curve shows that the scatter-air ratio for a circular field of this radius is 0.136. This means that if the dose in air at point P were 1.0, then the dose due to scatter at a depth of 5 cm on the axis of a circular beam of radius r_4 would be 0.136.

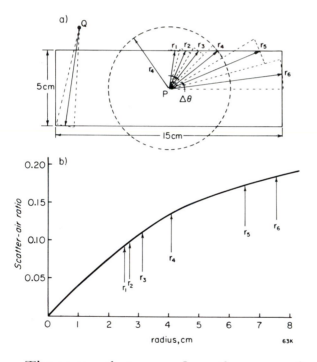

Figure 10-24. Diagram illustrating the use of scatter-air ratios to calculate the dose at two points. (a) Point P is inside the beam and receives both primary and scattered radiation. Point Q is outside and receives only scattered radiation. The dashed circle indicates a circular beam of radius r_4, one sector of which is considered to be part of the rectangular field. (b) Scatter-air ratio plotted against radius for a depth of 5 cm. The arrows indicate the radii of sectors in a.

The scatter that comes from the sector of angular width $\Delta\theta$ in the circular beam of radius r_4 would be 0.136 ($\Delta\theta/2\pi$). The amount of radiation reaching point P from the sector of angular width $\Delta\theta$ and radius r_4 but in the rectangular beam shown would be very similar to this. A similar argument can be made for each of the sectors r_1 through r_6 in Figure 10-24a. These 6 sectors cover one quadrant of the beam and the total dose at point P due to scatter would be:

$$D_{scat} = \frac{\Delta\theta}{2\pi} \sum_{i=1}^{n} S(d,r_i) \tag{10-19}$$

where n is the number of sectors required to cover the entire area of the field, that is $n\Delta\theta = 2\pi$.

Although point P was chosen to be at the center of the field for the above example, the procedure applies equally well to the calculation of the amount of scattered radiation at any point either in or out of the field. Points such as Q outside of the field, however, require some special treatment, because for each sector, two radii are involved, one from the point to the first reached boundary of the field, the second for the second boundary. The scatter from the former must be subtracted and from the latter added. The total dose at point P will be:

$$D_p = D_{prim} + D_{scat} = D_{X'} \left[f(x) \cdot T(d,0) + \frac{\Delta\theta}{2\pi} \sum_{i=1}^{n} S(d,r_i) \right] \tag{10-20}$$

where $f(x)$ is a factor allowing for attenuation of primary by a filter. Two examples will illustrate such calculations.

Example 10-6. Using scatter-air ratios, calculate the tissue-air ratio for a 4×15 cm field at a depth of 10 cm in a water phantom. Use $10°$ intervals over one quadrant, as shown in Figures 10-6 and 10-24.

Angles $= 5°, 15°, \ldots 85°$.

radii, $r_i = 2.01, 2.07, 2.21, 2.44, 2.83, 3.49, 4.73, 7.73, 7.53$

$S(10,r_i) = .076, .078, .082, .090, .104, .124, .155, .211, .208$

$T(10.0)$, the zero area tissue-air ratio $= .534$ (Table B-5d).

$f(x) = 1.0$ on the beam axis

Tissue-air ratio $= .534 + 4 \times \dfrac{1}{36} \sum_{1}^{9} S(10,r_i) = .534 + .125 = .659$

Example 10-7. Calculate the dose at a point 2 cm outside of a 4×15 cm field at a depth of 10 cm relative to the dose at the same depth on the axis. Assume cobalt radiation and take the point to be opposite to the central ray and adjacent to the long side of the field.

radii, $r_i = 6.02, 6.21, 6.62, 7.32, 8.49, 9.16, 8.28$ ($10°$ intervals)

$S(10,r_i)_1 = .182, .185, .193, .204, .222, .232, .219$ (Table C-1c)

radii, $r_i = 2.01, 2.07, 2.21, 2.44, 2.83, 3.49, 4.73$

$S(10,r_i)_2 = .076, .078, .082, .090, .104, .124, .155$

$\dfrac{2}{36} [\Sigma S(10,r_i)_1 - \Sigma S(10,r_i)_2] = \dfrac{1}{18} (1.437 - 0.709) = 0.040$

assume transmission through the collimator = .02

total $= 0.02 \times 0.534 + 0.040 = 0.051$

Tissue-air ratio on beam axis $= T(10, 4 \times 15) = 0.661$

relative dose $= 0.051/0.661 = 0.077$

10.14   LATERAL ELECTRONIC EQUILIBRIUM

The establishment of electronic equilibrium at the anterior surface of a phantom was discussed in section 7.03, and in section 7.14 we showed that there is a disruption in the pattern of electron tracks and a loss of equilibrium between kerma (energy lost by photons) and absorbed dose (energy lost by electrons) wherever there is a sharp boundary between different absorbing materials. In this section we show that this can also alter the shape of the edge of a beam, with the result that the beam penumbra (described in the previous section) appears to be increased.

Figure 10-25 depicts a beam of high energy photons incident on a phantom. The photon beam is considered to be infinitely sharp, that is, it has zero penumbra. Its profile is depicted below in Figure 10-25. Electrons are set into motion by photon interactions, and electron tracks are indicated. These electrons travel predominately in the forward direction but the tracks may be several cm long and will tend to spread out sideways due to electron scattering processes. Point A is well within the beam and will receive an equal number of electron tracks from the left and the right of it. Point B is still within the photon beam; it will receive electron tracks from the left but only a few from the right. The dose at point B would therefore be decreased due to the loss of electron tracks. Point C is completely outside of the photon beam but is close enough to it to still receive electron tracks, and the dose there would be increased. The result is that the effective beam penumbra is increased. This effect can extend over several mm for a high energy photon beam and should be taken into account when specifying the properties of high energy photon beams.

10.15   DETERMINATION OF ISODOSE CURVES

The measurement of isodose curves for an isotope machine is relatively simple because the radiation beam does not suffer from erratic fluctuations in dose rate. The simplest procedure for producing an isodose chart consists of moving a probe by a remote control mechanism across the beam in a water phantom. Three typical dose profiles, measured this way, are shown in Figure 10-26 for depths 1, 10, and 20 cm in a 10×10 cm cobalt 60 beam. The curves may be constructed either by taking readings about every cm in the region where the dose is essentially constant and every 1 or 2 mm in regions of high dose gradient or by coupling the output of the dosimeter to an x-y plotter and recording

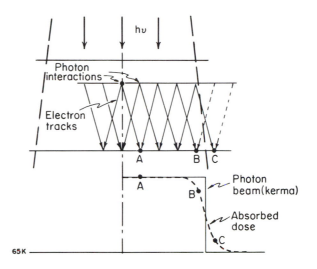

Figure 10-25. Diagram depicting loss of electronic equilibrium near the edge of a high energy photon beam. Point A receives electron tracks coming from all directions. Point B is inside the photon beam but receives fewer electron tracks than does A. Point C is outside of the photon beam but still receives some electron tracks.

the dose profile directly. For this type of measurement, a cylindrical chamber of small diameter should be used to approximate measurement at a point. To obtain the desired sensitivity, the chamber may be made rather long, since there is practically no dose gradient in a direction at right angles to the page. A chamber 3 mm in diameter and 20 mm long has reasonable dimensions for this type of study. A satisfactory probe may also be made using solid state detectors described in section 9.08. Transits of the kind indicated are made at 4 or 5 depths. The width of the 20%, 30%, 40%, etc. isodose curves for each depth may then be taken directly from graphs (like Fig. 10-26) and plotted. Finally, points of equal dose are connected to give the desired isodose curves. This is a task that can conveniently be done by a computer. At the present time, devices are available commercially that move a probe to any given point in a water phantom under computer control. They may also capture the dose values automatically and compile a table of dose values at chosen coordinate points. Various computer programs have been written to process and interpolate these numbers for direct use in computerized treatment planning.

10.16   DEPTH DOSE DISTRIBUTIONS FOR HIGH ENERGY ELECTRONS AND HEAVY PARTICLES

With the development of betatrons and high energy linear accelerators capable of producing electron beams, it is feasible to treat certain tumors with electrons. Such treatments are being carried out in a number of the larger centers. The depth dose curves for electrons as determined by Laughlin (L7) are shown in Figure 10-27 for electrons with 4 different energies. With the 6.2 MeV beam the dose rises from some 85% at the surface to maximum of 100 at about 1 cm and then falls linearly to almost zero at a depth of about 3 cm. The curves for the higher energies

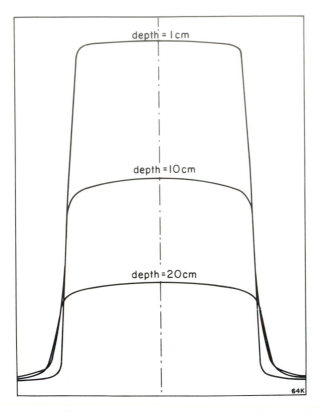

depth = 1 cm

depth = 10 cm

depth = 20 cm

64K

Figure 10-26. Dose profiles for a 10 × 10 cm beam for depths 1, 10, and 20 cm.

are similar, except now the surface dose is slightly higher, the maximum dose is at a greater depth, and the reduction of dose is not nearly as linear.

On the same graph is shown the depth dose curve for 190 MeV deuterons as determined by Tobias (T5). This curve has very attractive features, since the surface dose is small and the maximum occurs at a depth of about 13 cm. This curve is known as a Bragg curve. At the surface the high energy deuteron beam loses energy rather slowly. As it enters the phantom the rate of energy loss increases slowly as the particle's velocity decreases. Near the end of the range when the particle has little energy and is traveling slowly, the rate of energy loss suddenly increases and then falls to zero as the particle comes to rest. A lower energy deuteron beam would have its peak at a lesser depth.

The shape of the depth dose curves for electrons and for deuterons given in Figure 10-27 is quite different. The deuterons, because of their large mass, tend to travel in straight lines, giving a beam with sharp edges. On the other hand, electrons with smaller mass tend to be scattered more, so the edges of the beam are diffuse. This scattering results in some electrons being lost from the beam and in a continuous reduction in depth dose. In addition, the electrons lose some of their energy by bremsstrahlung production giving a beam with less well defined range.

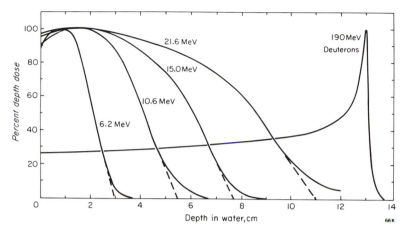

Figure 10-27. Depth dose produced by electrons from a betatron for incident energies of 6.2, 10.6, 15.0, and 21.6 MeV. Circular field 9.5 cm in diameter. Plotted from data of Laughlin (L7). Data for a beam of 190 MeV deuterons by Tobias (T5) is also shown for comparison.

The peak of the Bragg curve for deuterons is too narrow to encompass most tumors. It is conceivable that a tumor could be scanned by deuterons of different energies to yield a uniform distribution over a range equal to the tumor dimension. However, if several energy beams are required to yield a wide enough peak to cover the tumor, the differential between the net tumor dose and the net surface dose will largely be lost. In any case, the production of such high energy deuterons requires very expensive equipment with a large staff, and it is difficult to see how such machines can ever be used routinely in radiotherapy.

Figure 10-28 shows typical isodose curves for electrons with energies of 15 and 25 MeV for 10 × 10 cm beams. This type of distribution is useful in treating large tumors near the skin surface.

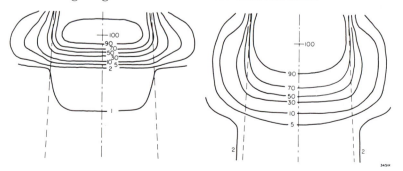

Figure 10-28. Isodose curves for 15 and 25 MeV electron beams from a linear accelerator. Field size is 10 × 10 cm.

10.17   **SUMMARY**

Before *accurately* controlled radiotherapy can be carried out, the following measurements and calculations must be made concerning cobalt or x ray machines.

1. Identify the beam quality. For a cobalt unit this is known. For a low energy x ray machine it is necessary to measure the half-value layer for a selection of filters and decide which filters should be used to get the required half-value layers (see sec. 8.03). It is convenient to adjust the filtration to obtain an integral half-value layer so that depth dose tables etc. may be used directly without interpolation. For a high energy linear accelerator or betatron, it will be better to measure a few points on the depth dose curve in a water phantom or equivalent.

2. From the known beam quality obtain tables of backscatter factors, percent depth doses, and tissue-air ratios as required for use in the department.

3. Calibrate the output of the machine in terms of exposure rate in air for a low energy x ray machine and in terms of absorbed dose rate at a reference point in a phantom for a cobalt unit and a high energy x ray machine (see secs. 7.11, 7.12, 7.13, and 9.13). For a cobalt unit it may also be useful to calibrate in terms of exposure rate in air or dose rate in free space (see sec. 7.11). For all machines the output should be measured for a range of field sizes. This is necessary because the output changes with field size due to scattering from the collimators and a number of other factors, and this effect will be peculiar to the design of the individual machine.

4. Obtain an isodose chart for each of the field sizes that will be used. Frequently such data may be obtained from the manufacturer of the treatment unit.

5. If a computerized treatment planning system is being used, the data as required must be entered into the computer. Instructions for doing this must be obtained from the vendor of the computer system.

PROBLEMS

1. A tumor at a depth of 8 cm is irradiated with a cobalt 60 beam having dimensions 6 × 8 cm at the tumor. The dose rate at this position in free space is 1.12 Gy/min. Find the dose rate at the tumor. A tumor dose of 2 Gy is to be delivered each day. How long should each treatment last?
2. If the source-to-tumor distance for problem 1 is 80 cm, what is the field size at the position of maximum dose and what is the daily tissue dose at this point?
3. Find the backscatter factor for a 6 × 10 cm field at HVL 1.0 mm Cu, assuming the thickness of the underlying tissue is great enough to supply full backscatter. Use Table B-1a. Compare with the entry in Table B-1b.
4. Explain why the variation of backscatter with HVL is as indicated in Figure 10-7.

5. A patient is to be treated on a cobalt unit with three 6 × 10 cm beams which intersect at T, the center of a tumor. The point T is 80 cm from the source and the dose rate in free space at this point is 0.85 Gy/min. The depths of tissue above T for the 3 fields are 8, 12, 15 cm respectively. Determine the dose rate at the tumor from each of the fields. Determine also the dose rate and beam size at the position of dose maximum for each of the fields.

6. Each of the 3 beams of problem 5 is to be left on for the same length of time. What is the total treatment time required to deliver 2 Gy to the point T?

7. If each of the 3 beams of problem 5 is turned on long enough to give the same tumor doses, determine these times, the total time, and the maximum dose given each field. Comment on the advantages and disadvantages to this arrangement.

8. The same beam arrangement as in problem 5 is used on the same machine to treat at a fixed SSD of 80 cm, using three 6 × 10 cm beams, the field sizes now being specified at the surface. (a) Calculate the dose rate in free space at the dose reference point (depth 0.5 cm); the dose rate with backscatter; the dose rate at the tumor for each beam. (b) If the given doses (dose just below the surface) are made equal, what is the total time required to deliver 2 Gy to the tumor? (c) If the tumor doses are now made equal, calculate the required given doses.

9. Using the data of Figure 10-4 for a zero area, determine the linear attenuation coefficient for cobalt 60 radiation in water and compare with the value in Table A-3b. Obtain also an effective attenuation coefficient for a beam area of 400 cm² and discuss reasons for the difference.

10. Determine the tissue-air ratio for a point on the edge of a 14 cm diameter circular field of cobalt 60 radiation using Clarkson's method and the data plotted in Figure 10-6.

11. Determine the tissue-air ratio at the corner of a 10 × 10 cm field. This can be done by the method used above or very simply by considering this field to be a fraction of a larger field. Use radiation parameters of problem 10.

12. Calculate the dose to a point which is at a depth of 10 cm and is 5 cm outside of the beam along one of the axes of a 15 × 15 cm cobalt field. Do the calculation for 1 Gy on the beam axis at the same depth. Use scatter-air ratios.

13. Calculate the percentage depth dose at a depth of 12 cm for cobalt radiation for a field that is 12 × 20 cm at a patient's surface, which is 130 cm from the source.

14. From data in Table B-5d calculate the tissue-phantom ratio for a 10 × 10 cm beam of cobalt 60 radiation for a depth of 12 cm. Use 5 cm as the reference depth and compare with the data in Table B-4a.

15. Using Table 10-4 giving equivalent squares, determine the square field equivalent to a 4 × 20 cm field. Find the 10 cm percentage depth dose for cobalt radiation for this square field by interpolation from square field data in Table B-2e and compare with the accurate value of the percentage depth dose given in the same table.

Chapter 11

TREATMENT PLANNING—SINGLE BEAMS

11.01   **DIRECT PATIENT DOSE CALCULATIONS**

The process of planning a course of radiotherapy involves the choosing and arranging of radiation beams around a patient in order to provide a high dose at the site of the tumor and as low a dose as possible everywhere else. The functions that were discussed in the previous chapter were derived for the purpose of facilitating the calculation of the dose to the tumor and to other tissues that are inevitably irradiated. These functions and the isodose curves that go with them were derived from measurements made in a water phantom. Their use provides a very good approximation to the dosage pattern that will be produced within an actual patient. The shape and composition of the patient does affect this pattern, however, and in many cases allowance for this must be made in dosage calculations.

In this chapter we will discuss the use of single beams. In the next chapter we will discuss the combination of beams to produce desired dosage patterns.

Figure 11-1 shows identical cross-sectional views of a head with a tumor in the tonsillar region. The diagram on the left shows an isodose chart for a beam from a fixed SSD cobalt unit superimposed on it while the diagram on the right shows the dose pattern for a beam from an isocentric cobalt unit superimposed on the same anatomical structure. We will first discuss a number of terms that are useful in treatment planning. For the moment we neglect any effects on the isodose distribution of surface shape or air cavities (the pharynx) or bones (the mandible and vertebra). With this simplification, doses to the various tissues may be obtained from the diagram directly.

REFERENCE DOSE. The concept of a reference dose was discussed at some length in Chapter 10. For Figure 11-1a the reference dose is the dose at point R, which is a point just below the skin (0.5 cm) on the axis of the beam. It is given the value 100% in this diagram. Sometimes, for a fixed SSD technique this dose is also called the *given dose*. Its actual value for a treatment is calculated from the calibration data of the machine and all other doses are determined relative to it (see example 11-1). For the isocentric technique shown in Figure 11-1b, the reference dose is the dose at R now located at the isocenter of the machine. The term "given dose" can be confusing if applied to an isocentric technique and maximum tissue dose should be used instead.

382

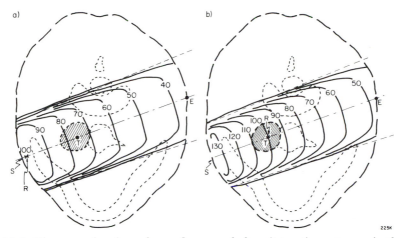

Figure 11-1. Diagrams showing a beam from a cobalt unit treating a tumor in the region of the tonsil. (a) is for a fixed SSD technique and (b) is for an isocentric technique.

TUMOR DOSE. Before discussing tumor dose we must introduce the concept of *target volume*. The target volume contains the tumor but because the edges of the tumor can rarely be located with certainty, the target volume is made larger. It therefore inevitably contains a certain amount of healthy tissue, which will be irradiated. The concept of target volume is discussed in detail in ICRU Report 29 (I8). In this book we will not distinguish between the tumor and target volume. It will be assumed the "tumor" contains the safety margin. The cross-hatched region of Figure 11-1 is then the target or tumor. The *tumor dose* usually refers to the dose at the center of the tumor although some other value can be used. In Figure 11-1a, the *tumor dose*, at point T, is 76%. The *maximum* tumor dose is 82% and the *minimum* is 70%. In Figure 11-1b the *tumor dose* is 100% with a *maximum* of 110% and a *minimum* of 92%. The simple arrangements of Figure 11-1 would not be suitable for treating the tonsil because the maximum tissue dose is much greater (more than 130%) than the tumor dose. The situation may be rectified by adding more beams directed toward the tumor. How this is done will be discussed in the next chapter.

SKIN DOSE. The term *skin dose* is used to describe the dose that actually occurs at a point on the surface of the patient. This is labelled S in Figure 11-1. For low energy x rays this would coincide with the peak dose. For beam energies corresponding to that of cobalt or greater, where there is skin sparing, the actual skin dose may not be well known. In a well-designed treatment unit it should be less than 50% of the reference dose but in a badly designed unit it can actually be greater. Leung (L2) has made an extensive study of this question in cobalt units.

Some of these ideas will now be illustrated by examples.

Example 11-1. A cobalt unit is calibrated using a water phantom at SSD = 80 cm and a 6 × 6 cm beam is used in the manner shown in Figure 11-1a to produce an absorbed dose rate of 1.16 Gy/min at a depth of 0.5 cm. The tumor dose is to be 1.33 Gy each day of treatment. Calculate the dose rate at the tumor and the daily treatment time. Calculate also the daily maximum and minimum tumor doses.

Given, or peak, dose rate = 1.16 Gy/min

Tumor dose rate = 1.16 Gy/min × 76/100 = 0.88 Gy/min

Daily treatment time $= \dfrac{1.33 \text{ Gy}}{0.88 \text{ Gy/min}} = 1.51$ min

Maximum tumor dose = 1.33 × 82/76 = 1.44 Gy

Minimum tumor dose = 1.33 × 70/76 = 1.23 Gy

Example 11-2. An isocentric cobalt unit is calibrated in air and gives a dose rate of 0.95 Gy/min at the isocenter for a 10 × 10 cm beam. Calculate the tumor dose rate and the daily treatment time for the dose prescription of example 11-1. The depth to the tumor center is 5.0 cm. The output factor relative to a 10 × 10 field in air for this machine for a 6 × 6 cm beam is 0.975 (see also Fig. 10-14).

Dose rate in air for 6 × 6 cm beam = 0.975 × 0.95 Gy/min
= 0.926 Gy/min

Tissue air ratio, 6 × 6 beam at 5 cm = 0.862 (Table B-5d)

Tumor dose rate = 0.926 Gy/min × 0.862 = 0.80 Gy/min

Daily treatment time $= \dfrac{1.33 \text{ Gy}}{0.80 \text{ Gy/min}} = 1.66$ min

The *exit dose* is the dose at the point E where the axis of the beam emerges from the patient. Reading this dose from the isodose chart (Fig. 11-1b), a figure of about 48% of the tumor dose is obtained. In actual fact, the dose at this point will be less than this because E will receive no scatter from the distal region outside the patient. This will be discussed in section 11.04.

The calculations made in the above examples have taken no account of the patient shape or composition and would be satisfactory for this example since their perturbing influence would be small. In many treatment planning situations, however, this is not good enough. The problem is in fact very complex. We will now discuss some practical methods that may be used as part of treatment planning procedures to allow for these effects.

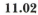

11.02 **ALTERATION OF ISODOSE CURVES**
BY CONTOUR SHAPE

In Figure 11-2 a 10 × 10 cm beam from a cobalt unit is shown irradiating a body section with a curved surface. The dashed lines show the isodose pattern obtained from measurements made in a water phantom where the surface S'S' was flat. The chart is for an isocentrically mounted cobalt unit and the axis of rotation is at point X. The source-axis distance is 80 cm. Consider first the point P, which is on the dashed 100% isodose line and 3 cm off the beam axis. It is at a depth of 8.3 cm below the fictitious surface S'S' but only 6.6 cm below the real surface SS measured along the ray line OP. 1.7 cm of tissue is "missing" along this ray, and therefore the dose at P would be increased. Table 11-1 gives approximate values for the attenuation per cm of various radiations, with 5% for ⁶⁰Co. This would suggest that the depth dose at point P should be increased by 1.7 × 5% = 8.5%.

In a similar way the dose at point Q, which has 0.8 cm of "extra" tissue above it, would be decreased by 0.8 × 5% = 4%.

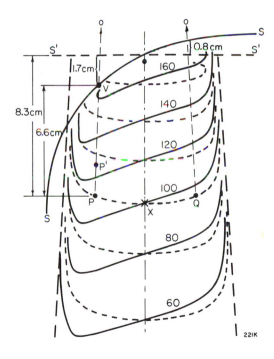

Figure 11-2. An isodose chart for a 10 × 10 field from a cobalt unit. The dashed lines are as determined in a water phantom. The solid lines show the distortion of the isodose pattern produced by the curved contour surface.

There are a number of ways of correcting the depth dose to allow for surface shape. The one just described is the simplest and is known as the *effective attenuation coefficient method.* It can only be approximate because it takes no account of the field size and scattering conditions. It is nevertheless useful when an estimate is required quickly. Clearly an "effective attenuation coefficient" can really only apply to a particular beam size

TABLE 11-1

Parameters Useful in Correcting Isodose Patterns for Air Gaps

Radiation	SSD (cm)	Attenuation (per cm)	k
x rays up to 1 MV	50	10%	0.8
cobalt 60	80	5%	0.67
x rays from 1 to 5 MV	100	4%	0.7
x rays from 5 to 15 MV	100	3%	0.6
x rays from 15 to 30 MV	100	2%	0.5
x rays above 30 MV		2%	0.4

Derived from data for 10 × 10 cm fields. Values for k taken from van der Giessen (V4).

and depth. The entries in Table 11-1 are calculated for a 10 × 10 field and a depth of 10 cm.

A somewhat more precise but still simple calculation may be made using tissue-air ratios. Consider again point P at a depth of 8.3 cm below the phantom surface. If the point were on the central ray of the beam the tissue-air ratio for it would be 0.775 (by interpolation in Table B-5d). The same table shows that the tissue-air ratio for a depth of 6.6 cm is 0.843 and the adjustment factor to the dose would be their ratio (C = 0.843/0.775 = 1.088), which is very close to the value calculated by the effective attenuation coefficient method. The *ratio of tissue-air ratios method,* should be better than the effective attenuation coefficient method because it at least takes into account the size of the beam.

A similar calculation can be carried out using percent depth dose data in a procedure known as the *effective SSD method.* Consider again point P, at a depth of 6.6 cm below the patient surface. The percent depth dose at this point as read from the isodose chart is 100%. We now shift the isodose pattern down the ray line OP until the line S′S′ reaches V. The value on the isodose chart at P′ is, by interpolation, 114. This value must next be adjusted by the inverse square law to allow for the fact that the chart has been moved away from the source. The correct factor for this example is $(80 + 6.6)^2/(80 + 6.6 + 1.7)^2 = 0.962$ and the corrected dose at point P is 114 × 0.962 = 109.7. This is close to, but slightly higher than, the value given by the tissue-air ratios method. The last two methods are equally precise and take account of the beam size and the depth of the point but neither take account of the change in scattered radiation resulting from the curvature of the surface. This can, in some extreme cases, be important, as will be illustrated by the following example.

Figure 11-3 shows a tangential irradiation of a curved surface (such as a chest wall) by a 12 × 15 cm beam from an isocentric cobalt unit. The isodose curves shown as dashed lines were produced from an isodose chart for this beam by the (effective SSD) method just described. The solid lines were produced using methods described in section 10.13 but modified* to take account of the absence of scattering material on the left side of the beam. Point Y on this diagram is the isocenter. The detailed calculation indicates that the relative dose at this point is 96% instead of 100%. This example illustrates that the calculation of dose, when the scatter conditions are very different from those in the water phantom, is difficult and the simple methods already described, although useful, must be used with some degree of caution. For complicated situations such as the chest wall, some experimental checks are very desirable. This can be done most conveniently using a number of TLD chips placed at points of interest in an anatomical phantom.

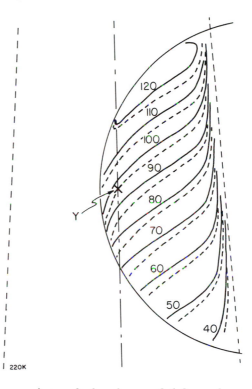

Figure 11-3. Isodose curves for tangential irradiation with a cobalt beam. The dashed isodose curves were produced by the effective SSD method. The solid lines were produced by methods that take the two dimensional scattering configuration into account.

All of the methods described so far are intended to be useful for calculating doses at designated points. Frequently, however, one needs to draw isodose curves for a specific patient contour without the aid of a computer. The following procedure can, in such cases, be used with satisfactory results. Refer to Figure 11-4. The dashed lines are from an isodose chart for a 10 × 10 cm cobalt beam at an SSD of 80 cm. In this example we are assuming that a treatment applicator is in use and its edge

---

*Program CBEAM, computerized treatment planning system, TP-11, Atomic Energy of Canada Ltd. (AECL).

makes contact with the skin at point A. For the ray through B, the air gap is "h." If the isodose chart is slid down along the ray through B by an amount k × h, where k is a fraction less than 1, the altered intersection of the isodose lines with this ray can be read off directly as shown. For ^{60}Co radiation, k is usually taken to be 2/3 and this is used in the example shown. The fraction k is different for each radiation quality and strictly speaking, for each beam size, depth of interest, and SSD. Suggested values for k are given in Table 11-1. One can determine doses along a series of ray lines like that through B and then drawn in the isodose curves. The method, called the isodose shift method, is practical but should be used with great caution for points near the surface. Although our example is for a fixed SSD unit it is equally applicable for both fixed SSD and isocentric techniques, although in this latter case the reference surface becomes a virtual surface and will not in general coincide with that for which the isodose curves were drawn.

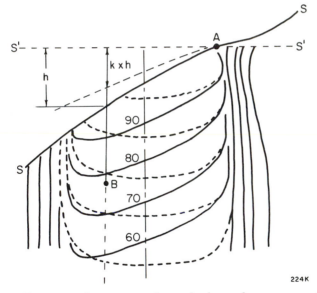

Figure 11-4. Diagram to illustrate how a standard set of isodose curves can be altered to take surface curvature into account. Isodose chart (dashed lines) is for a 10 × 10 cm beam from a cobalt unit operating at an SSD of 80 cm.

It must be remembered that the external shape of the patient is three-dimensional in nature. In making the above corrections it is assumed that the contour (for example, the dashed line of Fig. 11-1) has the same shape in front of and behind the plane in which the calculations are being made. Although this is a good assumption, in most cases it is not always so. The most notable exception is in the head and neck region where a beam might be used to treat the lower part of the head, the neck, and the upper part of the thorax. Calculations made for the neck could underestimate the dose by as much as 4 to 5%. The simplest way of assessing this is by making measurements using TLD in an anatomical phantom.

11.03   **BOLUS AND COMPENSATING FILTERS**

There are many occasions where one wishes to preserve the shape of the isodose curves and not have them altered by the patient's surface. This is particularly useful when two or more beams are combined to form a resultant distribution. One way of doing this is by the use of bolus (tissue-like material) as indicated in Figure 11-5b. Perhaps the simplest form of bolus is small cloth bags containing a mixture of 60% rice flour and 40% sodium bicarbonate. Paraffin wax mixed with approximately an equal amount of beeswax is also very useful. A very thorough discussion of tissue substitute materials is given by White (W7).

The use of bolus material for high energy radiation has the disadvantage that the skin-sparing properties will be lost because the buildup of dose will occur within the bolus. In order to preserve the skin-sparing properties a compensating filter should be placed some distance from the patient's skin but designed to duplicate the role of the bolus (Fig. 11-5d). For convenience, the compensator is frequently made of a heavy material such as Pb or a Pb alloy. Its dimensions therefore must be reduced (compared to the bolus) in the lateral directions to allow for the diverging rays and in thickness to allow for the higher attenuation in the filter material. The reduction of the primary beam is the most important factor, but scattered radiation must also be considered. The ratio of thickness (along a ray) of compensator to bolus material is approximately the inverse ratio of the linear attenuation coefficients of the two materials, but because of the altered scattering conditions, the compensator should be made 10% or so thinner than would be predicted on this basis alone. The actual ratio depends on beam size, depth of interest, and thickness of bolus material being represented. True compensation, therefore, can only take place at one depth; below this the doses will be slightly higher than predicted, above, slightly lower. A user adopting a system is strongly urged to make a few experimental checks comparing predicted doses with careful measurements.

There is a geometric relation between the size of the compensator and the size of the bolus it replaces. These sizes are directly related to their respective distances from the source. When the source-to-axis distance is constant, the source-to-skin distance may be different for each beam and this therefore makes the use of compensating filters rather complicated for isocentric techniques.

The principles and techniques for constructing compensating filters are discussed by Hall and Oliver (H12), Van de Geijn (V5), and Sundbom (S15). A semiautomatic machine for cutting filters is described by Cunningham et al. (C9), and a simple device for making compensating filters for large field irradiations is described by Leung et al. (L8).

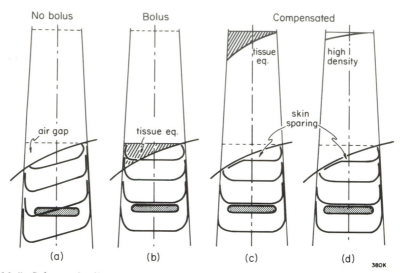

Figure 11-5. Schematic diagrams to illustrate the use of bolus and compensating filters.

11.04   DOSE AT EXIT SURFACE

Near the exit surface of the patient there may be insufficient material to provide full scattering conditions, and the dose will actually be somewhat lower than that derived from an isodose chart or from depth dose data. A guide to the expected dose can be obtained by dividing the dose by the backscatter factor as illustrated in the following example.

Example 11-3. A 6×6 beam from a fixed SSD cobalt unit is used to irradiate the head of a patient as shown in Figure 11-1a. Point E on the exit surface is at a depth of 14.5 cm. Determine the depth dose at this point.

Uncorrected percent depth dose at P = 36.6 (Table B-2e)

Field size at point P = $6 \times 94.5/80.0 = 7.1$ cm square

Backscatter factor for this field size = 1.025 (Table B-5d)

Corrected depth dose at P = 36.6/1.025 = 35.7

The depth dose calculated this way will still always be too high because scattered radiation at a depth is always greater than at the surface. The error is very small for the field size of the example but it can be considerable for very large fields. Van Dyk (V6) has for example shown that for the fields used for whole and half body irradiations the error can exceed 10% and is detectable as much as 10 cm in front of the exit point. Legaré (L9) has studied this problem for lower energy radiation where the scattered component is greater.

11.05   DOSE CORRECTIONS FOR TISSUE INHOMOGENEITIES

Inhomogeneities within an irradiated body alter the dose in a very complicated way. Some of the considerations may be discussed by referring to Figure 11-6. This diagram depicts a beam irradiating a water-like (relative density, $\rho = 1.0$) body that contains a low density structure ($\rho = 0.25$) shaped somewhat like a lung. Point A, which is in front of the low density region, receives primary photons that are not altered by the inhomogeneity but the backscattering of secondary photons to it will be reduced, bringing about a slight decrease in the dose at point A. This is not unlike the effect at the exit surface discussed in the previous section.

Point B is in the low density region and there will be an increase of dose at B because of the decreased attenuation of primary photons. On the other hand there will be a decreased amount of scattering from the low density material in its vicinity and this will tend to decrease the dose to B. Depending on the lateral extent of the inhomogeneity and the depth within it the decrease in scatter can more than compensate for the increase in primary with the result that the dose at point B can be unaltered or slightly reduced.

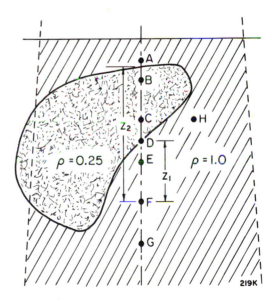

Figure 11-6. Diagram depicting an inhomogeneous phantom irradiated by a beam. Dose calculations are to be made at points A to G, which are at depths 1, 2, 4, 5, 6, 8 and 10 cm respectively.

Point C is well within the low density region and the dose there will be increased because of an increased amount of primary reaching it. Point D is beyond the low density region but is just at the surface of the high density ($\rho = 1.0$) material. This point may suffer a loss of electronic equilibrium leading to a slight reduction in dose. The effect is very complicated and no practical method has yet been devised to deal with it in a general way. Points E, F, and G all have their primary components increased by the same amount, but the scattered radiation to each will be different. Doses to all these points will be increased by the inhomogeneity. For point H there will be no alteration in the primary radiation but there will be a small decrease in the amount of scatter.

Because of the obvious complexities it has not yet been possible to derive a method that is both rigorous and practical to allow for inhomogeneities in dose calculations. In most cases, particularly with high energy radiation, the effect of inhomogeneities is so slight that it is in fact not necessary to take them into account explicitly. There are some regions, however, where they cannot be ignored, the most notable being the chest, containing the lungs. In this region dosage errors of 20% or more can be made if the low density regions are not taken into account.

The dose should be calculated first assuming water equivalence for all tissues within the external contour and then corrected for the presence of the inhomogeneities. The first step is important because it forms the link with previous clinical experience. The dose, at each point where it is required, is then corrected for the presence of the inhomogeneities by evaluating a correction factor.

As a first approximation, the methods described in section 11.02 for correction for incident surface shape can also be applied within the contour. The most direct method is to use a ratio of tissue-air ratios, giving a dose correction factor:

$$C = T_a(d',r_d)/T_a(d,r_d) \tag{11-1}$$

where d is the physical depth below the contour surface, d' is the equivalent thickness in wholly water equivalent material, and r_d describes the field size at the depth of the point.

Example 11-4. For Figure 11-6, determine the correction factor for points C and F which are at depths 4 cm and 8 cm respectively. The distance from the surface to the inhomogeneity is 1.5 cm and its thickness (along the central ray) is 3.5 cm. The radiation is a 10×10 cm beam from a cobalt unit.

For point C, d' = 1.5 + (2.5 × .25) = 2.125

$T_a(4, 10 \times 10) = .940$, $T_a(2.125, 10 \times 10) = 1.00$ (Table B-5d)

Correction factor = 1.00/940 = 1.064 (eq. 11-1)

For point F, d' = 1.5 + (3.5 × 0.25) + 3 = 5.375

$T_a(8, 10 \times 10) = .787$, $T_a(5.375, 10 \times 10) = .891$ (Table B-5d)

Correction factor = .891/.787 = 1.13 (eq. 11-1).

Although correction factors evaluated in this way are very useful, the method does have a number of obvious shortcomings. For example, for point A, no account would be taken of the presence of the large low density structure behind it. For points B to G, no account would be taken of the lateral dimensions of the inhomogeneity and for points E to G no account would be taken of its distance in front of the points. A correction factor that takes account of the distance between the point and the inhomogeneity was proposed by Batho (B14, Y3) and extended by Sontag (S16); this leads to:

$$C = \frac{T_a(z_1, r_d)^{\rho_1 - \rho_2}}{T_a(z_2, r_d)^{1 - \rho_2}} \qquad (11\text{-}2)$$

where ρ_1 is the density of the material in which the point lies and z_1 is the distance, along a ray, from the point to the anterior surface of that material; ρ_2 is the next, or overlying material; and z_2 is the distance to its anterior surface. The use of this factor is illustrated by the following example.

Example 11-5. Evaluate the correction factor using equation 11-2 for points C and F of Figure 11-6. For point C, $z_1 = 2.5$, $\rho_1 = .25$, $z_2 = 4$, $\rho_2 = 1.0$. For point F, $z_1 = 3.0$, $\rho_1 = 1.0$, $z_2 = 6.5$, $\rho_2 = 0.25$.

$T_a(2.5, 10 \times 10) = .989$ and $T_a(4, 10 \times 10) = .940$ (Table B-5d)

Correction factor $= 0.989^{-0.75}/.940^{0.0} = 1.01$

$T_a(3.0, 10 \times 10) = 0.974$ and $T_a(6.5, 10 \times 10) = 0.847$

Correction factor $= 0.974^{0.75}/0.847^{0.75} = 1.11$

Equation 11-2 reduces to a simple ratio of tissue-air ratios when the inhomogeneity is an air gap at the surface of the patient and corrections are being made for surface curvature.

This correction method, which is sometimes known as the *power law method*, gives very good results in most situations but it does not take account of the shape of an inhomogeneity. For example, it would not allow for the loss of scattered radiation to points A or H of Figure 11-6.

Sontag and Cunningham (S17) have suggested a modification of equation 11-1, whereby the shape and proximity of structures may at least be taken approximately into account. For example, for point A of Figure 11-6, the field size used for the tissue-air ratio in the numerator would be reduced somewhat to account for the nearby low density region. This method, known as the *effective tissue-air ratio method*, is especially adaptable to use with CT images in CT aided treatment planning. Figure 11-7 shows a CT image of the chest. The patient is being treated with a beam from a cobalt unit as shown in the insert. The isodose curves shown in this diagram were drawn assuming water equivalent for the whole section, that is, account was taken of the curved anterior surface of the patient but not the internal structures. The uncorrected dose at the point

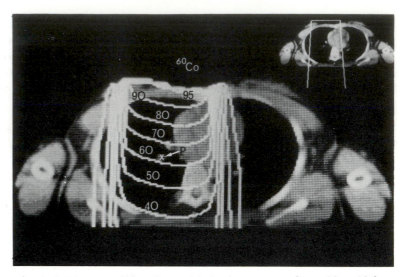

Figure 11-7. A CT image of the chest with isodose curves for a 12 × 10 beam from a cobalt unit superimposed. The placement of the beam is shown in the insert. The isodose curves have been obtained by allowing for the curvature of the patient's anterior surface but neglecting the structures inside of the chest.

labelled P in this diagram is 62%. This point is at a depth of about 8 cm but over 6 cm of this is in lung. Using a density of 0.25 for the lung, the water equivalent depth is 3.5 cm and the dose correction factor given by equation 11-1 is $C = T(3.5,12)/T(8,10) = 0.969/0.806 = 1.20$. One way of allowing for the shape of the internal structure is to change the field size used to determine the tissue-air ratio for the numerator of equation 11-1. This idea, based on a scaling theorem first proposed by O'Connor (O1), forms the basis of the "effective tissue-air ratio" method. For the example of point P of Figure 11-6, the dose correction factor would be given by:

$$C = \frac{T(d',\hat{r})}{T(d,r)} \qquad (11\text{-}3)$$

where d and d' have the same meaning as for equation 11-1, r is the radius of an "equivalent" circular field, and $\hat{r}$ is the radius scaled to allow for the way the scattering structures are configured around the point. The problem is how to determine $\hat{r}$. Sontag and Cunningham (S17) suggested the following procedure:

$$\hat{r} = r \cdot \hat{\rho} \qquad (11\text{-}4)$$

where $\qquad \hat{\rho} = \sum_i \sum_j \sum_k w_{ijk} \cdot \rho_{ijk} \Big/ \sum_i \sum_j \sum_k w_{ijk}$

is an effective density determined by choosing weighting factors w_{ijk} for the volume elements in the vicinity of P. It appears that the actual values of the w_{ijk} are not very critical but they must be such that the regions in front and near to the point of calculation are given the greatest importance. The summations in equation 11-4 are to be carried out over the irradiated volume, at least in the vicinity of the point of calculation. This involves a volume integration for each point of dose calculation and is not yet practical. Sontag and Cunningham (S17) have suggested an approximate method for reducing the volume integration to an area integration, making the procedure practical for CT aided treatment planning.

Figure 11-8 shows the dose distribution of Figure 11-7 corrected for the internal structures by means of the effective tissue-air ratio method. Point P is again shown and now can be seen to receive a relative dose of 70% compared to 62% as indicated in Figure 11-7. This is the result of a correction that for this point was calculated to be a factor of 1.13. The effective field size evaluated using equation 11-4 for this point was 5×5 cm, considerably smaller than the unscaled field size for equation 11-1.

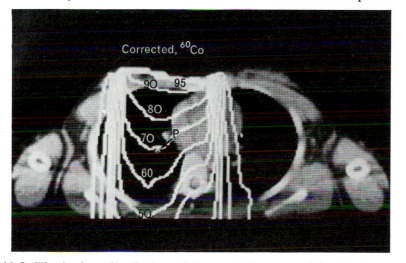

Figure 11-8. The isodose distribution of Figure 11-7 corrected for the tissue inhomogeneities of the chest. Eight CT images were used and dose correction factors were obtained using equations 11-3 and 11-4.

Rather extensive testing by Sontag et al. (S18) has suggested that use of the equivalent tissue-air ratio method can be expected to produce results that are accurate to better than ±5% and that simpler methods cannot be expected to be even this accurate.

A more detailed discussion of methods to deal with tissue inhomogeneities is given elsewhere (C10).

A group at the Ontario Cancer Institute is attempting to measure and calculate the change in dose at any point, P, resulting from an inhomogeneity at any other point (A6). This work has not yet resulted in a practical system of dose calculation.

11.06   WEDGE FILTERS

In the previous sections we have discussed methods of calculating the dose at a point. In this section we discuss the possibility of adding a filter so as to produce a desired value of a dose at a point. Specially shaped isodose curves have many clinical applications. Isodose curves that are flat at the surface of the phantom, flat at a certain depth, or angled to the axis may be created by suitably designed filters.

Figure 11-9b shows a set of isodose curves resulting from the addition of a wedge shaped attenuator to a cobalt beam. The wedge is usually made of a dense material such as lead or one of its low melting point alloys and is placed at least 15 cm from the skin so that electrons ejected from it will not contaminate the photon beam and eliminate the dose buildup effect at the patient's surface. It may have a straight sloping surface or be curved slightly so that the isodose lines are straightened. The wedge is designed to tilt the isodose curves through an angle known as the "wedge isodose angle." The most commonly used angle is 45° as shown in Figure 11-9b.

When such a distribution is combined with an identical one at right angles to it, a region of homogeneous dose is produced, as illustrated in Figure 11-9c. Such distributions are discussed more fully in the next chapter. Wedge filters have wide applications in high voltage radiotherapy, so a method for their design will now be given.

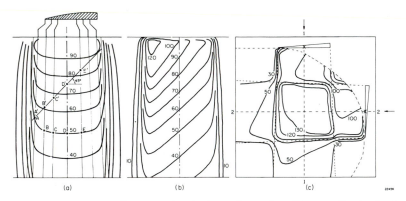

Figure 11-9. (a) Diagram to illustrate the design of a wedge filter to tilt the isodose lines through 45° for an 8 × 8 cm beam from a cobalt unit. (b) Isodose chart for the wedge of a. (c) Dose distribution produced by combining two wedged beams at right angles to produce a region of uniform dose.

Figure 11-9a shows how to design a wedge filter for an 8 × 8 cm cobalt 60 beam. On the chart a series of lines, which are rays from the source, have been drawn and their intersections with the 50% isodose curve are indicated by the points A, B, C, D, E. The ray through A is near the penumbral region but not in it. A line has been drawn through

A so that it makes an angle of 45% with the axis. This line intersects the various rays at A′, B′, C′, D′, E′. We would like to filter the beam so that the 50% isodose curve is made to lie more or less along AE′. This means that, for example, along the line DD′ enough material should be introduced to reduce the dose from 75 to 50, i.e. give an attenuation of $50/75 = 0.665$. We then determine x so that $e^{-\mu x} = 0.665$, giving $\mu x = 0.41$. If the wedge is to be constructed from lead and used for cobalt 60 radiation, $\mu = 0.63$ cm^{-1} and x becomes 0.65 cm. The same procedure may be followed for as many other ray lines as desired to make up a thickness profile of the filter.

The above considerations allow only for primary radiation. The effect of radiation scattered within the patient is such that the isodose lines are tilted less than expected. This can be allowed for by making the filter, in the case of Co-60, about 10% thicker than that predicted by the above procedure. Assuming the filter is to be placed about 20 cm away from the skin, its shape must be reduced laterally to allow for the diverging beam. This reduced lateral dimension is shown at the top of Figure 11-9a. After the wedge has been constructed, its isodose pattern should be checked by measurement.

11.07   ENERGY ABSORPTION IN BIOLOGICAL MATERIAL

In section 11.05 we discussed the alteration of percent depth dose data and isodose curves by tissue inhomogeneities. This alteration was brought about by the different photon attenuation and scattering properties of the different tissues. For a more precise characterization of the dose, however, it is necessary to consider the way in which the energy from the radiation is absorbed locally. To do this it will be helpful to remember that, as was discussed in section 7.02, energy absorption is a two-stage process: first, electrons are set into motion by the interaction of the photons; then, the electrons travel through the material and lose their energies by ionizing atoms along their paths. The first interaction is called kerma and the second is called absorbed dose. It was shown in section 7.03 that it is possible to calculate kerma (if the photon spectrum is known) but not absorbed dose. It is, of course, possible to determine absorbed dose by measurement, and it can also be inferred from kerma provided that there is an equilibrium between the production of the electrons and the stopping of them. This is called electronic equilibrium and is discussed in section 10.06. If this condition is fulfilled and an absorbed dose is determined in a water phantom, it can be converted to the value it would have in tissue (at the same depth and field size) by multiplying by the factor $(\overline{\mu}_{ab}/\rho)^{tis}_{wat}$.

$$D_{tis} = D_{wat} \cdot (\overline{\mu}_{ab}/\rho)^{tis}_{wat} \tag{11-5}$$

$(\overline{\mu}_{ab}/\rho)^{tis}_{wat}$ is the ratio formed by averaging the mass energy absorption coefficients for tissue and water over the photon spectrum at the point. This ratio is really a ratio of kermas and compares photon interactions in tissue to water. (See equation 7-12.)

Values for it for muscle,* fat, and bone for the photon spectra described in Table 7-2 are given in Table 11-2. From the data in this table it may be seen that the energy absorption in muscle is very close to that in water. Except for energies in the superficial therapy (or diagnostic radiology) range it is within 1% and even for these low energies the absorption in water is within about 4% of that in tissue. This confirms the use of water as a phantom material for soft tissue. Fat, on the other hand, has a lower effective atomic number than water, namely 6.46 compared to 7.51 (see section 7.10 and Appendix A-3) and shows lower energy absorption than does water for both low and high energy photon beams, because of the way photoelectric absorption and pair production vary with atomic number.

TABLE 11-2

Values of $(\overline{\mu}_{ab}/\rho)^{tis}_{wat}$ for Muscle, Fat, and Bone and $(\overline{\mu}_{ab}/\rho)^{mus}_{med}$ for Polystyrene, Lucite, and A150 Tissue-Equivalent Plastic Determined Using Equation 7-12 for the Photon Spectra Listed in Table 7-2

Photon Spectrum	$(\overline{\mu}_{ab}/\rho)^{tis}_{wat}$			$(\overline{\mu}_{ab}/\rho)^{mus}_{med}$		
	Muscle	Fat	Bone	Polystyrene	Lucite	A150
1. 60 kV$_p$	1.040	0.607	4.796	2.617	1.687	1.176
2. 100 kV$_p$	1.035	0.653	4.409	2.227	1.572	1.085
3. 250 kV$_p$	0.995	0.973	1.294	1.071	1.051	1.004
4. 270 kV$_p$	0.997	0.964	1.391	1.089	1.062	1.008
5. 270 kV$_p$	1.011	0.861	2.486	1.317	1.194	1.038
6. 400 kV$_p$	0.994	0.988	1.098	1.044	1.034	1.003
7. ^{137}Cs	0.991	1.000	0.957	1.023	1.020	1.001
8. ^{60}Co	0.992	1.001	0.954	1.024	1.049	1.002
9. ^{60}Co	0.992	0.996	0.995	1.029	1.024	1.002
10. 6 MV	0.991	0.998	0.959	1.026	1.021	1.003
11. 8 MV	0.990	0.995	0.962	1.028	1.022	1.005
12. 12 MV	0.990	0.987	0.979	1.039	1.029	1.014
13. 18 MV	0.989	0.980	0.993	1.047	1.033	1.022
14. 26 MV	0.989	0.973	1.004	1.055	1.038	1.029
15. 26 MV	0.990	0.981	0.991	1.047	1.034	1.022
16. 35 MV	0.989	0.965	1.019	1.068	1.044	1.039
17. 45 MV	0.989	0.961	1.027	1.073	1.047	1.044

Bone, with an effective number of 12.3 is just the opposite. It shows a very high energy absorption at low photon energies and just slightly elevated absorption at very high energies. In the middle energy range, from ^{137}Cs to 6 to 8 MV, the energy absorption per unit mass in bone is slightly less than that in water, because it has fewer electrons per unit mass than does water.

*The composition used for these materials is described in the introduction to the appendix.

For low energy photons the electron tracks are so short that the absorbed dose takes place just where the photons interact and equation 11-5 will always describe the dose in tissue compared to water for the same photon beam. At higher energies, where the electron tracks may be long (mm or even cm), the energy is carried away from the site of the photon interactions and the situation is more complicated because in a patient the photons may interact in one anatomical structure and the electrons they set into motion may be stopped in another.

It was shown in section 6.12 that the absorption of energy from electrons is described by the stopping power of the material. It was further shown, in section 7.14, how the dose might be expected to change in crossing an interface between two different materials. Stopping powers depend on atomic number and so if electrons cross an interface from tissue-to-bone, or the reverse, there will be a loss of electronic equilibrium. Before discussing the implications of this it will be useful to examine some of the relevant properties of bony structures.

Structure of Bone

The term *bone* is used for a particular kind of tissue (bone tissue) and also for any structure that is made from this kind of tissue. For example the femur is a "bone" and it is made out of bone tissue.

A typical long bone, for example the femur, consists of a shaft and two ends. The shaft is tubular and its walls are thick and composed of a dense type of bone tissue called "compact bone." The shaft is flared at each of its ends and the walls are thinner. The lower end of a femur is shown in Figure 11-10.

The flared ends of the long bones have internal support in the form of a scaffolding of connecting bars and narrow plates of bone termed "trabeculae." The spaces between these trabeculae usually contain the red bone marrow, which is engaged in producing blood cells. The trabeculae in man vary in thickness from 0.06 to 0.1 mm, while the bone marrow spaces between them range from 0.1 to almost 1 mm. A representative bone marrow cavity is shown in Figure 11-10d. It is 0.4 mm in diameter with walls about 0.1 mm thick.

The "compact bone" of the shaft is also riddled with small structures, some of which contain blood vessels (the Haversian canals), others contain cells called osteocytes (the lacunae), and still others allow the diffusion of tissue fluids to the living osteocyte cells. The lumen of the shaft of the long bones is filled with fatty (yellow) marrow, which is not involved in forming blood cells.

From this it can be seen that bone is a very complicated structure, the nature of which will affect the dose to bone, or the dose to tissues within the bone.

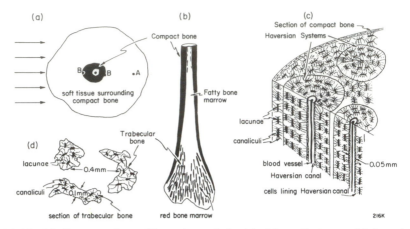

Figure 11-10. (a) Cross section of long bone imbedded in soft tissue. (b) Longitudinal view of lower end of femur. (c) Schematic diagram of Haversian system adapted from Ham (H13). (d) Cross section of trabecular bone.

Dose to Bone

When we consider bone from this microscopic point of view, we must consider the range of the electrons set in motion as is illustrated in Figure 7-3. From this diagram, it is clear that there may be a rapid gradient of dose near the interface. The absorbed dose in the calcified matrix of bone (mineral bone) itself may be calculated using equation 11-5, using $(\overline{\mu}/\rho)_{wat}^{bon}$, provided we are dealing with radiation that produces electron tracks that are short compared to the thickness of the bone structures. If the electron tracks are very long compared to the thicknesses of bone, we would have to use the equation:

$$D_{bon} = D_{wat} \cdot (\overline{\mu}_{ab}/\rho)_{wat}^{tis} \cdot \overline{\overline{S}}_{tis}^{bon} \qquad (11\text{-}6a)$$

where $\overline{\overline{S}}_{tis}^{bon}$ is the ratio of averaged stopping powers discussed in section 7.04. Values for $(\overline{\mu}_{ab}/\rho)_{wat}^{tis}$ for a number of photon beams are given in Table 11-2 and values for $\overline{\overline{S}}_{tis}^{bon}$ can be derived from data in Table 7-2. An example will help to illustrate these ideas.

Example 11-6. Nodules on the chest wall are being treated by 270 kV$_p$ radiation, HVL 2 mm Cu, to a surface dose of 45.0 Gy. Assume the anterior surface of a rib is 1.0 cm below the skin. The field size is 6 × 6 cm. Estimate the dose to the rib at this point.

Percent depth dose = 96.9   (Table B-2c)
Dose to water at 1 cm = 45.0 × 0.969 = 43.6 Gy
Max. electron range in water ≈ 0.05 cm   (Table 6-3)
Max. electron range in bone ≈ 0.05/1.6 = 0.03 cm
Upper limit to dose to bone = 43.6 × 1.39 = 60.6 Gy (Table 11-2)

The thickness of the trabeculae lie within the range of electron track lengths. This means that even with this low energy radiation, electronic equilibrium will not be established. The dose to bone will be somewhat less than 60.6 Gy but will certainly be greater than 43.6 Gy. This example is chosen to illustrate the difficulties in determining dose to such complex structures.

Dose Near a Bone Interface

The expected pattern of dose near a muscle–bone interface is shown in Figure 7-13 for cobalt 60 and 50 keV radiation. Spiers (S10) has examined this problem in some detail and showed that, for low energy photons, the dose to tissue right at the interface is high (because of the high photoelectric absorption in the bone) but that it falls rapidly due to the limited range of the photoelectrons. For high energy photons, the differential at the interface is not great (and may be lower rather than higher) but the fall in dose is much more gradual because of the greater range of the electrons. Aspin and Johns have made a rather careful study of the dose to tissue within small cylindrical cavities in bone (A7). For very high energy radiation, the dose to bone and near it is not very different from that to tissue and for most practical purposes in radiotherapy it may be considered to be the same.

Air Cavities

Epp et al. (E3) and Nilsson and Schnell (N5) have shown experimentally that there is a reduction in surface dose on the far side of air cavities in phantoms irradiated with beams from cobalt units and linear accelerators. The effect is analogous to the buildup of dose that occurs at the surface of an irradiated body. The reduction in dose depends on cavity dimensions, field size, and the depth of the cavity in the phantom and is greater for small fields, large cavities, and greater depths. For air cavities encountered in actual clinical practice, such as the larynx, the effect is not great; Epp estimates 10% or so. The reasons for this behavior are very complex and are not well understood—certainly they are related to the shape of the individual cavity.

Lung

Lung tissue has an effective atomic number very similar to that of the tissues that surround it but differs considerably in density. According to Fano's theorem* (F4) this should not upset the electronic equilibrium. This means the absorbed dose should be dependent only on the photon

---

*In a medium of given composition exposed to a uniform flux of primary radiation, the flux of secondary radiation is also uniform and *independent of the density* of the medium as well as of the density variations from point to point.

flux even in the vicinity of a lung-tissue interface and the correction methods described in section 11.05 should be sufficient.

The truth of this is not self-evident but it is made more apparent if one considers two materials, one of relative density 1.0 and another of relative density 0.5; although there would be twice as many electrons set into motion per unit volume of the first, they would travel twice as far in the second. This would serve to maintain the electron fluence at the same value.

11.08   **INTEGRAL DOSE—ENERGY IMPARTED**

When the beam of radiation enters the patient, energy is absorbed not only in the tumor region but also in many other places. The total energy absorbed from the beam by the patient is called the energy imparted and was defined originally by Mayneord (M11) as "integral dose." It is desirable to keep this quantity small while an adequate tumor dose is being delivered. An ideal situation, which can never be achieved, would be one in which all the absorbed energy was concentrated in the tumor with none elsewhere. This would give the minimum energy imparted for a given tumor dose.

The energy imparted to a mass of tissue, which is also called the total energy imparted, is the product of the mass of tissue and the dose it receives. The unit of energy imparted is the joule.

This concept is easily understood. Suppose, for example, a 10 g block of tissue is given an absorbed dose of 1.0 Gy, then the energy imparted is $1.0 \text{ Gy} \times 0.01 \text{ kg} = 1.0 \text{ J/kg} \times 0.01 \text{ kg} = 0.01 \text{ J}$.

Figure 11-11 shows a part of the isodose distribution for a 6 cm circular field for a cobalt 60 field at SSD 80 cm. For a given dose of 1 Gy, all the mass enclosed by the 90% isodose curve is raised to an average dose of 0.95 Gy. The energy imparted is consequently the product of 0.95 and the mass enclosed. The region between the 90 and 80% surface is raised to an average dose of 0.85 Gy, so the energy absorbed by this region is the mass enclosed times this number. The total energy imparted is found by adding together the contributions between successive isodose surfaces. The evaluation of the energy imparted by this method is not easy because of the difficulty of calculating the masses enclosed between successive isodose surfaces. In the case of the circular field of Figure 11-11 the surfaces are found by revolving the diagram about the axis and the volume enclosed may be found graphically. This has been done and the results are shown in Table 11-3. Column 2 gives the mass enclosed; column 3, the mean dose; and the final column, the product of columns 2 and 3, giving the total energy imparted. The total energy to a depth 22 cm is 0.383 J. It should be noted that contributions to the total energy imparted between successive isodose surfaces are almost constant.

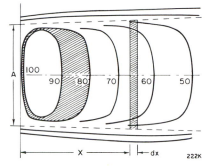

Figure 11-11. Part of the isodose distribution for a 6 cm circular field, cobalt 60, SSD 80 cm, to illustrate the meaning of energy imparted or integral dose.

TABLE 11-3

Total Energy Imparted to Depth 22 cm for 6 cm Circular Field (Area 28.3 cm²) at SSD 80 cm for a Given Dose of 1 Gy, to the Surface Using Cobalt 60

(1) Isodose Surfaces %	(2) Mass Enclosed g	(3) Mean Dose Gy	(4) Integral Dose J
100-90	42	0.95	0.040
90-80	40	0.85	0.034
80-70	44	0.75	0.033
70-60	52	0.65	0.034
60-50	63	0.55	0.035
50-40	81	0.45	0.036
40-30	120	0.35	0.042
30-20	200	0.25	0.050
20-10	210	0.15	0.031
10-5	240	0.075	0.018
5-0	estimated only		0.030
			Total = 0.383

This method of calculating total energy cannot be easily applied to a rectangular field because of the difficulty of estimating the volume between the surfaces. However, an approximate method due to Mayneord (M11) is accurate enough for most purposes. In this method, it is assumed that the isodose surfaces are flat from one edge of the beam to the other, that the dosage rate decreases with depth according to an exponential law, and that the size of the beam is of constant area A. Under these simplified conditions, the dose D_x at depth x can be written $D_x = D_0 e^{-\mu x}$ where D_0 is the dose at the surface. The total energy received by the rectangular shaded volume of mass $A\rho \cdot dx$ (Fig. 11-11) is $D_x \cdot A \cdot \rho \cdot dx$. The total energy to a depth d is given by the integral dose, Σ, where Σ equals

$$\Sigma = \int_0^d D_x \cdot A \cdot \rho \cdot dx = \int_0^d D_0 e^{-\mu x} \cdot A \cdot \rho \cdot dx = \frac{D_0 A\rho}{\mu}(1 - e^{-\mu d})$$

$$(11-7)$$

The student may show that if $d_{1/2}$ represents the depth of the 50% iso-dose surface, then $d_{1/2}$ can be considered as the half-value layer and is related to μ by the equation $\mu = 0.693/d_{1/2}$ or $1/\mu = 1.44\ d_{1/2}$. Substituting this value for μ, we obtain:

$$\Sigma = 1.44 \cdot D_0 \cdot A \cdot d_{1/2}\rho\,(1 - e^{-.693d/d_{1/2}}) \tag{11-8}$$

This expression takes no account of the spread of the beam but can be corrected for this effect to give as a first approximation:

$$\Sigma = 1.44 \cdot D_0 \cdot A \cdot d_{1/2}\rho\,(1 - e^{-0.693d/d_{1/2}})\left(1 + 2.88\,\frac{d_{1/2}}{f}\right) \tag{11-9}$$

where f is the source-to-skin distance. This expression gives the total energy imparted for a patient d cm thick. If, however, the patient is thick enough to absorb most of the radiation, i.e. d is much larger than $d_{1/2}$, then the bracketed term involving the exponential in equation 11-9 becomes 1.0. This condition is usually satisfied for low energy radiation. Under these circumstances, the energy imparted is given by:

$$\Sigma = 1.44 \cdot D_0 \cdot A \cdot d_{1/2}\rho\left(1 + \frac{2.88\ d_{1/2}}{f}\right) \tag{11-10}$$

These expressions will now be used in an example.

Example 11-7. Calculate the energy imparted when a 6 × 6 cm field of cobalt 60 radiation delivers 1.0 Gy at the maximum. The SSD is 80 cm.

$\quad$ $d_{1/2} = 10.5$ $\quad$ (Interpolation in Table B-2e)

$$\Sigma = 1.44 \times 1.0 \left(\frac{36 \times 10.5}{1000}\right)\left(1 + \frac{2.88 \times 10.5}{80}\right) \qquad \text{(eq. 11-10)}$$

$$= 0.54\,(1 + 0.38) = 0.75\ \text{J}$$

This result overestimates the energy because it assumes the exit dose in zero. If we use the more accurate expression of equation 11-6, we must multiply the above value by the factor:

$$1 - e^{-0.693 \times 22/10.5} = 1 - e^{-1.45} = 1 - 0.24 = 0.76$$

The energy imparted to the 22 cm depth is thus $0.75(0.76) = 0.57$ J.

Total energy imparted may be calculated in a completely different way using the concept of energy fluence as related to absorbed dose. We now focus our attention on the energy flowing in the radiation beam, and thus incident on the patient. If all of the energy incident is absorbed, then the energy imparted is obtained immediately. To illustrate this we redo example 11-7.

Example 11-8. Calculate the energy imparted for example 11-7 using the concept of energy fluence:

Dose at maximum = 1.0 Gy

Dose in air at same point = 1.0 Gy/1.022 = 0.978 Gy   (Table B-5d)

Energy fluence = $D/(\mu_{ab}/\rho)$ = 0.978 Gy/0.00297 m²/kg = 329.3 J/m²
(Table A-3b and eq. 7-8)

Incident energy in 6 × 6 beam = $329.3 \dfrac{J}{m^2}$ × 36 × 10^{-4} m² = 1.19 J

From Example 11-7 we saw that 24% of the beam emerged from the patient, so a better estimate would be 1.19 (0.76) = 0.90 J.

This result is a good deal larger than 0.57, obtained in example 11-7. The actual value will lie between these two. The first answer is too low because we have neglected radiation scattered sidewise from the beam, while the latter answer is too large because we have assumed that all scattered radiation is absorbed. These two examples illustrate the difficulty of making a precise determination of the total energy imparted.

A precise determination of total energy imparted is not usually required. Equations 11-7 through 10 are only approximate. For radiations up to 300 kV, equation 11-10 is usually accurate enough, but for more penetrating radiations, equation 11-9 should be used. When the peak of the buildup curve is some distance below the skin, as for 25 MV radiations, a procedure similar to that followed in compiling Table 11-3 is required.

From the above is it evident that the total energy imparted increases rapidly with increase in field size. If the field size is doubled, the area A is doubled and $d_{1/2}$ is increased, so the energy is more than doubled. When small fields are used, the energy imparted is usually not important. With large fields, however, the total energy absorbed, rather than the absorbed dose in a specified volume of tissue, may become the limiting factor in a given treatment.

We have already indicated that the total energy imparted should be kept as small as possible in treating a tumor. In tumors on the skin surface, this will be achieved by using radiation with a small percentage depth dose so that the energy absorption beyond the tumor will be small. The small depth dose can best be achieved using a short SSD. To avoid differential effects between bone and soft tissue, it is usually advantageous to use hard radiation such as is produced by cesium, cobalt, or some type of high energy machine.

Choice of Energy of Radiation

When the tumor is below the surface of the skin, the minimum energy imparted will be achieved using hard radiation. Figure 11-12 shows calculations for a point P at the center of a patient of thickness d. In this

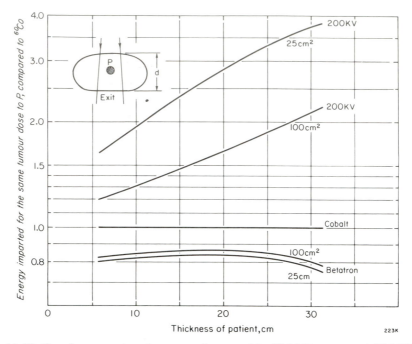

Figure 11-12. Graph comparing the energy imparted by 200 kV x rays and 25 MV radiation with that resulting from cobalt 60. Results are shown for 2 sizes of field as a function of the thickness of the patient. The energies imparted have been compared on the basis that for the 3 cases the same tumor dose is given to the point P at the center of a patient (see insert) (W17).

diagram, the energy imparted has been calculated for unit tumor dose at P and the values have been compared with cobalt 60, which is given the value 1.00. The energy imparted is plotted against patient thickness for two field sizes. For betatron radiation, the energy imparted is about 80% of that for cobalt regardless of the size of the patient and of the field. With 200 kV radiation, especially using small fields, the energy imparted may be 4 times as great as for cobalt. The advantages of high energy radiation in this regard are obvious. This point is discussed again in section 12.11.

FIELD POSITION. In general, the tumor is treated by several beams of radiation. From the point of view of energy imparted, the field that has its entrance point closest to the tumor will deliver the minimum integral dose per unit tumor dose. Unless there are clinical reasons against them, such fields are preferred.

PENUMBRA. The integral dose also depends on the penumbra. When a beam has a large penumbra (see section 10.13), the field size must be increased to encompass the tumor in a region of uniform dose. The total energy imparted to the patient is then increased greatly and much of the advantage of high energy radiation is lost.

Effects of Total Energy Imparted

The effects of radiation are very complicated and many changes that are observed in the patient's blood picture do not correlate as closely with the total energy imparted as one might hope. In the concept of energy imparted, no distinction is made between energy absorbed in soft tissue or fat and that absorbed in tissues of high radiosensitivity such as lymphatic tissue and bone marrow. This probably accounts in part for the lack of a good correlation. It has also been shown that the energy imparted in total body irradiations does not correlate with the severity of radiation sickness. Energy imparted can only be considered as a rough guide to constitutional effects to be expected following irradiation.

11.09   WHOLE BODY IRRADIATION

In certain blood disorders (leukemia, polycythemia vera), the patient is treated with a radiation bath to the whole body. Under these circumstances there is no specific tumor site, so a tumor dose cannot be specified. A skin dose also has limited meaning, for two different techniques yielding the same skin dose will produce widely different constitutional effects if the qualities of the radiation are very different.

The intent is to deliver a uniform dose to the whole body. The dose may be given by means of one or two large beams or with various types of combinations of smaller beams administered either sequentially or by using a number of sources simultaneously. No matter what the technique, calculations of the dosage should be made for various points in the irradiated volume to check for uniformity. Wherever possible, the calculations should be accompanied by measurements in phantoms. The use of radiation energies below that of cobalt 60 should be avoided. Because treatment distances will be large and will tend to be nonstandard, the simplest way of carrying out dosage calculations is by the use of tissue-air ratios or tissue-phantom ratios. This will be illustrated by an example.

Example 11-9. A large beam is used as part of a whole body treatment. The patient's anterior surface is at a distance of 225 cm from the source. The beam size at this distance is 70 × 50 cm. The dose rate, as measured in free space in a small mass of tissue at a distance of 80.5 cm is 1.0 Gy per minute. Calculate the maximum dose from this beam, the midline dose, and the exit dose for the trunk of a patient 24 cm thick. If the same beam is used for a posterior field, check dosage uniformity throughout the patient, each beam being applied for one minute.

> For this type of irradiation the field size is larger than the patient, and the field size that should be used is the area of the patient's trunk, which would be about 35 × 60 cm. However, since the in-

crease of the tissue-air ratio with area beyond 35×35 is small, we will make a negligible error in extrapolating slightly beyond the tissue-air ratio entry of 35×35 cm given in the appendix Table B-5d.

Dose rate in free space at anterior surface $1.0 \left(\dfrac{80.5}{225}\right)^2 = .128$ Gy/min

Tissue-air ratio for surface for a very large field = 1.09 (extrapolated, Table B-5d).

Maximum dose rate = $0.128 \times 1.09 = 0.140$ Gy/min

Dose rate in free space at midline = $1.0 \left(\dfrac{80.5}{237}\right)^2 = 0.115$ Gy/min

Tissue-air ratio for depth 12 cm = .81 (extrapolated, Table B-5d)

Dose rate at midline = $0.115 \times .81 = 0.093$ Gy/min

Dose rate in free space at exit surface = $1.0 \left(\dfrac{80.5}{249}\right)^2 = 0.104$ Gy/min

Tissue-air ratio = .53 (extrapolated, Table B-5d)

Dose rate at exit surface = $0.104 \times .53 = 0.055$ Gy/min

Surface dose (depth 0.5 cm) = $(0.140 + 0.055) \times 1.0 = 0.195$ Gy

The midline dose = $(0.093 + 0.093) \times 1.0 = 0.186$ Gy

A full examination of dose uniformity must include points off the central ray, and this is quite difficult to do. One may always use scatter-air ratios and the sector integration technique described in section 10.13. A simpler procedure using tissue-air ratio data for sets of rectangular beams that will give fairly good answers can be explained by the following example.

Example 11-10. For the large field treatment of example 11-9, estimate the dose rate in the midplane at a point, Q, which is 5 cm in from the side of the patient. The depth to this point is 8 cm for the anterior beam and 11 cm for the posterior beam.

Dose in free space at Q $= \dfrac{0.115 \times 237^2}{237^2 + 12.5^2} = 0.115$ Gy/min

To calculate the dose at Q, we consider the field to be equivalent to the average of a 10×60 cm field and a 25×60 cm field.

Tissue-air ratio for 10×60 beam, depth 8 cm = 0.843 (Table B-5)

Tissue-air ratio for 25×60 beam, depth 8 cm = 0.912 (Table B-5)

Dose rate at Q for anterior beam $= .115 \left(\dfrac{.843}{2} + \dfrac{.912}{2} \right)$

$$= 0.100 \text{ Gy/min}$$

Tissue-air ratio for 10×60 beam, depth 11 cm $= 0.736$ (Table B-5)

Tissue-air ratio for 25×60 beam, depth 11 cm $= 0.820$ (Table B-5)

Dose rate at Q from posterior beam $= 0.115 \left(\dfrac{0.736}{2} + \dfrac{0.820}{2} \right)$

$$= 0.089 \text{ Gy/min}$$

Dose at point Q $= (0.100 + 0.089) \times 1.0 = 0.189$ Gy

This calculation indicates that the dose at point Q is very nearly equal to the midline dose, suggesting that in this treatment the dosage is quite even throughout the treated region. It is frequently found, however, that for individual patients considerable dose variation will be observed and bolus or tissue compensators will be required. For a more detailed discussion of this problem the reader is referred to a paper by Rider and Van Dyk (R5).

At the Ontario Cancer Institute the problem of providing very large fields is considered to be so important that cobalt units have been designed or adapted specifically for this purpose. They are described in papers by Cunningham and Wright (C11), Van Dyk (V1), and Leung (L10).

PROBLEMS

Difficult problems are marked with an asterisk.

1. A tumor at a depth of 10 cm is irradiated with a cobalt 60 beam having dimensions 8×8 cm at the tumor. The dose rate at this position in the absence of the patient is 0.73 Gy/min. Find the dose rate at the tumor and find the treatment time to yield a tumor dose of 2.0 Gy.

2. A ^{60}Co beam, 10×10 cm, SSD = 80 cm, is directed obliquely into a patient at an angle of 30° from the normal. Use the isodose shift method to produce an appropriate isodose distribution. Compare the results with the solid lines of Figure 11-2.

3. Use the ratio of tissue-air ratios method to estimate the relative dose at point Q of Figure 11-2.

*4. Using scatter-air ratios estimate the dose correction factor for point Y of Figure 11-3. Assume the beam is 12×15 cm, that Y is on the isocenter, and that it is at a depth of 4 cm.

*5. Given that the HVL in Pb of cobalt radiation is 11 mm, calculate the thickness of lead required to compensate the dose at a point at a depth of 6 cm below an air gap of 2.5 cm in a 10×10 cm beam.

6. Assume point G of Figure 11-6 is at the exit side of a patient and is at a depth of 15 cm. In exiting from the patient, the beam encounters no scattering material. The beam is from a cobalt unit and is 10×10 cm at the entrance surface. Neglecting any inhomogeneities, estimate the percent depth dose at this point. Take SSD = 80 cm.

7. For problem 6 assume the inhomogeneity in front of point G has a thickness of 10 cm, a relative density of 0.3, and that point G is 3 cm behind the low density region. Estimate the depth dose at this point by at least three different methods.

8. Complete the design of the wedge filter for Figure 11-9. If facilities are available, construct the filter and determine its isodose pattern.

9. A pregnant woman is to be treated by a cobalt unit with a 10 × 10 cm field at 80 cm SSD. The tumor dose is to be 40 Gy at a depth of 5 cm. Estimate, using scatter-air ratios, the dose to a point at this depth 3 cm outside of the edge of the beam. Would external shielding decrease this dose?

10. A lead block, 5 cm thick, is placed on the axis of a 15 × 15 cm beam. The block casts a shadow that is 5 × 5 cm. Estimate the dose under the block at a depth of 10 cm relative to the dose at the same point with the block removed. Assume cobalt radiation.

*11. A region of a patient containing a steel pin 1 cm in diameter receives a dose from a cobalt unit which is calculated to be 40 Gy, neglecting the pin. Estimate the dose to tissues in contact with the incident and exit surfaces of the steel.

Chapter **12**

TREATMENT PLANNING—COMBINATION
OF BEAMS

12.01   **OPPOSING PAIRS OF BEAMS**

R adiation fields may be combined in a very large number of ways, and
hundreds of articles have been written on this subject. Here the discussion will be confined to the basic principles, and these will be illustrated by suitable distributions that are useful in treating tumors in different sites.

The simplest combination of two fields is achieved by directing them
along the same axis from opposite sides of the patient. Figure 12-1 shows
how the resulting dose distribution may be obtained. Both diagrams are
for cobalt beams, the one on the left is for fixed SSD, the one on the right
for an isocentric arrangement. The isodose curves for the individual
beams are shown as dotted and dashed lines. The solid curves are obtained by joining the points of intersection of appropriate curves. For
example, in the left hand diagram the 100 isodose line is found by joining A(30,70), B(40,60), C(50,50), D(60,40), and E(70,30). Similarly the
110 isodose curve is found by joining F(40,70), G(50,60) etc. Outside
the geometric edge of the beam, it is more difficult to find points of intersection of the appropriate isodose curves, but the resulting curve may be
located approximately. For example, the 40 curve passes through (20,20)
and then falls *outside* the 20 curve from one field and *inside* the 20 curve
from the other field. Sometimes it is convenient to sketch in some extra
isodose curves midway between the ones shown. For example, the 100
isodose curve will pass through the points (35,65) and (45,55), as well
as the ones shown.

Although the isodose pattern for Figure 12-1b appears at first sight
rather different from that of Figure 12-1a, closer scrutiny shows that they
are almost identical. The difference in appearance arises because they
are normalized in very different ways. For Figure 12-1a 100 is the maximum dose from each beam while for Figure 12-1b, 100 is the dose from
each beam midway between the entrance surfaces. For example, if
one were to trace the "199" isodose curve on Figure 12-1b it would
have an "hour glass" shape like the "110" isodose curve of Figure 12-1a.

Dose Along Axis of Two Opposing Beams

The variation in dose along the axis of Figure 12-1 is small, yielding
an almost uniform dosage from one beam entrance to the other. How-

411

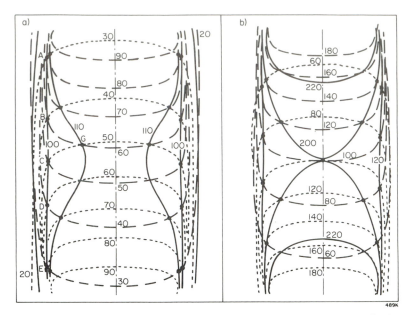

Figure 12-1. Isodose distribution obtained by combining two opposing radiation beams. Both are for 10 × 10 cm beams of cobalt radiation and the entrance surfaces are separated by 20 cm. (a) Fixed source-skin distance with dose values expressed relative to 100 at the maximum of each beam. (b) Isocentric arrangement with dose values expressed relative to 100 midway between the surface from each beam.

ever, when the fields are farther apart this is not the case, as is illustrated in Figure 12-2 where the dose along the axis has been plotted for typical low, high, and very high energy radiation beams. Graphs of dose versus depth are shown for field separations of 10, 20, and 30 cm plotted from data in the appendix (Tables B-2c, 2d, and 2i).

With 25 MV radiation, the dose rises from a low value on the surface to reach its maximum at a depth of 4 cm and then remains almost constant regardless of the field separation. For cobalt 60, the rise in dose occurs more rapidly below the skin and reaches its maximum at a depth of about 5 mm. Beyond this point the dose falls to a shallow minimum midway between the fields. This minimum is very shallow for a 10 cm separation but increases with the separation. At 20 cm the minimum dose is about 85% of the maximum dose and for 30 cm separation it is even less. For separations of from 10 to 20 cm, the minimum is only slightly less than the maximum, and we may consider the dose almost uniform from one maximum to the other.

For 200 kV radiation, the dose falls from a maximum at the skin surface to its minimum midway between the fields. This minimum becomes more and more pronounced as the field separation increases and at 20 cm separation it is about 55% of the maximum.

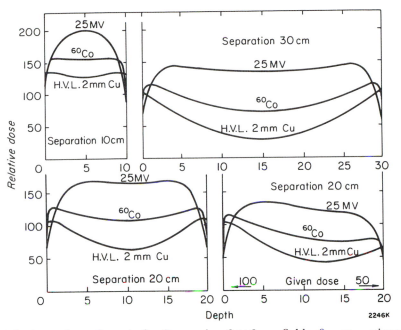

Figure 12-2. Dose along the axis for 2 opposing 6 × 8 cm fields, for separations of 10, 20, and 30 cm, 25 MV radiation at SSD 100 cm; cobalt 60 at SSD 80 cm; 200 kV radiation, HVL 2.0 mm Cu SSD 50 cm. The 3 symmetrical diagrams were calculated for given doses of 1 Gy to both fields, while the graph in the lower right hand corner results when the given doses are 1 Gy to the left and 0.5 Gy to the right.

Figure 12-2 also shows the effect of giving unequal doses to the opposing fields. In the graph shown, the left-hand field is given 1.00 Gy for 0.50 Gy to the right field. With 200 kV radiation we find, as before, a region of minimum dose between the fields; this minimum is now shifted towards that skin surface which was given the smaller dose.

Because of the widespread use of high energy radiation we will compare, in more detail, distributions for cobalt 60 with 10 MV and 25 MV radiation. Figure 12-3a shows relative depth doses for a single 10 × 10 cm beam with the doses normalized to 100 at a depth of 15 cm. Two curves are shown for cobalt radiation. The solid line is for a source-axis distance of 80 cm and the dashed line is for 100 cm. Diagram b gives the relative doses for opposed pairs with a separation of 30 cm. Graphs c and d are for opposing beams with 20 cm and 10 cm separation. In each case the doses are normalized to 100 at the midpoint.

From all of these diagrams and from the above discussion it should be possible to visualize the dose distributions that result from the use of opposing beams and some conclusions can be drawn. Such an arrangement is often used when it is required to treat a tumor that is situated approximately midway between two more or less parallel surfaces. If the separation is less than about 10 cm, cobalt radiation might be preferable as

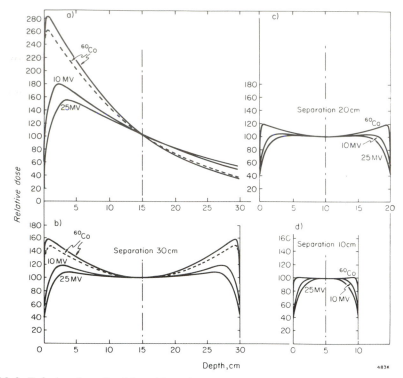

Figure 12-3. Relative dose for 10 × 10 cm beams of cobalt, 10 MV and 25 MV radiation. (a) Single beams with doses normalized at a depth of 15 cm. The dashed line for cobalt is for SAD = 100 cm, the solid line is for SAD = 80 cm. (b) As in a but an opposing beam is added with a separation of 30 cm. (c) and (d) Opposed beams with separations of 20 and 10 cm.

it would raise a rectangular column of tissue to a quite uniform dose and yet provide skin sparing. With separations much greater than this, however, higher energies must be used to avoid the dip in the middle. 10 MV radiation would be useful for separations up to about 20 cm. For still larger separations, 25 MV radiation is an advantage.

DISTRIBUTION IN THREE DIMENSIONS. The student should note that the dose distribution is three-dimensional in character. To aid in visualizing this the dosage pattern in a plane at right angles to the axis of the beam of Figure 12-1a is shown in Figure 12-4a. This diagram is for cobalt radiation. Figure 12-4b shows the corresponding pattern for 25 MV radiation.

Example 12-1. Estimate the shape and size of the 100 isodose surface when two 15 × 6 cm cobalt 60 fields are placed in opposition 20 cm apart. Use the isodose curves of Figure 10-18 and assume the treatment is to be at a fixed SSD.

From the isodose chart, we find that the depth dose at 10 cm is about 55%. Hence the dose midway between the fields is 110. The 50%

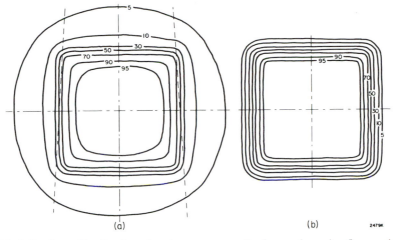

Figure 12-4. Isodose distributions in planes perpendicular to the axis of opposing fields of (a) cobalt-60 and (b) 25 MV radiations. The beams are isocentric, 10 × 10 cm and the separation is 20 cm.

isodose line crosses the 10 cm depth about 7.5 cm from the axis in the direction of the 15 cm dimension and about 2.5 cm in the direction of the 6 cm dimension. The shape of the 100 isodose curve in a plane midway between the two surfaces and parallel to these surfaces is thus a rectangle with rounded corners having dimensions 15 × 5 cm. The 100 isodose surface will be like the surface of a rectangular box with dimensions 20 × 15 × 5 cm but with rounded corners.

When a dosage pattern is calculated for any actual treatment situation, we must take account of the external shape of the patient because this may alter the shape of the pattern. These adjustments must first be made for each beam in the treatment plan and only then can the doses be added to form the composite distribution. Methods for doing this for single beams were discussed in section 11.02. Figure 12-5 illustrates the alteration in the isodose curves that take place when an opposing pair of beams is used to irradiate sloping surfaces. In the diagram on the left (Fig. 12-5a), no account is taken of the patient's contour, and the pattern is essentially the same as that of Figure 12-1b. When the patient contour, represented by the line labelled C, is taken into account the dose pattern shown in Figure 12-5b is the result. The pattern is no longer symmetric about the beam axes and the dose is higher on the left where the patient is thinner.

It is unlikely that the dosage distribution shown in Figure 12-5b would be acceptable clinically and methods such as the use of tissue compensators (section 11.03) should be used to provide a more uniform dose.

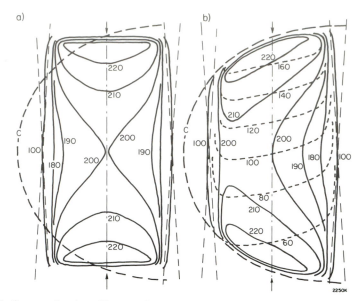

Figure 12-5. Opposed pairs of beams from a cobalt unit. The diagram on the left is similar to Figure 12-1b. The distribution on the right has been corrected for contour shape, the dashed curves being the distribution from the top beam corrected for patient contour as discussed in section 11.02.

12.02   COMBINATIONS OF OPPOSING PAIRS
Opposing Pairs at Right Angles

One useful arrangement of four fields is to place the opposing pairs at right angles (as shown in Fig. 12-6a). A combination of two such pairs of fields (6 × 15 cm) at right angles is shown in Figure 12-7b. The combined isodose curves are obtained in essentially the same way as was illustrated in Figure 12-1. First, the resulting distribution from two opposing pairs was obtained. One set of these is shown in Figure 12-7a. Then isodose curves for the opposing pair were laid over these and points of intersection located as before. It will be noted that the region of highest dose, as expected, is the portion that is common to all fields. This varies from 360 near the edge of the square-shaped section to 400 at the center. For this particular example the axis of the unit was placed at the center of the tumor and the depth to it was 12.5 cm for each field. If the tumor were the size and shape indicated by the hatched area, the minimum tumor dose would be 360 and the average would be about 380.

The fall-off in dose at right angles to the plane of the paper in Figure 12-7 can be judged from isodose curves in the 15 cm dimension of the field. For example, at a distance of 6 cm above the plane of Figure 12-7, the dose on the axis of rotation would be 90% of its value at the isocenter. This would be just over 360 in the composite distribution. With the use of 4 cobalt beams we have thus achieved a remarkably uniform dose in

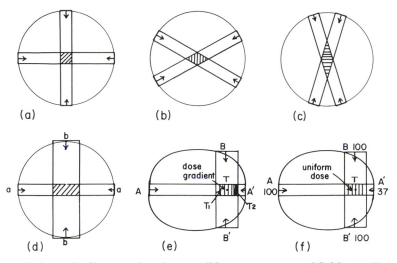

Figure 12-6. Schematic diagram showing possible arrangement of fields. (a) Two opposing pairs at right angles. (b) Two opposing pairs at 120°. (c) Two opposing pairs at 35°. (d) Two opposing pairs of different widths at right angles. (e) Two opposing pairs at right angles treating an off-center tumor. (f) Two opposing pairs at right angles treating an off-center tumor with field A' being given 37% of the amount given the other fields.

the region of the tumor. The greatest dose elsewhere would be (from Fig. 12-7b) just over 280, which is 70% of the tumor dose. Such an arrangement is useful for treating centrally located lesions, such as cancer of the esophagus. It would have to be remembered, however, that the esophagus is curved and it is necessary to make sure that it is contained within the three-dimensional shape of the isodose surfaces.

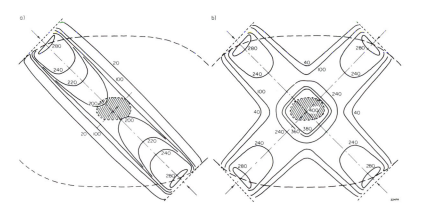

Figure 12-7. (a) Isodose curves for an opposing pair of 6 × 15 beams from a cobalt unit. (b) A second pair added at right angles to a. The dose at the isocenter is 100 from each beam. The source-axis distance is 80 cm. Such an arrangement could be used in treating cancer of the esophagus.

Opposing Pairs at Other Angles

In the above example, the region of uniform dose is essentially a rectangular block $6 \times 6 \times 12$ cm. Under certain circumstances the radiotherapist may wish to irradiate a rhombic-shaped block of tissue rather than a square one. This can be done by placing the opposing pairs at angles other than 90° as shown in Figure 12-6b and c. In one case a flattened type of rhomb, and in the other a rhomb with the points vertical, is obtained. The dose within the region of intersection in both cases will be essentially constant and will be approximately the same as in Figure 12-7. The resulting distributions are shown in Figure 12-8. Which is best will depend on clinical considerations such as the shape of the tumor and the position of critical tissues in the neighborhood of it. If we assume that the contour of Figure 12-8a is for the chest, the beams would be directed to the tumor through a minimum of lung but the high dose region would extend on to the spinal cord. Damage to the lung would be minimal but some might be inflicted on the spinal cord. In Figure 12-8b the fields are placed at a much larger angle to the vertical. This will serve to protect the spinal cord completely but will irradiate more lung tissue. From this simple discussion, it is clear that the shape of the high dose region can be altered at will merely by changing the angle of intersection of the opposing pairs.

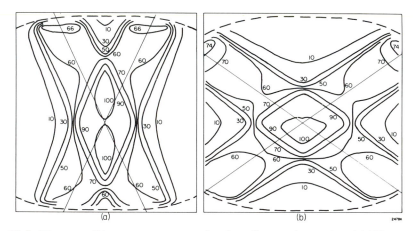

Figure 12-8. Two possible arrangements of pairs of opposing pairs. (a) The angle between the pairs is 50° and (b) the angle is 110°. Both are for 6×15 cm beams of cobalt radiation.

Three Sets of Opposing Pairs

Figure 12-9 shows a dose distribution resulting from three sets of opposing pairs. The distribution is more complicated because there are now regions that are irradiated by two of the six beams, yielding about

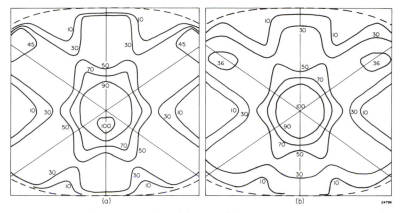

Figure 12-9. Dose distributions obtained by combining 3 sets of opposing pairs. (a) Cobalt-60, 6 × 15 cm beams, (b) 25 MV.

33% of the tumor dose, four of the six beams yielding about 67%, and all six yielding 100%. This arrangement provides over twice as much energy to the tumor as to any large section of normal tissue; however, the dose to the spinal cord could be as much as 65% of the tumor dose.

The production of complete sets of isodose curves such as those shown in Figures 12-5 to 12-9 is very time-consuming without the aid of a computer programmed to make such calculations. Fortunately this is not always necessary in routine radiotherapy. If the field arrangement has been used before and has been drawn up (for example, for a previous patient), it may only be necessary to calculate the dose at the isocenter. The method of calculating this dose can best be illustrated by a simple example.

Example 12-2. Using the six field arrangement of Figure 12-9b it is desired to give a tumor dose of 60.0 Gy in 6 weeks (30 treatment sessions). Use fields 6 × 15 cm of 25 MV radiation, SAD = 100 cm, and assume one opposing pair of fields is to be used each day. The treatment machine is calibrated at the isocenter to give a dose rate of 2.06 Gy per monitor unit at a depth of 5 cm in a water phantom for a 6 × 15 cm field. Calculate the number of monitor units required for each field as used each day. Deliver equal tumor doses from all fields.

Daily tumor dose = 60/30 = 2.0 Gy
Daily tumor dose per field = 1.0 Gy
Equivalent square for 6 × 15 field = 8.5 cm   (Table 10-4)
Calculations are outlined in Table 12-1. Steps for beam #1 are explained.
Tissue phantom ratio for 8.5 × 8.5 cm field, d = 14.2 cm = 0.823 (Table B-4b)
No. of monitor units/day for field #1 = 1.0/(0.823 × 2.06) = 0.59

TABLE 12-1

Beam No.	Angle, deg*	Depth, cm	Tissue-Phantom Ratio (Table B-4b)	No. Monitor Units for 1 Gy
1	−55	14.2	0.823	0.59
2	125	12.4	0.861	0.56
3	0	11.0	0.890	0.55
4	180	9.0	0.433	0.52
5	55	14.2	0.823	0.59
6	−125	12.4	0.861	0.56

*Angles are measured from the vertical (pointing down is zero), clockwise are positive.

Skin Dose

With the common use of high energy radiation today, skin dose is usually of limited concern. In Figure 12-7 the isodose curves have been drawn assuming that unit density bolus material has been placed against the skin to effectively make the surface of the patient flat. This raises the dose at the skin and for the opposing pair in Figure 12-7a would produce a skin dose of just over 280. This dose is made up of two components, 40 due to the exit dose from one field and about 240 as an entrance dose from the other. If no bolus material were used, the entrance dose from the upper field would be about 30% of the peak dose, depending on the amount of electron contamination in the beam. The total skin dose would then be $0.3 \times 240 + 40 = 112$. This calculation clearly shows the advantage of keeping the skin free of bolus material.

The biological effect of the radiation on the skin cannot, however, be determined by the dose to the surface of the skin, because the most superficial layer is inert keratin. Any observed skin reaction therefore depends upon the dose at some depth. When the dose rises very rapidly with depth, as it does for cobalt radiation, the effective skin dose is greater than the value that would be measured for the actual surface. Its exact value is frequently unknown. This must be taken into account when attempting to accurately correlate skin reaction with dose. With high energy radiation and good treatment planning, skin reactions are not usually a limiting factor in radiotherapy. However, unusual and severe skin reactions do sometimes occur and when this happens the dose under the actual conditions of treatment should be determined experimentally using dosimeters such as TLD.

Two Sets of Opposing Pairs of Different Sizes

In most cases the opposing pair of fields are of the same size but under some circumstances the second pair, which is to be added at right angles to the first, may have one dimension of a different size as illustrated in Figure 12-6d. Here one pair has dimensions a × c, where c is the dimension perpendicular to the page, and the other pair has dimensions b × c. The volume treated will be approximately a × b × c. It is clear that the fields should have one common dimension. In the above example, this common dimension is c, which is perpendicular to the page. The fields should be chosen so that they cover the tumor with an ample margin of safety around it.

Sets of Opposing Pairs for Off-center Tumors

At times the tumor may not be near the center of the body and the symmetry obtained in Figures 12-7 to 9 will not be present. This is shown schematically in Figure 12-6e and f. Here the tumor T is being irradiated by one pair of opposing fields A and A′ and another pair of opposing fields B and B′ at right angles. The depths to the tumor for fields A and A′ are very different, and if equal tumor doses are given from each field, the dose near the entrance surface of field A will be high and could well exceed the tumor dose. Such a situation would not be acceptable; it is imperative that the maximum tissue dose be determined for each treatment plan.

Two Split Fields

Figure 12-10a shows a split field for cobalt 60 consisting of two 4 × 10 openings with an opaque section in the middle of dimensions 4 × 10. This type of field may be made from a 12 × 10 field by placing a rectangular block of lead about 5 cm thick across the center of the field. Such a field is frequently used in treating the parametria and the pelvic wall after irradiation of the cervix with internal sources. Figure 12-10b shows two such fields in opposition. This combination raises two slabs of tissue, including the inner rim of the pelvic wall, to a uniform dose while sparing the uterus on the midline, which has already received adequate radiation from brachytherapy (see Chapter 13). If the uterus is off center or tilted, it may be advantageous to move the position of the central piece of lead in an appropriate manner to shield the uterus in its actual position rather than in its hypothetical one. In using this type of treatment, however, it must be remembered that anatomical structures can shift and change shape during the course of treatment. Precautions must therefore be taken to make sure that during the external beam treatment the shielded region does actually contain the desired structures.

In Figure 12-10a the isodose curves for the 12 × 10 cm field without the shielding block are shown as dashed lines. From this we can see how the block alters the isodose pattern. The isodose values are expressed relative to the reference dose on the axis of the unblocked field. Figure 12-10b shows isodose curves for a pair of split fields in opposition. Doses are relative to the midline dose for an unblocked pair.

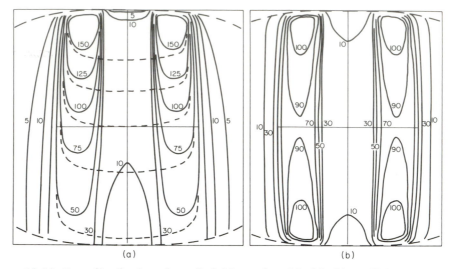

Figure 12-10. Dose distributions for split fields produced by blocking off the central portion of 12 × 10 cm cobalt 60 fields. The block is made of Pb, is 5 cm (approx. 5 HVL) thick, and blocks a region 5 cm wide at the isocenter. The SAD is 80 cm. (a) Single field with isodose curves for unblocked field shown as dashed lines. (b) Opposing pair.

It is often necessary to estimate the dose at specific points under shielding blocks such as these, and procedures for doing this are given in section 10.13.

12.03   ANGLED FIELDS AND WEDGED PAIRS

When it is desired to irradiate a small tumor through one skin surface, two angled fields may be directed as indicated in Figure 12-11a. Here two beams angled at 30° from the vertical are directed towards a point P, 8 cm below the surface. Figure 12-11a shows the resultant distribution for cobalt radiation using 6 × 6 cm fields. Although the fields are directed towards the point P, the high dose region occurs much nearer the surface. In fact, it occurs just below the intersection of the edges of the beams. This diagram illustrates the very important principle that when fields are directed through one side of a patient towards a tumor, they should be aimed considerably below it. This is sometimes referred to as "past pointing."

It is seen that in the region where the beams intersect, the resultant dose distribution appears somewhat like a single beam oriented midway between the other two. This has been called an "internal field" (P7) and is a useful concept for treatment planning. It might be possible, for example, to apply two more identical beams toward point P in a plane at right angles to the plane of the paper or a opposing pair of wedged fields also at right angles to the plane of the paper. These latter fields would have to be wedged so that their dose gradient was equal and opposite to the dose gradient produced by the "internal field."

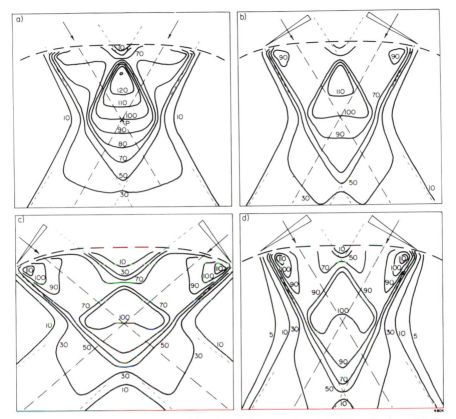

Figure 12-11. Angle fields produced by 6 × 6 beams of cobalt-60 radiation. (a) Beams at 30° from vertical and crossing at point, P, 7 cm below the contour surface. (b) Same as a but with 45° wedge filters added. (c) Same as b but angle increased to 50°. (d) Same as b but with 60° wedges.

Figure 12-11b to d illustrates the use of wedged fields, which were discussed in section 11.06. In Figure 12-11b, 45° wedge filters have been added to the beams of Figure 12-11a. Although this improved the dose uniformity within the region of beam overlap it would not be acceptable for treating a tumor that occupies the greater part of the overlap region. For angled beams like this to produce a uniform dose region it is necessary that the isodose curves for each of the beams be tilted so that they are parallel to the line that bisects the angle between the beam axes. In this case this would be a vertical line. The distribution of Figure 12-11b could therefore be improved either by increasing the angle between the beams or by increasing the wedge angle. Figure 12-11c shows the former, with the beams now directed at an angle of 50° from the vertical. (The use of 45° wedges suggests 45° but the slope of the contour surface would tend to counteract the wedge and the angle has been increased to allow for this.) The dose uniformity is better but now the maximum tissue dose, under the thin parts of the wedges, exceeds the tumor dose, and this

distribution would not be acceptable. Figure 12-11d shows the use of 60°
wedges and beams angled 30° as in b. Dose uniformity is again fairly good
but again the maximum tissue dose exceeds the tumor dose.

The behavior of the dose pattern achieved with the use of wedge filters
is well illustrated by these examples and indeed the arrangement of
Figure 12-11b might be used to treat lesions of the vertebral bodies. An
illustration of the use of wedges is shown in Figure 12-19.

12.04   **THREE-FIELD TECHNIQUE**

The inhomogeneity of the dose in the region of the tumor in Figure
12-11 may be overcome by directing, towards the point P, a third beam
from the opposite side of the patient. Such an arrangement is shown in
Figure 12-12.

The addition of field 3 neutralizes the falling off of the internal field
resulting from beams 1 and 2. We now have a dose distribution that is
fairly uniform in the region of the tumor. The maximum tumor dose
for this arrangement is 105% and the minimum is 94%. This degree of
dose uniformity might be acceptable but it could be improved still further by the use of tissue compensators.

For the isocentric arrangement of Figure 12-12, the tumor doses are
made equal for each beam. For such arrangements it is necessary to make
sure that no tissue outside of the tumor will receive too high a dose. Two
examples will illustrate this procedure.

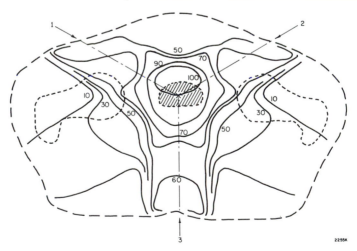

Figure 12-12. Isodose distribution for three 6×6 cobalt 60 beams at SAD 80 cm directed
toward a bladder tumor. The beams are symmetrically arranged at 120° to each other.

Example 12-3. Determine the maximum tissue dose outside of the target volume for the three-field treatment of Figure 12-12 using cobalt 60.
The distances from the isocenter to the surface for beams 1, 2, and 3 are
10.0, 9.5, and 10.5 cm respectively. Plan the treatment so that each beam

provides a tumor dose of 20.0 Gy.

> The maximum dose will be for field 3 since it has the greatest depth.
> Tissue-air ratio for depth 10.5 cm = 0.636   (Table B-5d)
> Field width at the max for this beam = $6 \times (80 - 10)/80 = 5.3$ cm
> Tissue-air ratio for 5.3×5.3 cm field, depth = 0.5 cm ≈ 1.02
> Inverse square adjustment to dose rate from 80 to $(80 - 10)$ cm is $(80/70)^2 = 1.31$
> Peak dose for this beam = $(20.0 \times 1.31 \times 1.02)/0.636 = 42.0$ Gy.

This is considerably lower than the tumor dose but would have to be taken into consideration as part of the treatment planning. A quick estimate of the peak dose could be made by using relative depth doses as given, for example, in Table B-3a. The relative dose for a 6×6 beam, SAD = 80 cm, 10 cm above the isocenter is 228.1. This would indicate a peak dose of $20.0 \times 2.28 = 46$ Gy that, as discussed in section 10.06, would be an overestimate.

Example 12-4. For example 12-3, determine the maximum tissue-dose when the tumor of Figure 12-12 is treated using 25 MV radiation from a linear accelerator with an SAD of 100 cm. Again assume 20.0 Gy from each beam.

> Depth of peak dose for each field = 4 cm
> Tissue-phantom ratio for depth 10.5 cm = 0.897   (Table B-4b)
> Field width, depth 4 cm = $6 \times (100 - 10.5 + 4)/100 = 5.6 \times 5.6$ cm
> Tissue-phantom ratio for 5.6×5.6 cm, depth 4 cm = 0.995
> Inverse square factor = $(100.0/93.5)^2 = 1.14$
> Peak dose for beam 3 = $(20.0 \times 1.14 \times 0.995)/0.897 = 25.3$ Gy
> Using relative doses the solution would be $20.0 \times 1.36 = 27.2$ Gy (Table B-3b)

The peak dose outside of the tumor for this energy is very much lower than for cobalt radiation. This very clearly illustrates the advantage of the high energy. The distribution of Figure 12-12 could also be improved by adding 3 more beams in direct opposition to fields 1, 2, and 3. By this means the tumor dose would still be 60 Gy but the maximum dose to any point outside of the tumor would be only slightly more than 20 Gy. This advantage would have to be balanced against the fact that a larger volume of healthy tissue would be irradiated to this dose.

The three-field technique shown in Figure 12-12 is one that has many applications as it is simple and results in a homogeneous dose about the tumor. When the fields are all directed at 120° to each other, the distribution is symmetrical, and maximum homogeneity of dose results. If anatomical considerations require fields at angles other than 120°, the distribution will still be good provided the angles do not differ greatly from 120°. For example, the anterior fields could be placed at 50° to the vertical rather than 60 and still yield a good distribution. Where possible, some symmetry should be retained by directing one of the fields along the bisector of the angle between the other two.

12.05   **BEAM DIRECTION**

When small radiation fields are used in treating a tumor, it is essential that these beams be directed accurately towards it, otherwise the high dose region will be displaced from the tumor position. Many devices have been designed to aid in the accurate direction of a radiation beam.

Backpointer

A most useful type of beam director for the fixed SSD technique is the backpointer illustrated schematically in Figure 12-13. It consists of a rigid tubular support, which may be fastened to the machine. In some installations it is fastened to a rack bar that carries either the backpointer or the pin and arc to be described in the next section. It is convenient to have the rack bar mounted on a ring that may be rotated about the axis of the beam so that it may be used at the angle that interferes least with the patient. The rigid support carries a sleeve through which passes an adjustable pointer, which lies along the axis of the beam. Before the backpointer may be used, a point must be located on the patient where the central ray of the beam is to enter the patient and a point where it is to exit. These points are placed so that a line drawn through them passes through the tumor. The patient is then positioned in front of the machine with the entrance point at the center of the treatment cone and the exit point aligned with the back pointer. Care must be exercised in the use of such a backpointer because even the most rigidly made device can be distorted if the patient is allowed to lean against the adjustable pointer. The correct alignment of the device may be tested by rotating the backpointer about the axis. If it is correctly aligned, the pointer will remain fixed in space on the axis of the beam as the device is rotated.

Pin and Arc

Another type of beam-directing device is the pin and arc illustrated in Figure 12-14. The pin and arc has three scales, an angular scale marked on the arc, a linear scale marked on the pin, and a linear scale marked on the rack bar that is connected to the machine. The pin is arranged so that it can be moved along the arc and also moved in the direction of its length while the arc is arranged so that it can be moved parallel to the beam by a sliding mechanism or a rack and pinion device (J6).

To use the pin and arc, the technician needs only one skin mark at the point P directly above the tumor and a knowledge of the distance d of the tumor below this point P. The technician first sets the pin to a depth

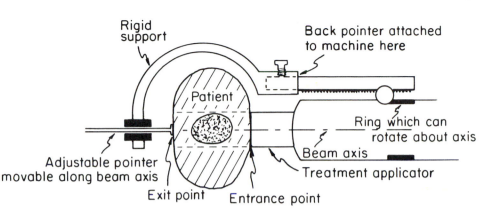

Figure 12-13. Schematic diagram showing a backpointer beam director. 1339L

corresponding to the distance d. (In the example shown the pin is set to a depth of 10 cm.) The pin is then slid along the arc until it is at the predetermined angle θ selected by the radiotherapist. (In the example, this angle is 45°.) The technician then rotates the treatment machine until the pin is vertical. This condition can be recognized by a spirit level on the top of the pin or by using an auxiliary angular scale on the machine. The rack is then moved to a reading of about 1.5 d (in this case 15 cm) and the machine is lowered until the pin touches the patient's skin at P. The treatment machine is then adjusted to the patient until the pin makes contact at P and the treatment cone touches the skin surface simultaneously. Under these circumstances, the distance, y, from the end of the treatment cone to the tumor is the reading on the scale on the rack bar and the beam is aligned to pass through the tumor.

The proper adjustment of the beam the first time the patient is "set up" requires some care but once the reading y has been obtained, beam direction with the pin and arc is very rapid. When the patient is set up for treatment the following day, the pin is set to the required depth and angle and the rack bar is adjusted to the setting y. The machine is then lowered so that the pin touches the skin marking at P, which will bring the treatment cone in contact with the skin.

A little study of Figure 12-14 will show that the arc must have its center on the axis of the beam and the rack bar must be parallel to the axis. The index for the scale on the pin must be arranged so that when the pin is set to zero, the end of the pin is on the axis of the beam. The index for the scale on the rack bar must be arranged so that when it is set to zero, the pin touches the end of the treatment cone. Testing of these two adjustments may be most readily carried out with the arc set to 90°.

The beam directing devices that have just been described are for fixed SSD setups and are not relevant for isocentric techniques. An isocentric

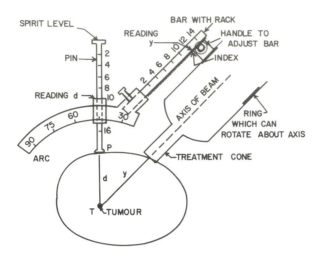

Figure 12-14. Schematic diagram of pin and arc. The pin and arc is shown arranged to treat a tumor d cm below the mark on the patient's skin at P, with the beam directed to the tumor at an angle of 45° to the vertical. The distance y from the skin surface to the tumor may be read directly from the scale on the rectangular bar.

machine is a large pin and arc device in itself and such additional attachments are not necessary.

Plaster of Paris Molds

When 250 kV radiation was used almost exclusively in the treatment of tumors, many fields directed towards the tumor were necessary to build up a sufficient tumor dose. Under these circumstances, the use of plaster of paris casts to help in beam direction was very valuable. These techniques were developed primarily by the Manchester School of Radiotherapy (P7, C12). Today, such molds have more limited application because simpler arrangements of fields are possible with high energy radiation. It is a well-known fact, however, that skin markings may move considerably with respect to the underlying tissues. When a patient is placed in some type of fitted mold, motion of this kind cannot take place and more accurate beam direction is possible.

Figure 12-15 shows a plaster cast to be used in the treatment of cancer of the esophagus using a 6-field technique. The steps in the production and use of such a cast are as follows:

1. Using plaster of paris bandages, a cast is made of the patient's thorax and is extended to include his shoulders. The cast is then cut along the midline on the anterior and posterior surface and the cast removed from the patient. The halves are then fitted with some type of clip so that it may be fastened securely on the patient for each treatment.

2. Lead markers are placed every cm along the anterior and posterior midline and the patient, wearing the cast, is radiographed while swallowing barium. Lateral and AP films are taken. The lateral film will show the position of the tumor, the lead markers, and the angle of the esophagus with respect to the line of markers. The AP film will show the position of the eosphagus with respect to the plane of the midline.

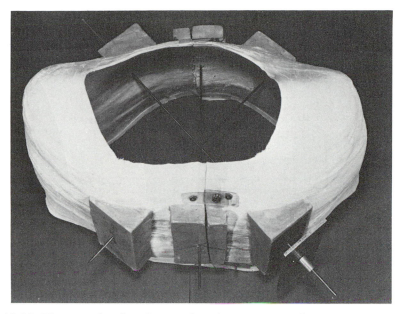

Figure 12-15. Photograph of a plaster of paris cast arranged to treat a cancer of the esophagus using 6 cobalt 60 fields with bolus.

3. A line is drawn on the lateral film through one of the lead markers, through the center of the tumor, and through a point on the posterior surface, as illustrated in Figure 12-16. The distances a and b from the inner anterior surface to the inner posterior surface and to the center of the tumor are measured on this film. The entrance and exit points as located on the film may be transferred to the cast from the position of the lead markers.

4. The cast is removed, reassembled, and a sharp-ended bicycle spoke calibrated in cm is thrust through the cast in the exact position of the line drawn on the film. The anterior-posterior diameter of the cast along this line, c, can be measured by reading the scale on the spoke. This is less than a, because of the magnification of the x-ray image. The actual position of the tumor is then bc/a from the cast and can be located on the spoke. When the center of the tumor is not exactly on the midline as seen from the AP film, this spoke should be moved laterally the appropriate distance.

5. Two other spokes are then inserted through the cast from the posterior side and directed towards the tumor at the chosen angle. For an esophagus this might be 45°, as illustrated in Figure 12-15.

6. Wooden or aluminum replicas of the end of the treatment cone are placed on the spoke in contact with the plaster cast, as illustrated in Figure 12-15. On a surface such as the chest wall, it will make contact at only one point and the rest of the air gap is filled with soft wax. This

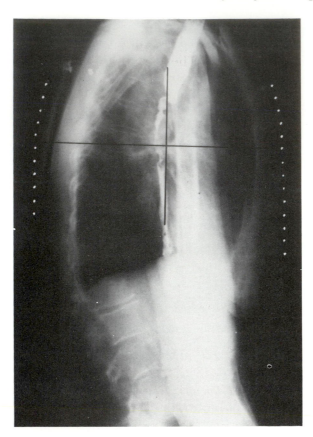

Figure 12-16. Lateral film of a patient wearing a plaster of paris cast, showing the lead markers and the position of the tumor.

wax mold provides a flat surface against which the treatment cone can be brought into contact and the exit point on the far side of the mold provides a point to which the backpointer can be adjusted in setting up the patient for treatment. Wax seats are provided for each field.

7. After the wax has been put in position, the measurements required for dosage calculations may readily be made with the calibrated spokes. The distance from the entrance field to the tumor for each of the fields may be read off directly and the distance from the entrance field to the exit point may also be determined in case one wishes to determine the skin dose. With cobalt 60 this would not usually be necessary. Calculations would then be carried out to determine the given dose to each of the fields to produce the desired tumor dose.

8. It is desirable to take a barium x-ray of the patient with the cast in position through one of the oblique entrance ports using a diagnostic machine with a field equal in size to the one planned for the treatment. If the planning has been carried out carefully, the film will show the esophagus centered in the treatment field.

The cast provides two main advantages over skin markings. First, it enables one to direct the beams accurately towards the tumor. This may be more difficult than it seems, especially when the esophagus is at an angle to the axis of the patient. The second big advantage is appreciated when the patient is set up for treatment. The plaster cast provides a method for reproducing the treatment set up precisely each day, for the entrance and exit points are clearly marked and a flat surface is provided as a seat for the treatment cone.

Casts may also be made from clear plastic by using vacuum molding techniques. The procedures used are as varied as the workers making them. A useful discussion of mold room techniques is given by Dickens (D8).

In many circumstances, particularly when high energy radiation is used, the use of bolus should be avoided since it eliminates the "skin sparing" advantage. Molds or casts are still useful, however, for beam direction and immobilization of the patient. Figure 12-17 shows a cast used in a way that illustrates a number of the features that have been discussed so far. The cast encloses the head and neck of the patient and is in use for a treatment of cancer of the larynx. The cast is made in the same way as described above, but instead of using wax seats to provide a surface with which the treatment applicator may be brought into contact, a hole is cut for each of the fields. Walls are built up around the holes to provide a receptable into which the treatment applicator is inserted. The skin dose is thus kept small and the maximum dose for each field occurs well below the surface. In the example shown in Figure 12-17, a tissue compensator, as discussed in section 11.03, is mounted in a slot in the base of the treatment applicator.

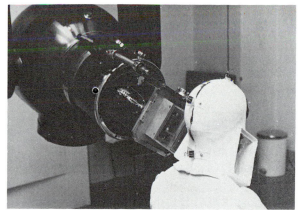

Figure 12-17. Photograph of a patient being set up on a cobalt unit for a treatment of cancer of the larynx. A plaster cast encloses the head and neck and recepticals are provided for the treatment applicator. No bolus is used but tissue compensators are provided to allow for the shape of the patient's surface.

Figure 12-18 shows a compensating filter being inserted into the base of the treatment applicator. The filter is mounted about 20 cm from the end of the applicator and is designed in such a way that it can be inserted into the base with the correct orientation. Only the correct size applicator will fit the receptacle in the cast and this applicator is interlocked with the collimator so that only the correct field size can be chosen.

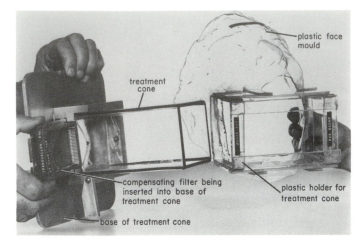

Figure 12-18. Photograph showing a plastic face mold, a treatment applicator, and a compensating filter being inserted into it. The treatment is for an intraalveolar carcinoma of the mandible and uses an opposing pair of cobalt 60 beams in a fixed SSD setup.

Figure 12-18 also shows a plastic face mold worn by the patient during treatment as an alternative to the plaster casts described above.

12.06   **SPECIAL FIELDS**

Wedge Fields

Wedge fields were introduced in section 11.06 and discussed also in 12.03. Their use is illustrated by one further example. Figure 12-19a shows the isodose curves for two wedge fields directed approximately at right angles to each other through an enlarged metastatic node in the region of the neck. The individual isodose curves are shown dotted and run at an angle of about 45° to the axis of each beam. These isodose lines are nearly parallel to one another and the falling off of dose with depth from one field is neutralized by the other field so that the combination gives a large volume of uniform dose.

In this particular treatment, wax seats were used, and a photograph of the cast is shown in Figure 12-19b. The thickness of the wax bolus appears excessive but examination of Figure 12-19b will show that in some places it is actually quite thin. This illustrates the point that when a treatment applicator is held against an irregular surface large gaps may occur. These will produce inhomogeneity of tumor dose unless bolus or tissue compensators are used. Since, in this case, one wishes to treat a volume next to and including the skin, bolus should be used. If, however, the tumor were well below the surface, it would be advantageous to avoid

Figure 12-19. Two wedge fields at right angles to treat an inoperable metastasis of the neck using a plaster cast and wax seats for the treatment cones. The lead wedges, shown here schematically, are located in the base of the treatment applicator as shown in Figure 12-18.

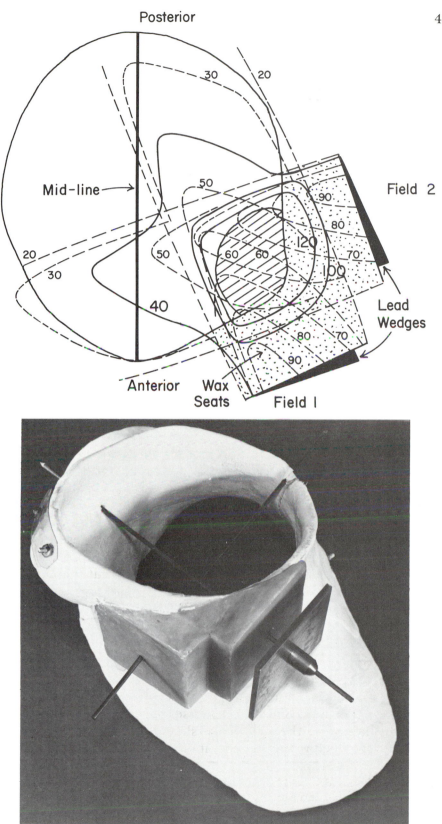

Posterior

Mid-line →

Field 2

Lead Wedges

Anterior   Wax Seats   Field 1

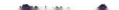

bolus and so achieve skin sparing. Such considerations also apply when one wishes to treat the skin to full dose as in the postoperative treatment of the chest wall as discussed by Bush and Johns (B15); in these cases, full or partial bolus should be used. Report 24 of the ICRU (I7) discusses many of these problems.

12.07   USE OF CT IN TREATMENT PLANNING

One of the greatest obstacles to accurate treatment planning has been the difficulty in obtaining precise information about the nature and location of anatomical structures. The availability of CT (Computed Tomography, section 16.19) to radiotherapy has solved this problem. Precise and highly detailed images of actual body cross sections can now be obtained. Examples were shown in section 11.05 where dose corrections for tissue inhomogeneities were discussed. The greatest contribution CT makes to treatment planning is in the delineation of the target and sensitive structures and the placement of radiation beams. The body section of Figure 11-7 is shown again in Figure 12-20 where 3 beams from a 25 MV linear accelerator are used to irradiate the mediastinal structures. The insert shows the outlines of the beams superimposed on the CT image and it can be seen how precisely the beam edges can be located with respect to these structures. One can locate sensitive structures, such as the spinal cord, with equal precision. It must be remembered, however, the all of these structures are three-dimensional and so such examinations must be carried out on several images so that the whole of the irradiated volume is studied. The isodose distribution shown in Figure 12-20 has not been corrected for the inhomogeneous tissues. The corrected distribution is shown in Figure 12-21. Each individual beam has been corrected using the equivalent tissue-air ratio method discussed in section 11.05. The corrections were greatest for the two posterior oblique beams because of the large amount of lung traversed. The dose at the isocenter, the center of the target volume, is 315 compared to 300, a correction of only 5%. This small correction is typical of such high energy radiation.

Such corrected dose distributions can now be obtained on a routine basis and treatment planning could be carried out using them exclusively (V8). It is recommended, however, that uncorrected dose distributions, such as that shown in Figure 12-20, be used as the basis for dose prescriptions. This is important because clinical experience has been obtained over the years with such data. The corrected distributions should be considered as additional information that will, in the course of time, when coupled with careful clinical analysis, serve to allow all aspects of the treatments to be more precise.

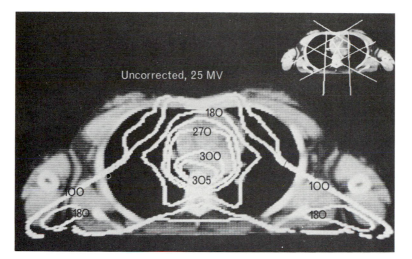

Figure 12-20. Diagram depicting CT and treatment planning. The insert shows 3 beams irradiating structures in the mediastinum. The placement of the beams can be determined precisely because of the accuracy and detail of the image. The radiation is from a 25 MV linear accelerator and the isodose curves have been obtained without taking account of the tissue inhomogeneities.

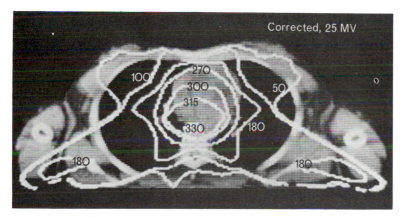

Figure 12-21. The isodose distribution of Figure 12-20 corrected for tissue inhomogeneities. The radiation beams are 10 × 10 cm from a 25 MV linear accelerator. The dose at the isocenter is altered from 300 to 315, a correction of only 5%.

12.08 ROTATION THERAPY—TUMOR DOSE CALCULATIONS

A logical extension of multiple beam therapy is to use one beam, have it directed towards the tumor, and cause the machine to rotate about an axis through the tumor, or keep the machine fixed and rotate the patient about this axis. Either technique is referred to as moving beam therapy or rotation therapy.

When the radiotherapist was limited to the use of 250 kV x rays, it was very difficult to get enough radiation into an internal tumor such as a cancer of the esophagus by using fixed fields in a cross-fire technique. As a result, many workers developed rotation techniques, as depicted in Figure 12-22a, with the patient strapped to a rotating chair and the beam directed at the tumor as the patient is rotated.

At the same time, special rotation x ray machines were developed in which the source moved around a stationary patient, as illustrated in Figure 12-22b. Alternatively, machines have been built to move in a circular path and to simultaneously transverse horizontally to cover the surface of a cylinder, as depicted in Figure 12-22c. Both types of machines could be made to move over any portion of the circle or cylinder. Converging beam units were developed in which the x ray head was made to move about a spiral with the beam always directed to one point below the surface (as depicted in Fig. 12-22d).

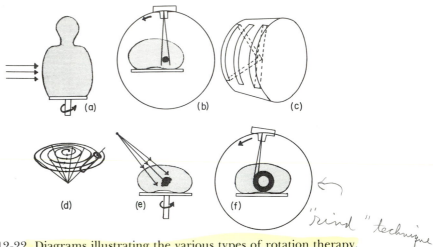

Figure 12-22. Diagrams illustrating the various types of rotation therapy.

"rind" technique

Another arrangement that has been used is depicted in Figure 12-22e, where the patient lies on a couch that rotates about a vertical axis. Isotope machines have been developed to be used in rotation therapy in a variety of ways, but usually as depicted in Figure 12-22b.

In certain circumstances, as in the irradiation of the chest wall, it is convenient to offset the beam from the axis of rotation as depicted in Figure 12-22f. This type of rotation therapy will place energy into an annular ring about the center of rotation.

Many workers have developed systems of dosimetry for rotation therapy. They are all somewhat similar, and space does not allow a discussion of them. The methods to be described here are based largely on work by the authors. An atlas of dose distributions produced by the International Atomic Energy Agency is devoted to rotation therapy (T6).

Tumor Dose Calculations

In fixed field therapy the depth of the tumor below the skin surface for each field is required. Likewise in rotation therapy, the depth of the tumor below the skin is required for a number of positions of the patient with respect to the beam. The use of the tissue-air ratio in treatment planning will be illustrated for an esophagus using the arrangement of Figure 12-22b.

Example 12.5 It is required to treat the bladder of Figure 12-12 to a tumor dose of 60 Gy in 6 weeks (30 treatments) using 360° rotation with a 6 × 6 cm cobalt 60 field. If the dose rate in free space at the axis of rotation is 0.8 Gy/min, find the treatment time per day.

The patient is placed so that the tumor is on the axis of rotation and the distance from the axis to the patient's skin is measured at evenly spaced angular positions of the machine. Intervals of 20° are satisfactory, and these are shown in column 2 of Table 12-2. The angles were measured clockwise from the vertical, starting at the anterior surface. Since the tumor is symmetrically placed, measurements need be made over only half of the 360°.

The tissue-air ratios are then obtained from Table B-5d (in the appendix) for a 6 × 6 cm beam and are given in column 3 of Table 12-2. These are totaled (5.463) and averaged to give a tissue-air ratio of .607. The average depth is found to be 11.5 and the tissue-air ratio corresponding to it is 0.636. This differs appreciably from the average tissue-air ratio, showing that where the depths are not almost all equal it is necessary to find the individual tissue-air ratios and average these rather than determine the tissue-air ratio for the average depth.

TABLE 12-2
Measurements for Treatment of Bladder Using Rotation Therapy
The Contour was Taken from Figure 12-12

Angle	Depth, cm	Tissue-Air Ratio (Table B-5d)	
10	7.5	.757	
30	7.7	.749	Dose rate in free space at axis = 0.80 Gy/min
50	8.6	.711	Average dose rate at tumor = 0.80 × 0.607
70	11.4	.602	= 0.486 Gy/min
90	14.9	.488	Total dose required = 60 Gy
110	14.4	.503	Dose per treatment = 60.0/30 = 2.0 Gy
130	14.7	.494	Time per treatment = 2.0/0.486 = 4.12 min.
150	12.9	.550	
170	11.2	.609	
Total	103.3	5.463	
Average	11.5	.607	

This calculation is based on the assumption that during the treatment, the patient or the machine performs an integral number of rotations. However, for practical purposes, this is unnecessary, provided several rotations occur during the treatment time. In this example, 4 to 5 turns would be quite sufficient. It should also be noted that source-to-skin distance was not used in this problem and that the same calculation would be valid for any source-to-axis distance. This calculation could be made equally well using tissue-phantom ratios. The procedure would be exactly the same. The isodose distribution for this treatment is shown on the left in Figure 12-24.

Partial Rotation

Suppose the radiotherapist wished to avoid treatment over a 40° angle, at which time the beam is directed through the spinal cord. In performing the calculations, the last measurement of Table 12-1 (angle 170°, depth 11.2 cm) would be excluded from the calculation. In this particular example this would not alter the average nor the treatment time very much.

When full 360° rotation is used, the isodose curves tend to be circles about the tumor. If partial rotation is used, this symmetry is lost and the region of highest dose is shifted from the axis of rotation away from the missing sector. The highest dose region may be brought back to the tumor region by placing the axis of rotation below the tumor towards the missing portion. If the missing sector is a small fraction of the 360°, the effect is negligible. As the portion becomes larger the distortion also becomes larger. If large sectors are missing, a detailed analysis of the resulting isodose distribution should be made before the partial rotation is used.

Treatment Planning in Rotation Therapy

From the above discussion it is clear that the radiotherapist requires the distance from the skin surface to the tumor for a number of angles of entry. Many machines are equipped with an optical distance indicator that can be used to obtain this information. A special pointer that moves along the beam axis can be constructed to read these distances directly by making the scale read zero when the pointer is pulled out so that its end is at the axis of rotation. This method is accurate and easy to use. A less reliable method involves the use of a piece of lead solder, which may be bent to follow the patient's contour. This may be transferred to a large sheet of paper. On this contour the tumor position is located and measurements made with a ruler.

12.09   ROTATION THERAPY—ISODOSE DISTRIBUTIONS

Isodose distributions for rotation techniques may be obtained by either calculation or measurement. The measurements may be performed in a number of ways. The most extensive sets of measurements are those of Dahl and Vikterlof (D9) and of Hultberg et al. (H14), who used many small ion chambers placed in Masonite® phantoms. For the high radiation energy, where the response of photographic film is independent of the energy of radiation, films placed between layers of phantom material may be used to provide a rapid qualitative assessment of the radiation dose distribution. If considerable care is used with the development of the film and if the response versus dose characteristics of the film are known, quantitative conclusions may be made as well. Lithium fluoride capsules (sec. 9.09) may also be used for the measurement of rotation distributions.

Calculations of rotation distributions are generally based on the superposition of single beam isodose charts. Charts normalized to 100% at the axis of rotation are most useful for this purpose (see Figs. 10-16b and 12-23).

The total dose at a point in a patient is obtained by adding together the contributions to that point from a series of fixed fields spaced at equal angular intervals around the axis of rotation. This procedure was followed for the calculation of the dose on the axis of rotation in example 12-5. The computation of dose for a point off the axis will be illustrated by using the same case. The appropriate single beam isodose chart, for a beam with cross section 6 × 6 cm at the axis of rotation, is shown in Figure 12-23.

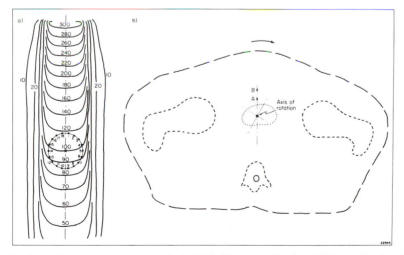

Figure 12-23. Isodose pattern for a cobalt 60 field normalized to 100 at a depth of 15 cm. Source-to-skin distance 65 cm, source-to-axis distance 80 cm, field size at axis 6 × 6 cm. The right side of the diagram shows the contour of the patient, the axis of rotation, and the points A and B at which the dose is to be determined.

Example 12-6. The bladder of Figure 12-12 is to be treated by a rotation technique as described in example 12-5 to a tumor dose of 2 Gy per treatment. Calculate the doses to points A and B, 2 cm and 3 cm respectively, anterior to the axis (see right side of Fig. 12-23).

We will first calculate the dose to point A. On the chart we construct a circle with center on the axis and with a radius of 2 cm, and locate on this points numbered 1 to 18, spaced at 20° intervals starting at 10°. Point A in the patient will in turn occupy positions 1 to 18 with respect to the isodose pattern as the rotation takes place. The steps in the calculation are shown in Table 12-3. Column 1 gives the position of the point A with respect to the isodose pattern, and column 2 the corresponding angle. Column 3 gives the depths from the contour to the axis of rotation, and column 4 the corresponding tissue-air ratios. These entries in columns 3 and 4 are the same as those of Table 12-2 and enable us to calculate the dose on the axis for each angle of entry. The relative doses for points 1 to 9 are read from the chart (Fig. 12-23) and entered into column 5. The products of columns 4 and 5 divided by 100 appear in column 6 and give the dose to A for 1 gray on the axis in free space for each position of the beam. Since the patient's contour is symmetrical about the anterior-posterior line, we need only consider points 1 to 9 and can omit the calculations for points 10 to 18. The entries of column 6 are totaled and averaged to give 0.614. This should be compared with the axis, which has a tissue-air ratio of 0.607. When the axis receives 2.0 Gy, point A will receive 1.99 Gy.

TABLE 12-3
Calculation of Dose at Off Axis Points A and B (Fig. 12-23)
Full Rotation with a Cobalt 60, 6 × 6 cm Field

(1) Position Fig. 12-23	(2) Angle	(3) Depth to Axis	(4) Tissue-Air Ratio for Axis	Calculations Point A (5) Percentage of Axis Dose	(6) Dose at A	Calculations Point B (7) Percentage of Axis Dose	(8) Dose at B
1	10	7.5	.757	118.	.893	127	.961
2	30	7.7	.749	115.	.861	122	.914
3	50	8.6	.711	109.	.775	108	.768
4	70	11.4	.602	103.	.620	75	.452
5	90	14.9	.488	96.	.468	53	.259
6	110	14.4	.503	92.	.463	68	.342
7	130	14.7	.494	89.	.440	80	.345
8	150	12.9	.550	87.	.479	81	.446
9	170	11.2	.609	86.	.524	79	.481
	Total		5.463		5.525		5.018
	Average		.607		.614		.558

Dose to axis 2.0 Gy   Dose to A = $\frac{.614}{.607} \times 2.0 = 2.02$ Gy   Dose to B = $\frac{.558}{.607} \times 2.0 = 1.84$ Gy

The calculations for point B are performed in exactly the same way. We locate points 1 to 9 on a circle of radius 3 cm (see Fig. 12-23) and read off the relative doses that appear in column 7. The products of entries in columns 4 and 7 appear in column 8. These are averaged to give a dose of 1.76 Gy to point B.

The dose to point B is about 12% less than the dose to the axis because for some angles of entry the point is very near the edge of the beam. If we had calculated the dose for a point 4 cm from the axis, the dose would have been very much less.

The method described in this example gives an accurate determination of the dose for points in the region of the tumor, i.e. near the axis. It is not useful in determining the dose near the skin surface for there the isodose pattern of each individual field overestimates the dose.

It is clear from this example that dosage calculations for rotation therapy are lengthy and time-consuming. Fortunately these distributions are relatively insensitive to variations in patient contour and it is frequently possible to reuse previously calculated (or measured) distributions from similar cases or to work from atlases of prepared distributions. An extensive atlas of moving field isodose charts has been prepared by Tsien et al. (T6) by applying computer methods to the procedure outlined in example 12-5. Most computer-based treatment planning systems now also include programs for producing dose distributions for rotation therapy.

Although dose distributions for rotation therapy are rather insensitive to the shape of the patient, it is instructive to see how the dose pattern does depend on various irradiation parameters.

Effect of Energy of Radiation on Rotation Distributions

Figure 12-24 shows the rotation distribution for a treatment of cancer of the bladder using a well-collimated cobalt 60 beam having minimal penumbra with a 6 × 6 cm field at the tumor. The diagram on the left is for a source-to-tumor distance of 80 cm. On the right is shown the distribution obtained with 10 MV photons at a source-to-tumor distance of 100 cm. In both cases the isodose curves are elliptical in shape with the long axis of the ellipse in the direction of the short axis of the patient. This is typical of the distribution about a tumor placed near the center of the body. For both it is seen that the nominal skin dose is less than 20%. In actual fact, when buildup is taken into account, the skin dose may be less than 10% of the tumor dose.

A comparison of the two sides of the diagram shows that the distributions are very similar. The 10 MV distribution is slightly better, showing somewhat lower doses outside of the tumor, but the difference is so slight that this could not justify a choice between these two radiations.

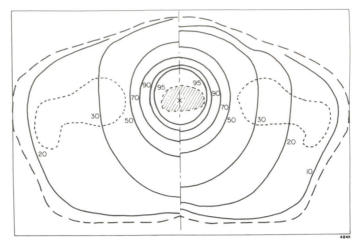

Figure 12-24. Isodose distributions for 360° rotation technique in treatment of cancer of the bladder using 6 × 6 cm field at the tumor. Left-hand side, cobalt 60 with a source-to-axis distance (SAD) of 80 cm. Right-hand side, 10 MV linear accelerator radiation, SAD = 100 cm. These isodose distributions were calculated by the method described in Example 12-6 and by Tsien et al. (T6).

Effect of Arc Angle

Figure 12-25 shows dose distributions for two different angles of arc. The one on the left half of the diagram is for 270° and the one on the right is for an arc of 120°. The most distinctive feature of dose distributions for arc therapy is the shift of the maximum dose away from the center of rotation toward the bisector of the arc. This is true no matter what the shape of the contour. It can be judged, from the right side of Figure 12-25, that the size of the high dose region also decreases as the arc angle decreases. It is also true, as pointed out by Tsien et al. (T7), that as the degree of rotation becomes less than 360°, the isodose curves are deformed in such a way that the lower portions (the side opposite the beam entrance surface) become flatter with the decrease in the arc angle. When the arc angle is 180° or less, however, the isodose curves tend to be pinched in at the sides and the lower portion again moves further from the axis. Both these effects may be observed in the diagrams of Figure 12-25. Arc angles of less than 180° should be used only after careful consideration of the distribution desired.

Effect of Beam Penumbra on Rotation Distributions

In Chapter 10 it was emphasized that a large penumbra should be avoided in irradiation. Two beams with the same parameters other than penumbra are compared in Figure 10-20. We now inquire into the type of rotation distribution these two beams will produce. Figure 12-26 shows the resulting isodose pattern when a cylindrical phantom of 20 cm

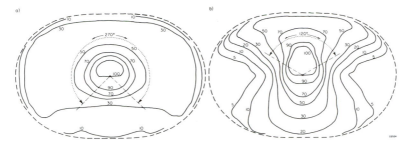

Figure 12-25. Isodose distributions for two angles of arc on an oval phantom. The one on the left is for 270° and the one on the right is for 120°. Both are for cobalt 60 radiation. The high dose region is moved toward the bisector of the arc; the smaller the arc, the greater is this shift.

diameter is irradiated by cobalt 60 in rotation therapy using 6 × 6 cm fields. The pattern on the left results from the use of the small penumbra, while the one on the right corresponds to the large penumbra. The difference is not great but the distribution using the small penumbra shows a more rapid fall off of dose outside the tumor region and a more even dose within the tumor region. The difference is more pronounced when yet smaller beams are used.

Source-to-tumor distance has little influence on rotation dose distributions. However, when this distance is small, the penumbra is likely to be large and this affects the distribution as described above. The limiting diaphragm cannot be placed closer than 35 cm from the axis or it will strike the patient when an eccentrically placed tumor is being irradiated, and this usually sets a limit on how small a penumbra can be obtained.

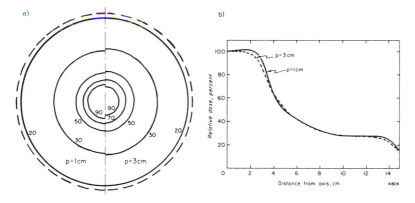

Figure 12-26. (a) Isodose distributions resulting from the irradiation of a cylindrical phantom 30 cm in diameter using a 6 × 6 cm field of ^{60}Co. The distribution on the left is for a penumbra at the axis of 1.0 cm. The penumbra is defined in Chapter 10. The right-hand distribution is for a penumbra at the axis of 3.0 cm. The source-axis distance (SAD) is 80.0 cm for both diagrams. (b) Dose profiles showing the effect of penumbra. The curves are dose versus distance from the axis of rotation.

Effects of Field Size on Rotation Distributions

The length of the field (perpendicular to the plane of rotation) has little effect on the shape of the isodose curves in the plane of rotation. This means that an isodose distribution for a square field can be used for rectangular fields, provided that the field size in the plane of rotation is kept constant. A change of field width in the plane of rotation, however, has important effects on the dose distribution (as illustrated in Fig. 12-27). This shows dose profiles for 360° rotation about a circular contour for fields of different widths. As the field width increases, the dose delivered to the region outside of the target volume increases markedly. In general, rotation therapy is not recommended when a large tumor is involved so that wide fields must be used.

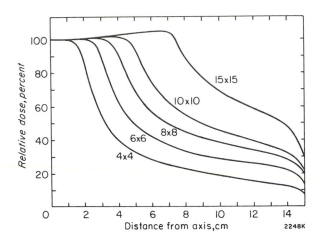

Figure 12-27. Dose profiles for 360° rotation about a 30 cm diameter cylindrical phantom for field sizes from 4 × 4 to 15 × 15 cm.

12.10   **COMPARISON OF FIXED FIELD AND ROTATION THERAPY**

Figure 12-28 shows a comparison of the treatment of cancer of the bladder by fixed field and rotation therapy. On the left is shown the result of directing four 6 × 6 cm fields at a SAD of 80 cm towards the tumor and on the right is the distribution resulting from rotation with the same field size. The rotation distribution is identical with that of the left side of Figure 12-24. It is evident that with rotation therapy the skin dose (about 15) is less than with fixed field therapy (40%) because rotation therapy is equivalent to using 8 to 12 fields. In addition, the isodose curves for rotation therapy tend to be smoother in shape and circular around the tumor region. In contrast, with fixed field therapy, unwanted "horns" resulting from the "pinch spots" between adjacent fields are present.

It is very difficult to compare the clinical results of these types of treat-

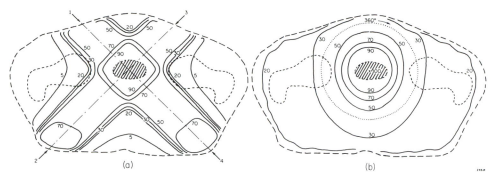

Figure 12-28. Isodose distributions for the treatment of cancer of the bladder using cobalt 60. Left side, distribution for four 6 × 6 cm fields at a source-to-axis distance (SAD) of 80 cm. Right side, rotation therapy using a 6 × 6 cm field at the tumor, also with a source-to-axis distance (SAD) of 80 cm.

ment, the choice being largely a matter of opinion. In fixed field therapy certain regions of the body receive virtually no radiation, but some tissues outside the tumor region receive a higher dose than they would with rotation therapy. In rotation therapy, on the other hand, all points outside the tumor region receive some dose. In particular, in this example, the femurs and pelvic walls are completely spared when fixed field therapy is used, but some other areas are raised to a relatively high dose; whereas in rotation therapy, all the surrounding structures receive some radiation.

A lower energy will be imparted in fixed field therapy provided that the fields are directed towards the tumor through the skin portals closest to the tumor. This difference will not likely be of clinical significance.

There are those who claim that patients may be set up for rotation therapy more quickly. This is probably true. However, there are those who believe that greater precision of beam direction can be achieved with fixed field therapy and the use of molds (sec. 12.05). It is evident that in rotation therapy, with a tumor such as in the bladder, the patient must be held firmly in place in the beam throughout the whole treatment.

Another comparison of fixed field and rotation dose distributions is shown in Figure 12-29. The treatment is for cancer of the larynx. The distribution on the left uses two wedged fields and the one on the right uses 360° rotation. Both distributions are for 6 × 6 beams from a cobalt unit.

In the rotation treatment all of the neck is irradiated to some dose while with the fixed fields some of the neck, for example the spinal cord, is not irradiated while other regions receive a relatively high dose. It is a matter of clinical judgment as to which of these two treatments is the better. It would also be possible to treat this tumor with 180° rotation or with a parallel and opposed pair.

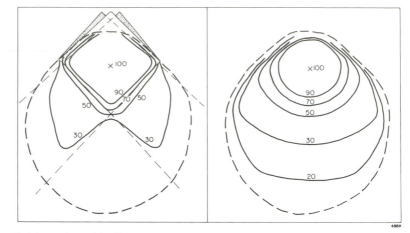

Figure 12-29. Isodose distributions for cobalt 60 in the treatment of cancer of the larynx. Left, two wedge fields at right angles using bolus. Right, 360° rotation about the tumor.

Summary of Procedure on Rotation Therapy

1. Place tumor on axis of rotation. This may be done from radiological findings or localization technique using an x ray tube in the head of the unit. Obtain the setting on some type of beam-directed device so that the treatment set-up may be reproduced accurately at subsequent treatments.

2. Rotate the machine, or patient, slowly and measure the skin-to-tumor depths for angles of entry spaced at equal angular intervals over the range of rotation. Generally, intervals of 20° to 30° are small enough.

3. Calculate the tissue-air ratio for each angle of entry and average.

4. Calculate the average dose rate at the tumor and determine the treatment time per session.

5. Adjust rate of rotation so that at least 4 complete rotations occur per treatment.

6. If the tumor is near one skin surface, the maximum skin dose should be estimated.

12.11   TREATMENT PLANNING—SOME
GENERAL CONSIDERATIONS

In planning radiation treatments, it is necessary to satisfy a number of criteria. One must deliver a high and uniform dose over a target volume, but as low a dose as possible to all structures outside of the target volume. It may also be necessary to protect certain sensitive structures so that they receive an especially low dose. Finally it is necessary to choose a dose fractionation scheme that favors the destruction of the tumor and the repair of the damage that will still be inevitably done to some healthy tissues.

The question of delivering a uniform dose over the target volume is largely one of geometry and is usually a matter of combining beams so that the falloff in dose due to one beam is exactly compensated by an opposite dose gradient from another beam or combination of them. Beam arrangements are discussed in the earlier sections of this chapter.

The protection of sensitive structures is also a matter of beam arrangement—making sure that beams do not irradiate these structures or, if they must, only after passing through the tumor.

Fractionation is a clinical and radiobiological question and is dealt with at some length in Chapter 17.

The question of minimizing dose to tissues outside of the target is partly a matter of beam arrangement but, more importantly, is concerned with the choice of beam energy. One way of quantitating this is to define a "figure of merit" as:

$$\text{figure of merit} = \frac{\text{Energy imparted to the target volume}}{\text{Total energy imparted to patient}}$$

All other things being equal, the best treatment plan would be the one that gave the highest value to this ratio. In a plan consisting of a number of beams, the best would be the one for which this figure of merit had been maximized for each beam individually.

To show what is meant by the figure of merit, consider the two depth dose curves for two very different beam energies plotted on a linear scale in Figure 12-30. They are for HVL 2 mm Cu (curve 1) and 10 MV x rays (curve 2). The depth dose data have been simplified somewhat by fitting them to simple exponentials of the form $e^{-\bar{\mu}x}$, where $\bar{\mu}$, the effective attenuation coefficient, is taken as 0.142 cm^{-1} for curve 1 and 0.480 cm^{-1} for curve 2. The curves are also adjusted to have a value of 1.0 at point P, which we will assume to be at the center of the tumor. They thus could represent the dosage pattern that would result from beams directed from the left side of the diagram. The tumor is imagined to extend a distance z above and below P as indicated by the shaded region labelled T. The region A is irradiated by the beam before irradiating the tumor, and C, after. Region B is the part of A that is spared because of the buildup of dose in the high energy beam. The figure of merit:

$$f = \Sigma_T/(\Sigma_A + \Sigma_T + \Sigma_C - \Sigma_B) \tag{12-1}$$

where the symbol, Σ, stands for energy imparted as defined in section 11.08. Since these curves are simple exponentials they can be integrated to give:

$$f = (e^{\bar{\mu}z} - e^{-\bar{\mu}z})/(e^{\bar{\mu}d_1} - e^{-\bar{\mu}d_2}) \tag{12-2}$$

For $z = 2$ cm, $d_1 = 9$ cm and $d_2 = 9$ cm, f equals 0.17 for the lower ener-

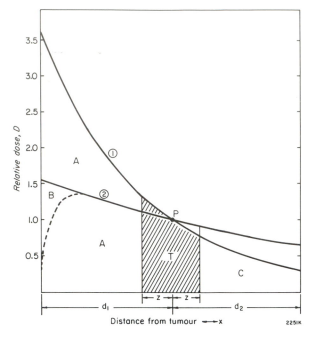

Figure 12-30. Relative dose curves representing depth dose data for a low energy photon beam (curve 1, 2 mm Cu HVL) and a high energy beam (curve 2, 10 MV x rays). They are plotted as simple exponentials with effective attenuation coefficients, μ, of 0.480 cm^{-1} and 0.142 cm^{-1} respectively. Region T represents a target volume containing a tumor. A, B, and C represent regions of healthy tissues.

gy and 0.22 (and more if buildup were considered) for the higher energy, showing that the higher energy delivers much less radiation outside of the tumor.

Of course, for this example we would know that the low energy is unsatisfactory because of the very high dose to region A. The choice is not so obvious, however, if the tumor is closer to the entrance surface and equation 12-1 gives a means of choosing beam energy. Using these ideas it can be shown that high energy radiation is always better than low energy radiation for tumors that are deeper than the depth of dose maximum for the radiation chosen.

Finally, it is also desirable to assess the energy imparted for the combination of beams that are used in a plan. Such an evaluation could be carried out for the beam arrangements shown in Figure 12-31. This figure shows two 4-field distributions as used by Allt (A8) in comparing the results of treatment of cancer of the cervix using cobalt radiation and betatron radiation. It can be seen at a glance that although both plans deliver substantially the same dose to a target volume, the distribution using the high energy delivers considerably less radiation to the rest of the patient. The figure of merit for these two plans are 0.14 and 0.17 for the cobalt and high energy respectively.

In the Allt study, a number of factors in addition to energy imparted differed between the two groups of patients, and the implications are less clear cut than would be desired. Nevertheless the fraction of patients alive after 5 years was very much greater (almost by a factor of 2, 60% compared to 34%) for the high energy group showing very clearly that

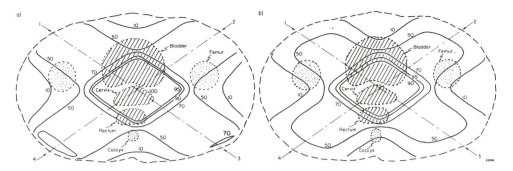

Figure 12-31. Four field dose distributions used by Allt (A8) in treating cancer of the cervix. The left hand diagram is for cobalt radiation and the right hand diagram is for a 22 MeV betatron. Both irradiate the tumor uniformly but the high energy beams deliver considerably less radiation to healthy tissues.

the use of high energy radiation with its improved dose distribution with careful treatment planning is an important life-saving procedure (see also section 17.16).

12.12 TREATMENT PLANNING AND RECORDING

A summary of the basic principles discussed in this chapter may be useful. Radiation fields should be arranged in number and direction so that the following principles are followed and the following statements concerning dosage may be made.

1. The field size should be selected to cover the tumor and a safe margin of at least 1 cm around it. If possible, enough of these fields should be used to make the tumor dose at least 50% larger than any other tissue dose. These fields in general should be arranged to maintain symmetry. Intersecting pairs or opposing pairs are useful. The shape of the high dose region may be altered by changing the angle of intersection of the fields. The beams should be directed to avoid critical normal tissues.

2. An homogeneous dose is given to the tumor including an adequate safety margin around it. Complete homogeneity can never be achieved, so the maximum and minimum tumor dose should be evaluated and recorded.

3. For low energy radiation, the skin dose, including any dose contributions by other fields, should be stated. For high energy radiation, the dose at the maximum, including any contribution from other fields, should be stated. For high energy radiation, the determination of a precise skin dose is difficult and is often not recorded because it is usually small.

4. Care should be taken that no region of high dose occurs outside the tumor. Likely regions of high dose are the pinch spots between angled fields.

5. With low energy radiation, bolus should be used and when casts are

employed, they should be fitted with wax seats. For high energy radiation, bolus should be avoided. Corrections to the tumor dose for lack of bolus should be made.

6. If the tumor is small, some type of accurate beam direction should be used.

7. If possible, corrections of the tumor dose for bone and air cavities should be made.

8. The number of fields, their size, and their arrangements should be recorded on a diagram. For routine work, a complete isodose distribution is not necessary.

9. The way the dose is administered is very important in determining the biological effect. Hence, the overall treatment time, the number of treatments, and the number of fields treated per day should be recorded. It is generally agreed that fractionation of the total dose over a period of from 3 to 5 weeks gives better results than treatment by a single massive dose. For small superficial tumors, fractionation over 1 to 2 weeks is common. Since the biological effect of a given amount of radiation depends on the fractionation, a statement that a tumor was given a dose of 50 Gy is meaningless unless the overall period between the first and last treatment and the number of exposures is stated. It is generally agreed that, for the range of dosage rates used in clinical practice, the biological effect is independent of dosage rate. Hence, dosage rate need not be specified.

10. The source-to-skin distance and the half-value layer or energy of the radiation should be recorded. These factors are involved in determining the tumor dose, so in this sense their inclusion is redundant. However, there is evidence to indicate that the biological effects of radiation depend to a slight extent on the energy of the radiation (see section 17.08).

11. The treatment should be planned to give a specific tumor dose. This plan may have to be altered by clinical considerations before the treatment is finished.

12. Other clinical considerations being equal, the technique that delivers the minimum energy imparted should be used.

PROBLEMS

Many of the following problems require specific isodose patterns. These or similar ones should be in the department. If they are not they should be obtained (see Chapter 10).

1. Obtain isodose curves for 2 typical high energy beams in use in the department and combine them in opposition with a separation of 20 cm.

2. Repeat problem 1 using identical 200 kV fields with HVL in the range 1.0 to 3 mm Cu. Discuss the differences between the resulting distributions.

3. Two opposing 15 × 6 cm fields with a separation of 20 cm are applied to a patient and each is given a dose of 1.0 Gy at the maximum. Find the dose on the axis at depths of 0.5, 1.0, 5.0, and 10 cm for:
   a. radiation with HVL 2.0 mm Cu, FSD 50 cm (Table B-2c).
   b. ^{60}Co radiation at SSD 80 cm (Table B-2e).
   c. 25 MeV linac radiation SSD 100 cm (Table B-2i).

4. Using appropriate isodose curves for a 15 × 4 cm ^{60}Co field at SSD 80 cm, estimate the shape and size of the 120% isodose surface when two 15 × 4 cm fields are applied in opposition 16 cm apart and are given equal doses of 1.0 Gy at the maximum.

5. Two 10 × 15 cm ^{60}Co fields at SSD 80 cm are arranged in opposition 20 cm apart and are given absorbed doses at the maximum of 1.0 Gy and 0.5 Gy respectively. Find the resultant dose along the axis for depths of 1, 5, 10, 15, and 19 cm measured from the entrance point of the field given the larger dose. Use data from Table B-2e.

6. The arrangement of fields shown in Figure 12-9a is used to treat a tumor midway between the AP fields, which are separated by 16 cm. The tumor is symmetrically situated between the oblique fields, which are 20 cm apart. ^{60}Co radiation at SSD 80 cm and field size 6 × 20 cm is used.
   a. Assuming each field is given the same dose, find the given dose to each field to yield a tumor dose of 60 Gy. Calculate the dose at a point 0.5 cm below the skin under the AP and the lateral fields.
   b. What dose should be given each field in order that the total skin dose be the same for all 6 fields and the tumor dose be 60 Gy? Evaluate the skin dose at a depth of 0.5 cm.
   c. By which of the techniques (a or b) will the smaller amount of energy by given to the patient? Discuss.
   d. What dose should be given each field in order that the dose contribution to the tumor from each of the fields be the same and the total tumor dose 60 Gy? For this arrangement calculate the total skin dose under the AP and lateral fields. Evaluate at a depth of 0.5 cm.

7. Two ^{60}Co fields 6 × 6 cm SSD 80 cm are directed at 60° to each other towards a point 10 cm vertically below the skin (as illustrated in Fig. 12-11a) and each given 1 Gy. Find the dose at the intersection of the axes and the maximum dose. Locate the position of the maximum dose.

8. Repeat the calculations of problem 7 using no bolus. Use the isodose shift method described in Chapter 11.

9. Three ^{60}Co 6 × 10 cm fields at SSD 80 cm are used to irradiate a tumor using a geometry similar to that of Figure 12-12. The distances from the entrance fields to the tumor are 10, 12, and 15 cm respectively. Find the given dose to each field to yield a tumor dose of 60 Gy,
   a. assuming each field is "given" the same dose.
   b. assuming the doses are balanced at the tumor.
   c. assuming each beam is "on" for the same length of time.

10. Combine 2 wedge fields like that of Figure 11-9 so that the axes intersect at a depth of 5 cm. Perform the combination with the axes at 60°, 90°, and 120°. Discuss your results from the point of view of homogeneity of dose in the region where the beams overlap.

11. Two parallel opposing 6 × 15 cm ^{60}Co fields 20 cm apart are used to treat the chest wall tangentially. Assuming the chest wall can be approximated by a cylindrical contour and that the fields are arranged so the top edges of the beam are 1 cm above the cylinder, determine the approximate isodose pattern.

12. A Farmer type ionization chamber is used to measure exposure rate on the axis of a

rotational cobalt 60 unit. The instrument gives readings of 61.0 for a 35 second exposure and 6.5 for 5 seconds when irradiated with a field size of 10×10 cm. The temperature and pressure were 25° C and 98.6 kPa at the time of measurement. The exposure calibration factor, as supplied by a standardization laboratory, is 1.025 R per scale reading. The factor to convert from exposure to absorbed dose in tissue is 0.00963 Gy/R and the attenuation factor for an equilibrium thickness of tissue is 0.985. Determine the dose rate in Gy/min in a small sample of soft tissue placed on the axis of rotation in a 4×15 cm beam. Take the output for this field compared to that of a 10×10 cm field to be 0.985.

13. The bladder described in Table 12-2 is to be treated to 60 Gy in 6 weeks (30 treatments) using rotation therapy with a 4×15 cm beam from the cobalt unit calibrated in problem 12. Find the average tissue-air ratio and the treatment time per day.

14. Repeat the treatment time calculation of problem 13 but for a 25 MV linear accelerator calibrated to give a dose rate on the axis of rotation of 2.4 Gy/min at a depth of 5 cm in a water phantom when irradiated with a 10×10 cm field. Take the dose rate at 5 cm depth in a 4×15 cm field to be 0.91 of that for the 10×10 cm field.

15. Following the method outlined in Table 12-3 and using an isodose distribution like that shown in Figure 12-23 for a 6×12 cm cobalt beam, draw an isodose distribution for complete rotation about a circular phantom having a diameter of 20 cm. Take the axis of rotation to be coincident with the center of the phantom. Note that this distribution will be a series of concentric circles. If every point within a cylindrical volume, having diameter 5.5 cm, were to be given a dose of at least 5.5 Gy, what must the axis dose be?

16. From the diagram produced for problem 15, find the dose at the geometrical edge of the beam expressed as a percentage of the axis dose.

17. From the dose distribution produced for problem 15, estimate the total energy imparted to the phantom. Assuming the target volume is the circle of diameter 5.5 cm, what fraction of the total energy imparted is delivered to the target?

18. Derive equation 12-2 from equation 12-1.

Chapter **13**

BRACHYTHERAPY—INTERCAVITARY AND INTERSTITIAL SOURCES

13.01   **INTRODUCTION**

$\mathbf{A}$lmost immediately after the discovery of radium by Marie and Pierre Curie in 1898, it was used to treat cancer by placing it near or in contact with a tumor. Treatment in this way is called brachytherapy, which means "short distance" therapy (as opposed to teletherapy, or "long distance" therapy). In brachytherapy the radioactive sources may be inserted into the body in direct contact with the malignant tissue so that a very high radiation dose can be delivered just where it is needed. For years these procedures were performed using radium. With the advent of the nuclear reactor many new isotopes have become available, and now even though other isotopes have largely supplanted radium, the procedures have remained those that were designed for it. In this chapter we will discuss the procedures and the use of a number of isotopes for brachytherapy. We will, however, begin with radium and will introduce other isotopes only after the system of dosimetry has been described.

13.02   **RADIUM AND ITS RADIOACTIVE SERIES**

Radium is the sixth member of the naturally occurring uranium series, which starts with $^{238}_{92}U$ and ends with stable $^{206}_{82}Pb$. Radium disintegrates with a half-life of 1622 years to form radon, $^{222}_{86}Rn$, which is a radioactive gas. If the radon is prevented from escaping, by being sealed in a capsule, there will be a buildup of several daughter products that form the radium series, consisting of seven radioactive isotopes: $^{218}_{84}Po$, $^{214}_{82}Pb$, $^{214}_{83}Bi$, $^{214}_{84}Po$, $^{210}_{82}Pb$, $^{210}_{83}Bi$, and $^{210}_{84}Po$. Some of these isotopes decay by means of an α particle and some via a β particle. One can tell the type of decay by noting the change in the atomic number. Two of those that decay by ejecting a β particle ($^{214}_{82}Pb$ and $^{214}_{83}Bi$) also emit γ rays. The encapsulation is thick enough to stop the α and β particles but not the γ rays and they can be used for the irradiation of tumors. The spectrum of these γ rays is discussed later in this section.

The growth of daughter products and radioactive equilibrium was discussed in section 3.16. When a sample of radium is placed in a sealed container, because it is undergoing radioactive decay, all of its decay products will be produced and in due course radioactive equilibrium will

453

be established. Under these conditions, each element in the chain disintegrates at the same rate as it is being produced. If N_1 is the number of parent atoms present with decay constant λ_1, then the number which disintegrate per second will be $N_1\lambda_1$. Initially, there will be no daughter atoms present but as the parent decays the number of these daughters, N_2, will increase until the rate at which they in turn decay ($N_2\lambda_2$) is equal to the rate at which they are produced. From this time on, the daughter will decay with the half-life of the parent and equilibrium between them is established with $N_1\lambda_1 = N_2\lambda_2$. After a period of time, long compared with the half-lives of the daughters, all of them will be in equilibrium and will decay with the half-life of the parent. Under these conditions:

$$N_1\lambda_1 = N_2\lambda_2 = N_3\lambda_3 = N_4\lambda_4 \text{ etc. or}$$

$$\frac{N_1}{T_1} = \frac{N_2}{T_2} = \frac{N_3}{T_3} = \frac{N_4}{T_4} \tag{13-1}$$

where the second equation is obtained from the first by using the relation between half-life T and decay constant λ (eq. 3-5). Equation 13-1 indicates that when a member of the series has a short half-life, the number of atoms of this type will be small, and conversely if the half-life is long, the number present at any time will be large.

Example 13-1. A sealed container holds 1 mg of radium. Find the number of atoms of ^{214}Bi present after equilibrium has been established.

> About one month after the source is sealed the amounts of radon, ^{218}Po, ^{214}Pb, and ^{214}Bi will be in equilibrium with the radium because one month is long compared with the longest half-life (3.83 days). The radon present has an activity of 1 mCi, or 3.7×10^7 Bq. (See section 3.03.)
>
> $\therefore 3.7 \times 10^7 = N_1\lambda_1 = N_2\lambda_2 = N_3\lambda_3$ etc.
>
> The half-life of ^{214}Bi is 19.7 min = 1180 s and
>
> $$\lambda = \frac{0.693}{1180s} = 0.587 \times 10^{-3} \text{ s}^{-1}$$
>
> $$\therefore N = \frac{3.7 \times 10^7}{0.587 \times 10^{-3}} = 6.3 \times 10^{10} \text{ atoms of } {}^{214}\text{Bi}.$$

When radium is sealed in a container, equilibrium is established and the active deposits decay with the half-life of radium, which is 1622 years. Because this is so long, a source of radium may be considered as being constant in strength over many years.

The Gamma Ray Spectrum of Radium

Radium in equilibrium with its decay products emits a number of gamma ray lines, one from radium itself, three from ^{214}Pb, and eight

TABLE 13-1
Principal Gamma Ray Lines from Radium and Its Active Deposits

Transition	Energy of Gamma Ray (MeV)	Relative Number
Radium → Radon	0.18	0.012
$^{214}Pb \rightarrow {}^{214}Bi$	0.241	0.115
	0.294	0.258
	0.350	0.450
$^{214}Bi \rightarrow {}^{214}Po$	0.607	0.658
	0.766	0.065
	0.933	0.067
	1.120	0.206
	1.238	0.063
	1.379	0.064
	1.761	0.258
	2.198	0.074
		2.290

from ^{214}Bi. These twelve lines are listed in Table 13-1 together with the relative numbers of each for one alpha ray disintegration of radium. It is seen that on the average each alpha disintegration of radium is followed by 2.29 gamma rays.

The complicated spectrum can, for many purposes, be considered as equivalent to two lines of energy 0.55 and 1.65 MeV. Their mean energy is quite similar to that from cobalt 60 (1.25 MeV). From the point of view of protection, however, radium requires thicker barriers than does cobalt because of the presence of higher energy gamma rays. After passing through a thick barrier, the softer components from the radium are filtered out leaving only the more penetrating components such as 1.76 and 2.2 MeV, and these are much more difficult to stop than the most penetrating component from cobalt 60 (1.33 MeV). An attenuation factor of 50 may be achieved for both radiations by 7 cm of Pb, but a factor of 10^4 requires 16 cm of Pb for ^{60}Co and 20 cm of Pb for radium.

13.03   ACTIVITY AND SOURCE SPECIFICATION
Radium

The quantity of radium in a source is always specified in mg or g of radium element. The first radium standards were prepared by Mme. Curie in the form of chemically pure salts and these standards are stored near Paris. Secondary standards are now available in most of the National Laboratories. Although radium sources are expressed in mg, they are measured by comparing their activity with that of a standard source containing a known mass of radium. In this comparison, the standard and the unknown are placed in turn near an ionization chamber and the ionization currents compared. This is a sensible way to measure radium sources because it is the emitted γ radiation that is of interest not the number of mg.

Because the gamma rays from a radium source arise mainly from the daughter products, new preparations of radium must be stored long enough (about 1 month) to establish equilibrium before the comparison can be made in the standardization laboratory.

Early experiments with radium indicated that one gram of radium underwent 3.7×10^{10} disintegrations per second. This became the reference for the first unit of activity, the curie (Ci). Later it was determined that one gram of radium produced in fact fewer disintegrations per second, closer to 3.61×10^{10}, but the number 3.7×10^{10} was retained for the unit. When other isotopes came into common use, the definition of the curie was extended to include them, as discussed in section 3.03. The present (SI) unit of activity is the becquerel (Bq) and is 1 disintegration per second. One millicurie is thus equal to 3.7×10^7 Bq or 37.0 MBq. One curie is equal to 37 GBq.

Radon

For some applications, it has been convenient to seal radon gas into a small hollow gold tube, called a gold seed, and use it instead of radium. The strength of such a source is measured in millicuries (now becquerels). Since the gamma activity of radium arises from decay products further down the decay series than radon (mainly ^{214}Pb and ^{214}Bi) and since the amounts of these active deposits depend upon the amount of radium or radon present, a 1 mCi radon seed will emit the same radiation as a 1 mg radium needle. As in the case of radium, the strength of a radon seed is measured by comparing its gamma activity with that of a known source of radium.

Radon as a useable brachytherapy source is obtained from radium in a radon plant (H15) wherein the radium salt in solution is kept in a vacuum-tight vessel in a safe surrounded by lead. As the radium disintegrates, the radon gas is liberated from the solution and collects above it. This gas is pumped off, purified, and then forced into gold tubing or into a small glass bulb. There are very few radon plants still operating because other isotopes are more convenient and less dangerous to use.

Suppose a radon plant contains 100 mg of radium. Then, if the radon is allowed to collect until equilibrium occurs, 100 mCi of radon could be pumped off and loaded into seeds. The radon that has been removed will start to decay with half-life 3.83 days, and in the meantime, the amount of radon in the plant will again increase as it is produced from the radium parent. The total radon activity in the seeds and in the plant must together total 100 mCi at all times. Therefore, the growth of radon activity in the plant will follow a growth curve like the one shown in Figure 3-13. This growth curve will be exactly the same shape as the radon decay curve but will be inverted starting at the origin, reaching 50% after 1 half-life (3.83 days), 75% after 2 half-lives, 87.5% after 3 half-lives.

13.04   **EXPOSURE RATE AND DOSE RATE FROM**
                     RADIUM AND RADON SOURCES

It is useful to relate the activity of a radioactive source to the exposure rate it produces at a specified distance. A quantity designated as Γ and discussed in section 7.15 has been used for this purpose. This quantity has been redefined and altered slightly a number of times. It has been called the "K factor," the "specific gamma ray constant," the "exposure rate constant," and the "air kerma-rate constant." Γ for radium has been obtained by experiment rather than calculation. The experiment is performed by placing an ionization chamber of known volume at a known distance from a standard radium source and measuring the exposure rate. This was carefully measured by Attix and Ritz (A9), who obtained a value of 8.26 ± 0.05 R hr^{-1} mg^{-1} for a distance of 1 cm. This is not an easy experiment to perform and in spite of great care there is still an uncertainty of ± 0.05 (0.6%) in this important constant, and a rounded off figure of 8.25 will be used in the calculations in this chapter. The following important relation is the basis of all radium dosimetry:

> *The exposure rate 1 cm from a 1 mg source of*   (13-2a)
> *radium filtered by 0.5 mm Pt is 8.25 R/hr*

The exposure rate constant is:

$$\Gamma_{Ra} = 0.825 \text{ R m}^2 \text{ hr}^{-1} \text{ Ci}^{-1} \qquad (13\text{-}2b)$$

A simple example will illustrate the use of these statements.

Example 13-2. A 10 mg radium source is inadvertently left in an unshielded drawer for 7 hours. Estimate the exposure that would be received by a worker who remained at a distance of 20 cm from the source for this time. Use both 13-2a and 13-2b.

$$\text{Exposure rate from 1 mg Ra at 20 cm} = 8.25 \frac{R}{hr} \times \left(\frac{1.0}{20.0}\right)^2$$

$$= 0.0206 \text{ R/hr}$$

Exposure rate from 10 mg at 20 cm = 0.206 R/hr

$$\text{Exposure for 7 hr} = 0.206 \frac{R}{hr} \times 7 \text{ hr} = 1.44 \text{ R}$$

Alternatively, using equation 13-2b we obtain:

$$\text{Exposure} = \frac{0.825 \text{ R m}^2}{hr \text{ Ci}} \times \frac{10 \times 10^{-3} \text{ Ci}}{(0.2 \text{ m})^2} \times 7 \text{ hr} = 1.44 \text{ R}$$

Some filtration is necessary in any experiment to determine the Γ factor of radium, because the penetrating beta particles that are emitted must be prevented from emerging from the source. A filter of 0.5 mm Pt is standard and the exposure rate with other filtrations may be related to it by a simple correction factor as follows. The exposure rate should be increased by 2% for each 0.1 mm Pt filtration less than 0.5 mm Pt and decreased by the same percentage if the filtration is more than 0.5 mm Pt. For example, a radium source using 1.0 mm Pt gives an exposure rate 10% less than 8.25 R/hr per milligram.

The Γ factor for radium may be calculated using the ideas of section 7.15 and the spectral distribution of the photon energies given in Table 13-I. The Γ factor is obtained from Figure 7-15 for each gamma ray from radium, weighted by the numbers in the last column of Table 13-1 and each is corrected for the attenuation produced by 0.5 mm Pt. By adding these weighted corrected Γ factors, the total exposure 1 cm from a 1 mg source of radium may be obtained. Since this calculation depends upon a number of factors not known too precisely, such as the spectrum from radium, the effects of filtration, and the production of bremsstrahlung, it is more accurate to obtain the Γ factor for radium by experiment as described above. The results of calculation and experiment are, however, in fair agreement.

13.05   CONSTRUCTION AND CARE OF BRACHYTHERAPY SOURCES

The following section deals primarily with radium sources but applies also to sources that use other isotopes such as ^{137}Cs or ^{60}Co. Autoradiographs of radium sources are shown in Figure 13-1. These pictures were taken by clamping the radium needle firmly against a film for a few seconds and during this time making a short x ray exposure at about 30 kV$_p$. The needle casts a shadow in the x ray picture and the position of the radioactive material is shown by the blackening caused by the radiation. Radium, usually in the form of RaCl$_2$, is mixed with a filler and loaded into cells about 1 cm long and 1 mm in diameter, and these cells are sealed. These sealed cells are then loaded into a platinum or steel sheath, which in turn is also sealed. The cells can easily be distinguished in Figure 13-1. In such needles, there are two seals that must be broken before the radium can escape. The escape of radium creates a very serious contamination problem (G11).

All new needles should be tested radiographically, as in Figure 13-1, before being accepted from the manufacturer. A slight bunching of the activity can be seen in some of the needles of Figure 13-1. If the bunching is severe, the needles should not be accepted. In the top needle of Group B, there appears to be some active deposits between two of the cells, which probably means that some of the active deposit was left on the outside of the cell at the time of loading.

In spite of the best care, needles may become bent, and leaks develop. It is important that twice a year all brachytherapy sources be tested for

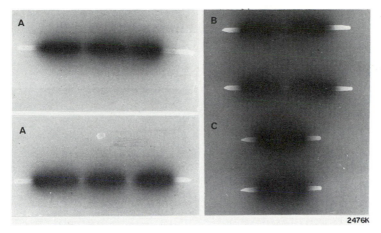

Figure 13-1. Autoradiograph and x ray picture of a selection of radium needles. A, 3 mg needles, active length 4.0 cm and actual length 6.0 cm. B, 2 mg needle, active length 2.9 cm and actual length 4.4 cm. C, 1 mg needle, active length 1.5 cm and actual length 2.8 cm.

leaks. It is necessary to have test equipment capable of detecting 0.2 kBq of radioactive contamination or for radium sources the leakage of about 40 Bq of radon in 24 hours. Radium sources can be tested as follows. About 6 sources of a given type are placed in a test tube with a wad of absorbent cotton on top and sealed with a stopper. A day later the cotton is tested for activity by holding it near a Geiger counter. If the needles have leaked, radon will have escaped and some of its active deposits will be in the cotton. If the group of needles contains a leaker, each should be placed in separate test tubes and tested again to find the faulty needle. The leaking needles should be returned to the manufacturer for repair.

Other sources must be tested by wiping each of them a few times with a pad of gauze and then testing the pad with a sensitive counter. If the count rate over the gauze is appreciably above background, contamination is indicated. Further investigation may be required, however, to determine whether it came from that source or from some other source that previously occupied the same storage location.

These tests are easy to perform but it is not always easy to interpret the results in absolute terms. Rawlinson (R6), using a liquid scintillation counter, designed a faster and more sensitive test for radon leakage. A number of sources to be tested are placed in a small closed container, containing also an open vial of the scintillating liquid. If radon is escaping, it will be entrapped by the fluid and may be detected by the counter. Exposure to the radon for an hour is sufficient. Exceedingly small leaks may be found in this manner and the leakage rate may be known in absolute terms. The above tests should be done routinely or after any incident that could result in source damage. If a source is bent or thought to be damaged, it should be segregated immediately and tested.

In order to achieve a uniform distribution of radiation in tumors, an adequate supply of needles with different linear densities of activity are required. It is difficult to distinguish at a glance needles that have the same external length but different activities. Most manufacturers are willing to gold plate a section of the needle for purposes of identification. This is more practical than numbering the needles, because small engraved numbers are soon illegible. In addition, the time consumed in attempting to read them constitutes an unnecessary radiation hazard.

When needles are purchased, the manufacturer specifies the activity, the active length, which is the distance between the extreme ends of the active deposits, the actual length, the diameter, and for radium the filtration. For reasons that will be discussed later, it is common practice to specify the activity of brachytherapy sources in terms of "radium equivalents." It is then not necessary to know the actual activity in, for example, a ^{137}Cs source. What is known is that it will produce the same dose rate (at the treatment distance) as a radium source of the specified activity. When sources are received, each should be measured by holding it for a reproducible length of time at a fixed point near some radiation measuring device. An electrometer and a large ionization chamber with a "well" in it is ideal but any sensitive ionization chamber can be used. It is an advantage if the response of the dosimeter is "air equivalent" (see Chapter 7). Variations from source to source will be present because it is impossible to load all sources with exactly the same activity. Any source that differs from the group by more than ±10% should not be accepted.

In specifying sources in terms of radium equivalent it is important to state the filtration that was used for the radium. For example, needles that are to be used for interstitial implants should be referred to radium filtered with 0.5 mm Pt, while tubes that are going to be used for gynecological insertions should be stated as equivalent to radium filtered with 1.0 mm Pt. The apparent inconsistency is unfortunate. It is maintained, however, to conform to long established procedures. This will be discussed more fully in the next section. The difference between the two specifications is about 10%.

STORAGE. Brachytherapy sources should be stored in such a way that every one is immediately accessible with minimum handling and yet be stored behind sufficient lead to be completely safe (see Chapter 15). Figure 13-2 shows a type of radium safe that has been in use for a number of years in 4 of the clinics of the Ontario Cancer Foundation (W8). In this safe the sources are stored in a series of vertical drawers, the tops of which are flush with the stainless steel working surface of the unit. Any one of the drawers may be raised by turning a selector valve to the proper position, which directs compressed air under that drawer. When the drawer is raised the ends of the needles are exposed and they may be removed by forceps. The insert shows, in greater detail, one of the drawers in its raised position. Holes in the lead block for individual needles may be seen. The drawer is then returned to its normal position with the unused sources. The large safe shown in Figure 13-2 has 29 drawers arranged in a rectangular array of 23 × 50 cm with a total working area of 60 × 180 cm. Separate drawers are used for each type of source. A few of the larger drawers are designed to store finished loaded molds or applicators. With such a safe, there is a minimum amount of transportation of the sources, for they can be sterilized and prepared for use on the working surface of the safe.

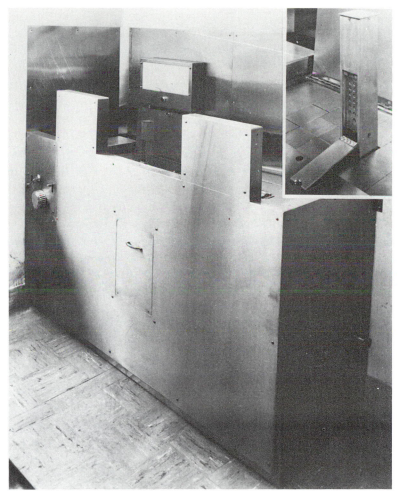

Figure 13-2. Photograph of radium safe and radium preparation surface in the Ontario Cancer Institute. Two barriers may be seen, behind which the technician may work. The insert shows the details of one of the drawers in its raised position. Lead glass eye shields may be added over each barrier if desired.

13.06 <mark>DOSE PRESCRIPTION IN</mark>
<mark>BRACHYTHERAPY TREATMENTS</mark>

During the early years of the use of radium a great deal of clinical experience was accumulated by a number of "schools" of radiotherapy. From this experience, rules were developed governing the arrangement of radium sources that were required to produce a desired clinical result. The rules were developed more or less by "trial and error" and were subsequently put into a systematic form. In this book we shall follow the "Manchester System" (M12, P8, P9) in which the sources are to be arranged in well-defined geometrical patterns. If the rules of source placement are followed for each treatment, the dosage pattern will be repeated and the dosage can be characterized by the product milligrams of radium multiplied by the time that it is left in place. This quantity, expressed as milligram hours, will be proportional to the total energy imparted (also called integral dose, section 11.08) to the patient. It does not tell anything about the distribution of the dose, although this can be calculated provided the details of the source strengths and placement are known.

The dosage system developed for radium has proved to be so useful that although other isotopes have now largely replaced radium, the radium system is still used and the strengths of the "radium substitutes" are given in "milligram equivalents" of radium. For example a ^{137}Cs tube used for gynecological purposes will be listed as equivalent to so many milligrams of radium filtered with 1.0 mm Pt. The equivalence is judged by equal dose rates at equal distances from the sources. The radium equivalent of a source of a known activity may be determined from the following relation.

$$Ra_{eq} = A \cdot \Gamma/\Gamma_{Ra} \qquad (13\text{-}3)$$

where A is the activity of the (radium substitute) source, Γ is its exposure rate constant, and Γ_{Ra} is the exposure rate constant for radium. Strictly speaking the right side of equation 13-3 should also be multiplied by the factor $(\bar{\mu}/\rho)/(\bar{\mu}/\rho)_{Ra}$, the ratio of mass energy absorption coefficients for the photon spectra of the two sources. This factor is so close to unity in most cases, however, that it is normally neglected.

The determination of radium equivalence is best carried out experimentally by measuring exposure rates a few cm distant from the source and repeating the measurements using a known radium source. These measurements are most appropriately made with an air-equivalent ionization chamber. Details are discussed by the NCRP (N7).

The radium equivalents for a few gamma ray sources important in brachytherapy, along with other relevant properties, are given in Table 13-2.

TABLE 13-2
Data for Selected Gamma-Ray Sources*

Radionuclide	Half-life	Photon Energies MeV	Exposure Rate Constant R m² h⁻¹ Ci⁻¹	Radium Equivalence mg Ra (0.5 mm Pt)
Cesium 137	30.0 y	0.662	0.328	0.398
Cobalt 60	5.26 y	1.17-1.33	1.307	1.58
Gold 198	2.698 d	0.41-1.09	0.238	0.288
Iodine 125	60.25 d	0.035	0.133	0.161
Iridium 192	74.2 d	0.136-1.06	0.400	0.485
Tantalum 182	115.0 d	0.043-1.45	0.782	0.948
Radium 226 in equilibrium and filtered by 0.5 mm Pt	1604 y	0.047-2.44	0.825	1.000

*Data from NCRP 41 (N7).

The usefulness of milligram hours in brachytherapy prescriptions is illustrated by the following example.

Example 13-3. A treatment of cancer of the uterus is to involve 5,000 mg hr using ^{137}Cs sources. The insertion is to be for 96 hours. Calculate the amount of cesium needed.

cesium required = 5000/96 = 52 mg Ra equivalent

When short-lived isotopes such as radon or ^{198}Au are inserted into tissue and left to decay, the number of milligram hours may be determined from the following expression.

$$\text{Ra milligram hours equivalent} = \text{Ra}_{eq} \times 1.44 \times T_{1/2} \quad (13\text{-}4)$$

where Ra_{eq} is the radium equivalent of the source as given by equation 13-3. In this expression the product $1.44 \times T_{1/2}$ is the mean life of the isotope (see section 3.04). The use of this relation may be clarified by an example.

Example 13-4. A certain treatment may be carried out in 5 days using 3.0 mg of radium. What amount of ^{198}Au would be required to produce the same energy imparted.

milligram hours of radium = 3.0 × 5 × 24 = 360 mg hr
Required gold 198 = 360/(1.44 × 2.698 × 24) = 3.86 mg Ra_{eq}
or, in activity = 3.86 × (0.825/0.238) = 13.4 mCi gold.

In the above example, the gold had an initial strength of 3.86 mg Ra equivalent (13.4 mCi). During the treatment it underwent decay but the total energy imparted would be the same as if it remained at its initial strength and was then removed at the end of its mean life of 93.2 hours (1.44 × 2.698 × 24).

For many years radium dosage was given in terms of "emitted dose" in mg hr. Statements of dose in this unit have meaning only when the geometric arrangement of the source is reproduced from patient to patient in exactly the same way. In the early 1930s the whole problem of radium dosage was placed on a rational basis by Paterson and Parker (P8, P9, T8) who devised a system of radium dosage called the Manchester System (M12), which enabled the radiotherapist to express the dose to the patient in "roentgens." The discussion that follows is based mainly on this system but is altered slightly so that the dose to the tumor may be expressed in terms of absorbed dose. In this system, the radiotherapist first decides on the dose to the tumor. He then calculates from tables and charts "R," the number of mg hr of radium required to deliver a dose of 10 Gy and finally the total number of milligram hours required for the selected tumor dose. Radioactive sources may be applied to tumors using surface applicators, interstitial single-plane implants, two-plane implants, volume implants, cylindrical implants, and as linear sources. Each of these methods will be discussed in detail, but first we will discuss the dosage pattern around a single linear radioactive source.

13.07   **RADIUM ISODOSE CURVES**

Isodose curves can be constructed for a radium source by joining points of equal dose rate. This is illustrated in Figure 13-3, where the isodose curves for a tube containing 13.3 mg of radium are shown. Such curves can be calculated for any linear source by the use of Sievert's integrals (S19) or obtained by direct measurement. The dose rate along the axis of the tube is less than it is at right angles because of the increased effect of oblique filtration. Very near the tube, in the region of high dose rate, the isodose curves will tend to be almost parallel to the source over its central region. Hence the isodose curves are more or less elliptical. At great distances, the isodose curves will tend to be circular for the source will behave as a point source. Along the axis the radiation will tend to be slightly more intense than along the line OB (Fig. 13-3). Along this line the oblique filtration of the platinum is a maximum, while exactly along the axis, part of the filtration of the encapsulation is replaced by the lesser filtration of the radioactive material itself. Consequently, there is a small cone of more intense radiation along the axis.

The distributions in space can be obtained by rotation of Figure 13-3 about the axis of the tube. Figure 13-3 may be used with reasonable accuracy for 5, 10, or 20 mg sources of the same length by multiplying the absorbed dose rates by the appropriate factors. The distribution of radiation when radium is placed in the uterus or cervix can be obtained by such isodose curves.

Computer methods have been extensively applied to the calculation

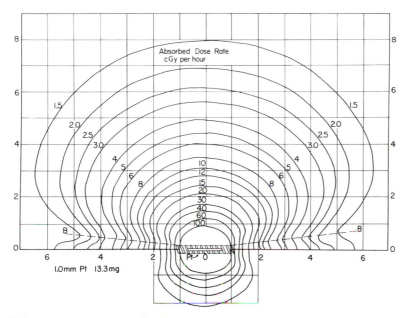

Figure 13-3. Dosage rate in cGy/hr from a 13.3 mg tube of radium of active length 1.35 cm, actual length 2.17 cm, and filtration 1 mm of platinum.

of radiation dosages around radium sources (Y4, S37). The calculation method most often employed is the repeated evaluation of the Sievert integral, which will now be described, although a number of programs use stored tables of numbers and look-up procedures.

Consider the radium source shown in Figure 13-4 with linear source density ρ and filtration d of platinum. The absorbed dose rate at P may be calculated as follows. The element of length dx of the source will contain ρ dx mg of radium and will produce at P a dose rate dD given by:

$$dD = \frac{\Gamma \, \rho \, dx \, e^{-\mu d/\cos\theta}}{r^2} \, f_{tis}$$

where $\Gamma \, \rho dx$ is the exposure rate in R/hr, 1 cm from the source of strength ρdx mg; r^2 corrects the exposure rate by the inverse square law; the exponential factor gives the attenuation produced by d/cos θ cm of the platinum sheath with linear absorption coefficient μ; f_{tis} converts exposure in air to absorbed dose to tissue. This expression may be integrated to give D, the dose rate from the whole source.

$$D = \frac{\Gamma \, \rho}{h} \, f_{tis} \int_{\theta_1}^{\theta_2} e^{-\mu d/\cos\theta} \, d\theta \qquad (13-5)$$

This integral cannot be evaluated analytically but has been determined using numerical integration by Sievert (S19).

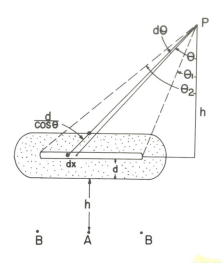

Figure 13-4. Diagram illustrating how the dose may be calculated at points near a linear source.

13.08   **LINEAR SOURCES**

Using equation 13-5, Paterson and Parker (P9) calculated the number of mg hr (R_L) in a source of active length L required to deliver an exposure of 1000 R to the point A (Fig. 13-4) h cm from the center of the source. Their results, converted to gray and allowing for an alteration* in the value of Γ for radium, are given in Table 13-3 (M12).

This table contains 2 parts, the first part for a filtration of 1.0 mm Pt and the second for 0.5 mm Pt. One table cannot be obtained from the other by a simple 10% correction factor because of the effects of oblique filtration. The correction will depend on the relative values of L and h. For small values of L, the effects of oblique filtration are small and the simple 10% correction factor is satisfactory (compare for example the entries for L = 0.5 and h = 2.0, which differ by 10%). However, for long active lengths and small values of h, the corrections are much greater (compare the entries for L = 20 and h = 0.5, which differ by over 17%).

Example 13-5. Three sources, each of 10 mg, filtration 1.0 mm Pt, active length 2 cm, actual length 3.0 cm, are arranged as a single line source. Find how long these should be left in the uterine canal to deliver a dose of 60 Gy to a point 1.0 cm from the center of the source.

> For this arrangement of sources, the distance between the extreme
>   ends of the active deposits is 8.0 cm.
> For L = 8.0   h = 1.0 R_L = 472 (Table 13-3)
> Required emitted radiation = 6 × 472 = 2832 mg hr
> Treatment time = 2832/30 = 94.4 hr.

---

*The original data was based on a value of 0.84 for the exposure rate constant for radium. The numbers were later multiplied by the factor C = 0.84/(0.825 × 0.957) = 1.064 (J12). The number 0.957 is the value of f_{tis} used at the time these tables were prepared. At the present time f_{tis} would be taken as 0.963. This would suggest a revision of the numbers by −0.6%. This is not significant, however, and so no further change has been made.

TABLE 13-3

Linear Sources

R_L—(mg hr to deliver 10 Gy) to a point h cm from the center of a linear source of active length L (point A, Fig. 13-5)

Active Length L	Treatment Distance–h cm						
	0.5	0.75	1.0	1.5	2.0	2.5	3.0
(a) Filtration 1.0 mm Pt							
0.0	35	79	140	317	562	878	1264
0.5	41	83	144	321	567	882	1267
1.0	49	91	153	330	576	889	1277
1.5	58	103	166	344	589	903	1293
2.0	69	119	183	362	609	922	1313
2.5	81	136	202	384	633	950	1341
3.0	93	153	224	411	662	983	1372
3.5	106	171	247	440	696	1019	1409
4.0	119	189	270	471	732	1059	1450
5.0	146	227	319	536	812	1146	1545
6.0	172	265	369	606	898	1242	1651
7.0	199	304	420	679	989	1347	1768
8.0	227	346	472	754	1084	1459	1890
9.0	255	387	527	830	1181	1574	2015
10.0	282	428	581	908	1277	1691	2149
12.0	337	511	688	1065	1479	1932	2431
14.0	394	594	798	1225	1683	2181	2724
16.0	449	678	909	1385	1894	2435	3022
18.0	505	762	1019	1549	2104	2692	3326
20.0	562	846	1128	1713	2317	2953	3633
(b) Filtration 0.5 mm Pt							
0.0	32	70	127	285	506	792	1139
0.5	35	74	129	289	509	795	1142
1.0	41	81	136	295	517	801	1151
1.5	50	91	147	305	529	813	1165
2.0	59	104	162	320	546	830	1185
2.5	69	118	179	340	569	851	1210
3.0	79	133	196	365	594	877	1237
3.5	89	148	214	391	620	908	1268
4.0	100	163	234	417	650	943	1300
5.0	123	195	274	471	718	1018	1377
6.0	146	228	316	530	789	1101	1466
7.0	169	260	359	588	864	1189	1564
8.0	192	292	404	651	944	1281	1668
9.0	213	325	448	714	1025	1375	1776
10.0	235	359	493	778	1109	1472	1887
12.0	280	427	581	908	1272	1674	2121
14.0	326	496	671	1038	1442	1882	2362
16.0	371	566	761	1170	1615	2096	2609
18.0	419	634	853	1302	1791	2309	2859
20.0	465	704	944	1438	1967	2523	3117

This table was prepared from the original by Meredith (M12) by multiplying his values by C = 1.064.

The dose at a point opposite the end of a needle (Point B, Fig. 13-5) depends only upon the ratio L/h. This dose, expressed as a percentage of the dose at point A opposite the center of the needle, is shown in Figure 13-5 as a function of the ratio L/h.

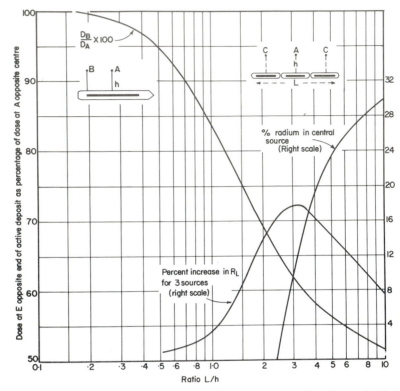

Figure 13-5. Upper left, graph showing the dose, D_B, opposite the end of the linear source (point B) as a percent of the dose, D_A, opposite the middle (point A). The graph is labelled $100 \times D_B/D_A$ and the points B and A are shown on the small diagram. Upper right, percentage radium required in central source to give the same dose to points A and C. The points A and C may be seen in the diagram showing the 3 tandem sources of total active length L. Bottom, percent increase in R_L for differentially loaded 3-source arrangement giving equal doses to A and C.

Example 13-6. Find the dose opposite the end of the linear source of example 13-5.

L = 8.0 cm, h = 1 cm and L/h = 8.0
From Figure 13-5, dose opposite end is 53% of dose opposite center.

Dose received at the end of source is $\dfrac{53}{100} \times 60.0 = 31.8$ Gy.

Differentially Loaded Linear Source

By arranging three sources in line (see insert of Fig. 13-5) with a weaker source in the middle, it is possible to achieve the same dose at points A and C. The amount of radium that should be placed in the central source expressed as a percent of the total is shown in Figure 13-5. Under these circumstances, an almost homogeneous dose from C to A to C may be achieved. For L/h less than 2.4, the central source should be omitted and an inactive gap left between the two outer needles. Under these conditions, a homogeneous dose from A to C cannot be achieved, the dose to A always being slightly higher than to C. When the radium is distributed with less radium in the central source, a larger number of milligram hours is required to deliver 10 Gy to point A. The percentage increase in R_L is given by the bell-shaped curve of Figure 13-5.

Example 13-7. From Example 13-5, calculate the percentage of radium that should be used in the central source and the total number of mg hr to deliver the same dose of 60 Gy to points A and C.

Since L/h = 8.0, radium in central source is 28.5% (Fig. 13-5)
Increase mg hr by 10% (bell-shaped curve of Fig. 13-5)
Required milligram hours = 2832 + 283 = 3115.

Calculations for linear sources may also be performed using Quimby's tables (Q1), which enable one to determine the dose at a whole series of points near a linear source.

Much more extensive data on the distribution of the radiation dosage in the neighborhood of radium sources has been provided by Young and Batho (Y4). They have used a computer to produce tables that enable one to know the dose rate at a large number of points on a rectangular grid around radium needles. The tables are made applicable to a very wide range of source lengths and strengths by using a reduced coordinate system where the coordinates of the grid are expressed in terms of the active length of the source. The advantage of this may be seen by referring to Figure 13-4 where the coordinates of point P are given by x and h as measured from the center of the source. If we write x = j L and h = k L, where L is the length of the active part of the source, then equation 13-5 may be written as:

$$D_P = \frac{\Gamma M}{L^2} \, f_{tis} \left[\frac{1}{k} \int_{\theta_1}^{\theta_2} e^{-\mu d/\cos\theta} \, d\theta \right] \qquad (13\text{-}5a)$$

In this expression we have also put $\rho = M/L$ where M is the radium content (for zero filtration) and L is the active length. The expression in the square brackets is, except for the filtration factor μd, independent of the dimensions of the radium source and depends only on θ, which in turn depends upon the coordinates j and k of the point P, and not on the length L. A separate table is required for each source diameter and filtration but not for each length, L. Batho (B16) and others have also evaluated the extent of reduction of dosage around a radium source due to tissue absorption and scattering. At a distance of 2 cm from the source, scattering nearly compensates for absorption and the dose rate in water is within about 2% of the dose rate in free space. On the other hand, at a distance of 10 cm the dose rate in water would be about 20% less than that in free space.

13.09   **INTERSTITIAL PLANAR IMPLANTS**

In cases where a tumor may be considered to be contained within a rectangularly shaped target volume, radioactive sources in the form of needles may be inserted directly into the tissues. The sources are generally placed in a plane at the center of this volume and if they are arranged properly a more or less uniform dosage will be delivered over the surface of the volume. In this section we will give a number of examples of such planar implants.

Rectangular Implants

In most cases of planar implants, especially where large areas are involved, rectangular arrangements are most readily achieved because long straight needles may be inserted to outline the tumor region. Typical arrangements of needles in implants are shown in Figure 13-6.

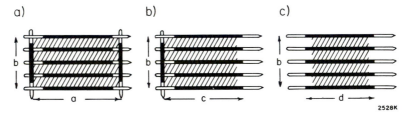

Figure 13-6. Diagrams showing arrangements of radioactive needles for planar implants. The shaded areas indicate the areas used for making dosage calculations.

The best type of implant is one in which both ends are crossed by needles as shown in Figure 13-6a. In this diagram, the regions of the active deposits are shown black and the inactive regions of the needles light. The area treated is a × b. Note that a and b are the separations between the extreme pairs of needles and correspond neither to the actual length of the needles nor their active lengths. It is necessary also to define the third dimension of the target volume—the distance away from the plane containing the needles. This has generally been called the "treatment distance," h. The treatment volume for Figure 13-6a would therefore be a × b × 2h.

Just as Table 13-3 gives the number of milligram hours required to produce 10 Gy for linear sources, in the same way Table 13-4 gives the number of milligram hours for radioactivity arranged over an area. Some examples will illustrate the use of this table and some of the rules for arranging the sources.

TABLE 13-4

Surface Applicators and Planar Implants

The table gives R_A, the number of mg hr required to deliver 10 Gy to muscle tissue for different areas and treatment distances. Filtration 0.5 mm Pt. The table may be used for planar implants by using a treatment distance of 0.5 cm.

Area cm²	Treatment Distance (cm)									
	.5	1.0	1.5	2.0	2.5	3.0	3.5	4.0	4.5	5.0
0	32	127	285	506	792	1139	1551	2026	2566	3166
1	72	182	343	571	856	1204	1625	2100	2636	3295
2	103	227	399	632	920	1274	1697	2172	2708	3349
3	128	263	448	689	978	1331	1760	2241	2772	3383
4	150	296	492	743	1032	1388	1823	2307	2835	3450
5	170	326	531	787	1083	1436	1881	2369	2896	3513
6	188	354	570	832	1134	1495	1938	2432	2956	3575
7	204	382	603	870	1182	1547	1993	2490	3011	3634
8	219	409	637	910	1229	1596	2047	2548	3067	3694
9	235	434	667	946	1272	1645	2099	2605	3123	3752
10	250	461	697	982	1314	1692	2149	2660	3178	3809
12	278	511	755	1053	1396	1780	2247	2769	3284	3917
14	306	557	813	1120	1475	1865	2341	2870	3389	4027
16	335	602	866	1184	1553	1947	2429	2968	3490	4131
18	364	644	918	1245	1622	2027	2514	3063	3585	4240
20	392	682	968	1303	1690	2106	2601	3155	3682	4341
22	418	717	1021	1362	1755	2180	2683	3242	3777	4441
24	444	752	1072	1420	1821	2252	2764	3326	3872	4540
26	470	784	1122	1477	1881	2328	2841	3405	3962	4634
28	496	816	1170	1530	1943	2398	2917	3484	4047	4730
30	521	846	1215	1582	2000	2468	2997	3562	4131	4824
32	546	876	1261	1635	2060	2532	3073	3639	4220	4915
34	571	909	1305	1688	2119	2598	3145	3713	4306	5000
36	594	935	1349	1743	2179	2662	3215	3787	4389	5089
38	618	967	1392	1793	2234	2726	3285	3859	4466	5174
40	642	994	1432	1843	2290	2787	3351	3931	4546	5258
42	664	1024	1472	1894	2344	2848	3421	4003	4626	5341
44	685	1053	1511	1942	2399	2908	3484	4071	4706	5422
46	708	1080	1550	1990	2452	2966	3548	4139	4781	5505
48	729	1110	1585	2037	2504	3025	3612	4207	4857	5586
50	750	1141	1619	2083	2556	3082	3676	4275	4929	5668
60	851	1283	1790	2319	2815	3362	3974	4605	5288	6054
70	947	1426	1944	2532	3059	3628	4257	4913	5632	6419
80	1044	1567	2092	2726	3301	3891	4532	5213	5958	6756

Filtration (mm Pt)	0.3	0.5	0.6	0.8	1.0	1.5
Correction to mg hrs	−4%	0	+2%	+6%	+10%	+20%

This table was prepared from the original by Meredith (M12) by multiplying his values by C = 1.064.

Example 13-8. An implant of the type shown in Figure 13-6a is designed using 5 long needles, 6 cm in actual length with active length 4.5 cm, and two crossing needles. The 2 outer long needles each contain 3 mg of radium (or equivalent) and the three central sources and the two crossing needles each contain 2 mg Ra. The total amount of radium is 16 mg. Determine the dose rate in a plane 0.5 cm from the plane of the implant and how long the sources should be left in place for a dose of 60 Gy. The dimension a is 5 cm and b is 4 cm.

Area of implant = $5 \times 4 = 20$ cm²
R_A from Table 13-4 = 392 mg hr/10 Gy
Dose rate = 10 Gy $\times$ 16 mg/392 mg hr = 0.41 Gy/hr
Time for 60 Gy = 6×392 mg hr/16 mg = 147 hr = 6 days 3 hr.

The dose distribution in the plane 0.5 cm away from the implant of Figure 13-6a and example 13-8 is shown in Figure 13-7a. The line representing 0.41 Gy/hr can be seen to include most of the area of the implant except for the corners, where the dose rate is well below the −10% expected. This is largely because of the gap in activity at the corners and could be eliminated if the active lengths of the crossing needles were greater.

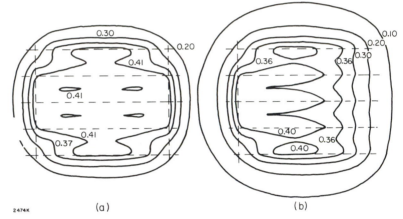

(a)   (b)

2474K

Figure 13-7. Isodose rate distributions in planes 0.5 cm away from the implants of Figure 13-6. The numbers are Gy/hr. The positions of the needles are indicated by the dashed lines. For a, both ends of the implant are crossed, for b only one end is crossed as in Figure 13-6b. (These isodose rate curves were obtained using program ISODOS, which is part of the Atomic Energy of Canada treatment planning system.)

In many anatomical situations, it will be impossible to cross one or both of the ends of the implant. When only one end is crossed (as indicated in Fig. 13-6b), the area that is treated should be considered as 0.90 b × c and when neither end is crossed the area treated is 0.80 b × d, that is, for each uncrossed end, the area treated should be taken as 10% less than the nominal area. Of course, care should be taken to insure that the shaded areas of Figure 13-6 amply include the tumor. After implants of this kind are made, radiographic examination is necessary to determine the actual dimensions of the implant.

Example 13-9. In attempting the implant of Figure 13-6a, it was not possible to cross the right hand end of the rectangle, resulting in the implant of Figure 13-6b. The implant now consists of two 3 mg needles 6 cm long, three 2 mg needles 6 cm long, and one 2 mg needle 4.5 cm long. The total amount of radium (or equivalent) is 14 mg and the dimensions a and b are 4.75 and 4 cm respectively. Determine the dose rate at a distance, h = 0.5 cm, and again the time for 60 Gy.

Area treated = $0.90 \times 4.75 \times 4.0 = 17.1$ cm^2
R_A (interpolation in Table 13-4) = 351 mg hr/10 Gy
Dose rate = 10 Gy $\times$ 14 mg/351 mg hr = 0.40 Gy/hr
Time for 60 Gy = 6×351 mg hr/14 mg = 150.4 hr = 6 days 6.4 hr

The dose distribution for the implant of Figure 13-6b and example 13-9 is shown in Figure 13-7b. The effect of the uncrossed end can be seen on the right side. The dose rate predicted by the Paterson-Parker system is 0.40 Gy/hr, and this can be seen to be representative of most of the area, although now a considerable portion of the treated area is lower than the -10% expected. The tables give a very good guide to calculation of the dose and timing, but for precise information about the dose distribution isodose curves are necessary.

DISTRIBUTION RULES. As can be seen from the above examples it is possible to achieve approximate dose uniformity at the "treatment distance." To do this, however, it is necessary to distribute the radioactivity in a planned way. The rules for rectangular implants are given in Table 13-5.

TABLE 13-5
Distribution Rules for Rectangular Planar Implants

Rectangles a × b	a < 2h arrange all radium on periphery
a = short side, b = long side	a > 2h add extra lines of radium parallel to
Linear density of the radium on periphery = ρ	longer side and spaced 2h
	If 1 line is added, use linear density $\rho/2$
	If 2 or more lines are added, use linear density $2\rho/3$

Elongation factor b/a	2	3	4
increase mg hr by	5%	9%	12%

Two-plane Implants

A single-plane implant can satisfactorily treat a block of tissue 1.0 cm thick. When a thicker block of tissue is involved, the activity should be distributed on two planes. Two-plane implants can satisfactorily treat blocks of tissue up to 2.5 cm. Calculations for a two-plane implant are illustrated in Figure 13-8.

Suppose the region involved has an area of 40 cm^2 and thickness 2.0 cm and is to be treated by placing the activity in planes A and B. The dose to the 3 planes D, C, and E may be calculated by using A = 40 and h = 0.5, 1.0 and 1.5, as indicated in Table 13-6.

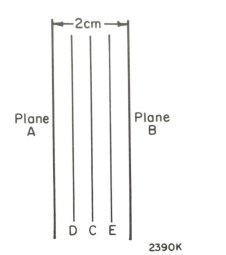

Figure 13-8. Diagram illustrating the calculation of dosage on planes C, E, and D between planes A and B of a two-plane implant.

994 mg hr are required to deliver 10.0 Gy to plane C. This amount of activity may be placed all on plane A or all on B as far as the dose to C is concerned but for homogeneity, it would be placed with 497 mg hr on each of the planes A and B. Now the doses to the other planes may be calculated as indicated in Table 13-6. It is seen that the dose to planes D and E is 12% higher than the dose to plane C. If the plane separations had been 2.5 cm, the minimum at the center would have been even more pronounced and hence not very satisfactory.

TABLE 13-6
Dose Calculations for a Two Plane Implant

	Plane D	Plane C	Plane E
	h = 0.5 cm	h = 1.0 cm	h = 1.5 cm
	$R_A = 642$	$R_A = 994$	$R_A = 1432$
Dose for 497 mg hr on plane A	7.74 Gy	5.0 Gy	3.46 Gy
Dose for 497 mg hr on plane B	3.46 Gy	5.0 Gy	7.74 Gy
Dose for 994 mg hr on A and B	11.2 Gy	10.0 Gy	11.2 Gy

In this example the number of milligram hours required to deliver 10.0 Gy to planes D or E is 994(10.0/11.2) = 887. Paterson and Parker (P9) calculate such an implant by placing h = 0.5 regardless of the plane separation and then increase the mg hr by 1.25, 1.41, and 1.52 for plane separations of 1.5, 2.0, and 2.5 cm. Such corrections are only approximate. Using this method, the number of mg hr to give 10.0 Gy to the "high" planes rather than to the central plane is determined. For this example $R_A = 642$ (A = 40, h = 0.5) and the corrected value is 462 × 1.41 = 905. This compares well with the value of 887 obtained above.

Surface Applicators and Seed Implants

Radioactive sources can also be used externally for treating lesions of the skin, and radioactive seeds can be inserted into tumors. Both can be arranged in circles or ovals as well as rectangles so more general distribution rules are required.

A surface applicator is shown schematically in Figure 13-9, where the area A is to be treated by distributing radioactive sources over an equal area A' in a plane separated from A by the distance h. By arranging the activity on the plane A' according to certain distribution rules, it is possible to achieve an almost uniform dose over the treated area A, as was discussed for the "treatment plane" using planar implants.

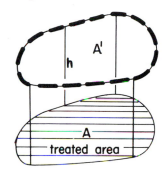

Figure 13-9. Diagram illustrating a surface applicator. The activity is arranged on plane A' to treat a plane of equal area A separated by distance h.

The distribution rules already described for planar implants also apply to surface applicators and seed implants but additional rules are required to look after the greater flexibility of placement that is possible. Rules for circular and oval surface applicators and seed implants are given in Table 13-7.

TABLE 13-7
Distribution Rules for Surface Applicators and Seed Implants

Distance between active ends should not exceed h

Circles with diameter d and treatment distance h. Arrange activity on outer circle, inner circle of diameter d/2, and as a central spot with percentage as indicated. For d/h = 2.83 the distribution is ideal.	d/h	1 to 3	3 to 6	6	7.5	10
	outer circle	100	95	80	75	70
	inner circle	0	0	17	22	27
	centre	0	5	3	3	3

Ellipses of small eccentricity may be used and considered as circles.

SMALL CIRCLES. In general, circular areas and circular distributions will tend to give the most uniform distributions. For small circles, whose diameter is less than 3 times the treatment distance (3h), all the activity should be placed around the periphery with not less than 6 radioactive foci. The distance between the active ends should not exceed h. A circle whose diameter is 2.83 h gives the optimum dose distribution over the treatment area and is referred to as ideal. Such an arrangement should be used whenever possible.

LARGE CIRCLES. For large circles and small h, the high dose will appear near the periphery of the treated region if all the activity is placed on the periphery of the area. In such cases, some of the activity is arranged as a central spot or on a circle of diameter d/2 with a central spot as well (illustrated in Fig. 13-10).

RECTANGLES. In many cases, circles or ellipses cannot be adapted to the region to be treated and square or rectangular arrangements may then be used. If a < 2h, all the activity should be put on the periphery but if a > 2h, extra lines parallel to the longer side should be added with the linear densities less than that of the periphery, as indicated in Table 13-5 and illustrated in Figure 13-10. Elongated rectangles require slightly more activity, as indicated in Table 13-5.

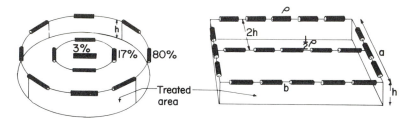

Figure 13-10. (a) Diagram showing the proper distribution of activity to treat a circular area of diameter d when the diameter of the circle is 6h. The percentage activity required in the 2 circles and at the center is given in Table 13-7 for d/h = 6. (b) Diagram showing the proper distribution of activity to treat a rectangular area a × b at a treatment distance h = a/4. Since a > 2h, an extra line has been added parallel to the longer side and spaced 2h as required by the distribution rule (Table 13-5).

Example 13-10. An area of 6.0 cm² is to be treated using radioactive sources placed on an equal area 1.0 cm away. Find the number of milligram hours of radium equivalent required to deliver a dose of 60.0 Gy in 5 days to the treated area.

R_A from Table 13-4 = 354 mg hr/10 Gy
mg hr for 60.0 Gy = 6 × 354 = 2124
Radium equivalent required = 2124/(5 × 24) = 17.7 mg.

DEPTH DOSE FROM SURFACE APPLICATORS. The depth dose d cm below the treated area may be obtained from Table 13-4 by comparing R_A for treatment distance h with R_A for treatment distance h + d. As an illustration, the depth dose 0.5 cm below the treated area of example 13-10 will be calculated:

From Table 13-4 for A = 6.0 cm² and h = 1.5 cm, R_A = 570 mg hr
From Table 13-4 for A = 6.0 cm² and h = 1.0 cm, R_A = 354 mg hr

Percentage depth dose $100 \times 354/570 = 62\%$
Dose to region 0.5 cm below surface $= 60.0 \times 62/100 = 37.2$ Gy

The percentage depth dose in this case is very small because the treatment distance is only twice as great as the depth of interest. If a larger depth dose is required, a large treatment distance should be used, in line with the discussions of Chapter 10. If the treatment distance were increased to 2.0 cm, the percentage depth doses would be $832/1134 = 73\%$.

13.10   VOLUME IMPLANTS

Where the region to be treated is more than 2.5 cm thick, the two-plane implant is not satisfactory because of the low dosage region midway between the planes. A volume implant in the form of a sphere, cube, or cylinder may then be useful. As in the case of all implants, there will be a region of high dose around each source. The number of mg hr to deliver 10.0 Gy (R_v) to a volume implant is given in Table 13-8 together with the distribution rules.

TABLE 13-8
Volume Implants

R_V—mg hr to give 10.0 Gy to volume implant: Radium equivalent for filtration of 0.5 mm Pt

Volume cm³	R_V mg hr	Distribution Rules
5	106	Volume should be considered as a surface with 75% activity and core
10	168	with 25%
15	220	
20	267	Rules for cylinders
30	350	
40	425	Belt—50% activity with minimum 8 needles
50	493	Ends—12.5% of activity on each end
60	556	Core—25% with minimum of 4 needles
80	673	For each uncrossed end, reduce volume by 7.5%
100	782	
140	979	$\dfrac{\text{Length}}{\text{Diameter}} =$ 1.5 2.0 2.5 3.0
180	1156	
220	1322	
260	1479	Increase mg hr 3% 6% 10% 15%
300	1627	
340	1768	
380	1902	

This table was prepared from the original by Meredith (M12) by multiplying his values by $C = 1.064$.

One of the most important types of volume implant is a cylinder (P10). When the cylinder is long compared with its diameter, the number of milligram hours must be increased as indicated by the elongation correction factors of Table 13-8. An example of a cylindrical volume implant will be given later. The distribution rules for other types of volume implants can be found in the original papers (M12, P8).

13.11   **RADIOGRAPHIC EXAMINATION OF**
                                RADIUM IMPLANTS

When surface applicators are constructed, there is no difficulty in placing the sources accurately on felt or sponge rubber of the required thickness. If this is done with care, the area A and the distance h can be controlled precisely and the dosage given the treated area accurately determined. There may, however, be difficulty in obtaining a proper distribution of activity with the limited variety of sources available in a department. For implants the sources can never be arranged exactly as the therapist plans, so some determination of the implant actually achieved is necessary. This can be done by taking anteroposterior (AP) and lateral x ray pictures of the implant and then recalculating it.

Figure 13-11 illustrates some of the geometrical considerations that are relevant. It shows projections of a radium needle in two planes at right angles as would be produced by a lateral and an AP radiograph. The needle has an actual length L but appears to have length a in the AP and length b in the lateral. It is apparent that a, c, and L form the sides of a right angle triangle so that $L = \sqrt{(a^2 + c^2)}$. The dimension c does not actually appear on the lateral but may be found from it by constructing the right triangle OEF. The length c is obtained by drawing a line on the lateral radiograph parallel to the direction of the beam for the AP radiograph. There is no difficulty in doing this on an actual radiograph because one can orient oneself from anatomical markings. Dimension c is combined with the apparent length a in the AP using $L = \sqrt{(a^2 + c^2)}$ to give the true length. It is clear from the diagram that the length may also be obtained by combining b in the lateral with the length d in the AP using $L = \sqrt{(b^2 + d^2)}$. The dimension d is found on the AP by a line in the direction of the x ray beam for the lateral.

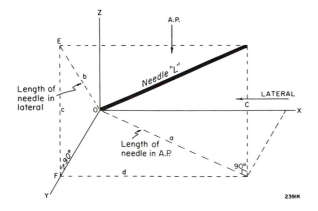

Figure 13-11. Diagram illustrating the appearance of a radium needle as observed by an anteroposterior and a lateral x ray film.

Figure 13-12 shows two radiographs (lateral on the left, and AP on the right) of a single plane implant in the tongue. Each of these images is magnified because the implant is closer to the focal spot than the film (see Chapter 16). The amount of magnification may be measured if a ring of known diameter (5 cm is a useful dimension) is placed on the patient the same distance from the film as the implant and radiographed with the implant. The ring can be seen near the left of the lateral and at the right side of the AP in Figure 13-12.

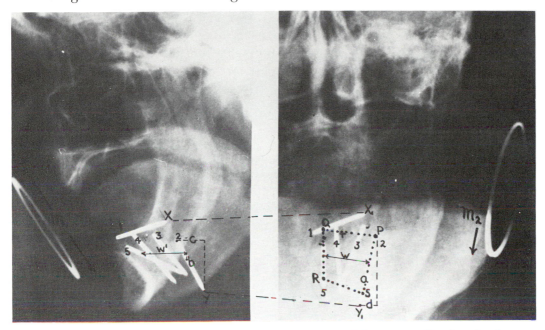

Figure 13-12. Lateral and AP radiograph of an implant of the tongue showing the ring gauge for magnification determination.

The radiographs should be oriented side by side (as in Fig. 13-12). Note that the ends of the needles in one picture should lie on the same horizontal line as the same end of the same needle in the other picture. Two such ends have been joined by the dotted line XX_1 and YY_1 to illustrate this. Because of slight differences in magnification, the lines may diverge or converge slightly as in Figure 13-12. It is important that the radiographs be lined up thus, otherwise erroneous conclusions may be drawn. If the radiographs have not been taken at right angles, this will become apparent when one tries to orient the films with respect to each other. In taking the two films, it is important that the patient remain fixed and the x ray source be moved through 90°. A jig to hold the films at right angles is useful. The only thing that is moved between radiographs is the magnification ring, which, in each case, must be placed the same distance from the film as the center of the implant. The respective needles should be distinguished by numbers as in Figure 13-12. Note that approximately parallel dotted lines could be drawn from the ends of each needle to the corresponding end in the other view. The ring should be measured in each view and the magnification determined. Let these be m_1 and m_2. To illustrate the principle, the length of needle 2 will be determined from the actual radiograph. The lengths a, b, c, and d of Figure 13-12 correspond to the lengths a, b, c, and d of Figure 13-11.

diam. ring in AP = 6.4 $m_1 = 6.4/5.0 = 1.28$
diam. ring in lateral = 5.5 $m_2 = 5.5/5.0 = 1.10$
length of needle in AP a = 3.3 cm a_c (corrected a) = 3.3/1.28 = 2.6
the right angle triangle is drawn on the lateral
the distance c, which is in the direction of the x rays in the AP radio-
    graph, is found, c = 1.2 c_c (corrected c) = 1.2/1.10 = 1.1
length of needle = $\sqrt{a_c^2 + c_c^2} = \sqrt{(2.6)^2 + (1.1)^2} = 2.8$ cm.

In a similar way, the length of the needle may be found using the expression $\sqrt{b^2 + d^2}$.

length of needle in lateral b = 2.8 $b_c = 2.8/1.10 = 2.55$
dimension d (taken from AP) = 1.1 $d_c = 1.1/1.28 = 0.9$
length of needle = $\sqrt{b_c^2 + d_c^2} = \sqrt{(2.55)^2 + (0.9)^2} = 2.7$

The actual length of the needle was 2.8 cm, in good agreement with the measured values.

In any actual calculation, there is no need to calculate the length of the needle, since this is known, except for purposes of checking. The method, however, may be used to find the size of the implant. This is also illustrated in Figure 13-12. The area of the implant should be drawn in as the dotted rectangle PQRS on the AP. This cannot be done precisely and the best that can be done is to make an intelligent guess. The lower edge of the implant is drawn as the line joining the lower ends of the active deposits of needles 2 and 5. These points are about 1/6 of the way along the needles. The upper boundary is more difficult to place. It obviously cannot be taken as needle 1, since this crossing needle is much too high. A compromise is shown in the diagram. It is now required to find the area of the rectangular shape PQRS. Its height may be taken as 5/6 of the length of needle 2 or 5/6 (2.8) = 2.33. The width is the distance w. The ends of the line w are located on the lateral and the length w' found on the lateral. The true width of the implant is now found by the methods discussed above.

distance w = 2.2   w (corrected for mag.) = 2.2/1.28 = 1.7
distance w' = 2.0   w' (corrected for mag.) = 2.0/1.10 = 1.8
true width of implant = $\sqrt{(1.7)^2 + (1.8)^2} = 2.5$ cm
true area of implant 2.5 × 2.3 = 5.75 cm^2

area corrected for uncrossed end (less 10%) = 5.2 cm²
The area 5.2 cm² should then be used to calculate the length of time
   the activity should be left in place to yield the required dose.

This implant is difficult to calculate for two reasons. In the first place, the plane of the implant is not parallel to the film for either of the radiographs. It would have been easier to interpret had the patient's head been angled so that the plane of the implant was parallel to the film for one of the pictures. The second difficulty arises because the pattern does not conform too closely to the idealized shapes required by the Paterson and Parker system. Without a computer there is no easy way to overcome this difficulty and all that can be done is to select the idealized rectangular shape that most closely corresponds to the actual implant. If the implant bears no relation to a Paterson and Parker distribution, the dose at a few selected points may be found by calculating the distance of these points from each of the needles, by the methods described above, and calculating the dose contribution from each needle using Quimby's data for linear sources (Q1).

Figure 13-13 shows radiographs of a tumor on the side of the neck that has been implanted with seven needles. In radiographing this implant, care was taken to turn the head so that the plane of the implant was parallel to the film for the lateral radiograph. Now the AP radiograph is hardly necessary except to show that the lateral is a true view. In addition, this is a good implant approaching closely the ideal Paterson-Parker arrangement. The area of the implant is ab × cd. The dimension ab may be found directly since it is 0.69 of the total length of the needle (4.2 cm). Hence, ab = 2.9 cm. Similarly, cd is 0.9 of the actual length of a needle or 0.9 × 4.2 = 3.8 cm. Hence the true area = 2.9 × 3.8 = 11.0 cm². In this case, no measurement of magnification is required and only the one radiograph is used.

In discussing Figure 13-13 some error is made because it was assumed that the x ray beam is normal to the film. This, of course, can only be true for one ray from the machine. For a small implant, the correction for this effect is usually small.

Steps Involved in Calculating an Implant

1. Immobilize the patient with the plane of the implant either horizontal or vertical.

2. Place the ring gauge the same distance above the film as the implant and take an x ray picture with the beam vertical.

3. Replace the ring gauge the same lateral distance from the film as the implant and take an x ray picture with the beam horizontal.

4. Develop the films and orient them side by side as in Figures 13-12 and 13-13. Check to see that the needles correspond by identifying each

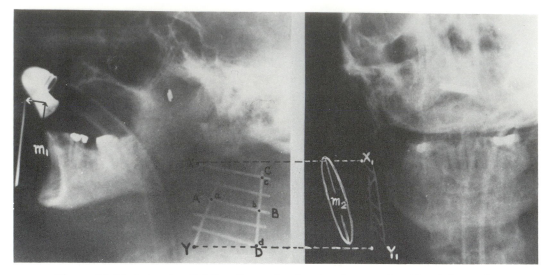

Figure 13-13. Lateral and AP radiograph of an implant on the side of the neck.

needle in both pictures by visualizing a system of parallel lines from the ends of all needles in one view to the corresponding ends in the other view. If they do not correspond, a mistake has been made in taking the radiograph.

5. If the implant was correctly oriented, as described in step 1, only one of the two films need be used for the calculation of a single-plane implant. For a two-plane or volume implant, both are needed.

6. Try to determine the dimensions of the implant using the needles of known length as the gauge. In some cases, this will not be possible and the dimensions must be calculated using the magnification gauge and both of the x ray films.

7. For a detailed calculation of the dosage pattern, use one of the many computer systems that are available.

13.12   **CLINICAL EXAMPLES OF**
                   BRACHYTHERAPY CALCULATIONS

In order to illustrate the methods described in this chapter, a number of typical examples will be discussed. It will be assumed that the department has available an unlimited number of radioactive needles of the specifications of Table 13-9 or their equivalents.

Example 13-11. It is desired to treat a neck node to 65.0 Gy with a permanent gold seed implant. The tumor measures 1 cm in diameter and it is decided to attempt an implant 2.0 cm in diameter.

Emitted radiation from 1 mCi gold = 26.9 mg hr equiv. (Eq. 13-4)
$A = \pi r^2 = 3.14$ cm^2 h = 0.5 R_A = 131 mg hr/10 Gy
Emitted radiation required = 6.5 × 131 = 852 mg hr

TABLE 13-9

Strength (mg)	Active Length (cm)	Length (cm)	Filtration mm Pt
3	4.5	6.0	0.5
2	4.5	6.0	0.5
2	3.0	4.5	0.5
1.3	3.0	4.5	0.5
1.0	3.0	4.5	0.5
1.0	1.5	2.5	0.5
0.5	1.0	2.0	0.5
13.3	1.5	2.0	1.0
10	1.5	2.0	1.0
3	1.5	2.0	1.0
3	1.0	1.4	1.0

Initial strength of gold required = 852/26.9 = 31.7 mCi

The ideal implant attempted is shown in Figure 13-14 and consists of 6 gold seeds around the periphery with a 5% central spot.

Activity of spot = 32 × 0.05 = 1.6 mCi

$$\text{Activity of each of the other seeds} = \frac{31.7 - 1.6}{6} = 5.02 \text{ mCi}$$

Seven gold seeds should be ordered with these activities. After the implant had been made, two x ray pictures taken at right angles and corrected for magnification revealed that the actual implant was elliptical with the dimensions shown in Figure 13-14.

Area treated $\pi ab/4 = \pi(2)(2.8)/4 = 4.4 \text{ cm}^2$

R_A (interpolation from Table 13-4) = 158 mg hr/10 Gy

Actual dose delivered after decay of gold =

$$\frac{32 \text{ mCi} \times 26.9 \text{ mg hr/m Ci} \times 10 \text{ Gy}}{158 \text{ mg hr}} = 54.5 \text{ Gy}$$

Figure 13-14. Diagram illustrating the gold seed implant attempted and the one actually achieved in the treatment of a rodent ulcer of the inner canthus.

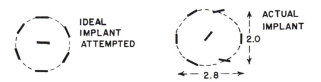

Note that this dose is less than that planned because the implant was larger than expected. If it was felt that this dose was not large enough to sterilize the tumor, a small x ray dose could be added to it. A single dose of 20 Gy (See Chapter 17) would be considered a lethal tumor dose. The extra dose required may be estimated thus:

Single x ray dose required = (65.0 − 54.5) (20.0)/65.0 = 3.23 Gy

In some cases the area of the implant would correspond more closely to the one planned and no extra x ray dose would be required. In others, the distribution might be even worse than the one illustrated, showing regions with no gold seeds. If the actual distance between any 2 seeds around the periphery were greater than 1.25 to 1.50 cm, an attempt should be made to introduce an extra seed to increase the dose in this localized area.

Example 13-12. It is desired to treat a lesion in the tongue by a single plane implant to 60.0 Gy in 8 days. The lesion measures 2×4 cm.

It was decided to attempt the implant shown in Figure 13-15a using four 6.0 cm needles (active length 4.5 cm) with the posterior ends uncrossed and one crossing needle of length 4.5 cm (active length 3.0 cm).

The arrangement follows closely the distribution rules since the parallel needles are spaced 1 cm apart (2h) and the central lines are 2/3 strength. After the implant had been made, the dimensions were found to be as shown in Figure 13-15a.

Actual area of implant 5.2 $(3.1 + 3.8)/2 = 18.0$ cm^2
Area corrected for uncrossed end (less 10%) = 16.2 cm^2
R_A (interpolation from Table 13-4 for h = 0.5) = 338 mg hr/10 Gy
60.0 Gy requires $6 \times 338 = 2028$ mg hr
Treatment time = $2028/(3 + 3 + 2 + 2 + 2) = 2028/12 = 169$ hr

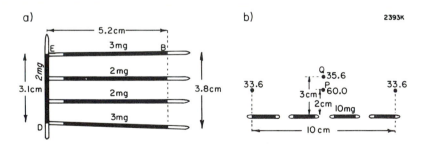

Figure 13-15. Arrangement of radium to treat (a) a tongue lesion with a single plane implant; (b) a carcinoma of the vagina with a linear tandem source.

Example 13-13. It is desired to treat a carcinoma of the vagina that has spread for 6 cm along the vagina using a linear source and an applicator that holds the vaginal wall into a cylinder 4.0 cm in diameter. The wall is to receive 60.0 Gy in about 8 days. In order to achieve a uniform dose over a length of 6 cm, the linear source should be longer than this to prevent the dose from falling off too rapidly near the ends. A linear source 10 cm long should be used.

L = 10, h = 2.0, R_L (Table 13-3) = 1277 mg hr/10.0 Gy
mg hr required = $1277 \times 6 = 7662$

Approx. radium equivalent required = 7662/(8 × 24) = 39.9 mg

Use four 10 mg tubes of active length 1.5 cm spaced as shown in Figure 13-15b so that the total length between the extreme ends of the active deposits is 10.0 cm.

Actual treatment time 7662/40 = 191.5 hr = 7 days, 23.5 hrs

Dose opposite end of source (Fig. 13-5) = (56/100) (60.0) = 33.6 Gy

Dose at Q (use h = 3.0, Table 13-3a) = (1277/2149) 60.0 = 35.6 Gy

Alternate Treatment. By using 3 sources in tandem with a weaker central one, the dose may be maintained constant over practically the whole length and the total length treated may be reduced to 6.0 cm.

L = 6.0, h = 2, L/h = 3, 10% radium central source (Fig. 13-5)

R_L (L = 6.0, h = 2, Table 13-3a) = 898 mg hr/10 Gy

% increase in R_L (Fig. 13-5) = 18%, corr. R_L = 1060 mg hr/10 Gy

Approx. radium (or equiv.) required = 6 × 1060/(8 × 24) = 33.1 mg

Use one 3 mg tube, active length 1.5 cm, for central source tube plus one 15.0 mg tube for each end source.

Space the three sources with a 0.25 cm gap so that the total length of active deposit is 6.0 cm.

Total radium = 15.0 + 3 + 15.0 = 33.0 mg

Treatment time = 6 × 1060/33 = 193 hr = 8 days, 1 hr

Another way to obtain an essentially uniform dose along the surface of the vagina is to insert into the vagina a hollow nearly cylindrical tube that has a larger diameter at the center than at the ends, and mount the radium along the axis of this applicator. By adjusting these dimensions to the proper value, the dose to all points of the vagina may be made almost the same. The shape of the hollow applicator should correspond to one of the isodose curves of Figure 13-3.

13.13 BRACHYTHERAPY IN GYNECOLOGY

Cancer of the uterus was first treated with radium in 1908. Since then many techniques have evolved, most of them developed from the patterns laid down by Regaud in Paris and by Forsell in Stockholm. These techniques, based primarily on clinical considerations, were developed long before the introduction of the roentgen and were of necessity empirical. It is remarkable that these two systems, which differed widely in the amounts of radium used and in the time schedule of their application, produced similar clinical results. Further, subsequent physical analysis has shown that they deliver essentially the same doses to important points in the pelvis.

In the 1930s the Manchester group analyzed the Paris technique from a physical point of view so that the dose at points in the pelvis could be expressed in roentgens. They further modified the Paris technique, using applicators designed to simplify dosage calculations. Space does not permit detailed discussions of the various systems. Some of the physical aspects of the Manchester system will be dealt with now (M12, P10, T8).

In the Manchester system, 1 to 3 radium tubes are placed in a rubber tube, which is inserted in the uterine canal. Simultaneously, radium tubes are loaded in appropriate-sized rubber ovoids, which are placed against the cervix and held at a constant separation by a rubber spacer. Figure 13-16 shows the intrauterine radium at positions U_1, U_2, and U_3 in the uterus and the intravaginal radium mounted in the spaced ovoids. In the Manchester system, a variety of lengths of intrauterine tubes and 3 sizes of ovoids are available to suit the particular anatomy in a given case. In the original system, radium tubes with the original Paris loadings of 13.3 and 6.6 mg were used. In the revised Manchester system (T8) radium in multiples of 2.5 mg are used.

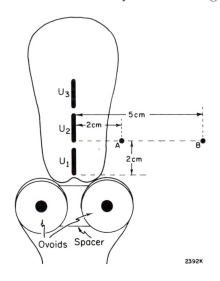

Figure 13-16. Schematic diagram of the uterus showing the use of intrauterine tubes and ovoids in the treatment of cancer of the uterus.

Tod and Meredith (T8) suggested that the point of limiting tolerance is point A situated 2 cm laterally from the uterine canal and 2 cm above the lateral fornix (Fig. 13-16). In addition, it is useful to know the dose at a point B on the pelvic wall opposite point A. In the average patient, this point B is about 5 cm from the uterine canal. When the uterine canal is shifted laterally due to disease, then of course the two points B on opposite sides of the pelvic wall will be different distances from the intrauterine radium. In the calculations given below, it will be assumed that the uterus lies along the midline and that both points are 5 cm from the intrauterine radium. Most experienced therapists feel that whatever other dose calculations are made, the dose at points A and B should be known in every case treated by a particular geometric arrangement.

The dose to points A and B for various combinations of radium are given in Table 13-10. The loadings shown in this table are those recommended in the revised Manchester system (T8) and are designed to give the same dose to A for the various combinations of intravaginal and intrauterine radium. From Table 13-10 it is seen that the dose rate to A is nearly the same whether 2 or 3 sources are used in the uterine canal and whether large, medium, or small ovoids are used in the vagina. This dose equalization is achieved by loading the large, medium, and small ovoids with 22.5, 20, and 17.5 mg respectively. The dose rates given in Table 13-10 for point B were obtained from Figure 13-3.

TABLE 13-10
Absorbed Dose Rate in Gy/hr at Points A and B of Figure 13-16

	Point A Gy/hr	Point B Gy/hr
(1) U_1—10 mg, U_2—10 mg, U_3—15 mg	.35	.088
(2) U_1—15 mg, U_2—10 mg	.35	.070
(3) Large ovoids with spacer—2 × 22.5 mg	.19	.090
(4) Medium ovoids with spacer—2 × 20 mg	.19	.082
(5) Small ovoids with spacer—2 × 17.5 mg	.19	.074
(6) Special loading U_1—20 mg	.28	.057

Data for point A was obtained from Tod and Meredith (T8) but adjusted to express the dose in Gy. Data for point B was obtained by calculation from Figure 13-3.

For the standard loadings, the absorbed dose rate at point A is .35 + .19 = .54 Gy/hr regardless of which of the uterine loadings, 1 or 2, and which of the vaginal loadings, 3, 4, or 5, are used.

In usual practice a total dose of about 75 Gy is delivered to point A in two weeks. The treatment is usually carried out in 2 sessions, each of about 3 days, with a week between treatments. With standard loading, the total treatment time is about 75.0/0.54 = 139 hours. The dose to point B depends upon the loading used. If arrangement 2 and 3 are combined, the total absorbed dose rate at B is 0.16 Gy/hr and the total absorbed dose is 22.0 Gy for 75.0 Gy to point A. For loading arrangements 1 and 3, the corresponding dose to B is 25.0 Gy.

The data of Table 13-10 strictly applies only as long as individual radium tubes of the strength indicated, or equivalent, are used. In most cases, through lack of sufficient radium stocks, it is necessary to bunch a number of tubes together in the intrauterine tube or ovoids, and this introduces uncertainties in dosimetry because of the effects of mutual filtration. When 2 tubes are placed together, an inhomogeneous dose pattern results because the extra filtration is present along the line joining their centers but is absent at right angles to this direction. Three equal sources bunched together give a good distribution and, for tubes with a filtration of 1.0 mm Pt, the 3 sources have an effective radium content 10% less than their actual content.

Dosage in Practical Cases

In any actual example, the dose to point A and B cannot be determined precisely by the above method, because the uterus may be eccentric for reasons of anatomy or as the result of disease. The uterine tube is therefore unlikely to be arranged in the idealized position of Figure 13-16. It is customary to check the localization of the sources by taking two radiographs at right angles by the methods described in section 13.11 or by taking two radiographs with a tube shift between exposures. In principle, the location of each of the sources in space, with reference to points of anatomical interest, is now determined and the dose to these points may be calculated from the radium isodose curves. The literature is filled with "easy" ways to carry out this type of calculation. The fact that there are so many "easy" ways is another way of stating that there is no simple way of performing such a calculation.

Recently, computers have also been applied to this task, and the methods for calculating doses around linear sources described in section 13.07 are used. Figure 13-17 shows isodose curves in 3 planes at right angles to each other for the source configuration indicated in Figure 13-16. The uterine sources are 10, 10, and 15 mg of radium respectively, the 15 mg tube being farthest from the cervix. The vaginal sources are each 20 mg and are spaced 3.5 cm apart. This corresponds to a combination of line 1 with line 4 of Table 13-10. Figure 13-17A is in the plane containing the uterine sources and would be a coronal plane except that it would normally be at a slant because of the angle of the uterus.

Points A are marked on this diagram and it can be seen that the dose rate there is about 0.52 Gy/hr, in agreement with data in Table 13-10. Dose rates of up to 0.8 Gy/hr are shown. Dose rates to tissues near to the sources are very much higher than this. Figure 13-17B shows a dose rate distribution in the saggital plane containing the uterine sources, and Figure 13-17C shows the dose rate distribution in the transverse plane containing the two vaginal sources. One of the potential complications with such treatments is radiation damage to the rectum or bladder. Isodose patterns such as those shown in Figures 13-17B and C are useful in this context because the locations of these structures can be determined with respect to the isodose lines and the doses to them estimated with a fair degree of accuracy.

Having calculated the dose to points such as A and B, and the bladder and rectum, the external field, if one is to be applied, should logically be adjusted for each individual patient in such a way as to deliver the required total dose to the points of interest. This procedure is by no means

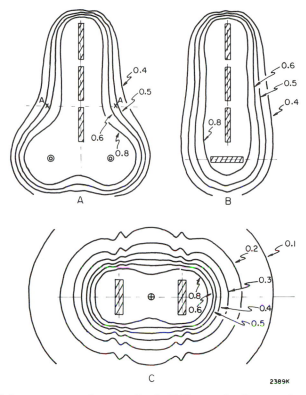

Figure 13-17. Isodose distributions in three perpendicular planes for the source arrangement of Figure 13-16. A is in the plane containing the uterine sources and points A and B, B is in the sagittal plane containing the uterine sources, and C is in a transverse plane containing the vaginal sources.

simple, for the external field must now be applied differently for each patient. No easy and accurate routine method for doing this has evolved. The problem would be greatly simplified if all of the treatment could be carried out using either brachytherapy alone or external irradiation alone. Brachytherapy alone provides good and adequate treatment for the average stage 1 (cancer confined to the cervix). When the cancer has spread beyond the localized region of stage 1, the dose distribution resulting from the use of internal sources alone is inadequate, and therefore external irradiation must be used. The problem of blending these radically different geometrical distributions to produce a homogeneous dose over the required volume is very difficult. The physics of the problem could again be simplified if the cervical canal and the vagina could be placed rigidly in a particular geometry with respect to each other and to the external markings of the patient. Again any device that forces these organs into a fixed geometry is unlikely to meet universal clinical approval and so this solution is not practical.

Another possible way of solving this problem may be to place the major emphasis on large volume external radiation therapy with or without the use of intracavitary sources in a simplified geometry.

Because of the difficulties of routine dose estimations, many clinics take radiographs to ensure that the sources have been introduced properly, but do not attempt accurate calculations based on them. Some clinics achieve some radiation control by making measurements in the bladder and rectum with a probe dosimeter at the time of the insertion. If the dose to these organs is unacceptably high, the internal sources are repositioned.

13.14   SPECIAL TECHNIQUES
Radioactive Gold Seeds

The use of radioactive gold seeds or grains as a replacement for radon in permanent implants was discussed in section 13.06. The Γ factors for radium and gold are 0.825 and 0.238 respectively (Table 13-2) and the following conversion factors are obtained (eq. 13-2).

$$1 \text{ mCi gold} = 0.288 \text{ mg Ra}$$

$$1 \text{ mg radium} = 3.47 \text{ mCi gold}$$

For use in permanent implants, however, the conversion should be made in terms of total emitted radiation (eq. 13-4).

$$1 \text{ mCi gold decayed} = 26.9 \text{ mg hr radium}$$

$$1 \text{ mg hr radium} = 0.0372 \text{ mCi gold decayed}$$

Generally, the supplier will state the activity of the seeds in mCi at a certain time on a certain day. If the activity is not known, the seeds may be "calibrated" by a direct comparison of the exposure (in roentgens) produced by the gold grains with that of a radium needle of known strength. A sensitive ion chamber with good energy-response characteristics is required for this purpose.

A gold grain introducer developed at the Royal Marsden Hospital (J13) is illustrated in Figure 13-18. The gold grains, which may be precision machined, are loaded into a cartridge and the whole assembly activated in a nuclear reactor. The activated cartridge is then loaded in the gun and is ready for use. The needle of the gun is inserted at the required spot and the trigger pulled once, which ejects one grain. The process is repeated until the complete implant is made. The gun is convenient to use and quite precise implants are possible.

Because the principal gamma ray emitted by gold is 0.412 MeV, in contrast to the penetrating spectrum from radium, protection problems with gold are much more easily solved, and radiation to personnel is minimized. Gold has one other advantage over radon. Although the major gamma activity of both gold and radon disappears after about 1 month, there is some gamma activity from radon for many years due to bremsstrahlung arising from the energetic beta particles from ^{210}Pb and ^{210}Bi.

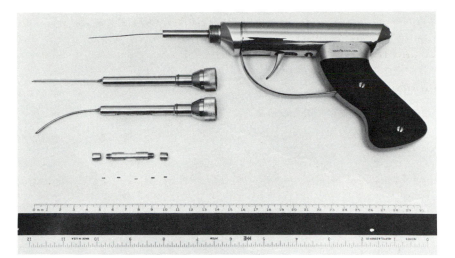

Figure 13-18. Photograph of gun for introducing gold seeds. A straight needle and a curved one are shown below the gun, along with a cartridge and a few seeds. The cartridge mounts in the barrel of the needle and when it is in place on the gun and the trigger pulled, the wire shown protruding from the gun is pushed through the center of the cartridge to expel the seeds one by one.

This activity can be measured with sensitive equipment 20 years after an implant is made and contributes a dose to an average implant of 1 to 3 Gy over a 10 to 20 year period (G12). It is suspected that chronic irradiation of this kind may have carcinogenic effects.

Plastic Tube and Afterloading Techniques

A number of investigators have evolved techniques using hollow plastic tubing that can be implanted in the tumor and then filled with the radioactive material, which may be in many forms: tantalum and iridium wire are the most important.

The usual procedure is to implant the tumors with a series of hollow needles following the Paterson-Parker distribution rules. The spacing of the needles will depend upon the strength of the ^{192}Ir (for example) at the time of implant. When all of the needles are correctly positioned, the radioactive wire is introduced into the hollow needles. To minimize radiation exposure to the operator, afterloading procedures may be used whereby radiographs, etc., are taken with the plastic tubing in place and only after calculations have been made are the actual sources inserted. There is no doubt that with this technique the sources can be more accurately positioned than when radioactive needles are used. This procedure also has the advantage that the sources are somewhat flexible and the implant is more comfortable to the patient. This flexibility, of course, decreases the precision of dose prediction.

Radioactive Solutions

Radioactive solutions may be introduced into body cavities to deliver radiation to the walls of the cavity. For this purpose, colloidal solutions of radioactive gold have been used extensively to treat tumors that produce ascites. Some 80% of all the gold used therapeutically is employed in this way. For intraperitoneal treatment, between 150 and 200 mCi of gold is injected into the peritoneal cavity and allowed to decay completely. For intrapleural injections, between 75 and 100 mCi is usually administered. During the first day, the gold is distributed in the cavity more or less uniformly. However, after 1 to 2 days, the colloidal gold particles are engulfed by the macrophages (scavenging cells) onto the surface of the cavity, thus increasing the absorbed dose rate on the surface (if physical decay is neglected). Because of these complexities, it is usual to administer gold on an empirical basis and not attempt dose calculations, although some monitoring of the activity is useful (M13). Since the beta particles have limited range, the dose is superficial, falling to about 20% in 1 mm.

Radioactive colloidal gold has also been used to treat tumors of the bladder. For this purpose, the gold may be introduced directly into the bladder or into an inflatable rubber bag within the bladder. The dose as a function of depth for the two cases is shown in Figure 13-19 adapted from Wallace (W9). When the solution is used directly, the radiation of the mucosa is by means of β and γ rays but, because of the limited range of the betas, the dose falls to about 20% in 1 mm. Such a distribution is fairly satisfactory in dealing with multiple small superficial papillary tumors, which often grow as processes towards the center of the bladder. The solution completely surrounds these processes. It has been suggested that ^{90}Y, with its higher energy beta ray, may be better than gold for this type of treatment. When an inflatable balloon is used, the betas are screened out by the rubber and the falloff of dose is much slower (50% in 6 to 7 mm), but now the high dose to the whole wall of the bladder carries a risk of the production of a contracted bladder and other radiation complications.

Bladder treatments have also been given using a centrally placed source of cobalt 60 or radium. The depth dose is even greater now (50% in 12 mm) as indicated in Figure 13-19. However, such a technique requires very careful control, for the source must be accurately centered in the bladder and maintained there during treatment. This is usually done by inflating a balloon inside the bladder and then introducing the source. The importance of accurate centering may be seen from the following calculation. Suppose the planned treatment distance is 2.5 cm (using a balloon with diameter 5.0 cm). An error of 0.5 cm in centering will increase the dose to one side of the bladder by the factor $(2.5/2.0)^2 = 1.56$

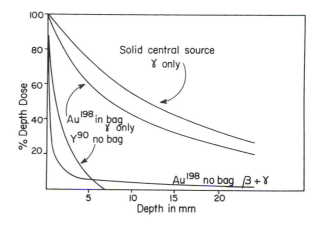

Figure 13-19. Percentage depth dose for radioactive solutions in a spherical cavity the size of the bladder. (Adapted from Wallace, W9.)

and reduce the dose to the remote side by the factor $(2.5/3.0)^2 = 0.7$. Special balloon catheters have been developed that inflate symmetrically and thus reduce the risk of misalignment of the central source. However it should be emphasized that because of these difficulties the central source technique should only be attempted by an expert.

Beta Ray Applicators

When radium is used for brachytherapy, all the alpha and beta particles are stopped by the case surrounding the radium salt, and only the gamma rays contribute to the biological effect. In the very early days of radium therapy, the containers often allowed some of the beta particles to escape in great enough quantities to give an excessive dose in the immediate neighborhood of the radium needle. Today all radium brachytherapy sources are surrounded with either 0.5 or 1.0 mm Pt, which removes all the alpha and beta particles. In the same way isotopes such as ^{60}Co or ^{137}Cs used as brachytherapy sources are encapsulated so that only γ rays are emitted from the source.

Beta ray applicators that are purposely made so that the beta radiation may be used are, however, useful for the treatment of certain very superficial lesions, especially those of the eye. For many years such beta ray plaques were made using radium. The radium was sealed into a shallow metal box, the back and sides of which were thick enough to cut off the beta rays while the front surface was made very thin to allow the beta particles to escape. At this surface some 95% of the ionization is due to beta particles and the rest due to gamma rays. At a depth of 5 mm most of the effect is due to gamma rays. Such applicators are not too satisfactory because of the presence of the penetrating gamma component. Radon was used for many years, sealed in a glass bulb whose walls are thin enough to allow the escape of the beta particles. Since it is impossible to produce glass bulbs with identical wall thicknesses, the beta ray dose from such applicators is hard to predict. Because of this and the presence of the unwanted gamma rays, radon applicators are not too satisfactory.

In 1952, ^{90}Sr, a long-lived fission fragment, became available for beta ray applicators. ^{90}Sr decays with a half-life of 28 years into ^{90}Y, which in turn decays with a half-life of 64 hours into ^{90}Zr. The maximum beta energy from the ^{90}Sr is 0.54 MeV, while the ^{90}Y produces a penetrating beta particle with maximum energy 2.27 MeV. ^{90}Sr, foil-bonded in silver, is covered with a polythene plastic to a thickness of about 0.5 mm, which is sufficient to stop the low-energy beta particles from the strontium. The back of the foil is usually covered with a layer of silver to absorb all the radiation. A group at the Royal Marsden Hospital (S20) have been mainly responsible for the development of the ^{90}Sr applicators. A summary of some of their measurements and those of Friedell et al. (F5) is given in Figure 13-20, which gives depth dose measurements for various beta ray applicators. The positions of the various components of the eye (cornea, aqueous humor, and lens of the eye) are shown along the horizontal scale. Curve 1 shows the depth dose from RaD + RaE (^{210}Pb + ^{210}Bi). It is seen that this drops to 10% at 1 mm and 1% at 2 mm. Curve 2 is the result obtained for radon, which drops to some 30% at 1 mm and 5% at 3 mm. Curve 3 shows the average percentage depth dose for a number of commercially available applicators. These give some 43% at 1 mm, 19% at 2 mm, 5% at 4 mm.

The group at the Royal Marsden Hospital (S20) have developed eye applicators in the form of spherical cups; 2 of these are shown in the diagram. The ^{90}Sr, silver backing, and the polythene shell can be seen. One of the applicators (A) is designed to treat the whole of the cornea, while the second (B) is designed to treat only part of it. In addition, they have developed 3 other applicators for special purposes. The percentage depth dose for type B, in which the ^{90}Sr covers a circular area 6 mm in diameter, is given by curve 3 and is similar to that obtained for commercial plane ^{90}Sr applicators (S21). Curve 4 gives the percentage depth dose for a large-plane applicator (diameter 1.6 cm). Finally, curve 5 gives the depth dose for the spherical applicator. Because of its curved nature, there is some "focusing" effect, so the depth dose along the axis is higher, giving 38% at 2 mm. Strontium applicators give an absorbed dose rate of about 1 Gy/min at the surface.

Automated Remote Afterloading Systems

The greatest source of radiation exposure to radiotherapy personnel has undoubtedly been the procedures used in handling sources and caring for patients undergoing treatments by brachytherapy. Afterloading procedures, already mentioned briefly, have greatly decreased the exposures to operating room personnel but have not altered exposure to

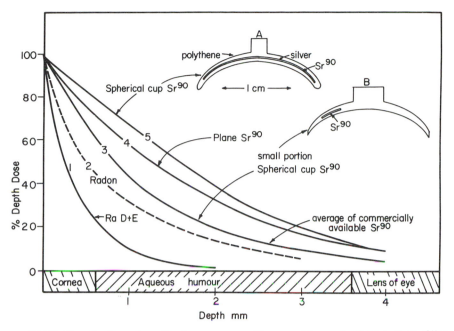

Figure 13-20. Depth dose data for beta ray applicators. Curve 1, RaD + RaE (^{210}Pb + ^{210}Bi), is taken from Friedell (F5). Curve 2, radon-average of 3 applicators, is from Friedell (F5). Curve 3, ^{90}Sr average of 9 commercially available applicators, is from Friedell (F5) and also results from Sinclair and Trott (S20) for their type 4, 6 mm circular spot on spherical shell. Curve 4, ^{90}Sr-plane applicator 16 mm diameter, is taken from Sinclair and Trott (S20). Curve 5 ^{90}Sr-spherical cup, 20 mm diameter, is from Sinclair and Trott (S20).

nurses and others who must care for the patient during the course of the treatment. It is relatively easy to keep exposure to both operating room personnel and nursing staff well below the "maximum permissible doses" (see Chapter 15) even without afterloading devices. Nevertheless, increased concern regarding radiation exposure and the ALARA principle has shifted the attention of physicists and engineers to remote afterloading systems.

These devices are used almost exclusively for brachytherapy in gynecology. The applicators, which are inserted into the patient, are usually connected by a long flexible tube to a well-shielded container in which the radioactive sources reside. The applicators, without sources, or with dummy sources, are positioned in the patient and radiographed and checked as needed. Then when all is ready and no staff are near the patient, the desired selection of sources is propelled down the tube and into place in the applicator. The device can also be interlocked to various interruption switches such as the door of the room so that whenever anyone enters, the sources are temporarily returned to the shielded container. A timer records and controls the time the sources are actually in the patient.

These machines have a number of advantages over the more manual methods in addition to their role in reducing radiation exposure. The sources are frequently small (for example small balls) and a great deal of flexibility in choosing source strength combinations is possible. This, coupled with computer calculation of dose distributions, allows much more tailoring of treatments to individual patient problems. In addition it also allows the possibility of using sources of much higher activities so that treatment times might be short, comparable to times used in external beam radiotherapy. The use of such high dose rates with its (for brachytherapy) unusual dose fractionation might be expected to involve unknown radiobiological effectiveness (see Chapter 17) so that without some experimentation the appropriate dose prescriptions are somewhat uncertain.

A number of remote afterloading devices have been made, both privately and commercially throughout the world and have been in use for many years. It should be emphasized that their role is a mechanical one, to automate the timing of the treatment and reduce staff exposure, but not to alter the nature of the treatment itself.

13.15   **SUMMARY**

The authors are aware that there are a number of satisfactory methods of treating the examples discussed in this chapter; however, they do illustrate the fundamental physical principles involved. For example, in treating cancer of the cervix, a variety of techniques such as those developed in Stockholm, Paris, Manchester, Houston, and elsewhere are in common use. They are all based on sound principles and the dosage received can be expressed in terms of the rad or the gray. Many radiotherapists have achieved very fine clinical results through years of experience without the use of the physical approach discussed herein, but it is difficult for such skills to be passed on to others without using a quantitative physical approach. Many of the differences in techniques are based on the assumption that dosage fractionation schedules are of great importance in determining clinical results. The authors are not prepared to enter into any discussion along these lines.

PROBLEMS

1. Radon gas is sealed in a gold tube and the source so produced is stored for several hours until equilibrium is established between radon and its gamma-emitting decay products. Find the number of atoms of ^{222}Rn, ^{218}Po (half-life 3.05 min), and ^{214}Pb present. Assume an equilibrium activity of 1 MBq.
2. Calculate the exposure rate at a point 10 cm from a short 20 mg radium needle filtered by 0.5 mm Pt. What is the significance of the assumption that the needle is short?
3. From the data given in Table 13-1, determine the mean energy for the spectrum of γ-rays from radium. Determine also the average or "effective" energy with respect

to exposure and determine the exposure rate constant for unfiltered radium. Discuss differences from equation 13-2b.

4. Plot the decay of ^{198}Au on semilog paper and find the residual activity of a source 4 days after it had an activity of 150 MBq.

5. Explain why the activity of a radon source cannot be measured immediately after it is prepared.

6. A mold contains 8 mg of radium and is worn for 7 days. How much gold should be used to deliver the same total dose in 7 days? What is the ratio of the initial dose rate delivered by the gold compared to that of the radium?

7. Determine the radium equivalent of 7.4 MBq of irridium 192.

8. Three cesium sources, each of 13.3 mg Ra equivalent (1.0 mm Pt), are arranged in a line to give a total active length 6.0 cm. Find how long the sources should be left in place to deliver 60.0 Gy to a point 2 cm from the line of the sources. For this treatment time what dose would be delivered to a point 1.5 cm from the source. Calculate also the dose opposite one of the (active) ends of the source, at a distance of 1.5 cm.

9. Two 13.3 mg radium tubes are arranged in a line with their centers 5.5 cm apart. A weaker source is placed midway between them. How much radium should be in this latter source to produce the same dose rates to points opposite each of the sources at a distance of 2.0 cm away from the line. Assume sources 1.35 cm active length 1.0 mm Pt.

10. Use the data of Table 13-3a to calculate the dose rate at a point 3.0 cm from a 13.3 mg needle of active length 1.5 cm and filtration 1.0 mm Pt. Compare with Figure 13-3.

11. A cesium needle appears 2.0 cm long in an AP radiograph with a magnification of 1.15 and 1.80 cm long in a lateral radiograph with magnification 1.25. The projection of the needle (length C in Fig. 13-11) in the lateral is 1.0 cm while the projection (length d in Fig. 13-11) in the AP is 1.45 cm. Calculate the actual length of the needle in two ways from these dimensions.

12. A single-plane implant with one uncrossed end, similar to Figure 13-6b, is to be used to treat a tumor 5 cm long and 4 cm wide. Design the implant, using radium from the list given in Table 13-9. The dose rate is to be approximately 10 Gy/day.

13. After the implant of problem 12 was made and radiographs taken, it was found that the width of the implant (measured from the centers of the outside needles, see also Fig. 13-13) was 3.8 cm and the length varied from 4.7 cm to 5.5 cm. Determine the required treatment time for 60.0 Gy.

14. It is required to treat a volume of tissues $5 \times 3 \times 2$ cm using a 2 plane implant separated by 2.0 cm. Select suitable sources from the list given in Table 13-9. After the implant was made it was $5.3 \times 3.4 \times 2.0$ cm. How long should the sources be left in place to deliver a dose of 55.0 Gy to a plane midway between the sources? Determine also the dose in the plane 0.5 cm from one set of sources and 1.5 cm from the other.

15. A cylindrical volume 5 cm in diameter and 5 cm long is to be treated with a cylindrical volume implant with crossing needles at one end. Select the appropriate sources from the list in section 13.12 and determine the treatment time to deliver 60 Gy in about 7 days.

16. The standard Manchester loadings for cancer of the cervix are given in Table 13-10. For an interuterine loading of 15, 10, and 10 mg and vaginal radium of two 22.5 mg sources placed 4 cm apart calculate the treatment time to deliver 70.0 Gy to point A. What dose will be given to point B?

17. A source of ^{198}Au has an activity of 15 MBq. What activity of ^{192}Ir will (a) give the same initial exposure rate; (b) give the same total dose?

Chapter **14**

NUCLEAR MEDICINE

14.01   **INTRODUCTION**

A wide variety of radioactive agents are now available to the clinician and their use in medicine has become very general. The field involving the clinical use of *nonsealed* radionuclides is referred to as nuclear medicine. Departments of nuclear medicine are to be found in most hospitals either as independent departments or as subdivisions of departments of diagnostic radiology. Most of them are primarily concerned with (a) the imaging of internal organs and (b) the evaluation of various physiological functions. To a lesser degree they may be involved in using various isotopes to treat specific types of disease. In this chapter we will deal with the physical principles underlying nuclear medicine and discuss in detail the dosimetry of administered isotopes.

The methods described in Chapter 7 for the detection and measurement of radiation are not suitable for radionuclides because they are not sensitive enough. The Geiger counter and scintillation detector are used almost exclusively for the clinical measurement of radionuclides. They are sensitive enough to detect the emission of a single particle arising from the disintegration of a nucleus. Geiger counters, which have been used for many years in this work, are now being replaced in most applications by the scintillation detector.

14.02   **GEIGER COUNTER**

The Geiger counter consists essentially of a cylindrical cathode with a fine wire anode along its axis. The device is filled with a special mixture of gasses at a pressure of about 10 cm of mercury. A Geiger counter (Fig. 14-1) appears schematically the same as an ionization chamber, and the student may wonder how they differ. To understand the differences, consider the behavior of the device when it is placed in a radiation field and increasing voltages are placed across it. The current or pulse scale of Figure 14-1 is linear from 0 to 1.0 and then logarithmic from 1 to 10^7. At low voltages the device is a simple ionization chamber and the current increases with voltage until saturation is achieved. Here all the ions produced in the gas are collected and the current or pulse is independent of the applied voltage. In this mode of operation the device is very insensitive. For example, an 18 keV beta particle from tritium absorbed in the device would deposit about 600 ions, that is a charge of about 10^{-16}

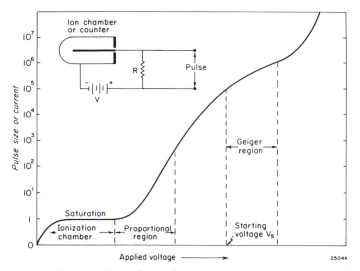

Figure 14-1. Graph showing the relation between the current or pulse from the ion chamber or counter as the voltage V applied between anode and cathode is increased.

coulombs, which would be impossible to detect. When we discussed ion chambers in Chapter 7 we were dealing with many thousands of such particles per second and thus achieved currents that could be measured.

As the applied voltage across the device is increased the ions produced are accelerated to high enough velocities to produce further ionization by collision. The current thus increases with voltage as illustrated by the proportional region of Figure 14-1 where gains of up to 10^3 are achieved. With the choice of the proper parameters for the gas, its pressure, anode construction, and the resistance (R), the device gives pulses proportional to the energy deposited by the particle. It is thus able to distinguish between the passage of one type of particle and another. Proportional counters have many applications in nuclear physics.

If the applied voltage is increased still more, a region is reached where the passage of each particle brings about a controlled avalanche of nearly fixed size and independent of the type of particle that triggered it. This is known as the Geiger region and extends for 100 to 200 volts above the starting value V_s. In this region gains of 10^5 to 10^6 are obtainable and individual ionizing particles can easily be detected. Now a single 18 keV beta particle would produce a short pulse of about 10^{-10} coulombs, which is easily detected. The Geiger counter can thus respond to individual photons, individual beta particles, or individual alpha particles, and a single disintegration of an atom can be detected with the device. If the applied voltage is increased beyond the upper limit of the Geiger region, uncontrolled avalanches will occur and the tube will break into continuous discharge much like a fluorescent lamp.

A given Geiger counter will operate properly only if the correct voltage is applied between the anode and cathode. The correct operating point may be found by placing the counter at a fixed distance from a radioactive source and observing the count rate as the voltage applied to the counter is gradually increased. At a certain voltage, which may range from 500 to 1500 volts, depending upon the construction of the counter, the Geiger counter will start to count. The rate of counting will increase rapidly from this starting voltage (V_s) and then more slowly as the plateau region is reached, as indicated in Figure 14-2a. In the plateau region the rate of counting is almost independent of the applied voltage. Plateaus have a slight slope, a typical value being about 5% per 100 volts. The plateau is often 150 to 200 volts long. It is usual to operate the counter at a voltage V_0 midway along the plateau. Although the counting rate is almost independent of the applied voltage, the size of the output pulses are not independent of voltage and increase as the voltage is increased (as indicated in Fig. 14-1).

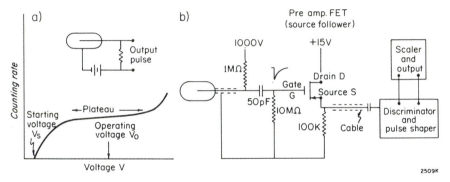

Figure 14-2. (a) Graph showing the counting rate as a function of anode voltage and the plateau for a Geiger counter. (b) Schematic diagram of circuit for Geiger counter.

Geiger counters may take many different forms depending on the purpose for which they are designed. Figure 14-3a shows one form of gamma counter. The anode is a fine wire sealed in a glass envelope and the cathode is a metal cylinder often made of lead. For optimum sensitivity, the cathode should have a thickness equal to the range of the electrons that may be set in motion by the gamma rays to be detected. When a gamma ray passes through such a counter, photoelectrons are ejected from the metal cathode and these initiate the discharge. Because most of the gamma rays pass through such a device without affecting it, gamma counters seldom have an efficiency of more than 5%.

In Figure 14-3b is shown a typical beta counter. The cathode consists of a very thin metal cylinder through which the beta particles can readily pass. The anode is a fine wire mounted in glass insulators to lie along the axis of the tube. When a beta particle enters this counter, it will almost always trigger the device so the efficiency is very close to 100%. For low energy beta particles the end window counter (illustrated in Fig. 14-3c) may be used. The anode consists of a fine wire with a small bead on its end while the cathode consists of a mica window metalized on the inside surface. Low energy beta particles can readily enter this counter through the thin window and so trigger the device.

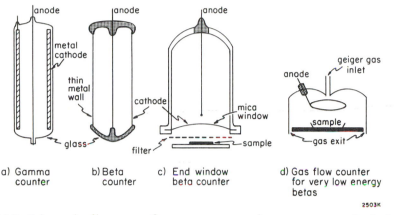

a) Gamma counter
b) Beta counter
c) End window beta counter
d) Gas flow counter for very low energy betas

Figure 14-3. Schematic diagrams of gamma counter, beta counter, end window beta counter, and gas flow-counter.

Finally, if *very* low energy beta particles or alpha particles are to be detected, it is advantageous to place the radioactive material *inside* the tube, thus avoiding the necessity of having the particles pass through the walls. After the sample is introduced into the counter, the counter must be flushed out with the special Geiger gas mixture and while measurements are being made, a slow flow of this gas through the device is maintained. Such counters are usually operated at atmospheric pressure. The high voltage is applied between the anode, which takes the form of a ring, and the cathode, which is the container of the tube. Gas flow counters are useful in detecting the very low energy beta particles from materials such as tritium.

Circuit Diagram. A schematic circuit diagram for a Geiger counter is given in Figure 14-2b. The anode of the counter is connected to the high voltage supply through a 1 MΩ resistor. When an ionizing particle passes through the tube the current through this resistor causes a rapid voltage drop, which appears as a negative pulse. This pulse is fed through the 50 pF condenser to the gate, G, of the field effect transistor (FET) of the preamplifier. This produces a negative pulse of about the same size at the source, S, of the FET. The effective internal impedance of the FET in this configuration is about 200 Ω, allowing the voltage pulse to be transmitted down a long cable to the discriminator and pulse-shaping circuits. The discriminator is a device to reject pulses that are smaller than a certain size and the pulse shaper is used to make all pulses the same shape regardless of their initial size. These uniformly shaped pulses are then introduced into a scaler or a count rate meter.

14.03   THE SCINTILLATION DETECTOR

The basic principles of the scintillation detector are illustrated in Figure 14-4. The device consists of a crystal, usually of sodium iodide, connected to a photomultiplier. The essential parts of the photomultiplier are the photocathode, 10 to 12 dynodes, and an anode. These components are mounted inside an evacuated glass envelope. When light strikes the photocathode, low energy photoelectrons are ejected from the surface. These electrons are collected by the first dynode, which is about 100 volts positive with respect to the photocathode. The electrons strike the first dynode with sufficient velocity to eject two or three secondary electrons from the surface, and these secondary electrons in turn are accelerated to the second dynode, which is 100 volts positive with respect to the first. At the second and succeeding dynodes each electron produces more electrons by secondary emission until a multiplication factor of about one million is attained by the time the final anode is reached.

Details of the scintillating crystal are also shown in Figure 14-4, where an x ray photon is shown interacting at a point 0. At this point a photoelectron is set in motion and the track of this photoelectron is represented by the heavy short line to P. As the photoelectron travels through the crystal, it excites and ionizes the atoms of the crystal and produces many flashes of UV or visible light. Some of these are shown by the light lines. These photons, which originate in the track, are emitted in all directions and are reflected diffusely in the magnesium oxide layer that surrounds the crystal. As long as they are not absorbed by this layer, they will finally emerge through the one *clear* side of the crystal and strike the photosensitive surface inside the photomultiplier. The crystal is usually coupled to the photomultiplier by silicone grease to prevent loss of these photons by reflection. The light photons, on striking the photosensitive surface, then eject low energy photoelectrons, which are collected and amplified, as described above.

The scintillation counter differs from the Geiger counter in one very important way. The number of electrons ejected from the photosensitive surface will be proportional to the amount of light that reaches this surface and this amount of light is in turn proportional to the energy absorbed from the photon beam by the crystal. Thus, the size of the pulse that emerges from the anode of the photomultiplier will be proportional to the energy of the photon absorbed in the crystal. The scintillation counter may therefore be used to distinguish between photons of different energy. It will be remembered that with the Geiger counter the pulse size was independent of the photon energy.

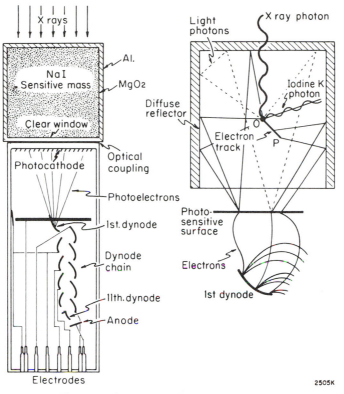

Figure 14-4. Diagram to illustrate the construction of a photomultiplier and the processes that occur within the crystal.

Although the energy of the output pulse is proportional to the energy of the photon that gave rise to it, there are number of effects that complicate this process. A monoenergetic photon gives rise to pulses of slightly different size due to the statistical variations within the crystal and photomultiplier. In the first place, the number of optical photons produced along the electron track has a statistical variation. In addition, there is a variable loss of these photons before reaching the sensitive surface, due to different path lengths and different numbers of reflections at the crystal surface. When the optical photons pass through the photosensitive surface, some will give rise to photoelectrons, while others will be transmitted unaffected. Further, some of the photoelectrons set in motion will be collected by the first dynode while others will escape. When the photoelectron is collected, it may or may not produce a secondary electron. Finally, there will be a variable efficiency of multiplication in succeeding dynodes. All of these effects combine to produce a gaussian spread of pulses about the mean value. This is illustrated in Figure 14-5a, which shows the spectra of gold 198 and cesium 137. These isotopes produce monoenergetic photons of energy 412 keV and 662 keV, respectively, and in a perfect detector would give rise to a single

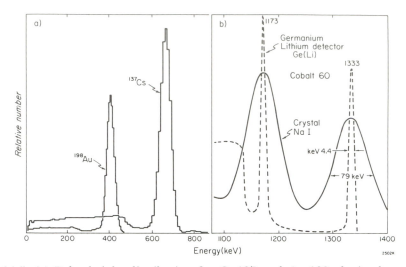

Figure 14-5. (a) Pulse height distribution for Cs-137 and Au-198 obtained on a 100-channel pulse-height analyzer using a 6 × 6 cm sodium iodide crystal. (b) Comparison of γ ray spectrum of Co-60 observed with a 3.5 mm-deep germanium lithium detector and with a 7.5 × 7.5 cm sodium iodide scintillation spectrometer.

narrow peak at these energies. Although each does show a prominent peak at the correct energy, not all the pulses are at this energy but are distributed about this energy for reasons given above.

In addition to the statistical spread of pulses about the peak, there are a number of low energy pulses distributed from zero to an energy near the peak. The low energy pulses are due to a different phenomenon. The photon of energy hν may interact with the crystal of Figure 14-4 by a Compton process rather than by a photoelectric process and the scattered photon of energy hν′ may escape from the crystal. The recoil electron with energy E′ = hν − hν′ will be absorbed and the light flash will be proportional to this energy rather than to hν and so appears as a lower energy pulse. When the incident photon has a high energy, the scattered Compton photons have a greater probability of escape. This effect is seen in Figure 14-5a, where the low energy tail for cesium appears much larger than for gold.

LIQUID SCINTILLATION COUNTER. In certain applications where extreme sensitivity is required and beta particles are to be detected, use may be made of the liquid scintillation counter. Here the sample to be counted is introduced into a glass vial filled with a scintillating fluid. This vial is then placed between two photomultipliers in a well-shielded lead castle. When a beta particle is ejected from the source, it produces an ionizing track in the surrounding scintillating fluid. The resulting scintillations are detected by the two photomultipliers. Usually the device is designed to count sequentially a large number of samples and record the activity of each. The device may be fitted with discriminators to reject particles of one energy and detect those of another. For high energy beta particles the device is nearly 100% efficient. For gamma rays the efficiency is determined by the fraction of the emitted gamma rays that interact in the scintillating fluid.

Basic Electronic Circuit

The basic circuit for the scintillation counter is illustrated in Figure 14-6. The photocathode, the dynodes, and the anode are connected to a resistor chain as indicated. When 1200 volts is applied to the chain, about 100 volts is produced between successive dynodes. When an electron is ejected from the photocathode by light, an amplified pulse of electrons is collected by the anode. The anode is connected to the inverting terminal, S, of the operational amplifier through the small coupling capacitor, C. With the operational amplifier connected as shown (see section 9.05) the terminal S is held at ground potential, so the pulse of electrons from the anode into S is exactly balanced by a flow from S through R_f to point O. The output terminal O thus rises by $V_0 = I\,R_f$ where I is the current pulse to the anode. This signal is independent of R_1, R_2, and C. The back-to-back silicon diodes connected to S protect the operational amplifier from transients by becoming conducting if the potential of S exceeds ±0.6 volts. The output pulse, V_0 is fed through a long cable to drive an amplifier and discriminator or pulse height analyzer. The discriminator is a device that excludes from the output circuit all pulses smaller than a preset value. For example, if in counting gold 198 (see Fig. 14-5a) the discriminator had been set at a value proportional to 300 keV, the only pulses that would be counted would be those with energy greater than 300 keV. The device would then count only those photons that were completely absorbed in the crystal and would reject photon interactions in which part of the energy escaped.

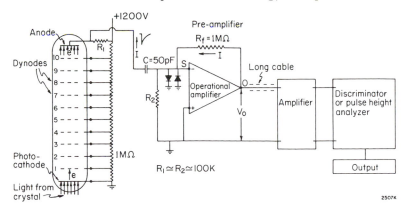

Figure 14-6. Schematic diagram of a circuit for a scintillation counter.

In some applications, it is necessary to count one radionuclide in the presence of another. When this is the case, more complicated discriminators, which have an upper and lower limit and which transmit through a so-called window, may be used. If it were necessary to count Cs-137 and Au-198 in the presence of each other, the window would be set to count first from 500 keV up (see Fig. 14-5a) (let this count due to cesium be represented by C); then the window would be set to count from 300 to 500 keV, which would count the gold plus a few counts from the cesium (let this count be G). Then the gold activity is G-fC, where f is the ratio of the counts from 300 to 500 keV to the counts from 500 keV up when cesium is counted alone.

For nuclear investigations, and in some clinical isotope work, the use of a pulse-height analyzer is indicated. The pulse-height analyzer is a device that sorts the pulses according to their size and stores the number of pulses of each size in a memory. At the end of the counting period, the information in the memory may be extracted in the form of either a numerical or a graphical record (Fig. 14-5). Instruments that sort the pulses into 400 or more channels are available. These yield far more information than a simple discriminator.

14.04   SEMICONDUCTOR DETECTOR

The semiconductor detector is a device for converting ionization produced in a crystal directly into an electrical pulse, which is amplified, sorted by a pulse height analyzer, and registered by a scaler. Essentially, the detector is a block of material with electrodes attached to opposite faces and a voltage maintained across the block. Ionization within the block produces the equivalent of the ion pairs produced in an ionization chamber. The only materials used successfully so far are silicon and germanium, which are nonconducting in their normal state, but which allow the ions produced by energy absorption to migrate rapidly to the collecting electrodes and produce an electrical pulse. It requires approximately 3 eV to produce the ion pair, compared to about 35 eV in a gas, and 1000 eV to produce a photoelectron at the photocathode of a scintillation counter. Since the statistical spread of pulses about a peak is proportional to the square root of the number of electrons initially produced, the spread for the semiconductor crystal is about $\sqrt{(3/1000)} = 1/18$ of that of the NaI scintillation counter. Figure 14-5b compares the γ ray spectrum of ^{60}Co observed with a germanium semiconductor 3.5 mm thick to that observed with a NaI crystal 7.5 cm thick. The remarkably sharp peaks from the semiconductor are evident. The width of the peak at half maximum is 4.4 keV for the semiconductor and 79 keV for the NaI crystal. The greater resolution of the semiconductor is a great advantage if one is interested primarily in detecting peaks from gamma rays whose energies are very nearly the same. From a sensitivity point of view, however, the crystal of NaI has the advantage, since its thickness can be made about 20 times as great and so will absorb a much larger fraction of the incident gamma rays. In addition, NaI crystals of large area (diameters up to 45 cm) can be grown, whereas the semiconductor is a device with a small area. Because of the insensitive nature of the semiconductor in comparison with NaI crystals, the former has not yet found much value in nuclear medicine. It is, however, useful in measuring the spectrum of x rays (see Chaps. 2 and 8).

14.05 STATISTICS OF ISOTOPE COUNTING

Radioactive disintegrations occur at random, and it is impossible to predict when a given atom will disintegrate. All that can be said is that during one half-life a particular atom has a 50:50 chance of disintegrating. Although little can be said concerning an individual atom, it is possible to predict the fraction of a large number of atoms that will disintegrate in a given time.

Suppose in an experiment with a source of long half-life, a counter records 10^3 counts in 1.0 minutes. If the source is again counted a number of times for a period of 1 minute, one will observe counts ranging from about 900 to 1100, with an average of 1000. The probability of observing a count N is given in Figure 14-7. Thus, for example, if the source is counted 1000 times, an answer of 940 or 1060 will be obtained 2.1 times; an answer of 960 or 1040, 5.7 times; and an answer of 1000, 12.8 times. The reason for the different experimental results is not due to any error made by the operator or by the counter but is due to the inherent statistical variations in the disintegration of the source. Indeed, if the same answer was obtained each time a measurement was made, one could conclude that the apparatus was *not* working properly.

POISSON DISTRIBUTION. The probability curve of Figure 14-7 is described mathematically by the expression:

$$P_N = \frac{a^N e^{-a}}{N!} \qquad (14\text{-}1)$$

where P_N is the probability of observing the value N when the expected value is a. The expected value a is the value one would observe if enough counts were taken and averaged to ensure a negligible error in the answer. N! is called factorial N, which is the product $N(N-1)(N-2) \ldots 1$. The sum of all the probabilities of Figure 14-7 can be seen by inspection to be about 1.00 since a rectangle of height .005 and width 200 would have about the same area. This Poisson distribution is applicable to many problems in biology and will be used to deal with the probability of cure in section 17.06.

STANDARD DEVIATION AND PROBABLE ERROR. It follows from the above that whenever a measurement is made, there is always associated with it a certain error due to these statistical fluctuations. The error is usually expressed in terms of the standard deviation, σ, or the probable error, p, which are defined as:

$$\text{Standard deviation} = \sigma = \sqrt{N} \qquad (14\text{-}2)$$

$$\text{Probable error} = p = 0.67\sqrt{N}$$

where N is the number of counts recorded. In the example illustrated in Figure 14-7, the number of counts observed in 1 minute is on the average 1000; hence the standard deviation is $\sigma = \sqrt{1000} = 32$ and the probable error $p = 0.67 \times 32 = 21$. The probability of observing a count in the range $N \pm p$ (in this case 1000 ± 21) is given by the area under the curve of Figure 14-7 between these limits. It can be shown that this probability is 0.50. This means that if many measurements of the number of counts are made, the observed number will lie outside the range 1000 ± 21 just as often as it will lie inside this range.

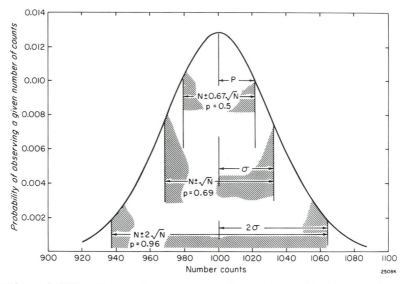

Figure 14-7. Probability of observing a given number of counts N when, on the average, 1000 counts are observed.

The standard deviation is larger than the probable error; hence, there will be a greater chance of observing a count within the range $N \pm \sqrt{N}$ than outside this range. It can be shown that the probability of finding the answer within the range $N \pm \sqrt{N}$ is 0.69 and outside the range is 0.31. Thus, a measurement will lie in this range 69 times out of 100. The probability of finding the measurement within the range $N \pm 2\sigma$ is 0.96 and the chances of obtaining a measurement outside this range is 4 in 100. These principles will be illustrated by several examples.

Example 14-1. Find the number of counts that should be taken to make the standard deviation in the measurement 2%.

Let N be the required number of counts.

Standard deviation $= \sigma = \sqrt{N}$

% error in standard deviation $= \dfrac{\sqrt{N}}{N} \times 100 = 2$

Therefore, $\sqrt{N} = 50$, $N = 2500$ counts, and $\sigma = 50$.

In this example, if 2500 counts are taken, the true value will lie within the range 2500 ± 50 in 69% of the measurements or in about 2 times out of 3. If greater confidence in the result is desired, more counts should be taken.

Example 14-2. Find the number of counts that should be taken to make the percent probable error in the measurement 1%.

$.67 \dfrac{\sqrt{N}}{N} = \dfrac{1}{100}$

$\therefore \sqrt{N} = 67$; $N = 4470$; $p = .67\sqrt{N} = 45$

This means if 4470 counts are taken the correct value will lie in the range 4470 ± 45 in half the measurements.

BACKGROUND. Any counter will show a small counting rate, even in the absence of a source, due to background radiation. The background may be taken into account as follows:

Let N_s be the sample counts measured in time t_s
Let N_b be the number of background counts in time t_b
The uncorrected activity is $A_s = N_s/t_s$
The background activity is $A_b = N_b/t_b$
The standard deviations in these activities are $\sqrt{(N_s)}/t_s$ and $\sqrt{(N_b)}/t_b$.
The true activity, A, of the sample is $A = A_s - A_b$.

We wish to determine the standard deviation in A. It can be shown that if two quantities have standard deviations σ_1 and σ_2 then the standard deviation in their sum or difference is:

$$\sigma = \sqrt{\sigma_1^2 + \sigma_2^2} \qquad (14\text{-}3a)$$

Hence the standard deviation in A is:

$$\sigma_A = \sqrt{\dfrac{N_s}{t_s^2} + \dfrac{N_b}{t_b^2}} = \sqrt{\dfrac{A_s}{t_s} + \dfrac{A_b}{t_b}} \qquad (14\text{-}3b)$$

Example 14-3. A sample counted in the presence of background gave 2700 counts in 3 minutes. In the absence of the sample the counter gave 300 counts in 3 minutes. Find the activity and its standard deviation.

$$A_s = \frac{2700}{3} = 900 \text{ min}^{-1}$$

$$A_b = \frac{300}{3} = 100 \text{ min}^{-1}$$

$$A = 900 - 100 = 800 \text{ min}^{-1}$$

$$\sigma_A = \sqrt{\frac{900}{3} + \frac{100}{3}} = 18.3 \text{ min}^{-1} \text{ (eq. 14-3b)}$$

$$\text{Percent standard deviation} = \frac{18.3}{800} \times 100 = 2.3$$

In determining the activity in this example a total time of 6 minutes was spent counting. The question could be asked what portion of the time should be spent counting background in order to achieve the maximum precision in a given total counting time? It can be shown that for maximum precision

$$\frac{t_s}{t_b} = \sqrt{\frac{A_s}{A_b}} \tag{14-4}$$

In the above example $t_s/b_s = \sqrt{(900/100)} = 3.0$ so that we should have counted the sample for 4.5 minutes and the background for 1.5 minutes. The reader may show that if this had been done the standard deviation would have been reduced from 18.3 counts/min to 16.3 counts/min.

14.06   RESOLVING TIME AND LOSS OF COUNTS

A Geiger counter is insensitive for a short period of time after each pulse has been received. This insensitive period depends upon the counter and its associated circuit but is of the order of 100 μs for most Geiger counters. Scintillation counters suffer from the same defect, although their insensitive periods are usually less than 10 μs. At high counting rates it is clear that some counts will be missed unless corrections for the effect are made.

Let N_o be the observed number of counts per second, N_c, be the corrected number of counts per second, and τ the insensitive period after each count. The total insensitive time in 1 second will be $N_o\tau$, and in this time $N_cN_o\tau$ counts will be missed. Therefore,

$$N_c = N_o + N_cN_o\tau \quad \text{or} \quad N_o = \frac{N_o}{1 - N_o\tau} \tag{14-5}$$

The resolving time may be measured experimentally by counting two sources of about the same activity separately and together. Source A is first placed near the counter and counted, then source B is placed beside source A and both counted and finally source A is removed and B counted alone. If N_A, N_B, and N_{AB} are the measured counts per unit time corrected for background, then:

$$\frac{N_A}{(1 - N_A\tau)} + \frac{N_B}{(1 - N_B\tau)} = \frac{N_{AB}}{(1 - N_{AB}\tau)}$$

Simplifying and neglecting terms in τ^2, one obtains:

$$\tau = \frac{N_A + N_B - N_{AB}}{2\,N_A N_B} \qquad (14\text{-}6)$$

In performing this experiment, high counting rates should be used, otherwise the difference between $(N_A + N_B)$ and N_{AB} will be very small and the numerator of equation 14-6 hard to determine precisely.

Example 14-4. In an experiment to calculate the resolving time, a Geiger counter gave 1182 counts per second for source A, 2063 counts per second for sources A and B together, with 1223 counts per second for source B alone. The background count was 2 counts per second and may be neglected in comparison. Calculate the resolving time and the corrected counting rate for source A.

$$\tau = \frac{N_A + N_B - N_{AB}}{2\,N_A N_B} = \frac{1182 + 1223 - 2063}{2\,(1182)\,(1223)} = 118 \times 10^{-6}\ s$$

Now using equation 14-5, we obtain for the corrected counting rate for source A.

$$N_c = \frac{N_A}{1 - N_A\tau} = \frac{1182}{1 - 1182 \times 118 \times 10^{-6}} = \frac{1182}{1 - 0.139}$$

$$= 1374\ \text{counts/s}$$

Thus, neglect of this correction would introduce an error of about 16% in the counting rate. With scintillation counters, the resolving time is small and corrections for loss of counts usually need not be made.

14.07 SAMPLE COUNTING—UPTAKE AND VOLUME STUDIES

In many diagnostic procedures it is necessary to determine the amount of radioactivity in a sample of blood, urine, feces, etc. The arrangement of the source and detector for the counting procedure is called the geometry of the set up. If, for example, a detector of area A cm^2 is placed r cm from a point source, then it will intercept a fraction $A/4\pi r^2$ of the radiations from the source. If the source has an activity of S μCi, then the counting rate will be:

$$\text{Counting rate} = (3.700 \times 10^4 \times S) \frac{A}{4\pi r^2} \cdot k \cdot \eta \cdot f \qquad (14\text{-}7)$$

In this expression, k is the number of detectable particles ejected per disintegration and is determined from the disintegration scheme (see Chapter 3), η is the efficiency of the detector for counting the radiations, and f is the fraction of the emitted particles that escape from the source. Now although equation 14-7 is simple in concept, it is of little practical value because of the difficulty in evaluating k, η, and f with any precision; hence, absolute determinations of activity are usually confined to standardization laboratories. In a nuclear medicine department, one solves the problem by a suitable comparison technique in which the unknown and a standard source are counted in the *same* geometry, as illustrated in the next section. Counting devices tend to be unstable, so it is essential that they be checked at frequent intervals. A constancy check, or stability check, is easily performed using a sealed sample of a long-lived radioactive material such as Co-60, Cs-137, or Ra-226.

Thyroid Uptake

One of the simplest measurements that may be carried out is the determination of the amount of iodine taken up by the thyroid gland in 24 hours. 10 μCi of I-131 as the sodium salt is given the patient orally, and an *equal* sample is set aside in a small test tube for use as the comparison standard. Twenty-four hours later the patient is positioned as in Figure 14-8a with the crystal of the scintillation counter about 25 cm from the thyroid. It is useful to have the patient lying down and to position the crystal over the patient by either a plumb bob or a pointer. The crystal should be provided with a conical diaphragm that excludes radiation from the region outside a 10 cm diameter circle, measured at the position of the neck of the patient. The crystal should be covered with a lead filter, A, 1.5 mm thick.

The counter is then positioned over a standard neck phantom, which may be a Lucite cylinder 12 cm in diameter with a hole drilled in it parallel to the axis 1 cm below the surface. This hole will take a 30 ml test tube containing the comparison standard. When measurements are made on it, the surface of this phantom is placed the same distance from the crystal as the surface of the patient's neck.

Four measurements are required for an uptake study.

1. With the crystal positioned as above, measure the activity of the thyroid in counts/min. Let this activity be P.

2. Cover the thyroid with a lead filter B (10 cm by 10 cm and 1.25 cm thick, see Fig. 14-8a) and obtain a background measurement P_b in counts/min.

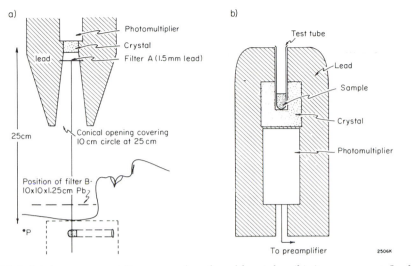

Figure 14-8. (a) Arrangement for measuring thyroid uptake. (b) Arrangement for blood volume determinations.

3. Position the phantom as described above and obtain the activity of the standard S in counts/min.

4. Cover the standard phantom with filter B and obtain a phantom background S_b in counts/min.

Sufficient counts should be taken to yield a precision of 2% or better. From these measurements, it follows that

$$\% \text{ thyroid uptake} = \frac{P - P_b}{S - S_b} \times 100 \qquad (14\text{-}8)$$

The difference between readings 1 and 2 gives the activity that came directly from the thyroid and excludes any activity arising from points in the patient remote from the thyroid. Likewise the difference between readings 3 and 4 corrects for the natural background of the counter and gives the counts that arose directly in the standard. If simple precautions such as these are not taken, very erroneous results may be obtained. There is no difficulty in measuring a thyroid with a very high uptake, but in a thyroid with a low uptake the activity from the rest of the patient can lead to large errors in the measured activity, unless the background measurement described in step 2 is carefully taken.

The filter A covering the crystal is designed to attenuate the softer scattered radiation from the patient. A still better arrangement used in many centers employs a discriminator that excludes all radiation below the photopeak. For iodine the prominent gamma ray is at 364 keV and the discriminator should be set at about 300 keV.

Example 14-5. In a thyroid uptake study, the activity as measured with filter B removed was 400 counts/min and with B in place 150 counts/min. The corresponding activities with the standard in position were 3000 counts/min and 160 counts/min respectively. Determine the percent thyroid activity.

$$\text{\% thyroid uptake} \atop \text{(eq. 14-8)} = \frac{400 - 150}{3000 - 160} \times 100 = \frac{250}{2840} = 8.8\%$$

If no account had been taken of the two background measurements, the % uptake would be incorrectly determined as:

$$\frac{400}{3000} \times 100 = 13.3\%$$

This illustrates the importance of taking background into account in dealing with a thyroid of small uptake.

Determination of Plasma Volume—Well Counter

An efficient way to measure the radioactivity of a sample is to use a well-type crystal, as illustrated in Figure 14-8b. Such a crystal almost completely surrounds the sample and most of the disintegrations in the sample give rise to pulses of light that are counted by the photomultiplier. Well counters are used when maximum sensitivity is required. The crystal and photomultiplier should be surrounded by a 10 cm wall of lead.

We will illustrate the use of a well counter by determining the patient's plasma volume. Serum albumin tagged with radioactive iodine (RISA) is available commercially. 10 μCi of RISA is injected intravenously into the patient and an equal amount saved as a standard. After 10 minutes to allow complete mixing in the patient, a sample of blood is removed and the red cells_are separated from the plasma by centrifugation. The radioactivity of the plasma is measured in the well counter. Since the normal patient's plasma volume is about 3000 ml, the activity of 1 ml of plasma will be about 1/3000 of the activity of 1 ml of standard. Thus, it is convenient to dilute the standard by placing it in 1000 to 2000 ml of water. The activity in counts/min of the diluted standard and the plasma sample are then determined in the same well counter. After corrections have been made for background, the plasma volume may be determined.

Example 14-6. In a plasma volume study about 10 μCi of RISA was injected intravenously and an equal amount diluted into 2000 ml of water for the standard. 10 ml of blood was removed and centrifuged to separate the plasma from the red cells. 3.0 ml of supernatant (plasma) was counted for 1 min giving 2470 counts. Then 3 ml of the standard solution was counted for the same time, giving 3,430 counts. The well counter had a background of 160 counts/min. Calculate the plasma volume.

Plasma activity = 2470 − 160 = 2310 counts/min
Standard activity = 3430 − 160 = 3270 counts/min
Therefore, plasma volume = (2000) (3270)/2310 = 2831 ml

14.08   IMAGING USING RADIOACTIVE MATERIALS

In the last section we discussed ways to measure the total activity in an organ. Often one requires a device that will allow one to visualize the distribution of activity in the organ; we will now discuss such devices.

Rectilinear Scanner

One of the simplest imaging devices consists of a scintillation counter in a radiation shield, which is moved slowly back and forth across the region of interest in the patient. The pulses from the crystal are amplified, scaled down by a suitable factor, and then made to operate a mechanical or electrical register, which produces a permanent record on a sheet of paper or a film as illustrated on the right of Figure 14-9.

Two types of collimating devices illustrated in Figure 14-9 are in common use. The simplest type (Fig. 14-9a) consists of a single hole in the lead shield, which allows a pencil of gamma rays from the thyroid to strike the center of the crystal. A typical thyroid scan with such a single hole collimator is shown in the upper right hand corner of Figure 14-9. Greater detail of visualization can be obtained using a focusing collimator shown in Figure 14-9b. In this collimator, the single hole is replaced by a number of tapered holes, all of which point to one point on the axis of the crystal. With such a device, smaller holes may be used and greater resolving power achieved (see scan B of Fig. 14-9). This scan shows greater detail than the former. Scans may be improved by rejecting gamma rays that have been scattered by the tissues surrounding the thyroid. These scattered gamma rays have lower energy and can be eliminated from the scaling circuit by either a discriminator or a pulse-height analyzer.

Both scans shown in Figure 14-9 are for a normal thyroid. When a thyroid carcinoma is present, the diseased region is usually nonfunctioning and so does not take up iodine. However, its presence may often be inferred because it crowds the normal thyroid out of its usual position. Thyroid scans are the easiest scans of all to perform because the thyroid takes up a high percentage of the administered activity and concentrates it into a small region near the skin. With modern techniques, good scans of many organs in the body can easily be obtained (see Fig. 14-11).

The Anger Camera

The gamma camera developed by Anger (A10, A11, R7) is an alternative type of device that can be used to obtain an image of the distribution of activity in an organ. It detects and records the activity in *all* parts of the organ within its field of view. Thus, it is particularly useful in studying the rate at which activity moves in and out of an organ. The basic

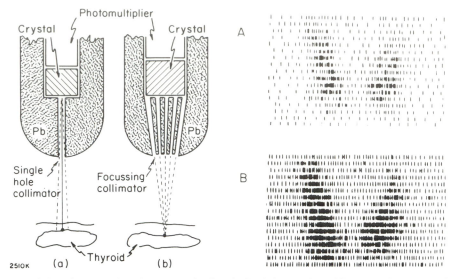

Figure 14-9. Diagram showing 2 methods of obtaining a thyroid scan using (a) a single hole collimator, and (b) a focusing collimator. Scans of normal thyroids are shown for the two types of collimators in A and B.

principles of the Anger camera are illustrated in Figure 14-10. The heart of the device is a NaI crystal about 30 cm in diameter and 1.2 cm thick mounted on a Lucite plate. This crystal is "looked at" by a large number of photomultipliers in an hexagonal array. Early cameras used 19 photomultiplier tubes each 7.5 cm in diameter. Recently, the trend has been towards the use of more tubes (37, 61, or 91) of smaller diameter. To increase the packing efficiency some units use hexagonal shaped photomultipliers. Light flashes from the crystal are transmitted to the photomultipliers by a Lucite coupling plate about 1.5 cm thick. The crystal is covered by a multichannel collimator made of lead containing thousands of parallel holes about 2 mm in size. The crystal photomultiplier assembly is surrounded by lead to exclude extraneous radiations. In use, the unit is usually held in a *fixed* position over the organ under study and the distribution of radioactivity in the organ is presented on the screen of a cathode ray oscilloscope.

When a gamma ray from a point P in the patient (see Fig. 14-10) is emitted in the vertical direction, it will pass through a hole in the collimator and produce a scintillation in the crystal. The X and Y coordinates of this scintillation will be exactly the same as the X and Y coordinates of the point P. The photomultipliers and associated electronic circuits are designed to determine these coordinates, X and Y. The electronic circuits are complicated but the principle of the device can be easily understood. When the scintillation occurs, flashes of light will go out in all directions and will excite all of the photomultipliers. The size of the signal

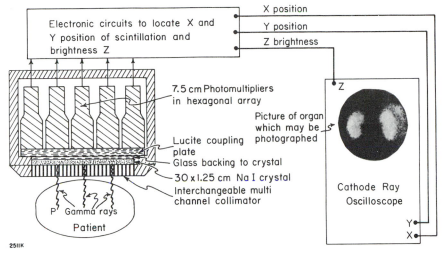

Figure 14-10. Schematic diagram to illustrate the Anger type camera.

received by each will depend upon its proximity to the flash. A voltage pulse is generated from the 19 pulses, which is proportional to the X coordinate, and this is applied to the X deflection plate of the scope. Similarly a voltage pulse proportional to the Y coordinate is developed and applied to the Y deflection plate. The sum of the 19 signals from the photomultipliers is also obtained yielding the Z pulse. If this Z pulse corresponds to the energy of the gamma ray emitted from the patient, the spot on the scope appears; if, however, it arises from a less energetic scattered photon, the signal is suppressed, thus preventing scattered photons from contributing to the picture. Hence, the device produces on the scope a single bright flash at coordinates X' and Y', which correspond to the coordinates X and Y of the position of origin of the gamma ray in the patient. The screen of the oscilloscope may be observed continually by a camera, so that each flash on the screen is recorded on film.

To increase its flexibility, the camera is provided with a series of interchangeable collimators of different thicknesses. The thick ones are necessary when penetrating gamma emitters are used, and the thin ones for low energy emitters. Also the multichannel collimator may be replaced with a pinhole collimator. This type of collimator is used to study a small organ, such as the thyroid gland, which is near the skin surface. This collimator has a single hole and is placed at a distance from the crystal so that an inverted image of the radioactivity in the patient is reproduced on the crystal and then transmitted to the scope.

The Anger camera is the most popular imaging device used in nuclear medicine today and as a result has been improved in many ways. Because most imaging today is done using technetium 99m, which emits a 140 keV gamma ray, shielding becomes a relatively simple task so that the collimators and the device can be made relatively light. The 140 keV gamma rays are readily absorbed in NaI so these crystals can be made quite thin, thus decreasing the spread of the light from the initial point of interaction and increasing the resolution. Modern cameras are designed to increase the precision in determining the coordinates X′ and Y′ and in making the device equally sensitive at all points within the large diameter of the crystal. To achieve this high performance, improved photomultiplier tubes, nonlinear transmitting light pipes, nonlinear preamplifiers, and microprocessors are used. In addition, devices that correct for blurring due to respiratory motion can be added to the camera. They are helpful for imaging an organ near the diaphragm such as the liver (B17).

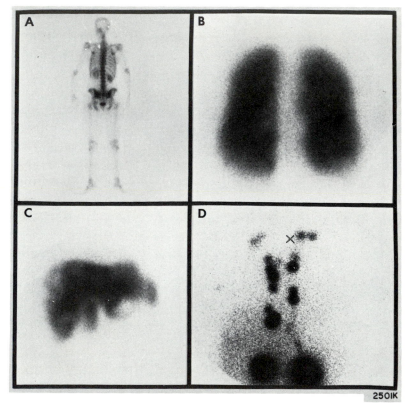

Figure 14-11. Typical Images from Anger Type Cameras. (a) Posterior skeletal scintigram imaged at 6 hours after an intravenous injection of 13.5 mCi of Tc-99m pyrophosphate. (b) Posterior scintigram of lungs imaged immediately after an intravenous injection of 2 mCi of Tc-99m macro-aggregated albumin. (c) Anterior scintigram of a liver imaged 30 minutes after an intravenous injection of 2 mCi of Tc-99m sulphide colloid. The scintigram indicates extensive disease of the liver. (d) Anterior scintigram of parasternal lymph nodes. The scintigram was made at 6 hours after an initial right subcostal injection of 0.5 mCi of Tc-99m antimony sulphide colloid and 3 hours after a similar left subcostal injection. The scintigrams were made with a commercial wide field of view gamma camera of the Anger type. The skeletal scintigram was imaged by slowly moving the camera or the patient during the imaging process.

Delay Line Scintillation Camera

Another form of Anger camera is one that uses two delay lines to determine the position of X′ and Y′ after each flash produced in the crystal. Each photomultiplier is connected through an amplifier to an X-delay line and through another amplifier to a Y-delay line. After a scintillation flash every photomultiplier sends a signal to the two delay lines where they are integrated to give a pulse with a peak at one position. These are transmitted down the delay lines and the time taken for the pulse to reach the end of each line determines X′ and Y′. If the sum of these two pulses corresponds to a legitimate pulse the pulses are accepted and a bright spot is produced at the appropriate spot on the oscilloscope. (For further details see R7.)

Positron Emission Tomography (PET)

The success of the CT scanner is diagnostic radiology (see section 16.19) has spurred a number of groups to develop a scanner that detects radiations emitted from the patient and creates a cross-sectional view of the activity in *a plane* through the organ of interest in the patient. The device makes use of the fact that when a positron is annihilated (see section 3.09) two gamma rays each of 0.511 MeV energy are emitted at the same point in time and at 180° to one another (B18). Imagine many banks of crystal photomultiplier tube assemblies placed around the patient as illustrated in Figure 14-12. Suppose a nuclear disintegration producing a positron occurs at some point P within the patient. If two counters (Q_1 and Q_2) receive a pulse at the same instant, i.e. register a coincidence, then we know that the point P must lie somewhere along the line Q_1Q_2. This information is stored in a computer. The counters are arranged to record coincidences between each counter in bank D with all of the counters of bank A. Similarly, coincidences between B and E and C and F are recorded. The coincidences are all stored and after the acquisition of enough data the computer is able to reconstruct the distribution of activity in the patient that must have been present to yield the observed coincidences. The principles involved in obtaining a visual display from the measurements is somewhat similar to the techniques used in obtaining an image from a CT scanner (see section 16.19).

An ideal camera should have enough crystal photomultiplier detectors that every annihilation photon is detected and matched up with the corresponding photon emitted at 180°. This is, of course, impractical since one would require crystals covering the whole of the surface of a sphere and the electronics to go with all these counters. Even with the limited number of detectors shown in Figure 14-12, the electronics is already complicated. This is a field that is developing rapidly, however, and new developments will undoubtedly appear (for example, see T9).

Positron cameras require the generation of positron emitting radioac-

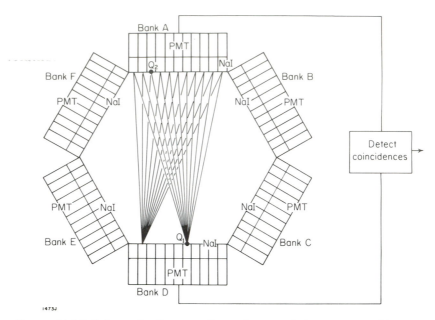

Figure 14-12. Schematic diagram of a positron emission tomographic camera.

tive materials. In general, these cannot be produced in reactors but require high energy protons or deuterons from a cyclotron. Since many of the available positron emitters have short half-lives, imaging with these really requires an in-house cyclotron, which is by no means a trivial installation. As of 1980 a number of companies are developing special cyclotrons for hospital environments. There is much interest in positron emitters of carbon, nitrogen, and oxygen such as carbon 11 (20.3 min), nitrogen 13 (9.97 min), oxygen 14 (71 s), and oxygen 15 (124 s). These can be activated in the gaseous state as CO, CO_2, NH_3 etc. and then quickly incorporated into various amino acids, which are required for protein synthesis, allowing one to study many physiological processes. There is no doubt that imaging with positron emitters will fill an increasingly important role in clinical investigations in the future.

14.09   STUDIES WITH RADIOACTIVE TRACERS

A few of the important isotopes used in nuclear medicine, with their half-lives and the energy of the photons emitted, are listed in Table 14-1. By far the most important isotope is Tc-99m. This tag can be incorporated into a variety of molecules or attached to various colloids. The isotope has a convenient half-life (6.0 h) and emits a 140 keV photon, which is easily detected outside the patient. This isotope is continuously available from a generator that consists of a long-lived parent Mo-99, from which the Tc-99m may be eluted as required (see section 3.16). The use of an isotope with a half-life of about 6 hours is a major advantage because it is long enough to follow most physiological processes and is short enough to avoid unnecessary exposure to the patient. For example, the student may show that 100 μCi of Tc-99m gives about the same dose after complete decay as 1 μCi of I-131. This means for the same dose one can prescribe over 100 times as much Tc-99m as I-131 and thus obtain a much better scan. Until the evolution of the short-lived radionuclides, liver, kidney, or brain scans took about one hour and could achieve resolutions of about 2 cm. With the short-lived radionuclides, much larger doses can be used and similar scans can now be made in a few minutes with a resolution of a few millimeters.

TABLE 14-1
Important Isotopes Used in Nuclear Medicine

Z	Nuclide	Half-Life	Principle Photon Energy (MeV)
6	carbon 14	5760 y	beta emitter
15	phosphorus 32	14.3 d	beta emitter
24	chromium 51	27.7 d	0.320
27	cobalt 57	270 d	0.014, 0.122, 0.136
27	cobalt 58	70.7 d	0.811, 0.864, 1.675 plus annihilation gammas
31	gallium 67	3.24 d	0.092, 0.184, 0.299, 0.393
43	technetium 99m	6.0 h	0.141
53	iodine 123	13.0 h	0.159
53	iodine 131	8.04 d	0.284, 0.364, 0.637, 0.723
50	xenon 133	5.2 d	0.081
79	gold 198	65.0 h	0.412, 0.676, 1.088
81	thallium 201	73.0 h	0.135, 0.166

A few of the most important tests in nuclear medicine are summarized in Table 14-2. The first column gives the test, the second the agent used, its form, the activity required, and the route of administration, which is usually intravenous (I.V.). The last column describes briefly the purpose of the test, how the test is carried out and the interpretation of the results of the test. The reader should note the importance of Tc-99m in today's practice of nuclear medicine.

14.10   BIOLOGICAL AND EFFECTIVE HALF-LIFE

When a radioactive nuclide is administered internally to a patient, the effect of the isotope decreases with time by two processes. The isotope is eliminated from the patient and undergoes radioactive decay. Let λ_b be the fraction of the isotope eliminated biologically per unit time, λ_p the fraction which decays physically per unit time, and λ_{eff} the fraction that disappears per unit time by both processes. Then λ_{eff}, which is called the effective transformation constant, is given by:

$$\lambda_{eff} = \lambda_p + \lambda_b \qquad (14\text{-}9)$$

TABLE 14-2
Important Tests in Nuclear Medicine

Test	Agent, Amount, and Route of Administration	Purpose, Method, Interpretations, and Indications
Plasma volume	Serum albumin tagged with I-131, 10 μCi I.V.	To determine plasma volume in patients with excessive blood loss, burns, cardiovascular disease, or renal disease. Inject albumin and determine dilution (see ex. 14-6). Normal plasma volume (40 $\pm$ 5 ml) per kg weight.
Red cell volume	Erythrocytes tagged with 50 μCi, Cr-51	To determine the red cell volume and the half-life of red cells in patient. Inject tagged red cells and determine red cell volume and their half-life. Normal red cell volume = (33 $\pm$ 5 ml)/kg weight, normal half-life 26-30d.
Vitamin B_{12} absorption	Vitamin B_{12} with IF tagged with Co-57, 5 μCi orally, and vitamin B_{12}, tagged with Co-58, 1.0 μCi orally.	To study the absorption of vitamin B_{12} and the effect of the intrinsic factor (IF) on this absorption. Inject (a) vitamin B_{12} combined with its intrinsic factor (IF) tagged with Co-58. Determine the activity excreted in urine. If the ratio of activity of Co-57 to Co-58 is greater than 1.7, the patient suffers from pernicious anemia.
Thyroid	I-131 as the Na salt, 50 μCi orally	To test thyroid function and, if necessary, plan radioiodine therapy. Inject I-131 and measure uptake 24 hours later (see ex. 14-5) 24 hour uptake in range 10-40% is normal.
Imaging of thyroid	Na^{99m}TcO$_4^-$, 2 mCi I.V.	To visualize areas of thyroid with increased or decreased uptake and shape of gland. Inject intravenously as the pertechnetate ion and scan 2 hours later or take picture with Anger camera.
Imaging the brain	Tc-99m glucoheptonate, 20 mCi I.V.	To study vascularity of brain resulting from physical injury or a tumor. Abnormal brain scan shows foci of increased radioactivity against a "cold" background.
Imaging liver and spleen	Tc-99m sulphur colloid, 2 mCi I.V.	To identify abnormality in liver and spleen. A sulphur colloid tagged with Tc-99m is injected into patient and an image obtained on an Anger camera 30 min later. Normal areas concentrate the colloid, diseased areas do not.
Kidney	Glucoheptonate tagged with Tc-99m, 10 mCi I.V.	To locate space-occupying lesions in the kidney. Organ is viewed by an Anger camera. The tracer is rapidly fixed in the healthy kidney. Diseased areas show reduced uptake indicating renal trauma, tumors, or cysts.
Lung	Albumin macroaggregates tagged with Tc-99m, 3 mCi I.V.	To locate regions of defective perfusion in lung. Because of the size of macroaggregates, they are trapped in the pulmonary capillary bed. "Cold" areas indicate defective perfusion.
Internal and mammary lymph nodes; internal iliac lymph nodes	Antimony sulphide colloid tagged with Tc-99m, 500 μCi.	To examine and localize internal mammary and pelvic lymph nodes. The colloid is injected interstitially into an appropriate tissue plane and the nodes are imaged a few hours later with Anger Camera (E6, E7).
Skeleton	Phosphates tagged with Tc-99m, 0.2 mCi per kg weight I.V.	To locate tumors of the bone, regions of trauma, or arthritic regions. Image skeleton with Anger camera or scanning device 2 to 4 hours after injection. The phosphate tracer behaves like calcium.
Tumors	Gallium-67 as the citrate, 3 mCi I.V.	To locate tumors and regions of inflammation. A positive scan indicates the presence of disease, but a negative scan does not preclude disease.

The 3 transformation constants are related to the corresponding half-lives by equation 1-27 so that we may write:

$$\lambda_{eff} = \frac{0.693}{T_{eff}}; \quad \lambda_p = \frac{0.693}{T_p}; \quad \lambda_b = \frac{0.693}{T_b} \tag{14-10}$$

where T_{eff}, T_p, and T_b are the effective, physical, and biological half-lives respectively. Substituting these values in equation 14-9 one obtains:

$$\frac{1}{T_{eff}} = \frac{1}{T_p} + \frac{1}{T_b} \quad \text{or} \quad T_{eff} = \frac{T_p \cdot T_b}{T_p + T_b} \tag{14-11}$$

This is the relation between the effective half-life, the biological half-life, and the physical half-life. T_{eff} is the half-life that is used in dosimetry problems. It is smaller than both the physical and the biological half-lives.

Example 14-7. In a thyroid study, the activity of the thyroid was found to decay with a half-life of 5.0 d as measured against a source of constant activity. Find the biological half-life.

The physical half-life for iodine is $T_p = 8.05$ d and the effective half-life is $T_{eff} = 5.0$ d; substituting in equation 14-11:

$$\frac{1}{5.0} = \frac{1}{8.05} + \frac{1}{T_b}$$

Therefore, $\dfrac{1}{T_b} = \dfrac{1}{5.0} - \dfrac{1}{8.05} = \dfrac{3.05}{(5.0)\,(8.05)}$

Hence, $T_b = 13.2$ d

In most studies it is usual to compare the thyroid activity with the decaying standard source of the same isotope. If this had been done, the thyroid activity would have appeared to decay with a half-life of 13.2 d.

RESERVATIONS CONCERNING THE BIOLOGICAL HALF-LIFE. In discussing the biological half-life, we have assumed that an organ or patient excretes the same fraction of its activity in each interval of time. This assumption leads to exponential elimination of the isotope in an analogous way to the physical exponential decay of a radionuclide. This is obviously a gross oversimplification as can be seen from the following discussion. Suppose a patient is given an oral dose of iodine. This iodine is first absorbed into the bloodstream from the gut. Once in the bloodstream, it is distributed to all tissues. The thyroid tissue continually removes the iodine and stores it. At the same time the kidney removes some of the iodine and excretes it. As the iodine level in the blood falls, tissues other than the thyroid return iodine to the blood. Thus the iodine is distributed into many compartments with varying rates of uptake and release. It is obvious then that this complex process cannot be represented by a single parameter such as the biological half-life. Some workers speak in terms of a series of half times, which are not equal. The biological half-life can at best describe a biological system in a very approximate way.

14.11   ABSORBED DOSE ARISING FROM
RADIONUCLIDES WITHIN THE BODY

In several of the earlier chapters of this book we have determined the dose to tissues arising from external beams of radiation. In Chapter 13 we dealt with the dose arising from the insertion of *encapsulated* sources of radiation into tissue in the form of implants. We now deal with the much more complex problem of calculating the dose to tissues in a given organ arising from radioactive material in the *same* organ or some *other* organ of the body. These calculations are important in the field of health physics since it is essential to know the dose to a critical organ arising from activity in some other organ. The numbers arising from these calculations are needed by those charged with the task of specifying maximum permissible doses to radiation workers. This aspect of the problem will be further dealt with in Chapter 15. Dose calculations are also required for patients who receive a radioactive isotope in the treatment of a diseased tissue, as for example in the treatment of thyroid cancer with radioiodine.

Since 1968, a committee of the Society of Nuclear Medicine called MIRD (*Medical Internal Radiation Dose*) has taken as its responsibility the creation of extensive tables so that dose calculations can be made for all the commonly used radionuclides (L1). The reader is advised to obtain these MIRD pamphlets for ready reference. The MIRD committee has reduced a very complex problem to manageable proportions. In this section we will discuss the physical principles behind the use of these tables and will use exerpts from them to solve a few specific problems.

NUCLEAR DATA. The starting point for any dose calculation requires detailed information on the physical factors involved in the decay of the radionuclides. Needed are the types of "particles" emitted, their relative numbers, and energy. These have been collected together in MIRD #10 (D1) for 54 of the commonly used radionuclides. To illustrate their use we present in Table 14-3 data from MIRD #10 for technetium 99m, the most commonly used isotope in nuclear medicine. The first column gives the transition; the second the mean number of emissions per disintegration; the third column the energy difference for the transition; the final column describes the nature of the transition in terms of nuclear symbols. From the first three columns one can calculate the energy emitted per disintegration, as shown at the bottom of Table 14-3, yielding the value $.2284 \times 10^{-13}$ J.

Before any further calculation of dose can be carried out, a detailed knowledge of the nature of the gamma transitions is required. These are described by symbols shown in column 4 such as E1, M3, M4 defining the multiplicity order of the transition. In addition the internal conver-

TABLE 14-3
Input Data for Tc-99m, Half-Life 6.03h*

(1) Transition	(2) Mean No. per Disintegration	(3) Transition Energy (MeV)	(4) Other Nuclear Data
gamma 1	.9860	.0021	E3
gamma 2	.9860	.1405	M1, $a_K = .104$, K/L conv. ratio = 7.7
gamma 3	.0140	.1426	M4, $\alpha_K = 23.0$, $\alpha_L = 9.21$
energy emitted per dis.		= (.9860) (.0021) + (.9860) (.1405) + (.0140) (.1426) = .1426 MeV	
		= (.1426) (1.602 × 10⁻¹³ J) = .2284 × 10⁻¹³ J	

*From Dillman and Von der Lage (DI)

sion ratios for the K or L shell (α_K, α_L) and the K to L conversion ratio are required. A knowledge of these parameters enables one to calculate the number of conversion electrons and the number of "holes" left in various shells. From the fluorescent yield one can determine the number and energy of the K or L characteristic radiation and the number and energy of the Auger electrons.

These details taken from MIRD #10 (D1) and called *output data* are given in the first 4 columns of Table 14-4. The first entry is for the

TABLE 14-4
Output Data for Technetium 99m

(1)	(2) Mean # per Dis.	(3) Mean Energy of Particle (MeV)	Total (4) g rads/ μCi.h	Total (5) J/dis × 10⁻¹³	Local (6) J/dis × 10⁻¹³	Remote (7)
(1) Gamma 1	.0000	.0021	.0000	.0000	.0000	.0000
(1a) Int. Conv. el-M	.9860	.0016	.0035	.0026	.0026	
(2) Gamma 2	.8787	.1405	.2630	.1980		.1980
(2a) Int. Conv. el-K	.0913	.1194	.0232	.0174	.0174	
(2b) Int. Conv. el-L	.0118	.1377	.0034	.0026	.0026	
(2c) Int. Conv. el-M	.0039	.1400	.0011	.0008	.0008	
(3) Gamma 3	.0003	.1426	.0001	.0001		.0001
(3a) Int. Conv. el-K	.0088	.1215	.0022	.0016	.0016	
(3b) Int. Conv. el-L	.0035	.1398	.0010	.0007	.0007	
(3c) Int. Conv. el-M	.0011	.1422	.0003	.0002	.0002	
(3d) Fluorescent $K_{\alpha1}$	.0441	.0183	.0017	.0013	.0013	
(3e) Fluorescent $K_{\alpha2}$	.0221	.0182	.0008	.0006	.0006	
(3f) Fluorescent $K_{\beta1}$	.0105	.0206	.0004	.0003	.0003	
(3g) Auger el KLL	.0152	.0154	.0005	.0004	.0004	
(3h) Auger el KLX*	.0055	.0178	.0002	.0002	.0002	
(3i) Auger el LMM	.1093	.0019	.0004	.0003	.0003	
(3j) Auger el MXY†	1.2359	.0004	.0011	.0008	.0008	
			.3029	.2279		
					.0298	.1981
(1)	(2)	(3)	(4)	(5)	(6)	(7)

*KLX = an Auger electron emitted from the X shell in which X stands for any shell higher than the L shell as a result of the transition of an L shell electron to a vacancy in the K shell.
†MXY = X and Y each stand for any shell higher than the M shell.

gamma 1 transition and we see from the second and third column that no gammas of energy .0021 MeV appear but that all of the gammas are internally converted in the M shell producing electrons of energy .0016 MeV. The next entry (#2) is for gamma 2, which does appear in 0.8787 of the disintegrations with the total transition energy of .1405 MeV and is in addition converted in the K, L, and M shells as shown by entries 2a, 2b, and 2c. Entries 3a, 3b, 3c are for gamma 3, which behaves somewhat the same as gamma 2. The rest of the table deals with the "holes" left by the conversion electrons leading to the entries for the fluorescent radiation and the Auger electrons resulting from gamma 3.

The fourth column gives the energy deposited in g rads per μCi h. It is called the equilibrium dose constant, Δ, because in determining it we assume the isotope is uniformly deposited in a large enough organ so that none of the gammas or fluorescent photons escape and so that in any given element of volume the same number of particles are emitted as are absorbed. In SI units the unit of cumulated activity is the Bq s, which is one nuclear disintegration, and the unit of energy is the joule or kg Gy. In these units the equilibrium dose constant is expressed in J/dis, and values determined in this way are given in column 5. The relation between these units is obtained thus:

$$1\ \mu\text{Ci h} = 3.7 \times 10^4\ \frac{\text{dis}}{\text{s}} \times 3600\ \text{s} = 1.332 \times 10^8\ \text{dis}$$

$$1\ \text{g rad} = 1\ \text{g} \times 100\ \frac{\text{erg}}{\text{g}} = 100\ \text{erg} = 10^{-5}\ \text{J} = 10^{-5}\ \text{kg Gy}$$

$$1\ \text{g rad per}\ \mu\text{Ci h} = 10^{-5}\ \text{J}/1.332 \times 10^8\ \text{dis} = .751 \times 10^{-13}\ \text{J/dis}$$

The use of these two units is illustrated by a simple example.

Example 14-8. Table 14-4 shows that gamma 2 has an energy of .1405 MeV and is emitted in .8787 of the disintegrations. Find the equilibrium dose constant, Δ, for this "particle" and express it in J/dis and in g rad/ μCi h.

$$\Delta = .1405 \times .8787 \times 1.602 \times 10^{-13}\ \frac{\text{J}}{\text{dis}} = .198 \times 10^{-13}\ \frac{\text{J}}{\text{dis}}$$

$$= .198 \times 10^{-13} \times \frac{1}{.751 \times 10^{-13}}\ \frac{\text{g rad}}{\mu\ \text{Ci h}} = 0.263\ \frac{\text{g rad}}{\mu\text{Ci h}}$$

These values appear in columns 5 and 4 of Table 14-4.

If we add up the equilibrium dose constants for all of the "particles" emitted by Tc-99m, we obtain .2285 × 10^{-13} J/dis, which checks with the value at the bottom of Table 14-3, showing that all of the energy has been accounted for.

CALCULATION OF DOSE. Imagine some source organ in the body containing a given amount of activity. We wish to calculate the dose received by a target organ due to this activity. The dose calculation will involve the detailed physical information given in Table 14-4 but will require in addition biological information such as the biological half-life, as well as anatomical information concerning the shapes and sizes of different organs, and the geometrical relationship between them. These sizes and shapes will vary from patient to patient. To create a system of dosimetry, the first task is to define a standard phantom, hopefully representing the "average man."

Figure 14-13 shows schematically the adult human phantom with the principal internal organs. The cross sections of the head and trunk are assumed to be elliptical and the shapes of internal organs are defined mathematically (see MIRD #5, S22). One can imagine each organ in turn being filled with a radionuclide and then, using the Monte Carlo technique (see section 6.10), determine the number and types of scattered photons that reach any other organ and thus determine the dose to this organ. Detailed calculations of this type can be found in MIRD #11 (S22), and a very small fraction of these results are presented in Table 14-5 for a few isotopes and a few source and target organs. In this table the dose is given in rad/μCi h and in Gy/Bq s. We illustrate this table by an example.

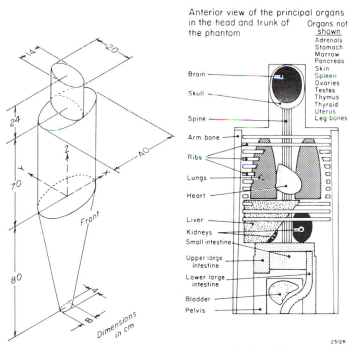

Figure 14-13. "Standard man" with internal organs developed by the MIRD committee #5 to make possible dose calculations for any organ due to the presence of radioactive material in any other organ. (Adapted from Snyder et al., S22.)

TABLE 14-5
Absorbed Dose per Unit Accumulated Activity*

Isotope	Half-Life	Source	Target	rad/μCi h	Gy/Bq s
Tc-99m	6.03 h	liver	liver	4.6×10^{-5}	3.45×10^{-15}
			ovaries	4.5×10^{-7}	3.38×10^{-17}
			testes	6.2×10^{-8}	4.66×10^{-18}
			red marrow	1.6×10^{-6}	1.20×10^{-16}
		thyroid	thyroid	2.3×10^{-3}	1.73×10^{-13}
		bladder	thyroid	2.1×10^{-9}	1.58×10^{-19}
I-131	193 h	thyroid	thyroid	2.2×10^{-2}	1.65×10^{-12}

$$1 \text{ g} \frac{\text{rad}}{\mu\text{Ci h}} = .751 \times 10^{-13} \frac{\text{J}}{\text{Bq s}}$$

$$1 \frac{\text{rad}}{\mu\text{Ci h}} = .751 \times 10^{-10} \frac{\text{Gy}}{\text{Bq s}}$$

*Data taken from MIRD #11 (S22)

Example 14-9. Calculate the mean dose to the liver and ovaries resulting from the intravenous injection of 1 μCi (3.7×10^4 Bq) of technetium attached to a compound that is completely and uniformly localized in the liver. Assume instantaneous uptake and a biological half-life large compared to the physical half-life (6.03 h).

Cumulated activity = $3.7 \times 10^4 \times 6.03 \times 3600 \times 1.44$
   = 1.16×10^9 dis

Liver (Table 14-5) Dose = $1.16 \times 10^9 \times 3.45 \times 10^{-15}$
   = 3.99×10^{-6} Gy = 4×10^{-3} mGy

Ovaries (Table 14-5) Dose = $1.16 \times 10^9 \times 3.38 \times 10^{-17}$
   = 3.92×10^{-8} Gy = 3.9×10^{-5} mGy

The simplicity of the absorbed dose calculations by the MIRD system is obvious. However, no claim can be made for great precision because the patient has been replaced by a model and simplifying assumptions have been made concerning decay.

It is instructive to make a dose estimation from first principles. We will calculate the dose to the thyroid for an accumulated activity of 1 dis in the thyroid of mass .020 kg. We must first decide which of the emissions of Table 14-4 will escape, and which will be absorbed. The gammas have an energy of 140 keV with a mass attenuation coefficient of 0.155 cm^2 g^{-1} in water (see Table A-4a). This corresponds to a linear coefficient of 0.155 cm^{-1} or a half value layer of 4.4 cm. This is large compared with the "radius" of the .020 kg thyroid (1.7 cm) so we can assume with fair accuracy that all the gammas escape.

The K_α fluorescent radiation has an average energy of about 18 keV with an attenuation coefficient of about 1 cm^{-1} (see Table A-4a) or an

HVL of about .693 cm. This is small compared with 1.7 cm so we can assume to a fair approximation that none of the fluorescent radiation escapes. All of the emissions that are locally absorbed are transferred to the 6th column of Table 14-4 and totalled to give $.0298 \times 10^{-13}$ J/dis. Now the gray is 1 J/kg so the dose to the thyroid is:

$$D = .0298 \times 10^{-13} \frac{J}{dis} \times \frac{1}{.020 \text{ kg}} = 1.49 \times 10^{-13} \frac{Gy}{dis}$$

This is slightly less than Monte Carlo calculation (Table 14-5), which gives 1.73×10^{-13} Gy/Bq s. Our calculation is too low because we assumed all the 140 keV radiation escaped.

We now consider a much more difficult problem: the calculation of the dose to the thyroid from technetium in a distant organ such as the bladder. We consider only the gamma emissions of Table 14-4 since all the others will be absorbed by the intervening tissues. The total of the three gammas is 0.1981×10^{-13} J/dis. From the standard man we estimate the thyroid to be 60 cm from the bladder. For the 140 keV gamma by interpolation we obtain from Table A-4a:

$$\mu = 0.155 \text{ cm}^2 \text{ g}^{-1} \qquad \mu_{tr} = 0.0271 \text{ cm}^2 \text{ g}^{-1}$$

An underestimate of the dose will be obtained if we calculate the attenuation of 60 cm of waterlike tissue using μ since this will neglect the buildup of dose due to scattered radiation. A realistic estimate of the effects of scattered radiation by analytical methods is almost impossible and it is for this reason that Snyder et al. (S22) used the Monte Carlo technique. In spite of this reservation we will continue the calculation to see how large an error is made.

The energy fluence at the thyroid will be reduced by the attenuation of 60 cm of tissue and by the inverse square law giving:

$$0.1981 \times 10^{-13} \frac{J}{dis} \cdot e^{-0.155(60)} \cdot \frac{1}{4\pi(60)^2 \text{ cm}^2} = 4.0 \times 10^{-23} \frac{J}{dis \text{ cm}^2}$$

and the energy absorbed in the thyroid is:

$$4.0 \times 10^{-23} \frac{J}{dis \text{ cm}^2} \times .0271 \frac{cm^2}{g} = .108 \times 10^{-23} \frac{J}{g \text{ dis}}$$

$$= .108 \times 10^{-20} \frac{J}{kg \text{ dis}}$$

$$= 1.08 \times 10^{-21} \text{ Gy/dis.}$$

The Monte Carlo calculation (see Table 14-5) gives 158×10^{-21} Gy/Bq s, which is larger by a factor of more than 100, again emphasizing the importance of scattered radiation and the use of the MIRD data rather than this simple calculation.

14.12   PERMISSIBLE DOSES IN NUCLEAR MEDICINE

No official upper limits have been placed on the organ dose or the whole body dose arising from the administration of radionuclides.

It is the feeling of most investigators that no firm rule should be laid down, but that the potential risks of any procedure should be evaluated in terms of the potential benefits and that this consideration should override all others. For example, if the potential risk of a brain tumor, with death in 6 months if not detected and treated, is weighed against the potential radiation risk of a brain scan, then a very large dose of radiation becomes diagnostically acceptable. The important principle that no more radiation be given than is absolutely necessary to establish the diagnosis has an important corollary. Enough radiation should be used to make an accurate diagnosis. A serious error in judgment would be perpetrated if, after weighing the risks and benefits, one decided to perform a brain scan using too small a dose of radioactivity.

From the above discussion it is clear that no firm permissible dose should be established for a diagnostic procedure. On the other hand, this does not mean that a clinician should be unconcerned with the absorbed dose. He should know the approximate absorbed dose for each of the procedures used. In this chapter, methods for calculating the dose have been presented.

The use of short-lived isotopes such as Tc-99m provide an enormous advantage, since large amounts of these nuclides may be used without delivering large absorbed doses to the organ.

PROBLEMS

1. By taking areas under the curve of Figure 14-7 between the limits $N \pm \sqrt{N}$ and $N \pm 0.67 \sqrt{N}$, show that the probabilities of finding a measurement in these ranges are 0.69 and 0.50 respectively.
2. A series of 30 measurements with a counter gave a mean value for an activity of 10,000 counts/min. How many of the observations should have been within the range 10,000 ± 100? 10,000 ± 67? 10,000 ± 200?
3. A counter with preset counts and preset time is arranged to stop after 10,000 counts or 10 minutes, whichever occurs first. What are the standard deviations and the percent standard deviations if the count rate is 2000 c/min? 200 c/min?
4. How many counts should be obtained to give a probable error of 0.5%? What will be the percent standard deviation?
5. In a preliminary experiment to measure a low activity, the background was found to be about 30 c/min and the sample plus background about 45 c/min. If 200 min is available for counting, how long should be spent in counting background and how long in counting the sample to give the maximum precision?
6. If the actual count rates in problem 5 were 30.0 c/min and 45.0 c/min, determine (a) the percentage standard deviation in the true activity that can be obtained using the optimum counting periods and (b) the percentage standard deviation that can be obtained if the two activities are each counted for 100 min. From this example it

will be apparent that it is unnecessary to select the counting periods with great precision.

7. Given that the percent standard deviation in the product or quotient of 2 numbers that have percent standard deviations of σ_1 and σ_2 is $\sqrt{(\sigma_1^2 + \sigma_2^2)}$, find the standard error in the plasma volume determination of example 14-6, neglecting the statistical uncertainty in the background.

8. A scintillation counter has a resolving time of 10 μsec. What count rate can be tolerated if the loss of counts must be kept less than 1%?

9. In an experiment to determine the resolving time of a counter, the count rates were 1050 c/s, 1500 c/s, and 2350 c/s for sources A, B, and A + B respectively. Determine the resolving time. With such a counter what is the corrected counting rate at an observed counting rate of 1000 c/s?

10. In a thyroid study, 0.6 MBq of I-131 is given the patient. If the biological half-life is 15 days, find the amount of activity left in the patient after 10 days.

11. A patient is given an injection of Na-24 (half-life 15.0 h) and blood samples are drawn and counted immediately. The 1-hour sample gave 2,700 c/min per ml and the 8-hour sample gave 1,290 c/min per ml. Determine the biological half-life of the Na-24.

12. A patient is given an injection of P-32, and 2-ml blood samples are taken at 24 hours and at 48 hours. Both samples were counted 50 hours after injection. The counting rate for the samples were 6,820 and 3,610 c/min respectively, including a background of 120 c/min. Calculate the biological half-life. What would the counting rates have been if the samples had been counted immediately after being taken?

13. Justify the statement made in section 14.09 regarding the relative doses of Tc-99m and I-131.

14. Use equation 14-1 to evaluate the probability of observing 1000 counts when the expected number is 1000 counts. This will present a problem on a small calculator since the equation involves the quotient of two very large numbers. The problem can be solved using Stirling's formula:

$$N! \approx (2\pi)^{1/2} N^{(N + 1/2)} e^{-N}$$

to evaluate factorial N for large values of N. Check your answer using Figure 14-7.

15. 2.0×10^9 Bq of Tc-99m is injected into a patient. Assume half the isotope is localized in the bladder, from which it decays with a biological half-life of 4 hours. Determine the dose to the thyroid.

Chapter **15**

RADIATION PROTECTION

INTRODUCTION

Τhe development of atomic energy has brought with it an awareness
and concern for the potential hazards of ionizing radiation. The
International Commission on Radiological Protection (ICRP) has dealt
with the hazards in a long series of publications; some are listed in the
references (I1-I11). In the 1960s the ICRP defined a maximum permissible dose (MPD) as the dose that in the light of present knowledge is
not expected to cause detectable body injury to a person at any time during his lifetime. MPD's are still specified but emphasis is now more
strongly placed on the idea that any exposure should be justified by some
benefit. They now state that all exposures should be kept as low as reasonably achievable, economic and social factors being taken into account.
This is called the ALARA principle (As Low As Reasonably Achievable).

   In the 1960s the emphasis of radiation protection tended to be on
genetic damage. Today it is more on the risks of producing cancer in
various organs of the body. The ICRP are now attempting to quantitate
these risks and relate them to the risks faced by workers in other industries. They recommend setting dose limits and interpreting these limits
in such a way as to make the hazards of working with radiation at least as
low as the risks of working in a so-called "safe industry."

15.02   **DOSE EQUIVALENT**

   In Chapter 9 methods for expressing the dose in grays were discussed.
Unfortunately, the problems of radiation protection are not this simple,
because a dose of one type of radiation may produce a much larger biological effect than the same dose of a different type of radiation. Therefore, to obtain a quantity that expresses on a common scale the damage
incurred by an exposed person the concept of dose equivalent has been
introduced:

$$H \text{ (dose equivalent)} = D \times Q \times N \qquad (15\text{-}1)$$

where D is the absorbed dose, Q is the numerical quality factor determined by the type of radiation involved in the exposure, and N is the
product of other modifying factors that determine the radiobiological
damage. We will discuss N later—for the moment we will take it as 1.0.
When the dose equivalent concept was first introduced, D was expressed

in rads and H in rems. These terms are still used but the ICRP now recommends that dose, D, be measured in grays and the dose equivalent, H, in sieverts (Sv) in honor of the Swedish scientist who for many years was active in the ICRP. The relation between these units is:

$$1 \text{ gray} = 1 \text{ Gy} = 1 \text{ J/kg} = 100 \text{ rads}$$
$$1 \text{ sievert} = 1 \text{ Sv} = 1 \text{ J/kg} = 100 \text{ rems}$$

(15-2)

Since Q is a numerical factor without dimensions, the dose equivalent in sieverts unfortunately has the same dimensions as the gray. The sievert (Sv) and the millisievert (mSv) will be used throughout this chapter.

Quality Factor (Q)

One physical parameter that describes the quality of radiation is the linear energy transfer (LET). The LET expressed in keV/μm gives the rate at which an ionizing particle deposits energy along its track (see sections 6.17 and 10.16). Heavy particles such as protons, neutrons (which indirectly ionize), and alpha particles produce dense tracks and have a large LET while electrons produce tracks with a small LET. Electrons with an energy of about 1 MeV have an initial energy deposition of 0.2 keV/μm in water. As the electron energy decreases, the rate of energy loss increases. Heavy particles such as alpha particles deposit energy at rates up to 200 keV/μm in water (see sec. 6.17).

Radiobiological experiments have shown that in general the dense tracks (high LET) produced by heavy charged particles produce a greater biological effect, for the same energy deposited per unit mass, than do low LET tracks produced by electrons. Thus Q is a function of LET. Q is closely related to the factor, RBE, discussed in section 17.08. RBE is used in radiobiology while Q is used for radiation protection. Both relate the dose required to produce a given biological effect from a reference radiation to the dose from the test radiation that produces the same effect, and both use 200 kV$_p$ x rays as the reference. Because radiobiological information is derived from much higher doses than apply to radiation protection, RBE is considered to be a more precise quantity than is Q. It is principally for this reason that Q is defined, especially for use with radiation protection.

Values for Q are given in Table 15-1. For example, a particle that loses energy at 23 keV/μm has a Q of 5. If a person were irradiated to a dose of 0.6 mGy by such radiation, the dose equivalent would be H = 5 $\times$ 0.6 = 3.0 mSv, and the biological damage would be equivalent to 3.0 mGy from low LET radiation.

In many situations the LET of the radiation will not be known. If this is the case the ICRP recommends the use of an average quality factor, $\overline{Q}$, given in the second part of the Table 15-1.

TABLE 15-1
Quality Factors to be used in Determining Dose Equivalents*

LET (keV/μm)	Q	Type of Radiation	$\bar{Q}$
3.5 or less	1	x rays, gamma rays, and electrons	1
7	2	neutrons, protons, and singly charged particles of rest energy greater than 1 amu of unknown energy and un-	10
23	5	known particles.	
53	10	α particles and multiply charged particles (and particles	
173	20	of unknown charge) of unknown energy.	20

*From ICRP Publ. 26 (I9)

There is a conceptual difficulty with these units. Suppose for example that the quality factor for a certain type of high LET radiation is 20, and that a tissue was given a dose of .05 Gy. This would mean that the dose equivalent is 1.0 Sv. Because the sievert has dimensions J/kg this would suggest *incorrectly* that the energy deposited in the tissue was 1.0 J/kg. In fact, the energy absorbed is .05 J/kg but this amount of radiation produces biological damage equivalent to that produced by 1.0 J/kg of low LET radiation.

MODIFYING FACTORS N. Equation 15-1 includes a term, N, which represents the product of a number of factors that may modify the biological damage. Biological effects depend upon many factors other than dose, such as dose rate, fractionation, tissue environmental factors such as oxygen, and spatial distribution of the dose pattern. For example, when isotopes are injected and deposited in bone, there may be regions of very high local concentration. If these produce an abnormally large biological effect, then N may be given a value greater than 1.0. By including the modifying factor N in equation 15-1, the concept of dose equivalent need not be altered as new radiobiological facts become available.

CALCULATION OF DOSE EQUIVALENT. If a person is exposed to a number of types of radiation at one time, then the total dose equivalent is found by summing the individual dose equivalents, thus:

$$H = \sum_i D_i\, Q_i\, N_i \qquad (15\text{-}3)$$

Example 15-1. A person is exposed to 0.2 mGy of radiation from Co-60 and 0.3 mGy of radiation from neutrons with an LET of 7 keV/μm. Determine the dose equivalent.

For neutrons with an LET of 7 keV/μm (Table 15-1), Q = 2
$\therefore$ H = 0.2(1.0) mSv + 0.3(2) mSv = 0.8 mSv

15.03   **BACKGROUND RADIATION**

In trying to assess the level of an acceptable dose we are greatly helped by the fact that the human race since the dawn of time has been exposed to radiation from natural causes. The average yearly dose to the whole body from background radiation is summarized in Table 15-2. It arises from three main sources: cosmic rays, external gamma rays, and internal radiation. Cosmic rays are heavy charged particles from outer space. They tend to be deflected away from the equatorial regions of the earth by the earth's magnetic field and funnelled into polar regions. Hence, their intensity is minimum near the equator and maximum near the poles, changing by about 20% in going from the equator to latitude of 50°. To reach the earth they must pass through the atmosphere, which acts as an absorbing blanket over the surface shielding us from these rays. Their intensity then depends strongly on altitude, changing by a factor of 2 in going from sea level to an elevation of 2 km. An average annual figure for the U.S.A. from these cosmic rays is 0.44 mSv (44 mrem).

TABLE 15-2
Estimate of Annual Whole-Body Dose Equivalents in mSv in U.S.A. (1970)*

Naturally occurring radiations		
Cosmic rays	.44	
External gamma rays	.40	
Internal radiation—^{40}K		
^{14}C, Radon dis. products etc.	.18	
Total natural radiation	1.02	
Man-made radiations		1.02
Global fall out		0.04
Nuclear power		0.00003
Diagnostic x rays (excluding fluoroscopy)		0.72
Nuclear medicine (radiopharmaceuticals)		0.01
Occupational		0.008
Miscellaneous		0.02
Total average whole body dose per year		1.82 mSv
Including fluoroscopy, this total will be rounded off to		2.0 mSv

*From the BEIR report (B19)

External gamma rays arise from the radioactivity in the earth's crust, which varies widely from place to place on the earth's surface. Activity tends to be high in regions of granite rocks. Since people spend most of their time indoors the radiation level to which they are subjected depends on the material used to construct their homes and the degree of ventilation of them. Persons living in stone houses will be subjected to higher doses than those living in wooden houses, due mainly to the radon that comes from small amounts of uranium in the granite rock. External gamma rays account for about 0.40 mSv (40 mrem). The exact value depends greatly on geography and varies from about 0.28 mSv to over 8.0 mSv (M14).

The human race is subjected to internal radiations arising from radioactive materials present in our bodies. K-40 occurs naturally and is present in all of us. It emits beta and gamma rays, which contribute to the whole body dose. Air contains radon at a concentration of about 1.1×10^{-2} Bq/l (.3 pCi/l) and so radon is continually entering and being expelled from our lungs. In this process the active deposits of radon (sec. 13.02) are trapped in the lung where they damage lung tissues mainly by α bombardment. When radon and its active deposits are *ingested*, the active deposits become concentrated in the skeleton and contribute to the whole body dose. The total effect of these internal emitters give a yearly dose equivalent of 0.18 mSv.

The sum of these three components is about 1.02 mSv and is the annual whole-body dose equivalent arising from natural radiation, averaged over the population of the U.S.A. It must be emphasized that this is an average dose. People in some locations receive more, others less. For example, people in Denver, Colorado (altitude 1.6 km) have an average yearly dose of 1.25 mSv, while about one sixth of the population of France is exposed to about 3.0 mSv per year (H16). It is interesting to note that a 5 hour jet flight contributes an extra dose equivalent of about 0.025 mSv to passengers and crew due to the increase in cosmic rays with altitude (N8).

To the natural background radiation all of us experience must be added the manmade radiations. These are also summarized in Table 15-2. It should be noted that diagnostic x rays, excluding fluoroscopy, contribute over 90% of the whole body dose by man-made radiations. If we add rather arbitrarily a figure of about 0.2 mSv for fluoroscopic x rays (a reasonable guess) we find the total of manmade radiations contribute about 1.0 mSv. Thus man-made radiations have to date doubled the radiation levels mankind had been subjected to for centuries.

A number of estimates have also been made of the gonadal dose per year. This amounts to about 0.90 mSv from our environment and in the U.S. between .18 and 1.36 mSv due to medical and dental radiology. Experience in various laboratories has shown that doses due to diagnostic x rays can be reduced below its present value by a factor of about 10 without loss in diagnostic information (T10, J14). If this were done universally it would make an important reduction in our radiation burden.

15.04   **TISSUES AT RISK**

In earlier publications of the ICRP, use was made of the idea of a critical organ and the maximum permissible dose to it. In publication 26, attempts have been made to assess the risks to all organs and arrive at a total risk of irradiation. Before discussing this it is essential to draw a distinction between stochastic and nonstochastic effects. A stochastic effect is one for which there is no threshold and for which the probability of occurrence depends on dose linearly down to zero dose but the *severity* of the effect is independent of dose. For example, cancer of the breast may result from radiation. The *probability* of a woman developing such a cancer may be proportional to the dose she receives but the severity of the disease is almost certainly not. This will depend much more on her ability to reject the cancer.

Nonstochastic effects are those that have a threshold value. A good example of such an effect is a cataract in the lens of the eye. Evidence suggests that these do not occur at low doses but can suddenly appear after a much higher, threshold dose. The severity of the effect then does depend upon the dose.

The ICRP over the last 20 years has studied this problem in detail; their findings are given in publication 26 (I9) and the major stochastic risks are summarized in Table 15-3. The first column indicates the type of risk involved, the second gives the number of the paragraph in publication 26 in which the risk is discussed, and the third column indicates the risk per Sv. For example, the risk of leukemia is shown as 2×10^{-3} Sv^{-1}. The sum of all the risks is 16.5×10^{-3} Sv^{-1}. The values in the table for all but the first item give the risk of death, not the risk of tumor induction. For example the value of 2.5×10^{-3} Sv^{-1} for breast is for death. Since about 50% of breast cancer is curable, the risk of induction of breast cancer by radiation is about 2 times as large as the value in the table. Since 97% of thyroid cancers can be cured, the risk of induction is about 30 times the value in the table. For leukemia, lung, and bone cancer the cure rate is small, so that risk of induction and death are essentially the same.

TABLE 15-3
Estimated Risk Factors for Mortality*

Organ	Paragraph in #26	Risk per Sievert	W_T—Weighting† Factor	H_L—Dose Equiv. Limits (Sv/y)
Hereditary effects	60	4×10^{-3}	.25	.2
Breast	57	2.5×10^{-3}	.15	.33
Red bone marrow (leukemia)	44	2.0×10^{-3}	.12	.4
Lung cancer	51	2.0×10^{-3}	.12	.4
Thyroid	56	$.5 \times 10^{-3}$	.03	1.65‡ (.5)
Bone cancer	48	$.5 \times 10^{-3}$	.03	1.65‡ (.5)
Remainder	59	5×10^{-3}	.30	.8‡ (.5)
Total risk		16.5×10^{-3}	1.00	whole body → .05

*Calculated from data in ICRP #26 (I9)
†These "weighting factors" are simply the fractions of the overall risk, i.e. entries in Col. 2 divided by 16.5×10^{-3}.
‡These are reduced to 0.5 Sv in order to limit the risk for nonstochastic effects (see discussion under dose equivalent limits).

Although the major concern of the ICRP is now with the risks of cancer, they are still, of course, concerned with hereditary effects of radiation. They estimate (see paragraphs 43 and 60 in ICRP-26) that the risk factor for hereditary effects as expressed in the first two generations is about $4 \times 10^{-3}/\text{Sv}$. This is about a factor of 4 smaller than the total risk given at the bottom of Table 15-3. The meaning and use of this table are illustrated by an example.

Example 15-2. Estimate the number of deaths from leukemia in a population of 1 million by background radiation to the blood-forming organs of 1.0 mSv/y.

From Table 15-3, risk of deaths from leukemia $= 2.0 \times 10^{-3} \text{ Sv}^{-1}$
Number deaths $= 10^6 \times 2.0 \times 10^{-3} \text{ Sv}^{-1} \times 10^{-3} \text{ Sv y}^{-1} = 2/\text{y}$

Since there are about 70 leukemia deaths per year per million people in Ontario, this calculation would suggest that 68 of these fatal leukemias were induced by factors other than background radiation.

The ICRP knows that these figures are at best only approximate and are subject to considerable debate since induction of cancer is dependent on age and sex, and many other factors. For example there is no specification of the area of the field or the volume of tissue irradiated. For lack of a better approach, we will assume for risk calculations that the mean dose to the organ is the important parameter. This mean dose is determined from the total energy imparted to the organ divided by the mass of the organ. We will now compare risks due to radiation exposure with other risks in society.

Risks in Industry

The ICRP has studied the risks of fatal accidents in industry and some of these results are given in Table 15-4.

From this table it is seen that workers in so-called "safe industries" have a risk of 10^{-4} of having a fatal accident per year due to their occupation. The risk to a miner is larger by a factor of 10.

TABLE 15-4
Accidental Deaths per Million People per Year in United States in 1972*

Trade	72 ⎫	Safe industries
Manufacturing	96 ⎭	
Service	120	
Government	131	
Transport	362	
Agriculture	657	
Construction	710	
Mining	1000	

*From ICRP #27 (I10)

It would seem logical, by limiting the dose, to attempt to make the risk for a radiation worker not greater than a worker in a "safe industry." If the dose to a radiation worker were limited to 5.0 mSv per y (500 mrem/y), i.e. 5 times background, then the total risk (see Table 15-3) would be:

$$16.5 \times 10^{-3} \text{ Sv}^{-1} \times 5.0 \times 10^{-3} \text{ Sv y}^{-1} \approx 10^{-4} \text{ per year}$$

and a radiation worker would be as safe as workers in safe industries.

For over 20 years the maximum permissible dose for radiation workers has been limited to 50 mSv per y (5000 mrem/y). Such radiation workers are monitored with film or TLD, and experience shows that the arithmetic mean of these doses is less than 5 mSv y^{-1} with very few doses approaching 50 mSv y^{-1}. Hence, although the dose limit has been set at 50 mSv y^{-1}, in actual fact, the dose average has been less than 1/10 this value. Radiation workers are thus as safe as workers in "safe industries." Of course to be logical one has to admit that the radiation worker is also subject to normal industrial risk.

Table 15-4 gives the number of *fatal* accidents per year in industry. The number of less severe accidents is larger by at least 100 (I10). Fatal accidents in industry lead to death instantly (or nearly instantly) while a radiation death from cancer usually occurs many years later, due to the long latent period for its induction, and a worker so exposed may still have 10 to 20 years of productive life. Comparing the risks in this way, therefore, overestimates the risks of radiation relative to other risks.

To put these risks in a more familiar context, there is a fatal risk of 10^{-4} for the following (P11):

40,000 miles of travel by air
6,000 miles of travel by car
75 cigarettes
Merely living 1.4 days for a man aged 60

Partial Exposure

Suppose a person receives a dose to one organ rather than to the whole body. This can happen, for example, when a radioactive isotope is ingested. If we follow through with the logic of the last few pages we would conclude that if one organ alone were irradiated it could be given a larger dose for the same total risk. Column 4 in Table 15-3 gives the weighting factors for the different organs. These weighting factors were obtained from the risk given in column 3. The total risk to all the organs is 16.5×10^{-3}; the risk to the gonads is 4×10^{-3}. If we divide the latter by the total we obtain 0.25, which is the weighting factor for the gonads. It appears in the 4th column and the sum of these weighting factors is of course 1.00.

Dose Equivalent Limits for various organs are not tabulated in publication 26 but they are there by implication. Perhaps the ICRP decided not to tabulate these doses because of their ALARA guideline that requires the protection officer at all times to find ways to reduce the dose by as much as is reasonably achievable. In this respect the dose limit is very different from a speed limit. Car drivers consider a speed limit as the speed that they should drive or slightly exceed. A dose equivalent limit on the other hand is an upper limit; at all times one should seek ways to reduce dose to as small a value as is reasonably achievable. The ICRP does state the dose equivalent limit for whole body irradiation as 50 mSv y^{-1} (5000 mrem y^{-1}) or 50 times average background. If we divide this figure by the weighting factor, we obtain a dose equivalent that should be allowed a particular organ assuming that *only this organ receives radiation*. For example, for the gonads the dose equivalent would be 50 mSv y^{-1}/0.25 = 200 mSv y^{-1} or .2 Sv y^{-1}. These values appear in the 5th column and are the dose equivalent limits we refer to as H$_L$.

However, the ICRP also feels that *at no time should the dose equivalent exceed 0.5 Sv y^{-1} in order that nonstochastic effects be limited*. Thus, the figures in column 5 apply provided they are *less* than 0.5 Sv y^{-1}. If they are over .5 Sv y^{-1} then the 0.5 Sv y^{-1} limit applies. Thus, for the thyroid the dose equivalent limit is not 1.65 Sv y^{-1} but 0.5 Sv y^{-1}.

The implications of Table 15-3 are, however, troublesome. For example, H$_L$ for irradiation of the breast alone is 0.33 Sv y^{-1}. If we multiply this by the risk of cancer for the breast (2.5×10^{-3} Sv^{-1}) we obtain 0.8×10^{-3} per year or about 1 in 1000 per year. Thus, a woman radiation worker would have 1 chance in 1000 of dying of cancer of the breast due to this radiation. This is not acceptable to her or to the protection officer. As soon as the film badge indicated the possibility that the annual dose would reach a level such as 0.33 Sv, steps would be taken to alter the worker's routine to reduce the expected dose by a factor of at least 10. Of course, this hypothetical case is rather extreme since it is hard to envisage a situation in which *only* the breast would be irradiated.

The reader may well ask why not reduce the whole body dose limit from 0.05 Sv by a factor of 10 to 5 mSv (5 times background). A change in regulations of this kind would cost millions of dollars because it would require the addition of a tenth value layer to every installation. Then, of course, the people who fear radiation at any level (without regard to perspectives such as have been drawn in this chapter) will say, let's add another tenth value layer and the problem never ends. The fact still remains that the present dose limits for radiation workers and the philosophy behind the way they are interpreted makes radiation one of the safest industries. The unnatural fear of radiation by some members of the public during the 1970s has seriously undermined the expansion of our nuclear energy program, which is absolutely essential to the survival of our civilization. It is to be hoped that governments will soon start to lead, rather than follow, and that energy policies will include expansion of the nuclear energy program.

The radiologists will also have to do their part in reducing the risk of radiation. Table 15-2 shows that 90% of our man made radiation risk comes from diagnostic radiology. Money should be spent on dose reduction as described in Chapter 16 rather than in the overprotection of many of our radiation facilities.

Dose Equivalent Limits for the Planning of Radiation Facilities

In planning radiation facilities we need to protect three classes of people: the radiation worker, the nonradiation worker, and the public at large; for this planning, dose equivalent limits must be specified. For the calculations given in this chapter we will use the following limits.

Radiation worker: $H_L = 5\text{mSv/y}$ i.e. $5 \times$ background
Nonradiation worker: $H_L = 0.5\text{mSv/y}$ i.e. $0.5 \times$ background   (15-4)
Public at large: $H_L = 0.05\text{mSv/y}$ i.e. $0.05 \times$ background

We now attempt to justify these limits.

RADIATION WORKERS: The dose equivalent limit of 50 mSv/y for the radiation worker is still in use but is not satisfactory for barrier calculations because of the ALARA principle, since a dose reduction factor of 10 can usually be achieved without too much difficulty. This leads to the figure of 5 mSv/y given in equation 15-4.

NONRADIATION WORKERS: In our context, these are persons who work in a hospital but do not work with radiation. Setting a dose limit for these is at best rather arbitrary. One approach to this problem, which has considerable logic, has been suggested by Adler and Weinberg (A12). Since background radiation varies quite widely over the earth's surface, and since there is no evidence of increased cancer in high dose regions of the earth's surface, and since people do not even take this into account in deciding where they will live, the dose equivalent should be placed equal to the standard deviation in background. This is about 0.2 mSv/y. This makes the value of 0.5 mSv/y for nonradiation workers stated above look "reasonable."

THE PUBLIC AT LARGE. There is one other class of people that should be protected—the public at large. These are people who might visit a hospital, or walk by a hospital, or live or work near one. The Atomic Energy Control Board of Canada has, for example, insisted that such persons be protected to 0.05 mSv/y (1/20 of background).* This level was arrived at from experience with nuclear installations, where it was shown that such a requirement could easily be met by such practical measures as moving the restraining fence far enough from the reactor. They have extended this rule to hospitals where achieving this level may at times be very difficult because most of the hospital itself is available to the public.

---

*This dose equivalent is equal to the extra dose received in a 10 hour jet flight.

In spite of this reservation, we attempt to design protection to reach this level.

DOSES AND BIOLOGICAL DAMAGE. In therapeutic and diagnostic radiology, relatively high doses may be necessary for certain procedures. To assess the risk of such doses one should be aware of the biological damage that may result. The doses required for a few types of biological damage are given in Table 15-5.

TABLE 15-5
Doses for Different Types of Biological Damage*

Induction of menopause and permanent cessation of fertility in women at age 40	3 Gy
Depression of sperm counts in males	0.25 Gy
Permanent sterility in males	~3 Gy
Cosmetically unacceptable skin changes	20 Gy
Threshold for lens opacification	15 Gy
There is other evidence (M15) to suggest that the threshold for lens opacification may be as low as 2 Gy.	

*From ICRP-26 (I9)

15.05   PROTECTIVE BARRIERS

In order to reduce the dose rate to the acceptable level at the position occupied by personnel, it is usually necessary to place barriers of lead, concrete, or some other material between them and the radiation source.

In section 15.02 it was shown that the dose equivalent was determined from the dose through the use of the appropriate quality factor. Since in this book we are primarily interested in x rays, gamma rays, and high energy electrons for which the quality factor is 1.0, the dose equivalent in sieverts is numerically equal to the dose in grays.

Figure 15-1a shows a possible configuration of high energy radiation therapy machine in a treatment room. It could be a cobalt unit or a linear accelerator. Since almost all units today use isocentric mounts, this type is illustrated in Figure 15-1, with the axis of rotation at OA. The source, S, moves in the vertical plane SS' and so the beam can be directed in any direction in this plane. Two positions for the source, S and S' are shown. We wish to determine the wall thicknesses required to protect radiation workers, hospital workers who are not involved with radiation, and the public at large. The wall thicknesses required will depend on the output of the machine, the type of radiation, the distance to a point such as C, the time the beam points in this direction, and the time persons occupy a region such as C. In making these calculations it is essential to consider three types of radiation from the source: *primary* radiation, *leakage* radiation, and *scattered* radiation.

PRIMARY RADIATION. This is the radiation from the source that emerges through the collimating system. In Figure 15-1 it is confined to

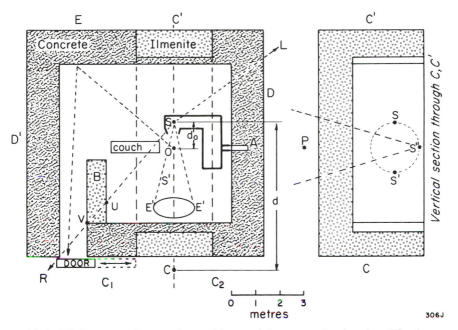

Figure 15-1. High energy isocentric machine and its protective barrier. The isocenter is at O and the unit rotates about axis AO. The walls are of concrete and ilmenite. Control panel is at C; Diagram on the right is a vertical section through line CC'.

the cone SEE'. The size of this cone is determined by the maximum field size of the unit. Since the machine can rotate, this cone of primary radiation can be directed in any direction within the vertical plane through SOS'.

LEAKAGE RADIATION. Leakage radiation from the source or target is always present. This is radiation that emerges from the head through its protective barrier in a direction such as SL. In a linac, radiation may be generated at a number of places along the beam transport system, but the main source will usually be near the spot where the electrons are focused to produce x rays or at each bending magnet. There is no universal agreement on maximum permissible leakage levels. The ICRP (I11) and NCRP (N9) have suggested that the leakage at 1 m should be limited to 0.1% of the useful beam also at 1 m. Their recommendations were originally directed towards x ray equipment operating at 250 to 400 kV, where the shielding thicknesses involved are a fraction of those for megavoltage radiation. When the same recommendations are applied to high energy linacs, it is difficult to meet this value without the addition of large masses of protective material, which may compromise the usefulness of the machine for radiotherapy. As a result of these considerations the IEC (International Electrotechnical Commission, I12) has suggested that a leakage of 0.5% is satisfactory. In the subsequent calculations we will protect external points on the assumption that the leakage is 0.1%.

SCATTERED RADIATION. Whenever an x ray beam strikes matter, scattered radiation will result. In a therapy unit the main source of this radiation will be the patient. Precise calculations of the scattered radiation are impossible but for most situations sufficient accuracy is achieved by assuming that the scattered radiation at 90°, 1 meter from the scatterer is 0.1% of the primary beam at the scatterer (NCRP #49—Table B2, N10). Obviously the amount of scattered radiation is dependent on field size. The 0.1% figure is about correct for the maximum field size. Scattered radiation also depends on direction, being maximum in a direction close to that of the primary beam. Protection from the primary beam is usually the most difficult so it will be dealt with first.

Protection from Primary Radiation

WORKLOAD (W). An intelligent design of the barriers must start from the workload. Linacs deliver very high dose rates to tissue of up to 5 Gy/min at 1 meter, but this does not mean the dose per 8 hour day is $8 \times 60 \times 5.0 = 2.4 \times 10^3$ Gy. A little thought will convince the reader that such a high output machine is *off most of the time*—while the patient is being set up. Experience shows that a group of technicians have to work very hard to treat 80 patients in an 8 hour day on one machine. Since the average treatment is about 2.5 Gy, the upper limit of the workload at 1 meter is about:

$$W_0 = 2.50 \; \frac{Gy}{pat.} \times 80 \; \frac{pat.}{d} \times 5 \; \frac{d}{week} \times 50 \; \frac{week}{y} \qquad (15\text{-}5)$$
$$= 5 \times 10^4 \; Gy/y = 5 \times 10^4 \; Sv/y$$

We will use the symbol W_0 to represent the work load at the isocenter of the machine. It is the dose delivered to this point per year under normal operation of the radiation source with no patient in the beam. For discussion on workloads see Table 2 in appendix C of NCRP #49 (N10).

It is important to distinguish between the dose rate when the machine is on and the average dose rate over an 8 hour day. For the linac discussed in the last paragraph, the former is 2.4×10^3 Gy per 8 hour day while the latter is $80 \times 2.5 = 200$ Gy per 8 hour day. These differ by a factor of 12.

INVERSE SQUARE LAW. The dose at a point such as C in the primary beam is less than the dose at point O by the inverse square law factor $(d_0/d)^2$ (ignoring for the moment the barrier in the diagram) where d_0 is the source to isocentric distance, and d is the distance from the source to the point being protected (d = SC, Fig. 15-1).

USE FACTOR (U). To determine the barrier needed between S and C we need to know the fraction of the treatment time during which the beam points at C. This factor could be determined by observing the operation of the unit during a typical day, but this is not very practical since we would like to know the factor *before* the installation is made. The American National Commission on Radiation Protection (NCRP) recommends the use factors in Table 15-6. For a therapy unit the use factor for a side wall is 1/4. Unfortunately, the NCRP has not stated a use factor for the ceiling, which in the age of isocentric therapy machines is an important barrier. Our experience indicates that the beam is pointed down 60% of the time, upward about 30% of the time, and 10% in each of the horizontal directions. These lead to the approximate use factors given in the last column of Table 15-6. All of these are conservative, since the 50% attenuation provided by the patient is not included.

TABLE 15-6
Use Factors for Primary Barriers*

	Radiographic	Therapeutic	Therapeutic—Our Experience with Isocentric Mounts
Floor	1	1	1/2
Walls	1/4	1/4	1/10
Ceiling	†	‡	1/4

*From Appendix C, Table 3, NCRP-49, page 64 (N10)
†Generally very low
‡Variable but usually taken to be less than 1/4

OCCUPANCY FACTOR (T). The dose to personnel at a point such as C depends on persons being at C while the machine is being operated. For a technician operating the unit one would assume 100% occupancy with $T = 1.0$. Occupancy factors for other situations as recommended by NCRP are given in Table 15-7. These are also very conservative, so more realistic ones will be used in calculating the protection for the public at large.

Let the required attenuation factor produced by the barrier be A, then:

$$\text{Dose per year to personnel at point in question} = W_0 \left(\frac{d_0}{d}\right)^2 \cdot \frac{UT}{A}$$

If we equate this dose to the dose equivalent limit H_L from equation 15-4, we may rearrange this equation to yield the required attenuation factor A:

$$A = \frac{W_0}{H_L} \left(\frac{d_0}{d}\right)^2 \cdot UT \qquad (15\text{-}6)$$

In protection work it is convenient to specify the barrier in terms of the number of *tenth value layers* (TVL). This may often be obtained from the value of A by inspection, or by taking the log of A to the base 10 thus:

$$\text{Number of tenth value layers} = \log_{10} A \qquad (15\text{-}7)$$

Tenth value layers for a number of materials and a number of high energy machines are given in Table 15-8.

TABLE 15-7
For Use as a Guide in Planning Shielding Where Other Occupancy Data Are Not Available

Full Occupancy (T = 1)	Work areas such as offices, laboratories, shops, wards, nurses' stations; living quarters; children's play areas; and occupied space in nearby buildings
Partial Occupancy (T = 1/4)	Corridors, rest rooms, elevators using operators, unattended parking lots
Occasional Occupancy (T = 1/16)	Waiting rooms, toilets, stairways, unattended elevators, janitors' closets, outside areas used only for pedestrians or vehicular traffic

*From Appendix C, Table 4, NCRP-49, page 65 (N10)

TABLE 15-8
Tenth Value Layers† (m) for Protection Calculations*

Material	Co-60 Scattered at 90°	Co-60	5 MV	10 MV	25 MV
Earthfill ~1600 kg/m³	.23	.34	.48	.57	.74
Concrete ~2400 kg/m³	.15	.23	.32	.38	.50
Ilmenite‡ ~4000 kg/m³	.074	.14	.19	.23	.24
Lead	.015	.042	.047	.052	.051

*Data from L11 and other sources
†1 HVL = .31 TVL; 1 TVL = 3.2 HVL
‡Ilmenite is the tradename for heavy concrete made using one type of iron ore as the aggregate.

TYPICAL CALCULATION OF PRIMARY BARRIER. We now illustrate these ideas by calculating the barrier required to protect radiation workers at position C of Figure 15-1, assuming our machine is a 25 MV linac with a work load of 5.0×10^4 Sv/y. For radiation workers at C, $H_L = 5$ mSv/y $= 5 \times 10^{-3}$ Sv/y and for these people the occupancy factor T = 1.0. For the side wall our experience suggests a use factor of U = 1/10. The distance $d_0 = 1$ m and the distance SC = 6 m.

$$A = \frac{5.0 \times 10^4}{5 \times 10^{-3}} \times \left(\frac{1}{6}\right)^2 \times \frac{1}{10} \times 1.0 = 2.8 \times 10^4 \qquad \log_{10} A = 4.45$$

This indicates that we will need 4.45 tenth value layers. From Table 15-8 we see that we require $4.45 \times 0.50 = 2.2$ meters of ordinary concrete or $4.45 \times 0.24 = 1.1$ meters of ilmenite. These are massive walls!

CALCULATION OF CEILING THICKNESS FOR PRIMARY RADIATION. In some positions of the source the beam points vertically upward. It is required to find the ceiling thickness to protect persons at P directly above the unit with $S''P \approx 5$ m (see Fig. 15-1). This region is to be occupied by hospital staff who are *not* radiation workers. For these people $H_L = 0.5$ mSv/y (equation 15-4). Occupancy factor will be taken as 1.0 and use factor $U = 1/4$.

Substituting in equation 15-6 we obtain

$$A = \frac{5.0 \times 10^4}{0.5 \times 10^{-3}} \times \left(\frac{1}{5}\right)^2 \times \frac{1}{4} \times 1.0 = 1.0 \times 10^6 \quad \log_{10} A = 6.0$$

We thus require 6.0 tenth value layers or $6.0 \times 0.24 = 1.44$ m of ilmenite. The width of this strip of barrier needs to be about 3 m to protect the region when the collimator is wide open. Since in use the collimator will be wide open only a small fraction of the time, most points above the unit will be overprotected most of the time.

Protection Against Leakage Radiation

Leakage radiation can be in any direction from the linac target; since it can be any place around the circle $S'SS''$, we will assume the source is at its average point O, the isocenter of the machine. The manufacturer guarantees that the dose rate 1 m from O is at most 0.1% of the primary,* so the work load is 50 Sv/y (equation 15-5). Consider a typical point such as D (4m from O) that is occupied by radiation workers with $T = 1.0$ and for which $H_L = 5$ m Sv/y. For these calculations we must use a use factor of 1.0, since leakage radiation may be emitted in direction D no matter which direction the machine is pointing. Substituting in equation 15-6, we obtain:

$$A = \frac{50}{5 \times 10^{-3}} \times \left(\frac{1}{4}\right)^2 \times 1.0 \times 1.0 = 6.2 \times 10^2 \quad \log_{10} A = 2.8$$

If we make the side walls of ordinary concrete, we require a wall thickness of $2.8 \times 0.50 = 1.4$ m. If ilmenite is used the required thickness is 0.7 m.

The space above the ceiling occupied by nonradiation workers must be protected to 0.5 mSv/y, so it will require 1 more tenth value layer than the side walls, i.e. 3.8 half-value layer or 1.9 m of ordinary concrete. Since the band of heavy concrete in the ceiling is 1.4 m thick it would make sense to make the whole of the ceiling 1.4 m thick with only heavy con-

---

*This number is for linacs, betatrons, and other electrical producers of radiation. For isotope machines, leakage is limited to .02 mSv/h average at 1 m.

crete in the band over the machine and with a composite layer of 0.9 m of ordinary concrete and 0.5 m of heavy concrete over the rest of the ceiling. The student may show that this will give adequate protection for leakage reduction. If the public will occupy the space above the linac of Figure 15-1, we would need one more TVL unless one could claim an occupancy of $T = 1/10$. If the space were used as an outpatient department or waiting room one could claim a $T = 1/10$ since relatives would not be present more than 1 month out of a year and then for at most a few hours per day. A similar claim could be made for a region such as D which could be a driveway or parking lot.

Scattered Radiation

Scattered radiation can be assumed to be less than 0.1% of the primary for even the largest fields. Since scattered radiation is softer than the primary or the leakage radiation, scattered radiation will be no problem if the walls and ceiling can cope with leakage radiation.

15.06   **DESIGN CONSIDERATIONS FOR PROTECTIVE BARRIERS**

The protective barriers for high energy machines are massive and can cost very large sums of money. It is, therefore, worthwhile to consider other alternative arrangements. The unit shown in Figure 15-1 is arranged to rotate about axis A and at times will point towards C. An alternative configuration is shown in Figure 15-2 with the axis along CO. This would reduce the barrier in direction C of Figure 15-1 or Figure 15-2 but increase the required barrier in direction D. To determine the "best" configuration one should explore both arrangements, taking into account the types of personnel that will occupy regions such as C and D.

PRIMARY BEAM STOPPER. To ease protection problems, some units are provided with a massive primary beam stopper, Q (Fig. 15-2), which is fastened to the machine. It is wide enough to intercept all the primary radiation from the unit. When such a primary beam stopper is used, the main radiation protection problem arises from leakage radiation and massive barriers may still be required. Such a beam stopper may interfere with "porting" the patient, so in some units this barrier is made retractable.

BAFFLES. High energy machines usually require a baffle, B, as illustrated in Figure 15-1 or 15-2. This baffle must be placed in such a way as to intercept any beam such as SR (Fig. 15-1) that can irradiate the door region—otherwise the door has to be as thick as the walls. It should be thick enough to make the distance VU equal or greater than the wall at C' (Fig. 15-1). Since this baffle wastes expensive space, it should not be made unnecessarily thick. It is often convenient to make the baffle of ilmenite blocks, which can be assembled into a baffle after the machine

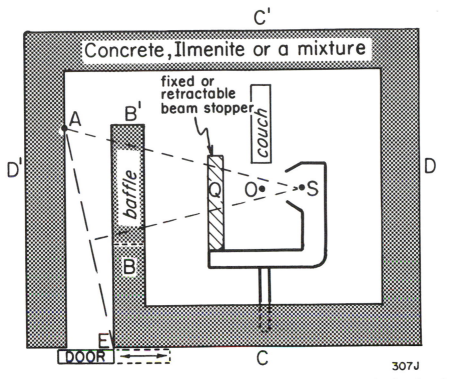

Figure 15-2. Schematic diagram of high energy machine and its protective barrier. Q is an optional primary beam stopper. The baffle could end at B or B′.

is installed. The thickness of the baffle and the distance it extends into the room can thus be tailor-made to the installation.

Door. The baffle may be thick enough to protect people outside the room for rays such as SR (Fig. 15-1) but the situation may still not be satisfactory since scattered radiation and neutrons will travel down the maze. The maze must usually be closed by a sliding or rotating door. The amount of scattered radiation that reaches the door will depend upon the number of rays of the type SAE shown in Figure 15-2. Primary radiation from S bombards concrete at A (assuming the beam stopper is not in place) which in turn scatters to E. Karzmark (K7) and Toy (T11) have measured the scattered radiation or albedos to allow the determination of the radiation scattered down the maze for a few photon energies. Unfortunately, data for linacs in the 10–25 MV range are not yet available.

The thickness of the door will depend upon the maze. If the baffle ends at B (Fig. 15-2) a thick door will be required but if the baffle reaches into the room to B′ then the protection built into the door may be essentially dispensed with. We have found a pneumatically operated sliding door made with a steel framework useful. It is initially hollow with a thickness of 30 cm and is mounted on an overhead track. After installation, measurements are made with a neutron detector and a photon detector in the door region and then the required amount of lead and concrete blocks are placed into the hollow door. Our 25 MV linac with a baffle similar to Figure 15-1 requires 2 layers of lead about 2 cm thick, between which is placed concrete blocks about 20 cm thick. Even with a long maze a door is required for protection. Interlocks should be installed on the door to prevent people from entering the radiation room while the machine is "on." A maze is cheaper to build than a massive sliding door but the maze has the disadvantage of adding many steps to the technician's working day and wastes space.

OPTIMUM DESIGN. The protective barriers for high energy machines are massive and can cost very large sums to install. In new installations it is wise to place these machines far enough underground to avoid radiation problems through the ceiling or the walls and also to avoid floor-loading problems that exist on higher level floors. If the protection has to be achieved in a completed hospital or in a new hospital a deep basement with a very thick ceiling is required. If a number of units are to be installed they should be clustered together so that the walls of one unit protect the next. To minimize costs, the rooms should be made as small as possible consistent with allowing enough space for setting up patients and servicing the machine. Judicious use of mirror walls can give the impression of spaciousness. Small rooms also reduce the distances technicians must walk. Manufacturers of high energy machines will usually want their unit to appear to advantage and often suggest larger rooms than are necessary. Often a few hours of design effort by the physicist can save many dollars. To achieve optimum design we require more information on the amounts of scattered radiation down mazes.

TELEVISION MONITORS. For high energy machines transparent viewing windows are not practical. The patient may be observed during treatment with a television camera and monitor.

PSYCHOLOGICAL HAZARD. After installation of the unit one should of course check for radiation leaks. This is most easily done using some type of ionization type survey meter calibrated in μSv/h. It should be noted that a Geiger counter may be unsatisfactory in monitoring pulsed radiation from a linac, because it may saturate in the pulse. If a survey meter is placed next to the control panel at C (Fig. 15-1) and the unit is turned on, the counter will count rapidly, especially if the unit is directing its beam horizontally towards C. This would not disturb a technician because the yearly dose would be less than 5 mSv. A problem, however, could well arise at a point such as A above the unit where a nonradiation worker could be 8 hours a day. Would such a person be satisfied that the *average* dose level was less than 0.5 mSv/y (i.e. 1/2 of background) when a survey meter at position A showed a high reading when the machine came on (see problem 6). Until radiation is considered as being no different from other hazards of life, this could create a problem. One of the major difficulties in dealing with radiation arises from the fact that we have instruments of such high sensitivity that the uninformed can easily measure levels of radiation far below "safe" values.

15.07   DIAGNOSTIC X RAY INSTALLATIONS

In general, the protection for diagnostic units is simple since these units normally are on a very small fraction of the time and the energy of the photons involved is much lower than for a therapeutic unit. The cheapest barrier can be made using 10 cm concrete building blocks covered with plaster, making a 15 cm wall. Doors are usually made using 1/16 inch of Pb glued to plywood. Technicians operating diagnostic units can often be simply protected by standing behind 1 inch plate glass walls. Table 15-9 gives typical tenth value layers for x rays generated at a few kilovoltages. These apply reasonably accurately after the beam has passed through the tube housing or has been filtered by protective material so that only the penetrating component remains in the beam. Measurements by Taylor (T10) show that exposures even on the inside of the walls of rooms rarely exceed 1 mSv/week and barriers for protection are not generally required.

TABLE 15-9
Tenth Value Layers*

Attenuating Material	Tube Potential kV$_p$										
	50	70	100	125	150	200	250	300	400	1000	2000
Lead (mm)	0.17	0.52	0.88	0.93	0.99	1.7	2.9	4.8	8.3	26.0	42.0
Concrete (cm)	1.5	2.8	5.3	6.6	7.4	8.4	9.4	10.4	10.9	14.7	21.0

*From NCRP 49, Table 27 (N10)

In the last two sections we have shown how protection can be planned for either an x ray or isotope installation and have emphasized the physics involved in these calculations. If a radiological department is being planned, the physicist is urged to obtain the relevant publication and to use these in protection planning. These give typical protection calculations for fluoroscopic, radiographic, dental, fluorographic, and therapy installations. The physicist should also take into account that the dose equivalent limits in use in his locality may *not* be the same as those of equation 15-4.

15.08   PROTECTION AGAINST RADIATION FROM SMALL SOURCES OF RADIUM, COBALT, AND CESIUM

Protection of personnel using small sources of radium, cobalt 60, or cesium 137 is usually a much more difficult task than protecting personnel using x ray units or high energy machines. Table 15-10 gives the

TABLE 15-10
Thicknesses of Lead Required to Reduce the Dose Rate to 1 mSv/40 Hour Week

Isotope	Exposure in R per hr at 1 m	HVL (cm Pb)	Required Thickness of Pb (cm) at		
			30 cm	1 m	2 m
100 mg radium	.084	~1.4	11.8	6.5	3.8
100 mCi Co-60	.135	1.2	11.6	7.4	5.0
100 mCi Cs-137	.039	0.6	6.1	3.8	2.6

thickness of lead required to reduce the dose rate to 1 mSv/40 hour week. The table may be used for other source activities using the appropriate HVL and for other distances using the inverse square law.

Example 15-3. Find the barrier required to protect personnel to 0.1 mSv/week situated 50 cm from a 400 mCi source of cesium 137.

> 3.8 cm of Pb protects to 1 mSv/week, 1 m from a 100 mCi source (Table 15-10)
> Extra attenuation required for distance is   2.0 HVL
> Extra attenuation required for source is   2.0 HVL
> Extra attenuation required to reduce dose by 1/10 is   3.1 HVL
> Extra attenuation required   7.1 HVL
> Extra lead needed = 7.1 × 0.6 = 4.3 cm
> Total lead needed = 4.3 + 3.8 = 8.1 cm

Hazards from Sealed Sources

Personnel must be protected from radiations arising from sealed sources such as radium needles, cobalt or cesium needles, and various types of beta ray plaques. A few guiding principles are given below, but for further details reference should be made to the appropriate handbooks.

1. To protect the hands from β and γ rays, reliance should be placed on distance. Manipulations should be carried out with long-handled forceps as expeditiously as possible.

2. During such manipulations the body should be protected from gamma rays using a suitable barrier. To protect the eyes from beta and gamma rays, the manipulations should be carried out by viewing the operation through a layer of lead glass.

3. The room in which sources of radioactive material are loaded for molds, etc., should be well ventilated to guard against inhalation of radon, which will escape if a radium source is broken. Radium storage rooms should be well ventilated for the same reason.

4. Radium sources should be tested periodically for leakage (see section 13.05).

15.09   **RADIATION SURVEYS**

After the installation of the radiation equipment, it is essential that a qualified expert carry out a radiation survey of the new installation. A number of points should be investigated.

1. If the protection has been designed on the basis of restrictions of the orientation of the x ray beam and limitations of the generator below its maximum rating, suitable interlocks should be provided to prevent the machine from being operated other than in the planned way. Often protection is designed on the basis that the tube not point towards the control panel. If this is the case, an interlock should prevent the machine operating under these conditions.

2. Interlocks should be provided to shut the machine off automatically as the door to the treatment room is opened. This is particularly important in teleisotope installations, which are silent in operation and would provide no warning to a person who might inadvertently enter the room while the machine is "on." It is wise to have a radiation monitor in a cobalt 60 room to sound an alarm if a source inadvertently remains "on" when the door is open.

3. With the machine operating at its full rating, the protection should be tested with a suitable type of radiation survey meter at points outside the room.

4. Neutrons may create a protection problem for linacs that operate above 20 MeV. The walls of concrete designed to protect against x rays will be satisfactory in stopping neutrons. Neutrons, however, will be scattered down the maze and must be finally stopped by the door to the treatment room. The measurement of these neutrons in the presence of x rays is not easy. One useful device is the Nemo® detector. It consists of a LiI crystal coupled to a small photomultiplier at the center of a 30 cm sphere of polyethylene. The incident fast neutrons are slowed down by the polyethylene and finally captured by the Li to yield one alpha particle and one triton, which are counted by the photomultiplier. This detector may be made insensitive to x rays if small pulses are rejected by the counting circuit. Its response is more or less proportional to dose equivalents in sieverts; that is, it takes into account the quality factor. A number of devices for measuring neutrons are available.

More data on the scattering of neutrons down mazes is needed to allow for the design of the optimum maze. Mazes are often overdesigned, leading to loss of valuable space and unnecessary costs.

5. Leakage radiation around a machine may be located by moving an ion chamber around the machine, which is operating with the shutter closed. The ion chamber will average the exposure over the area of its sensitive volume and so will not detect leaks confined to small gaps in the protective housing. These may be located with film and corrected

with the appropriate thickness of lead.

6. In cases where the beam from a therapy unit points in certain directions only a fraction of the time, as in a rotation unit, the protection may be measured using a film monitor. The film should be left at the point in question for 1 month during normal operation of the unit.

For further details concerning radiation surveys, reference should be made to the appropriate handbooks (N11, N12).

15.10   PROTECTION IN RADIOISOTOPE DEPARTMENTS

1. In handling unsealed sources, great care should be exercised to prevent the isotope from entering the body through inhalation, ingestion, or absorption through cuts. Ingestion will usually arise from the transfer of small amounts of activity from the hands to the mouth. Therefore, eating and smoking should not be permitted in isotope laboratories.

2. Manipulation of open isotopes should be performed under a fume hood with an external vent.

3. The spilling of activity on work surfaces should be avoided as much as possible through the use of trays, etc., as the decontamination of such surfaces, especially with long-lived isotopes, is very difficult.

4. All working areas, sinks, etc. should be monitored periodically for activity and decontaminated when necessary.

15.11   PERSONNEL MONITORING

Some type of personnel radiation monitoring should be used by all persons working with radiation facilities. The film badge method or TLD is convenient for determining the total dose of beta, x, or gamma radiation accumulated over a period of one to three months. To give some information concerning the quality of the beam, it is usual to cover the film partially by a filter or filters of different materials and thicknesses. Very soft x rays or beta rays will not affect the film covered by the filter whereas penetrating radiation will affect both parts almost equally. Film badges or TLD must be calibrated against known amounts of radiation of the same quality being measured. One serious disadvantage of this type of monitoring arises because personnel may not become aware of an overexposure until several months after the event, at which time they may be unable to remember how the radiation was received. They are, therefore, not in a position to avoid further radiation arising in the same way.

Pocket dosimeters are also suitable for personnel monitoring. They are capable of greater precision and suffer less from quality dependence than films. Their main advantage over film arises from the fact that an overexposure can be detected at once and the person is thus aware of the way in which the exposure occurred. He may then be in a position to avoid further exposures of the same kind. Pocket dosimeters are expensive and cannot readily be used routinely in a large department. They are particularly useful during periods when the person is aware that a radiation hazard exists, as when a teletherapy source is being loaded or large quantities of radioactive material are being dealt with. For these applications and for the identification of high exposure regions during fluoroscopy a dosimeter that "beeps" when placed in a radiation field is useful.

Very few firm rules can be made concerning protection. However, in all cases persons should avoid unnecessary exposure in the performance of their duties and protection facilities should always be overdesigned rather than underdesigned. To facilitate protection, it is essential that one person, called the protection officer, continuously supervise and check all procedures involving radiation hazards. Without such a person, rules firmly established at one time will gradually be disregarded. In the field of protection, continuous vigilance is essential.

15.12   SUMMARY

The authors are aware that this chapter may create as many problems as it solves, since there is no agreement as to whether maximum permissible dose should still be used or whether one should approach the problem through risk estimates as discussed in section 15.04. There is no worldwide agreement on this problem, and in fact, there is a great deal of controversy. Our concern in this book is the radiation worker in the hospital.

Certain groups of workers in hospitals tend to show relatively high doses on their monitors. These are the nurses who look after the radium and the nurses who look after patients who contain radioactive sources during the treatment of cancer of the cervix. In diagnostic departments there are also groups that tend to have high doses. These are involved in special angiographic diagnostic procedures in which relatively large doses may be given the thorax and the head and neck of technicians and radiologists. At the time of writing, one would find it nearly impossible to limit the dose to these workers to 5 times background (5 mSv); they should however, be limited to the former MPD of 50 mSv/y.

Protection regulations tend to be applied in the following way. If a radiation worker shows very little radiation on his radiation monitor over a period of time, and then suddenly receives 10 times as much, the work habits of this worker are studied, and the reason for the increased exposure determined. Radium nurses, and workers on special procedures in diagnostic radiology, may every week receive a much larger dose than the person mentioned above. This would be known by the radiation protection officer who would not alert the worker but would continue to seek ways to reduce the dose. The fact remains then that certain groups of people are being exposed and it is very difficult to see how this exposure can be reduced. It is for this reason that regulatory agencies do not want to reduce the legal limits from 50 mSv to 5 mSv. If such were done and the rules were followed literally, it could prevent certain very valuable diagnostic procedures and seriously interfere with the treatment of certain types of cancer. This suggests that as in other industries certain groups do accept extra risks in order to carry out a worthwhile task.

PROBLEMS

1. A person receives a dose of 0.10 mGy from x rays, .20 mGy from radiation with an LET of 7 MeV/μm, and .20 mGy from the recoil of heavy nuclei. Determine the dose equivalent in mSv.
2. Design a treatment room for a cobalt 60 unit similar to Figure 15-2. Assume the unit treats 40 patients per day. Make the room as small as practical. Design so that space C is occupied by radiation workers, while C', D, and D' are occupied by hospital workers who are not radiation workers.
3. Design a treatment room for a 10 MeV linac similar to Figure 15-1. Assume a work load of 50 patients per day and that radiation workers occupy spaces C, C', D, and D'.
4. Repeat the calculations of problem 3 for the configuration of Figure 15-2.
5. Find the barrier required to protect personnel to 0.1 mSv/week situated 5 m from a 400 mCi source of cobalt 60.
6. Find the instantaneous dose rate at point P immediately above the unit shown in Figure 15-1 when the machine is pointing upward.

Chapter 16

DIAGNOSTIC RADIOLOGY

16.01   **INTRODUCTION**

In the earlier chapters of this book we have been concerned with the amount of energy from an x ray beam that is absorbed by tissues *in the patient* during treatment. In diagnostic radiology we are interested in the beam of x rays which is transmitted *through* the patient. The different tissues in the patient attenuate the x rays to produce a shadow picture, enabling us to visualize the internal structures. In this chapter we will be concerned with methods for presenting this picture and for optimizing the amount of information in it. In an earlier era, the main concern in diagnostic radiology was how to get the best picture. Today we must also be increasingly concerned about the dose received by the patient. It must be realized that every x ray examination carries a risk and involves some damage to the patient.

It has been estimated (Table 15-2) that diagnostic radiology in the U.S.A. contributes a whole body dose equivalent averaged over the population of 0.72 mSv (72 mrem) per year. This should be compared with the whole body dose equivalent of 1.02 mSv received on the average by everyone from natural background.* The risks associated with both these sources must be similar but there is one major difference: we can reduce the dose from diagnostic radiology.

Individual patients are the ones who receive radiation from diagnostic radiology and their doses can easily be 1000 times as large as the average quoted above. Further, many patients have repeat examinations. We must conclude that diagnostic radiology does contribute to cancer deaths. Of course, diagnostic radiology contributes enormously to cancer cures. The philosophy today must be to minimize the deleterious effects of radiation and maximize the benefits. Thus, unnecessary diagnostic procedures should be avoided and those that are necessary should be performed with the minimum dose consistent with getting a good enough picture to allow a reliable diagnosis. We have evidence (T10) that the dose from diagnostic radiology can be reduced by a factor of at least 3 with little work and by a factor of 10 or more if all conditions are optimized. If such reductions became universal, diagnostic radiology could be made safer for patients.

---

*These numbers have been revised in Beir #3, 1980 (B20). The new numbers are about 20% lower than the values used here.

The clinical value of diagnostic radiology is such that in spite of the small hazards to man, there must always be eagerness to introduce new techniques for which sophisticated equipment is now becoming available. This has been particularly true in the 1970s when we have seen the rapid development of computer assisted tomography, angiography, and electrostatic imaging. Here we will present the physical principles upon which these techniques are based.

In earlier chapters of this book we emphasized absorbed dose and played down the importance of exposure. This was done purposely because in radiotherapy the focus of attention was on the *energy absorbed* in tissue. In diagnostic radiology on the other hand we are more concerned with the *radiation transmitted* to the sensing device after having passed through the patient. For this application exposure is more convenient and is used throughout this chapter.

Certain sections of this chapter require mathematical skills for a proper understanding of the contents. This is particularly true of sections 16.12 to 16.16. Students should not be discouraged by the complexity of these sections since subsequent sections return to a more qualitative approach.

16.02   PRIMARY RADIOLOGICAL IMAGE

Figure 16-1 illustrates the attenuation of an x ray beam by a patient made up of different tissues, resulting in a variation of the transmitted radiation. This variation of transmitted radiation is referred to as the *primary radiological image*. The pattern of transmitted radiation may be expressed in terms of variations in photon fluence, variations in energy fluence, or variation in exposure. Since the eye is insensitive to x rays, this image is converted to a visible image by a fluorescent screen, image intensifier, or film. The beam that emerges from the patient contains primary and scattered radiation. We saw in Chapter 10 that for beams with energies up to 150 kV used in diagnosis, and for thickness of tissue involved in patient examination, the scatter component is considerably greater than the primary. Since only the primary beam contains useful information about the object being examined, it is desirable to reduce the scattered radiation reaching the screen or film by means of a grid placed as indicated in Figure 16-1. This grid allows only that radiation which comes from the direction of the source to reach the imaging system. Grids will be discussed in detail in section 16.09. The scatter component may also be reduced by limiting the size of the x ray field to the region to be examined.

The beam that finally reaches the film or screen contains both useful information and noise. The imaging system can never increase the information but may well lose some of it, resulting in deterioration of image quality. By noise we mean variations of the intensity of the beam in the

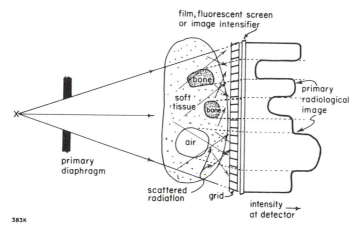

Figure 16-1. Diagram showing how the primary radiological image is produced.

image plane that are *not* due to corresponding variations in transmission of the beam by the patient.

IMAGES PRODUCED BY TISSUES. Fat, soft tissue, and bone can be distinguished from one another in an x ray image because they attenuate x rays in different ways. The mass attenuation coefficient for these tissues are given in Tables A-3c, 3d, and 3e in the appendix. Using the densities of Table 5-3, the linear coefficients were determined and are plotted in Figure 16-2. Also shown are the linear coefficients for two commonly used contrast media, containing iodine and barium. We illustrate the use of this data by an example.

Example 16-1. 10^7 photons generated at 65 kV$_p$ and filtered with 2 mm Al are directed toward an ankle. Calculate the number of photons that emerge through 5 cm of muscle and through an adjacent region containing 0.5 cm of bone and 4.5 cm of muscle. Will the bone be visualized?

> An approximate calculation of this kind can be performed by replacing the spectrum of x rays by monoenergetic photons of some mean energy. From the insert of Table 16-1, we note that a spectrum generated with a peak voltage of 65 kV$_p$ is equivalent to a monoenergetic beam of 34.2 keV. The beams are equivalent in the sense that both have the same HVL in Al.
>
> μ(muscle) = .32 cm^{-1} and μ(bone) = 1.18 cm^{-1} (from Fig. 16-2)
>
> Number photons transmitted through 5 cm muscle $= 10^7 e^{-5(.32)} = 10^7 e^{-1.60} = 2.02 \times 10^6$
>
> Number transmitted through 4.5 cm muscle plus 0.5 cm bone $= 10^7 e^{-[4.5(.32)+.5(1.18)]} = 10^7 e^{-2.03}$
> $= 1.31 \times 10^6$

The bone transmits about 66% as many photons as the adjacent area, so it will show an excellent shadow.

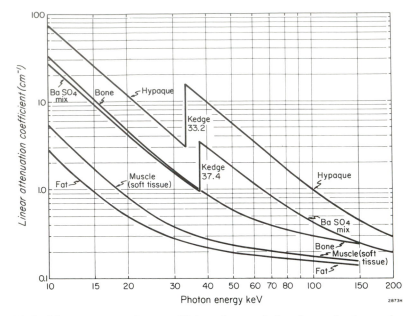

Figure 16-2. Linear attenuation coefficient in cm^{-1} for fat, soft tissue, bone, 75% Hypaque, and $BaSO_4$ "mix." The coefficients are the total less coherent scattering and were calculated using data in the Appendix. The compositions for fat, soft tissue, and bone are given in Table 5-3. 75% Hypaque contains, per cm^3, 0.25 g $C_{18}H_{26}I_3N_3O_9$, 0.50 g $C_{11}H_8I_3N_2O_4$, and 0.65 g water, giving a density of 1.40 g/cm^3. $BaSO_4$ "mix" consists of 450 g $BaSO_4$ in 2500 ml water to give a suspension of density 1.18 g/cm^3.

These calculations are not very accurate because one cannot replace a heterogeneous beam of x rays by an equivalent monoenergetic one, especially when one is concerned with a beam absorbed by the photoelectric process, which varies rapidly with energy. For more precise calculations, we require the spectral distributions of the radiations used in a diagnostic department, and a set of such data is presented in Table 16-1. This data was obtained by Epp and Weiss (E2) using a scintillation spectrometer by the method outlined in Chapter 9. The table also gives the normalizing factor required to give an exposure of 10 roentgens in air. For example, this table shows that when x rays are generated at 90 kV_p and filtered by 2 mm Al, for an exposure of 10 R, there will be a fluence of $9110 \times 4.68 \times 10^5$ photons/cm^2 in the energy range 39.5 to 40.5 keV. We will use this table to determine how well structures may be visualized. Tables of spectral distributions have been assembled by Birch (B21).

Images Produced by Contrast Media

To visualize many organs in the body, it is necessary to introduce into the patient a contrast medium that is deposited in the organ and that absorbs x rays either more or less than the surrounding tissues. Three types

TABLE 16-1
Relative Photon Fluence per Unit Energy Interval (photons/cm² keV) versus Photon Energy (keV)*

(1) Photon Energy (keV)	(2) Added Filtration 1 mm Al 45 kV$_p$	(3) 55 kV$_p$	(4) Added Filtration 2 mm Al 65 kV$_p$	(5) 70 kV$_p$	(6) 80 kV$_p$	(7) 90 kV$_p$	(8) 98 kV$_p$	(9) 105 kV$_p$
10	0	70	0	0	0	0	0	0
12	320	250	0	0	0	0	0	0
14	1320	870	80	0	100	30	120	0
16	3710	2500	480	490	460	360	440	260
18	6170	4950	1790	1390	1170	1050	1100	900
20	8170	6980	3350	3150	2370	2410	2160	2030
22	9920	8980	5630	5030	3950	4070	3850	3390
24	10500	10060	7450	7050	5860	5660	5540	5450
26	10350	10630	9180	8900	7820	7590	7560	7000
28	9250	10350	10590	10200	9550	9240	9000	8300
30	7690	9350	11030	10750	10260	10400	9760	9380
32	5670	8000	10390	10500	10340	10280	9830	9650
34	3880	6330	8910	9600	9700	9910	9750	9720
36	2630	5110	7720	8980	9250	9560	9640	9750
38	1630	4330	7000	8540	9080	9350	9500	9740
40	870	3650	6500	8100	8870	9110	9350	9700
42	290	2900	5890	7500	8560	8990	9180	9610
44	0	2160	5160	6780	8110	8810	8990	9560
46		1490	4410	6070	7570	8540	8780	9440
48		900	3610	5300	7000	8120	8550	9300
50		480	2820	4570	6390	7620	8220	9100
52		250	2140	3920	5760	7140	7860	8760
54		110	1600	3300	5190	6600	7460	8350
56		0	1100	2640	4600	6030	6910	7920
58			650	2140	4020	5460	6390	7430
60			370	1640	3500	6770	12120	20540
62			150	1310	2930	4300	5220	6410
64			0	850	2420	3620	4580	5930
66				500	1890	3070	4030	5400
68				240	1360	3100	5580	9740
70				0	950	1970	2910	4460
72					640	1510	2470	3980
74					390	1150	2060	3600
76					220	870	1710	3160
78					110	640	1420	2810
80					0	470	1150	2490
82						340	910	2150
84						220	700	1850
86						110	530	1570
88						0	380	1330
90							260	1050
92							150	800
94							100	560
96							20	370
98							0	210
100								60
102								0

Peak kV	Equivalent keV	Factor to deliver 10 R in air
45	25.5	4.43×10^5
55	29.1	4.44×10^5
65	34.2	5.39×10^5
70	37.1	5.10×10^5
80	40.6	5.00×10^5
90	43.4	4.68×10^5
98	46.1	4.42×10^5
105	49.3	4.11×10^5

*From Epp and Weiss (E2) and *Physics in Medicine and Biology*.

of contrast media are in common use: gas, compounds containing iodine, and compounds containing barium. Gas has negligible density compared to tissues and can be considered as absorbing no x rays. Gas cavities are easily distinguished from body tissues at all beam energies, since they transmit x rays without attenuation.

Barium and iodine absorb x rays very strongly, and so organs filled with these transmit very little radiation. The absorption data for barium and iodine are plotted in Figure 16-2 for suspensions of these materials as they are commonly used in diagnosis. Both show a sharp discontinuity in the absorption curve at the K edge. Iodine will cast a very dense shadow especially for energies just above its K edge at 33.2 keV, while barium shows the same effect just above 37.4 keV. We will now use this data to determine whether a 1 mm artery can be visualized by injection of Hypaque,® a contrast medium which contains iodine.

Example 16-2. In an examination of the arteries of the heart, Hypaque is injected into a coronary artery and an x ray picture taken at 90 kV$_p$, with an exposure of 50 mR. Assume the patient in the direction of the x ray beam is 13 cm of soft tissue (the patient would be thicker than this but much of the path is air). Will an artery 1 mm in diameter be visualized?

To solve this problem accurately we use the spectral data of Table 16-1 and the attenuation data of Figure 16-2. The values in column 7 of Table 16-1 when multiplied by 4.68×10^5 give the number of photons per cm^2 per keV interval for an exposure of 10 R. For an exposure of 50 mR, which is smaller by a factor of 200, the factor is $4.68 \times 10^5/200$ = 2340. To obtain the photon fluence per keV interval, we multiply each table value by $e^{-(\mu_{\text{soft tissue}} \times 13.0 \text{ cm})}$ and the factor 2340, yielding the curve A of Figure 16-3. The area under this curve is 2890×10^4 photons/cm^2. The corresponding fluence through 12.9 cm of soft tissue plus 0.1 cm of Hypaque is obtained in exactly the same way using the exponential factor $e^{-\{(\mu_{\text{soft tissue}} \times 12.9 \text{ cm}) + (\mu_{\text{Hypaque}} \times 0.1 \text{ cm})\}}$ yielding curve B of Figure 16-3. The area under this curve is 1752×10^4 photons/cm^2. This curve differs from curve A mainly in the region above the iodine K edge at 33.2 keV. The 1 mm iodine-filled artery reduces the photon fluence by 60.6% relative to the surrounding tissue. The artery would be easily visualized.

Most detectors of radiation do not "count" photons. If the detector is an air-wall ionization chamber, then the response in roentgens per keV may be obtained from Figure 16-3 by dividing each ordinate by the entries of Table A-2b in the appendix, which give the photon fluence per roentgen. For example, the fluence per keV at 40 keV is 62.0×10^4 photons/cm^2 keV. If this is divided by the appropriate entry in Table A-2, that is 2171×10^{11} photons/m²R, we obtain:

$$\frac{62.0 \times 10^4}{\mathrm{cm^2\ keV}} \times \frac{1\ \mathrm{m^2 R}}{2171 \times 10^{11}} = 28.6 \times 10^{-6}\ \frac{\mathrm{R}}{\mathrm{keV}}$$

yielding point P on curve C of Figure 16-3. The total area under this curve is 1112×10^{-6} R. In a similar way one determines curve D, which gives the distribution of exposure transmitted through 12.9 cm of soft tissue plus 1 mm Hypaque. The area under this curve is 662×10^{-6} R. Thus, the Hypaque-filled artery reduces the exposure by 59.5% relative to the region around the artery.

To see if these calculations are reasonable, we note that 13.0 cm of soft tissue reduces the exposure from 50 mR to 1.112 mR, i.e. by a factor of 45. If the beam were monoenergetic at 38 keV the attenuation factor would be $e^{(13.0 \times .285)} = 41$, suggesting that no major error has been made.

This problem has been dealt with in enough detail to illustrate the principles involved. In doing this calculation we have simplified the problem considerably since in any real situation the injected Hypaque might be diluted by the blood, so the effect would not be as pronounced as illustrated in Figure 16-3. It would also be less pronounced because of the effects of scattered radiation, which would reduce the contrast.

It is left as an exercise for the student to determine whether other structures in the body can be visualized (see problems 1 to 5).

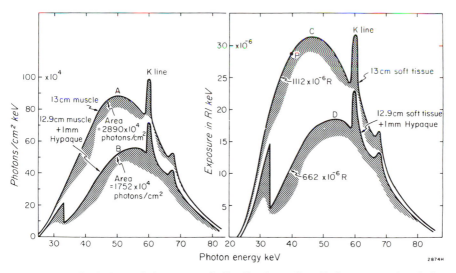

Figure 16-3. Calculation of the spectral distribution of radiation transmitted through 13.0 cm of muscle and through an adjacent area containing a 1 mm artery filled with Hypaque. Primary spectrum taken from Table 16-1 at 90 kV$_p$ at an exposure of 50 mR. Curves A and B represent the spectrum in photons/cm² keV. Curves C and D give the spectral distribution in roentgens/keV.

16.03   **RADIOGRAPHIC IMAGES**

The primary radiological image described in the last section includes the information concerning the patient the radiologist would like to obtain. However, this information is not in a useful form, and it is necessary to convert it by some type of imaging device to make it visible to the radiologist. This can be done in two important ways: by *producing an image on a film* and *by producing a visible image on the fluorescent screen of an image intensifier*. The latter may be viewed directly by the radiologist, or photographed by a camera, or observed by a television camera and presented on a television monitor (see Fig. 16-5). These two methods we now describe in detail. A new method of processing an image with a computer will be dealt with in section 16.19 on CT scanning.

Image Produced on Full Size Film

X ray films are relatively insensitive to x rays because only a small fraction of the incident x ray energy can be absorbed in a film. To overcome this lack of sensitivity the film is usually sandwiched between two fluorescent screens as illustrated in Figure 16-4. These screens absorb the x rays and emit visible and ultraviolet light, which exposes the film. The film consists of a plastic base coated on both *front* and *back* with a relatively thick emulsion. The front emulsion is exposed mainly by light from the front screen, and the back mainly by light from the back screen. Some light from the front screen reaches the back emulsion and some light from the back screen reaches the front emulsion, depending on the dyes in the film. This is referred to as "crossover."

INTENSIFYING SCREENS. Intensifying screens (Fig. 16-4) consist of a plastic base upon which is mounted a partially reflecting coating followed by a layer of fluorescent material mixed with a suitable binder. The layer is coated with a protective skin to prevent mechanical abrasion. The screens and film are held in a strong, light-tight cassette having a metal back but an x ray transparent front. The cassette is designed to squeeze the film between the two screens and to maintain intimate contact between the screens and film over their entire area. This is essential to avoid loss of resolution through spreading of the emitted light. To avoid loss of light emission the screens must be kept clean and should not be touched in the loading and unloading process. An educational booklet on screens is available from Kodak (K8).

RAPID FILM CHANGERS. In order to study movement in the body, for example, flow of contast media along arteries and veins, it is necessary to record pictures in rapid succession. This can be done by means of a mechanical film changer giving up to 6 films per second. The sequence of pictures is then obtained directly at full size on a series of x ray films. Each film will have the resolution and detail obtained in normal radio-

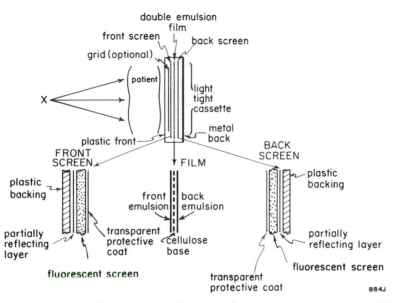

Figure 16-4. Diagram to illustrate how films and fluorescent screens are used in diagnostic radiology.

graphic work, so this method is often used when the highest detail is required. However, 6 pictures per second is frequently not sufficient to stop the more rapid motions of the heart, esophagus, etc., and in addition, the dose to the patient from such a technique is high. For example, in a sequence of 18 films of the pelvis, the patient may receive an exposure of 6 R. Furthermore, films are expensive and their storage represents a substantial and increasing cost. Techniques using intensifier tubes and TV systems have partially replaced rapid film changers.

Image Produced in an Image Intensifier

During the 1970s there was rapid development of image intensifiers and systems such as the one illustrated in Figure 16-5. In the configuration shown, the x ray tube is below the table and is rigidly connected to the image intensifier above the table. X rays passing through the patient impinge on a fluorescent screen inside the image intensifier. The light from this screen ejects electrons from the photocathode, which are accelerated by some 25 kV to produce a small but very intense visible image on a fluorescent screen at S. The radiologist may view the bright image at S in a number of ways, which we will now describe.

FLUOROSCOPY. Using the system of mirrors shown in Figure 16-5, the radiologist may observe the picture directly or may view it indirectly through a television chain. When he sees an image he wishes to record, a cassette loaded with film between two screens is automatically moved into the space between the patient and image intensifier and a picture is taken. Since the picture at S is bright, there is no need for the radiologist to dark adapt his eyes before carrying out fluoroscopy. In an earlier decade fluoroscopy was carried out by the radiologist viewing a large fluorescent screen in the place of the image intensifier. The screens were very dim and the radiologist was forced to dark adapt his eyes before examining the patient. The temptation to increase the current through the tube to make the screen brighter was always present. Because of the possible high doses to the patients, the direct fluoroscope has been made illegal in many countries.

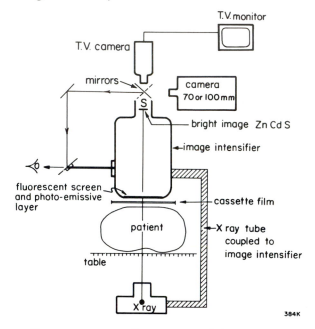

Figure 16-5. Schematic arrangement of an image intensifier with its accessories used to carry out fluoroscopy and other types of examinations.

RECORDING OF IMAGES ON 70, 100, OR 105 MM CAMERA. Because the image on screen S of Figure 16-5 is bright, the radiologist has many options to view the image other than fluoroscopy. One technique, of increasing popularity, is to photograph the output phosphor S with a 70 or 105 mm roll camera or a 100 mm cut film camera. Not only does this replace radiography using full sized films for many applications where the highest resolution is not required, but it also permits rapid sequences of images at up to 12 per second. This can be used for dynamic studies of the esophagus and for arteriography of the abdomen, head, and neck.

X ray exposures are automatically timed to occur while the camera shutter is fully open. Exposures used are about one-fifth of those required for a full size film screen combination. For example, a series of 18 images of the pelvis requires an exposure to the patient of only 1.2 R instead of 6 R. In addition x ray tube loadings are reduced, the tube life increased, and there is a substantial saving in the cost of film. This is clearly an important method of radiography in many kinds of dynamic studies, as well as in spot-filming in gastrointestinal studies.

CINE RADIOGRAPHY (35 MM CINE CAMERA COUPLED TO IMAGE INTENSI-FIER). For studies of the heart and coronary arteries, a 35 mm cine camera is mounted so as to photograph the output phosphor of the image intensifier. Since the response of the image intensifier to changes in fluence is fast, the cine camera may in turn be run at a high speed. Thirty or sixty pictures (or frames/s) are standard but speeds up to 200 frames/s may be achieved. The detail in each picture is limited by the unsharpness introduced by the image intensifier and by the quantum mottle due to the small exposure per frame. The obtainable resolution is 2 to 3 line pairs per mm (lp/mm) and exposures are 1/20 those for full size film screen combinations. See sections 16.04 and 16.15 for a discussion of quantum mottle, resolution, and noise.

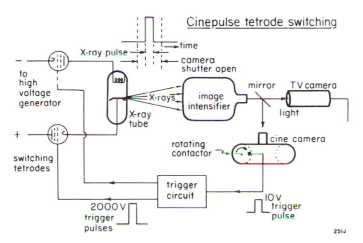

Figure 16-6. Schematic circuit for cine pulse tetrode switching.

Although the image intensifying system allows pictures to be obtained at a considerable reduction of patient exposure compared to the rapid film changer, the large number of frames still leads to substantial exposures. For example, a 10 s series of pictures at 60 frames/s will involve an exposure of about 10 R and as many as ten series may be required to study one patient. In order to minimize exposure to the patient, it is arranged for x rays to be emitted by the tube only when the film is stationary and ready for exposure. Since film movement normally occupies at least 50% of the total cine time, a saving in exposure of a factor of 2 is obtained. Modern equipment uses tetrode or triode switching of the high tension circuit to produce x ray pulses that are 1 to 4 ms long, delivered when the film is stationary. Figure 16-6 shows a typical system. The cine camera contains a rotating contactor that triggers the exposures with pulses of about 2000 V to make the tetrodes conduct and thus apply the high voltage to the tube. X ray exposure occurs when the camera shutter is fully open and the film stationary. This not only reduces patient exposure but also reduces movement blurring when recording high-speed motions. These pulsing techniques permit accurate exposure control. They are no longer confined to cine and are being increasingly used in other types of radiology.

RECORDING TELEVISION PICTURES. The electrical signals from the television camera may be stored on magnetic tapes or discs, which are then the permanent record. The surface of the disc or tape is covered with a layer of iron oxide, which may be magnetized by a magnetic field derived from the electrical television signal. A typical tape gives one hour of recording and can store some 100,000 television pictures. Tapes are used for lengthy dynamic studies when thousands of pictures must be stored in such a way that they can be replayed in rapid succession. When a few hundred pictures or just a single picture must be stored, and the same picture must be replayed over and over to allow for continuous viewing, it is better to use a disc since the recorded track on the disc is not damaged by continuous replay.

VIDEOTAPE RECORDING. This is often used as a backup for cine film. Recording on cine film has a disadvantage. The film takes time to develop, and the adequacy of the film record is not known until after processing is complete and the film viewed. Videotape recording overcomes this disadvantage, since the pictures are available for immediate replay on the television monitor. Thus, the adequacy of the investigation is determined instantly. This also allows the transmission of images to a distance, and gives the possibility of immediate picture processing, image enhancement, numerical analysis of the pictorial information (video-densitometry), and even continuous replay of a single picture. A disadvantage of videotape recording is the band-width, which is limited to about 10 MHz. This corresponds to a resolution of 2 lp/mm on the front face of a 25 cm image intensifier field. This is about half the resolution of the original intensifier image, so some useful information may be lost. Clearly, there is an urgent need for video recorders with a greater band-width. For a discussion of bandwidth, see section 16.08.

VIDEODISC RECORDING. Videodisc recording is used during fluoroscopy to reduce patient exposure. A pulse of x rays is used to record a single picture. This is played back continuously to the operator until he decides that he wants to see a new view of the patient. A second pulse of x rays then produces a new picture, which is stored on the next track on the disc and is again replayed continuously. Thus, the operator always sees a nonflickering picture but the patient is exposed intermittently to x rays. Savings of up to 10 times in dose during fluoroscopy are thus possible for some procedures.

PHOTOGRAPHING THE TELEVISION MONITOR. To record x ray images with extremely small exposures, a television camera may be focused on the output phosphor S (Fig. 16-5) to produce a visible image on the television monitor, which can then be photographed. The brightness gain of the television system allows one to obtain x ray images with exposures of the order of 20 μR on the front of the image intensifier. This is 1/20 of the amount required using a full-sized film screen combination. The resulting images will be very mottled but Hynes has shown (H17) that these images are adequate for many examinations in which contrast material is used. The technique is very flexible because when maximum resolution is required it can be achieved quickly and simply by boosting the x ray exposure and reducing the camera aperture to keep the light constant. In using the technique it is an advantage to employ high resolution television cameras and monitors.

ELECTRONIC EXPOSURE CONTROL. In recent years, the trend in diagnostic radiology has been towards the automatic control of x ray exposures using phototiming, as illustrated in Figure 16-7. One common arrangement on the left employs small (5 × 5 cm) fluorescent screens placed behind the grid and just in front of the film-screen cassette. The light emitted by the screen is transmitted to the photomultiplier by the "light" pipe, where it is converted to an electrical signal and amplified. The output may be used to terminate the exposure. Some units use a very large flat ion chamber in place of the fluorescent screen. Often a number of detectors, be they ion chambers or screens, are placed in the field so the exposure can be terminated when the exposures at different places in the field have reached the proper values.

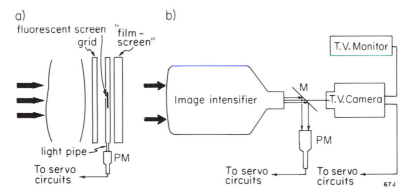

Figure 16-7. Diagram to illustrate how phototiming may be achieved (a) when "film-screen" techniques are used and (b) when image intensifiers are involved.

Figure 16-7b shows how phototiming can be achieved when image intensifiers are used. A small part of the light output is taken from the beam by the mirror M, directed onto a photomultiplier tube PM, and used to control the operation of the x ray tube. In some systems the control signal is taken from the output of the television camera. In fluoroscopy the output signal is used to adjust the viewing level by altering the kV or mA or both. Such a method has some inherent dangers, since faulty components or incorrect adjustments may increase the exposure to the patient to very high levels. Suppose, for example, that the sensitivity of the photomultiplier dropped to 10% of its original value; the servo mechanism would automatically increase the kV or mA of the x ray tube to compensate, and the patient would receive 10 times the dose. The increase in brightness of the intensifier output will be seen by the radiologist if he views the intensifier output directly, and he can therefore ask for the fault to be rectified. However, if he views the image on a television monitor he might not know that this had happened since television systems often adjust their sensitivity automatically to keep the monitor picture constant. Better ways to control patient dose are needed.

16.04   **QUALITY OF AN IMAGE**

The quality of an image can be described qualitatively by expressions such as density, brightness, unsharpness, resolution, contrast, fog, and noise. Many of these expressions have precise meanings, which can be quantitated, and which will be dealt with later in this chapter. Here we will discuss them in a qualitative way using Figure 16-8.

UNSHARPNESS. The object with sharp edges at A will usually produce an image with blurred edges at A'. This unsharpness may be due to the size of the focal spot, failure of the edges of the object to align with the direction of the beam, motion of the object during the exposure, blurring in the screen-film combination, and other factors.

RESOLUTION. The two objects B, a distance d apart, produce two images at B' with blurred edges. Since the images can be seen as separate images, the objects are said to be resolved. However, when the objects are moved closer together as in C, the images at C' blur into one another and are not resolved. Resolution is often quoted in line pairs per mm. Typical resolutions achievable in a diagnostic department are from 30 lp/mm for high detail x ray film to 1 lp/mm in television systems. This means simply that in a television system opaque objects 1 mm apart will just be resolved. The specification of resolution in line pairs per mm is, however, not as precise as it sounds, because the resolution will depend upon the attenuation of the object used in making the test and will be influenced by the conditions of viewing the image.

CONTRAST. Suppose the photon fluence at some reference point is Φ_0 and at an adjacent point is Φ_1, (Fig. 16-8). The contrast produced by the object at A can be defined as:

$$C(\Phi) = \frac{\Phi_1 - \Phi_0}{\Phi_0} \quad \text{or} \quad \frac{\Delta\Phi}{\Phi_0} \tag{16-1}$$

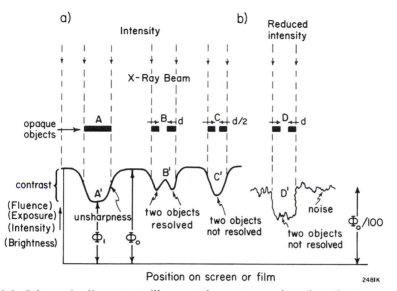

Figure 16-8. Schematic diagram to illustrate the terms used to describe image quality. The vertical scale could be given in any of the following units: photon fluence, energy fluence, intensity, density, brightness, depending upon how the radiological image is observed.

Contrast can also be expressed in terms of energy fluence or exposure. Although these three definitions will not give exactly the same numerical value, the differences usually will be small. For example, 1 mm of Hypaque used to visualize an artery (illustrated in Fig. 16-3) yields a contrast of $(2890 - 1752)/2890 = 0.401$ based on fluence or $(1112 - 662)/1112 = 0.405$ based on exposure.

Whether the eye can see a given contrast depends upon many factors. For example, a given contrast on a bright screen may be detectable whereas the same contrast on a dim screen may not. It also depends on how rapidly the contrast changes with distance along the film or screen. The contrast seen on a television monitor for a given examination will depend upon the particular setting of the electronic components in the television chain.

CONTROL OF CONTRAST AND DENSITY. The x ray image depends for its formation on differences in absorption by the various parts of the patient. In the energy range where photoelectric absorption is important (see Chapter 5), bone will absorb much greater amounts of radiation than soft tissue and will cast sharp shadows giving high contrast. As the energy is increased, the differential between bone and soft tissue will decrease and the radiograph will show less contrast. An x ray picture taken at high energy will thus appear "flat" compared with a similar picture taken with lower kV. In the extreme case of 2 MV radiation (see Fig. 5-12) the differences between bone and soft tissue disappear almost completely.

In general, contrast tends to decrease with increase in photon energy, to increase with increase in film development time, and to reach a maximum value under optimum development conditions. The contrast visualized also depends on viewing conditions: for optimum viewing, the illuminator should be of uniform intensity, of variable brightness, and masked to the region of interest on the film.

Density refers to the "blackness" of a film (it will be defined in sec. 16.07). For a small range of optical densities near 1.0 it is roughly proportional to the exposure for high contrast films commonly used in radiology. The exposure is proportional to:

$$\frac{mAs \ V^n}{F^2} \tag{16-2}$$

where mAs is the product of the tube current in mA and the exposure time in seconds, F is the focus-to-film distance, V is the kilovoltage, while n is a number between 2.0 and 4.5 that depends on kilovoltage, beam filtration, and thickness of patient.

Example 16-3. If the kilovoltage is increased from 80 to 90 kV_p and the focus film distance is increased from 100 to 150 cm while the tube current is held constant, calculate the factor by which the exposure time must be changed to yield films with the same exposure and hence the same density. Assume n = 3.

Factor to correct for change in focus to film distance $= \left(\dfrac{150}{100}\right)^2 = 2.25$

Correction for change in kV $= (80/90)^3 = 0.70$

Exposure time should be increased by factor $2.25 \times 0.70 = 1.58$

The choice of the optimum parameters for a given x ray examination is not easy. It is usual to first choose the kilovoltage from a consideration of the patient's thickness and the type of investigation, and then the mAs is adjusted to give the correct density. There is no question that a better choice could often be made to give as good a picture with a smaller dose (see secs. 16.16 and 16.21).

NOISE AND MOTTLE. In various sections of this chapter we emphasize the importance of reducing the dose to the patient. There is a fundamental principle, however, that prevents us from reducing the dose without limit. During an x ray exposure the film is bombarded by individual photons, and these photons will produce a mottled pattern much the same as do raindrops falling on pavement. After a few drops, the concrete looks mottled but as they continue to fall, they start overlapping and the mottle disappears. The same thing occurs when photons bombard film.

From section 14.05 we saw that the statistical error in counting a radioactive source depends upon the square root of the number of counts. Thus, if N counts were taken in a given time, the statistical error or noise is $\sqrt{N}$, and the noise represented as a fraction of the signal is $\sqrt{N}/N = 1/\sqrt{N}$. In dealing with radiological images, the relative noise in the image plane will depend upon the number of photons that strike a given area of the image plane and will, by analogy with the above, be represented by $1/\sqrt{\Phi}$. Clearly, we wish to minimize the relative noise in the same way we attempted to minimize the relative error in isotope counting. There are many other sources of noise, which we will discuss in 16.15.

These ideas are illustrated on the right side of Figure 16-8, where we have assumed that fluence is about 1/100 of the value for the left-hand part of the diagram. We have, however, increased the sensitivity of the scale by the same factor of 100 so that the signal may be seen. Although the noise is now 1/10 as large as it was before, it is 10 times as large relative to the signal and therefore gives the jagged contour. The effects of noise are also illustrated in the diagram, for now we see that two opaque objects d cm apart that were resolved (see B and B′ of Fig. 16-8) are now no longer resolved (compare D and D′). Noise will thus reduce resolution.

16.05   IMAGE INTENSIFIER TUBE

An intensifier tube is illustrated schematically in Figure 16-9. X rays from the source pass through the patient and enter the evacuated intensifier tube through the glass or metal envelope and an aluminum screen on which is deposited fluorescent material. This material absorbs some 60 to 70% of the x rays, converting their energy into fluorescent light. This light is absorbed by the photocathode, which ejects low energy photoelectrons into the evacuated tube. In a typical absorption of one x ray photon some 100 photoelectrons are emitted. These are accelerated and focused by the high voltage between the two ends of the tube to form a very bright image on the output phosphor or viewing screen. This image may be some 10,000 times brighter than the image on the input fluorescent screen for two reasons. In the first place, the image may be reduced in diameter from about 25 cm to 2.5 cm, that is by a factor of 10 in diameter or of 100 in area. Since the same number of electrons reach the output phosphor as leave the input phosphor, the number of electrons per unit area striking the output phosphor will be increased by 100 times. In addition these electrons are accelerated to a high energy within the tube and on striking the output phosphor will each produce 100 times as many light photons. Hence the total brightness gain is about $100 \times 100 = 10,000$. The viewing screen may be observed by an optical system that enlarges it for viewing to about the same size as the original. In this enlarging process no loss in brightness need occur provided the optical system transmits all the light it gathers.

Since the image intensifier is at the heart of the system depicted in Figure 16-5, it is instructive to discuss some of the parameters involved in its design. To yield the maximum signal for a given exposure, the fluorescent screen should be made thick enough to absorb most of the x rays and yet thin enough to insure that the light from the screen does not spread much before reaching the photocathode. To meet these conflicting aims the screen is made by growing needlelike crystals of CsI on the aluminum substrate. A photograph of a mosaic of such crystals is shown in the insert to Figure 16-9. With a needlelike structure, the CsI can be made thick enough to absorb most of the radiation and yet the light generated is carried to the photocathode without spreading by the needlelike crystals, which act as light pipes. With such a design one achieves both excellent absorption of the x rays and good resolution.

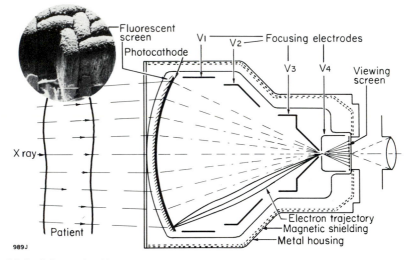

Figure 16-9. Schematic diagram of image intensifier tube. The insert shows a photograph of the CsI layer. This layer is in the form of many crystal light "pipes," which prevent the light from spreading and direct it towards the photocathode. (Diagram showing focusing electrodes adapted from CGR Ltee, Paris.) Insert courtesy of Philips (P12).

The first image intensifiers were made using a mixture of ZnS and CdS activated with silver. This material cannot be grown as needles and so does not lend itself to a light pipe configuration. Modern tubes using CsI activated with sodium are 3 to 4 times as sensitive and are rapidly replacing them.

The next step in the chain of conversions occurs at the photocathode. It should be chosen to efficiently convert the light from the screen into photoelectrons. Finally, the viewing screen of Figure 16-9 should be an efficient light emitter under electron bombardment and should emit light that is detected efficiently by the eye or the television camera.

In the late 1970s continual improvement of the image intensifier took place. By the addition of a number of electrodes within the tube it is possible to focus smaller areas of the input screen onto the 2 cm output phosphor, with a gain in resolution but a loss in output brightness. Manufacturers give the user the option of two or three discrete field sizes, such as 25 and 15 cm or 22.5, 15, and 10 cm. Recently, continuous variation of the field size has been introduced and the maximum size has been increased to 35 cm. In addition, by improving the electron optics of the intensifier, images with resolutions above 5 line pairs per mm out to the edge of the tube can be achieved with minimum distortion and much improved contrast. At least one company is developing fiber optics to carry the light from the output phosphor to the television camera. Improved coupling between the image intensifier and the television camera will improve the image. (Recent review papers on modern image intensifiers are K9, P13, V9.)

16.06   PHOSPHORS—FLUORESCENT MATERIALS

Fluorescent screens are at the heart of imaging techniques and since rapid development in this field is certain we will discuss them in detail. These screens are used to expose film, as the input phosphor of the image intensifier, as the output phosphor, and as the screen in the television monitor.

The conversion of x ray energy to light makes use of the fluorescence and phosphorescence of certain crystals by the mechanisms illustrated in Figure 16-10. This diagram shows the electronic energy levels for the fluorescent material. These energy levels are somewhat different from the discrete levels described in Chapter 1. In solid materials where atoms are close together, the possible energy levels for the electrons are a continuous band, which is shown in Figure 16-10 as the lower shaded area called the valence band. Electrons in this band are confined to atoms or groups of atoms. If they are excited by x rays, they can be moved up to the conduction band shown at the top of the diagram. Here the electrons are free to roam. In general, electrons cannot exist in the forbidden gap. However, if the otherwise pure crystal contains a small amount of impurity, discrete positions for electrons are produced in the forbidden gap. These are shown as small horizontal lines in the diagram. Impurity levels may trap electrons or release them to the conduction band by thermal agitation.

When a crystal absorbs x rays, most of the energy leads to excitation of the lattice by path A, causing an electron to move from the valence

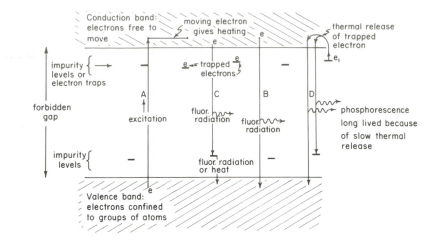

Figure 16-10. Excitation. Energy levels in materials that phosphoresce and fluoresce.

band into the conduction band. If the electron returns to the valence band by path B, a photon corresponding to this energy difference is radiated. This radiation is called fluorescent radiation. If the electron reaches an impurity level the crystal could stay in this state for an interval of time and then emit radiation, or it could emit the radiation very quickly. If the emission is prompt (10^{-10} sec) it is called fluorescence, if it is delayed it is called phosphorescence. Alternatively, the excess energy could be given up as heat. Electrons, such as e_1, can be trapped for an interval of time and then raised to the conduction band by thermal vibration of the lattice. Deexcitation of such an electron by paths D would give phosphorescence. The energy of the phosphorescence radiation may be different from the energy of the fluorescence radiation. In general, phosphorescence that gives a long-lived emission of visible light is a nuisance in diagnostic radiology, since the screen will continue to glow long after being exposed to the x rays. In the extreme a screen exposed once could fog the film when a second picture is being taken. The color of the light emitted in fluorescence depends upon the chemical composition of the material and is also very dependent on the presence of small amounts of chemical impurities that may be present in an otherwise perfect crystal lattice. For example, CsI : Na is a screen made from CsI with a small amount of Na impurity. This fluoresces over a broad range of wavelength with a peak fluorescence at 420 nm. If the Na impurity is replaced by Tl (Thallium) then the screen gives its peak fluorescence at 550 nm.

Fluorescent Materials

For many years calcium tungstate ($CaWO_4$) has been used by most companies as the basis of their screens. However, today many other materials are in use and the properties of some of these are summarized in Table 16-2. This list is by no means complete as new screens are becoming available each year. The table gives the trade names of some of these screens. Some of the screens, such as calcium tungstate or barium strontium sulphate, are used without the addition of impurities, while others such as gadolinium oxysulphide include a small amount of activator. This is indicated in the name by adding the symbol for the activator after the colon ($GdO_2S:Tb$).

To be useful as a screen, it must emit radiation in a region of the spectrum that is matched to the receptor. There are three main receptors that must be considered: blue sensitive film, orthochromatic film sensitive to green and blue light, and the eye. Their response curves are plotted in Figure 16-11. Blue sensitive film has its peak response in the range 400 to 450 nm (curve 2). $CaWO_4$ (curve 1), $BaSrSO_4$ (curve 3), and $BaFCl:Eu^{2+}$ (curve 4) emit radiation that is well matched to blue sensitive film. To the precision of Figure 16-11 curves 3 and 4 are identical.

TABLE 16-2
Fluorescent Materials

Material	λ max* (nm)	Remarks
$CaWO_4$	430	A common phosphor for blue sensitive film: typical screens are Dupont Detail, Par, and High Plus.
$BaSrSO_4$	390	Used with blue sensitive film: typical screen is Kodak-Regular.
$GdO_2S:Tb$	545	New rare earth phosphor—for green sensitive film: typical screens are Kodak Lanex; 3M Trimax α4, α8 and α12.
$LaOBr:Tb$	350-500	New rare earth phosphor—for blue sensitive film: typical screens are Agfa—MR 200, 400, and 600; and G.E. Blue Max 1 and 2.
$BaPbSO_4$	370	Phosphor for blue sensitive film: typical screens are DuPont High Speed and Kodak Xomatic Fine.
$Y_2O_2S:Tb$	350-600	For use with blue or green sensitive film—useful for mammography and low kV applications; typical screen is GAF.
$BaFCl:Eu^{2+}$	390	For use with blue sensitive film: typical screen DuPont Quanta II.
$(ZnCd)S:Ag$	~530	Originally used as input and output phosphors of image intensifiers—now used as output phosphor.
$CsI:Na$	420	Input phosphor for image intensifiers.

*Wavelength of maximum emission; where several peaks are present, a range of wavelengths is given.

Green sensitive film (curve 7) is sensitive in the green at 550 nm and in the ultraviolet (below 400 nm). This film was developed to match screens similar to $GdO_2S:Tb$, which emits a whole series of lines (curve 6) but with the main peak at 550 nm. Another useful screen is $LaOBr:Tb$, which emits a series of lines in the range of 380 to 450 nm that is well matched to blue sensitive film. It is obvious that judgment should be used in deciding on the screen-film combination. Care should be taken to ensure that they are matched. It would, for example, be foolish to use a

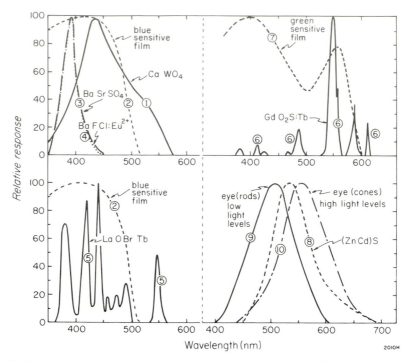

Figure 16-11. Emission spectra of various screens and response functions of films and the eye (see references B22, M16, S23, S24).

screen of $GdO_2S:Tb$ with blue sensitive film as this would lead to an insensitive combination.

We now turn to the eye. The physiology of the eye is very complex. Curve 9 of Figure 16-11 gives the response of the eye at low light levels. For dim light, vision is by the rods in the retina and the peak response is at about 500 nm. In earlier days when large fluorescent screens were viewed directly by the radiologists during fluoroscopy, a good screen to match the eye was $(ZnCd)S:Ag$. Nowadays, image intensifiers are used and we are interested in the sensitivity of the eye at high light levels where vision is by cones with peak response in the yellow green at 560 nm (curve 10). The output phosphor of the image intensifier (Fig. 16-9) is still made of $(ZnCd)S:Ag$ (curve 8), which lies between curves 9 and 10 for the eye, giving an excellent match to the eye for both high and low light levels.

As well as seeking a good match between the screen and the receptor, several other important properties should be considered in selecting a screen: the screen should efficiently absorb the x ray beam transmitted through the patient; it should concentrate the light on the film with a minimum amount of lateral spread; it should generate a minimum noise; and it should be durable under repeated use.

16.07 **RADIOGRAPHIC FILM**

When film is used in imaging in diagnostic radiology, it is almost always placed between two fluorescent screens and responds in reality mainly to the light emitted by the phosphor. The blackening of the film due to direct exposure by the x rays usually amounts to less than 2% of the total effect. Detailed discussions of the properties of film and development processes will be found in M17, H18.

DENSITY. After being developed and fixed, the film is viewed by placing it in front of a uniformly illuminated light box, where the exposed section appears black and the unexposed is white. If the brightness of the light beam from the illuminator is B_0 (see insert Fig. 16-12) and the amount transmitted is B, then the density, D, of the film is defined by:

$$D = \log_{10}\left(\frac{B_0}{B}\right) \quad \text{or} \quad B = B_0 e^{-2.203\,D} \tag{16-3}$$

On the right of Figure 16-12 the density scale is displayed adjacent to the light transmission scale, according to equation 16-3. Note that if the film transmits 1/10 of the incident light beam, then the ratio $B_0/B = 10$, and the density is 1.0. Similarly, a density of 2.0 corresponds to a transmission fraction of 1/100. From these scales, it can be seen that a density increase of 0.3 reduces the fraction transmitted by a factor of 2.0, regardless of the density chosen. (Density increases from 0 to 0.3, 0.3 to 0.6, 1.0 to 1.3, etc. all correspond to a twofold reduction in the fraction transmitted.) The reason for this choice of definition for density may be explained as follows. A film with density 1.0 transmits 1/10 the incident light. Two of these films in contact will transmit $0.1 \times 0.1 = 0.01$ of the light and so, from equation 16-3, will have a density 2.0. Now the two films have twice the quantity of reduced silver grains as the single film. Hence, it is reasonable to express the combined density of the films as 2.0. *Thus the density, defined in this way, is proportional to the amount of silver developed in the film.*

CHARACTERISTIC CURVES. The relation between the density of a film and the log of the exposure in mR is shown in Figure 16-12. These curves are called characteristic curves, or H and D curves (in honor of Hurter and Driffield who described them in 1890), and are the standard format used in displaying the properties of a film. These curves have four important regions. *The flat portion* at the extreme left where the density is independent of exposure is due to the density of the film base plus background fog: the density here is present whether the film is exposed or not. All films show some fog. Fog tends to increase if the film is old, especially if it has been stored at high temperatures. The next region is called the *toe* of the curve: in this region the density increases rapidly with exposure. This is followed by a straight portion where density increases linearly with the *log* of the exposure. Finally, the curve starts to flatten out and at high exposures, *saturation* sets in and there is no further increase in density. It is customary to use films in diagnostic radiology in the linear part of the graph at densities from 0.4 to about 2.0, preferably near 1.0. A film with density 0.4 appears light and one with density 2.0 appears black. Higher densities up to 3.0 and 4.0 may be used if an intense illuminator is available.

At very high exposures (not shown on Fig. 16-12), the optical density starts to *decrease* with increasing exposure. This reversal is used in diagnostic radiology when direct positive transparencies of radiographs are required. To produce these a radiograph is placed in contact with an unexposed film and exposed to a very bright light. This reverses the image, yielding a copy of the film, that is a positive, rather than a negative. This is referred to as solarization, since originally the reversal was accomplished with sunlight.

GAMMA. In an x ray film, image detail may be visualized when one tone stands out in contrast to an adjacent tone. The minimum difference in exposure that will be detectable will depend upon the slope of the characteristic curve. The slope of the straight line portion is referred to as the *gamma of the film,* where:

$$\gamma \text{ (gamma)} = \frac{D_2 - D_1}{\log_{10} X_2 - \log_{10} X_1} = \frac{D_2 - D_1}{\log_{10} (X_2/X_1)} \quad (16\text{-}4)$$

D_1 and X_1 are the density and exposure of one point Q on the graph and D_2 and X_2 are the corresponding values for another point P (see Fig. 16-12).

Example 16-4. Determine the average gamma between P and Q.

For point P, $X_2 = 3.0$ mR
$\qquad\qquad\qquad D_2 = 2.26$
For point Q, $X_1 = 1.0$ mR
$\qquad\qquad\qquad D_1 = 1.04$

Hence γ (eq. 16-4) $= \dfrac{2.26 - 1.04}{\log (3.0/1.0)} = \dfrac{1.22}{.477} = 2.56$

The calculation of γ involves taking the log of the ratio of two exposures. If the H and D curve is plotted so that the *distance* from density 1.0 to 2.0 is the *same* as 1 cycle on the log exposure scale then the student may show that

$$\gamma \text{(gamma)} = \tan \theta \qquad\qquad (16\text{-}5)$$

Figure 16-12 was plotted so that one cycle equals one density interval. Using a protractor, the student may measure the angle (about 69°); the

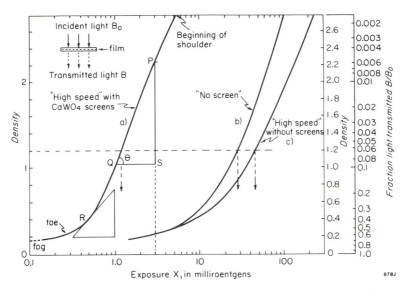

Figure 16-12. Typical characteristic curves of x ray films. (a) "high speed" film with calcium tungstate screen; (b) "no-screen" film; (c) "high speed" film without screen. The right hand scales show the density corresponding to the fraction of light transmitted. The horizontal scale is a logarithmic scale in mR. Curves a and b are replotted in Figure 16-13 using a linear exposure scale.

$\gamma = \tan 69° = 2.60$ in agreement with the above calculation. The slope of the characteristic curve at any other point, such as R, is called the gradient and may be evaluated by drawing a tangent.

LATITUDE. The exposure should be chosen to make all parts of the radiograph lie on the straight-line portion of the characteristic curve, thus ensuring the same contrast for all densities. The straight portion is known as the region of *correct exposure,* the toe the region of *under-exposure,* and the shoulder as the region of *overexposure.* The latitude is the range of exposures over which the densities will lie in the region of correct exposure. For curve a, this range is from about 0.6 mR to 6 mR, an exposure range of 10:1. It is clear that if a larger latitude is required, it can only be achieved by using a film with a smaller gamma.

SPEED OR SENSITIVITY. Speed of a film can be determined by finding the exposure required to produce a density of 1.0 greater than the density of the base plus fog. In Figure 16-12 the base plus fog is about 0.2 so we draw a horizontal line at density 1.2 and locate the exposures of 1.2, 30, and 50 mR for films a, b, and c respectively. The sensitivity of the three films are the reciprocals of these exposures, i.e. 0.83 mR^{-1}, 0.033 mR^{-1}, and 0.02 mR^{-1}. Film a has the highest sensitivity and the highest speed. Speed and sensitivity are almost synonymous. For practical purposes one can often neglect the density of the base plus fog.

FILM DEVELOPMENT. The characteristic curves of Figure 16-12 are very dependent on the way the film is developed. Modern x ray departments all use automatic processing. The film is passed through the system by a series of rollers, which transport the film at constant velocity through the developer tank, the fixing tank, the washing tank, and finally the dryer. The time for the whole process is about 90 seconds and this is usually not adjusted. Since each film uses up some developer and fixer, the concentration of chemicals is automatically kept constant by replenishing these at the time the film enters the machine.

The only parameter that is at the discretion of the user is temperature, which should be kept constant to about 0.2° C. In Figure 16-13a density is shown as a function of relative exposure for a particular film processed at three different temperatures. The main effect of a change in temperature is to alter the speed. For this case reducing the temperature from 34.4° C to 27.7° C reduces the speed by a factor of 2.0. It is also evident from the figure that increasing the temperature increases the fog. In general, there is an optimum temperature for which the speed is satisfactory, the fog is held to an acceptable level, and the gamma is high. For our case this occurs at about 31° C.

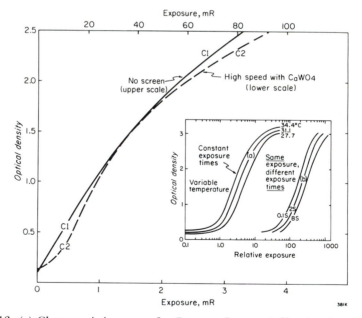

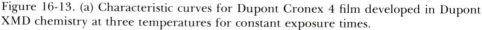

Figure 16-13. (a) Characteristic curves for Dupont Cronex 4 film developed in Dupont XMD chemistry at three temperatures for constant exposure times.

(b) Characteristic curves for Kodak X-omatic H film with Dupont Hi Plus screens given the *same exposure* but delivered in 0.1, 2, and 8 seconds. These three graphs illustrate reciprocity failure.

Curves C1 and C2 show the data of curves a and b of Figure 16-12 plotted using a linear exposure scale. Curve C1 is for a film exposed without a screen, while C2 is for a film exposed with a screen.

RECIPROCITY. It is usually assumed that the same density is produced in a film exposed to x rays, provided the kV on the tube is held fixed and the product of tube current (mA) and time (s) is constant. That is, an exposure of 1 s at 200 mA should give the same density as 10 s at 20 mA, or 0.1 s at 2000 mA. When this condition is satisfied we say that the reciprocity law is valid. Often, however, it will be found that when a given amount of radiation is delivered over a longer time the density produced is less; this is called reciprocity failure and is illustrated in Figure 16-13b. Three identical films with their screens were exposed to the same amount of radiation but for different lengths of times. The film exposed for 8 s is slower by a factor of 1.7 than the film exposed for 0.1 s. The explanation of reciprocity failure is not simple; a partial explanation is as follows.

In order to sensitize a silver bromide crystal so that it can be developed into a silver grain, the energy from 2 or 3 light photons must be deposited at a certain site in the crystal within a short period of time. At low exposure rates the energy from the first photon may be dissipated thermally in the crystal before a second photon arrives to make the sensitization permanent. Thus, part of the density that should have been produced is lost. This effect does not occur when the blackening is due to the absorption of x rays, as in "no screen" film, since the energy deposited by the interaction of one x ray photon is sufficient to ensure the development of the grains of silver.

It should be emphasized that reciprocity failure is an effect due to exposure rate. It is present for most radiographs, since exposure rate varies from one part of the image to another. This should not concern us as long as characteristic curves are determined for the same exposure time as for the radiograph. In principle, therefore, one should have a different characteristic curve for each exposure time employed. In practice, Figure 16-13b shows that the shape of the characteristic curve changes very little with intensity but its position on the exposure axis shifts considerably depending on the exposure time. This is of major importance in tomography, when exposure times of 6 s are used.

Reciprocity failure also occurs for a different reason when very *short* exposures are employed, but this is not usually a problem in diagnostic radiology.

COMPARISON OF FILMS USED WITH AND WITHOUT SCREEN. Although the characteristic curves a and b of Figure 16-12 look more or less the same shape when density is plotted versus exposure on a *logarithmic* scale, they are really exposed by quite different mechanisms. To illustrate this idea we have replotted the data of Figure 16-12 using a *linear* exposure scale in Figure 16-13 (curves C1 and C2). The "no screen" film shows a *linear* increase in density with exposure up to a density of about 1.0 and then gradually starts to saturate. In contrast, the response of the film used with a screen is sigmoidal. The difference can be explained as follows. The film without screen is exposed by x ray photons, each of which deposits enough energy to sensitize a single grain of silver, hence the initial linear relation; as the silver grains are used up the curve starts to show saturation.

When films are exposed with screens the x ray photons are absorbed in the screens, which emit visible and ultraviolet light. It is these light photons that cause 99% of the exposure to the film. Since it requires the absorption of several of these light photons to sensitize a single grain of silver, we obtain a sigmoidal response at small densities. In summary, when x ray photons interact with film a plot of density versus exposure on a linear scale should be used as in film dosimetry (Fig. 9-16). When light photons are responsible for the blackening, H and D curves using a logarithmic exposure scale are more useful.

DETERMINATION OF CHARACTERISTIC CURVES. With the increasing interest in doses delivered in diagnostic radiology, it is important that the total system from the x ray machine to the developed film be under strict control. When unsatisfactory films are produced, it may be due to any number of faults: the film may have been changed by the manufacturer without the radiologist's knowledge, the screens may have deteriorated or been altered, or the chemistry of the developer may have been changed.

To check on the speed and contrast of the film, one must determine the characteristic curve for a film-screen combination. It is necessary to keep the kV_p constant and vary the exposure by altering the mA or the time or the distance. Altering the distance is the accepted method, but in practice this is not so easy, as distances up to 10 meters may be required. If the mA and time are altered, then there may be some doubt as to whether the kV_p has altered with the changing mA. If time is altered then reciprocity failure may be present and this would have to be corrected for. Simple systems need to be developed to allow the technician to check the film, the screen, and the development in one simple test. One such device for determining characteristic curves has been developed in our laboratory.

COLOR FILM. Medichrome® (made by Agfa Gevaert) is a film that uses silver bromide as the sensitive element but that creates an image with blue dye. The film is processed in three stages. In the first, the blue dye in the film is coupled to the silver sites that have been activated. In the second, the silver coupled to the dye is removed from the film. Finally, the unaffected silver is dissolved in the fixer. Thus *all* the silver in the film is recovered at the time of development and can be used to create more film. This is a real advantage when one considers the dwindling supply of silver in the earth's surface and the rapid escalation of its price.

Present interest in this film also arises from the fact that it gives the radiologist a film with extended latitude. When viewed with white light the film has two parts to its characteristic curve. It has the normal high gamma portion for densities up to about 1.3 and then a long region of lower gamma up to density 3.0. The radiologist can view structures in bone, or vessels outlined by contrast media in the lightly exposed parts of the film under conditions where the gamma is high, and also see images in soft tissues at lower gamma in parts of the image that would normally be too black to see on a view box.

"No Screen" Film. These are used when speed is not a great problem, as in the radiography of body extremities, and when extreme detail is required. "No-screen" films are packed in light-tight paper envelopes ready for use or they may be loaded into a light-tight cardboard cassette. This cassette is often fitted with a thin sheet of lead foil that absorbs radiation backscattered from the region beyond the film that, if not intercepted, would cause a loss of contrast. For dental work, no-screen films are loaded in individual light-tight paper containers backed with lead and are immediately ready for use.

16.08   TELEVISION TECHNIQUES

Television techniques are becoming more and more important in radiology. In the very near future, it is likely that television will have as important a place as films have had in the past. The basic components involved in a television system are illustrated in Figure 16-14. X rays pass through a patient to strike the sensitive surface, P, of an image intensifier (see sec. 16.05) to form a bright image on the phosphor, Q. Light from this phosphor is focused by a lens system, L, onto the receptor, R', inside the television camera, which converts the light into an electrical signal. The electrical signal is transmitted through the cable from the examining room to the viewing station where it drives the cathode ray television tube to yield a picture that can be observed by the radiologist or photographed with a camera. The three basic devices that make the whole system possible are (a) the image intensifier, (b) the camera, and finally (c) the monitor. Billions of dollars have been spent in the perfection of components b and c for the entertainment industry. When correctly coupled they produce a very sophisticated imaging system. Radiologists are fortunate to have been able to take advantage of the outstanding technical developments of the television industry to improve their imaging methods.

Transmission of pictures takes place by (1) scanning the original light image one line at a time, (2) transmitting these picture lines down a cable as time variations of an electronic signal, and (3) rebuilding the picture line-by-line on the picture monitor. Consider first the television camera

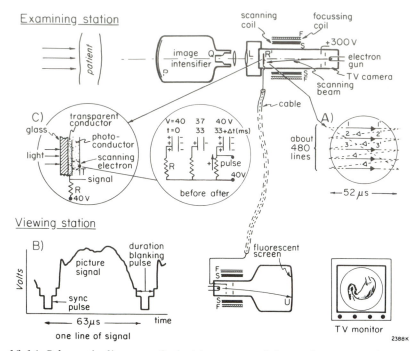

Figure 16-14. Schematic diagram of television system. It is not drawn to scale. The image intensifier is a device about 30 cm long and 15 to 30 cm in diameter. The camera is about 4 cm in diameter and 15 cm long. The monitor usually gives a picture 30 to 50 cm in diameter.

tube, the light sensitive face of which is shown in detail in insert C. The back of the receptor is scanned by a sharply focused electron beam. This beam is moved across the face of the camera by electrical signals applied to scanning coils placed around the camera tube. The scanning pattern is illustrated in insert A. The electron beam takes about 52 μs to travel from 1 to 1' across the face of the tube, when it is very rapidly returned to point 2. The beam then scans from 2 to 2' and then returns to 3, etc. 480 such lines are scanned before the scanning beam reaches the bottom of the picture. It is then returned rapidly to position 1, to repeat the previous sequence. A complete sequence takes 33.3 ms, so 30 complete pictures are transmitted every second. Since this repetition rate sometimes leads to a flickering of the picture when viewed by the eye, it is common practice to scan the odd-numbered lines first, then to scan the even-numbered lines next, giving two half pictures, each with every other line missing. These half pictures are then interlaced on the picture monitor to give the appearance of a single picture, but now the flickering is much reduced since the picture is scanned from top to bottom each 1/60 s, although the total picture is still produced in 33 ms. In North America, the standard number of lines in a complete picture is 525, although about 45 of these are wasted in returning the beam from line

480 back to line 1. In Europe the standard is 625 lines, with about 45 wasted. It is possible to use other numbers of lines for special types of work, but this requires considerable redesign of camera and monitor.

As the electron beam scans each line, an electrical signal is conducted out of the camera tube. The strength of the signal varies with the intensity of the light image focused on the face of the tube. Insert B of Figure 16-14 shows the electrical signal produced as the electron beam scans a single line. The variations of voltage are of course variations with time, but each point in time corresponds to a position in the original picture. The insert also shows that two other signals are present in the voltage variations that are transmitted from the camera to the monitor. The first is a synchronization pulse that occurs at the beginning of each line and ensures that the timing of the start of each line is precisely controlled in both the camera tube and the picture monitor. The second is a blanking pulse, which starts just before the synchronization pulse and ends just after it. The blanking pulse, which is about 11 μs long, cuts off the scanning electron beam in both camera tube and picture monitor during the time that the beam is returning from the end of one line to the beginning of the next. If this pulse is not present, bright retrace lines will be seen in the reconstructed picture. At the end of each picture field there are major synchronization and blanking pulses lasting about 1.4 ms, which return the beam to the top of the picture.

The electrical signals from the camera are transmitted to the picture monitor, where the synchronization signal is separated from the blanking and picture signals. The monitor (picture tube) contains an electron gun in which electrons are accelerated to about 20 kV to strike the fluorescent screen, which emits light. The amount of light emitted depends on the number of electrons in the beam, which in turn is controlled by the voltage variations from the camera that are applied to the grid of the television tube. Thus, as each line of the original picture is scanned on the camera tube face, a line is presented on the picture tube face. Since the time the electrical signal takes to travel from the camera to the picture monitor is very small, the original picture is thus instantaneously rebuilt on the picture monitor line by line.

TELEVISION CAMERA. Operation of the camera is illustrated in Figure 16-14C. The end of the tube consists of three layers: the glass envelope, a transparent conducting layer of tin oxide called the signal electrode, and a photoconductive layer. The photoconductive layer is an insulator that is rendered partially conducting when bombarded by light. When light strikes this, it produces regions of variable conductivity, which correspond to the regions of variable brightness on the fluorescent screen at Q. These are "read" sequentially by the scanning beam. A potential of about 40 volts is applied to the signal electrode. The scanning beam is produced by an electron gun in which electrons are accelerated by

300 volts and are focused on the photoconducting layer. The electron beam charges the photoconductor to cathode potential, as shown in Figure 16-14C, which illustrates an enlarged part of the photoconductor around T. We represent a small part of the photoconductor by a small parallel plate capacitor. The negative charges deposited on the photoconductor will produce a potential across the capacitor. As an example we show a potential of 40 volts at t = 0. This is the situation just after the scanning beam leaves the point T. During the next 33 ms, the charge will leak off the capacitor by an amount proportional to the average brightness of the screen during this interval. In the sketch we show the voltage having dropped to 37 V at time t = 33 ms. The scanning beam now passes T again and in a short increment of time, Δt, replenishes the negative charge to 40 volts. This induces a pulse of positive charge from ground producing an output pulse across the load resistor R that is proportional to 3 volts. Thus, each "point" in turn is "read," producing an output signal as a function of time corresponding to the brightness of the screen along one line.

Bandwidth is a parameter that can be used to describe the resolution of the television system. It is the maximum temporal frequency to which the system will respond. Typical values for closed circuit television used in x ray work are 10 MHz for a standard 525 line system and 25 MHz for a 1023 line system. Since the time per frame of either of these is fixed at 33 ms, this determines the horizontal spatial resolution on the monitor. Each television image lasts 33 ms and consists of 525 lines; hence, each line is scanned in 33 ms/525 = 63 μs. A 10 MHz bandwidth will allow the recording of 10×10^6 lp/s; the number of line pairs recorded per television line is $(10^7$ lp/s$) \times 63$ μs = 630 lp. If the field of view is 250 mm wide, the resolution will be 630 lp/250 mm = 2.5 lp/mm. A 25 MHz system with 1023 lines will have a correspondingly better resolution.

SUMMARY OF TELEVISION TECHNIQUES. Because of the cost of film and the increased concern regarding patient dose, television techniques will become more and more important in radiology. The television components usually do not have as high a resolution as the image intensifier. Increasing the bandwidth of the components to 25 MHz or higher will greatly increase the range of application of television techniques and will soon allow the same resolution as can be achieved with full size film-screen combinations. (Detailed description of television technology and its use in x ray work may be found in G13, Z1.)

16.09   **GRIDS**

When the beam of x rays passes through the patient (see Fig. 16-1), the beam is absorbed and scattered. A useful shadow is produced by the attenuated primary beam, while the scattered radiation from the patient will tend to mask the effects of the primary and spoil the radiograph. This scattered radiation may be removed by a grid placed between the film and the patient. The construction of a grid is illustrated in Figure 16-15. It consists of a series of lead strips of thickness c and of height h separated by spacers of low density material of width b. In a typical grid, the strips might be 0.05 mm thick, of height 2.5 mm, and separated by spacers 0.35 mm wide. The ability of the grid to discriminate against scattered radiation is measured by the grid ratio, defined as

$$\text{Grid ratio} = h/b \qquad (16\text{-}6)$$

Grids may be parallel or focused. They may be stationary or moving. Two grids may be combined to yield a crossed grid.

A parallel grid is illustrated in Figure 16-15a. It is seen that the primary beam will be cut off by the lead strips at a distance w, where w is related to the focus-to-film distance, f, thus:

$$\frac{w}{f} = \frac{b}{h} \quad \text{or} \quad w = f \times \frac{b}{h} = \frac{f}{\text{grid ratio}} \qquad (16\text{-}7)$$

Using this equation, the maximum width of field that may be radiographed for a particular grid may be calculated. For example, suppose a 12:1 grid is used with a focus-to-film distance of 1 meter, cut off will occur at a distance w = 100/12 = 8.33 cm from the normal ray. In fact, the radiograph will show a gradual reduction in density on both sides of the central ray before this cutoff point is reached. This means that large areas cannot be radiographed with a parallel grid. In this example, the width of the radiograph would be less than 17 cm.

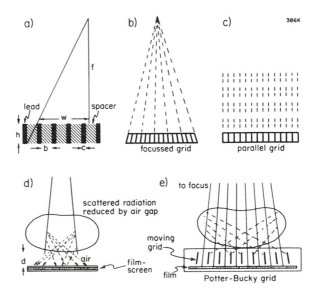

Figure 16-15. Diagram illustrating the different types of grids and the meaning of the grid ratio.

FOCUSED GRID. In a focused grid, the thin strips of lead are placed at an angle, all pointing towards the focus, as illustrated in Figure 16-15b. A focused grid shows no cutoff, provided the focal spot of the x ray tube is at the focus of the grid. However, errors in alignment both vertically and horizontally will lead to cutoff of the beam in the same way as in a parallel grid. In North America, the commonly used focus-to-film distance is 100 cm although distances from 75 cm to 180 cm are used for special procedures. Most focused grids are designed to be used at 100 cm.

CROSSED GRID. In order to obtain even greater discrimination against scattered radiation, it is possible to place 2 grids at right angles. If each has a ratio of 8:1 they will have a resultant ratio of 16:1. Actually, two crossed grids each of ratio 8:1 will give slightly better discrimination against scattered radiation than a single grid with ratio 16:1 because a single grid can never stop scattered radiation that occurs in the plane defined by the lead strips and the focal spot.

MOVING GRID. When a focused or parallel grid is used, each lead strip will appear on the radiograph as a very fine line. Modern grids can be obtained with as many as 40 lines per cm. Under these circumstances, the appearance of these fine lines causes little concern. However, they can be removed completely if the grid is moved during the radiographic exposure, as illustrated in Figure 16-15e. This is the principle of the Potter-Bucky grid. The grid in this case is usually focused and may be moved on a curved surface or in a plane. The grid may be made to oscillate or move continuously in one direction. The motion is timed by the exposure control of the diagnostic machine to start just before the x rays are turned on. The traveling period should be made greater than the exposure time, otherwise most of the exposure will occur with the grid displaced to one side, resulting in nonuniform exposure of the film. Since the output from the x ray machine comes in pulses, grid lines will appear on the film if the grid moves a distance equal to its spacing in the time taken for one pulse. Synchronization of this kind must be avoided.

AIR GAP. The use of a grid will always increase the exposure because it will absorb some of the primary radiation. Often enough discrimination against scattered radiation can be achieved by simply placing a 10 to 20 cm air gap between the patient and the detector, as illustrated in Figure 16-15d. Since the scattered photons travel at an angle to the primary beam they will disperse laterally in the space between patient and film and so be reduced in intensity. Such air gap techniques are often used in chest radiography.

EFFECTS OF GRIDS ON EXPOSURE. Table 16-3 indicates the increase in exposure needed when grids are used. For example, in imaging through 20 cm of water at 100 kV$_p$, an 8:1 grid reduces the primary by a factor of 1.8 and the primary plus scatter by 3.7. To obtain the same density on

TABLE 16-3

Grid Factors for Primary (P) and for Primary plus Scattered Radiation (P + S) for X ray Beams Passing through 20 cm Water

Grid ratio		60 kV	80 kV	100 kV	120 kV
8:1	P	1.9	1.8	1.8	1.7
	P + S	4.3	4.0	3.7	3.4
12:1	P	2.1	2.1	2.0	2.0
	P + S	5.3	5.0	4.8	4.4

the film the exposure would have to be increased by a factor of 3.7. This is called the grid factor.

In order to reduce exposures, grids with smaller ratios are being used more frequently. For example, one can use a 5:1 grid in front of the image intensifier during fluoroscopy and add to this a 5:1 grid at right angles when spot films are required. This gives a radiograph with good contrast. (For discussion on grids, see B23.)

16.10   FOCAL SPOT OF X RAY TUBE

The imaging properties of an x ray tube depend upon the focal spot. Hundreds of papers have been written on this subject because it is an easy problem to investigate experimentally and lends itself to theoretical analysis. However, in clinical practice the spot is usually small enough to have little effect on the clinical value of most radiographs. Nevertheless the problem will be discussed in some detail here in order to introduce and clarify the concepts involved in the theoretical analysis of the degradation of images. (A few of the papers dealing with focal spots and the use of Fourier transforms in studying their effects on image degradation are B24, B25, B26, B27, B28, C13, G14, M1, M18, M19, M20, M21, N13, P14, R8, R9, R10, R11, R12, S25, T1.) The focal spot may be studied by taking a pinhole picture of it or by taking a picture of a resolution test pattern. The second technique using a star pattern is becoming increasingly popular.

Pinhole Picture

Figure 16-16 shows a pinhole in a material opaque to x rays placed on the axis of the beam a distance F from the focal spot. A "no-screen" film or a film-screen combination is positioned at a distance (F + d) and a picture taken. After development the density pattern on the film may be determined. It will often show two linelike structures as illustrated in Figure 2-9. From such a picture the width, W′, and length, L′, of the blackened region may be estimated. From similar triangles the effective focal spot dimensions W and L are simply:

$$W = W'/m; \qquad L = L'/m; \qquad m = d/F \qquad (16\text{-}8)$$

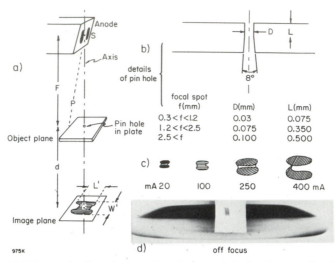

Figure 16-16. (a) Schematic diagram to show how a pinhole picture of a focal spot may be determined; (b) recommended dimensions and construction of pinholes for the investigation of different sized focal spots (NEMA, N13); (c) change in focal spot size with tube loading (adapted from Bernstein, et al., B25), (see also C13); (d) off-focus radiation determined in our laboratory.

where m is the magnification of the focal spot image as produced by the pinhole.

To obtain a good pinhole picture, the pinhole must be small compared to the focal spot being investigated. The table in Figure 16-16 shows the recommended dimensions of the pinhole for focal spots of different sizes. For example, to study focal spots in the range 0.3 to 1.2 mm, the hole should be 0.03 mm in diameter. Further, the hole must be in a dense material of high atomic number that is opaque to x rays, such as gold-platinum alloy (N13). Obtaining small holes in these materials is not easy.* When small holes are used to give one the proper resolution, intensity problems may appear. To get a satisfactory picture, long exposures may be required that may damage the x ray tube, especially if "no screen" film is used. Except for the smallest focal spot, a film-screen combination has sufficient resolution to give an acceptable picture, and the chance of overheating the target is avoided.

The size and shape of the focal spot depends upon the direction from which it is viewed relative to the axis. For example, in direction SP of Figure 16-16a the length of the source will be much smaller than L'. The focal spot size increases with tube current. This is illustrated in Figure 16-16c where the focal spot is shown for tube currents of 20, 100, 250, and 400 mA. From these remarks it is clear that the size of the focal spot is not a well-defined parameter.

OFF-FOCUS RADIATION. X rays are produced whenever electrons are stopped in material. In most tubes there will be regions in which stray

---

*Pinholes may be obtained from Nuclear Associates Inc., Carle Place, NY 11514.

electrons bombard parts of the anode other than the focal spot. If a pinhole picture is taken in such a way as to greatly overexpose the focal
spot region, then other regions of x ray production become visible. This
is illustrated in Figure 16-16d, where we see radiation being emitted
from the whole of the rotating anode. The radiation from the focal
spot is attenuated by a layer of lead placed on the film to intercept most
of it. In this particular case, 10% of the emitted radiation comes from
off-focus radiation, which degrades the image and increases the dose to
the patient. It should be minimized.

Focal Spot from Star Resolution Pattern

A completely different approach to the study of the focal spot is to use
a star resolution pattern,* a part of which is illustrated in Figure 16-17a.
This star pattern consists of an array of lead wedges about 0.03 mm
thick, arranged as the spokes of a wheel with gaps between the wedges of
the same width as the lead. The lead wedges are embedded in plastic
to make the device permanent. The bars have an angular width of 2°
as do the blank spaces between them, so that the pattern contains 90
tapered spokes of lead and 90 tapered spokes of plastic in a circle usually
of diameter 45 mm. The lead bar and the adjacent plastic bar are called
a line pair, so there are 90 line pairs in the full circle. At the periphery
of circumference 45π mm, there will be $90/45\pi = 0.637$ line pairs per
mm (lp/mm). At any smaller diameter D, the line pair frequency is
$(0.637)45/D$. Near the center where D = 2.25 mm the frequency is
12.74 lp/mm.

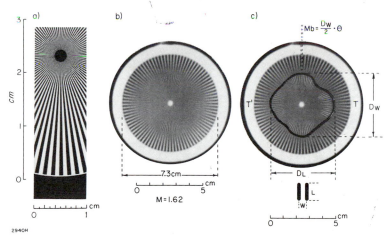

Figure 16-17. (a) Radiograph of test pattern *in contact* with the film 50 cm from the
source. (b) Radiograph of the test pattern at the same distance from the source but with
the film 81 cm from the focal spot. (c) The same picture as b but touched up to allow for
better reproduction. Relevant distances are given.

---

*These may be obtained from Funk Optik-Foto, Erlangen, West Germany, or Nuclear Associates
Inc., Carle Place, New York 11514.

If the test pattern is placed in *contact* with fine grain film and radiographed, the pattern shown in Figure 16-17a is obtained. In order to display this properly, the picture has been magnified as indicated by the vertical scale beside the picture. The bar pattern can be seen from the edge (0.64 lp/mm) into the center where the frequency is 12.7 lp/mm. Using the scale at the bottom of Figure 16-17a, the student can easily verify that at a radius of 11.2 mm (half way between center and edge) there are 1.27 line pairs in 1 mm.

Imagine now that the test pattern is placed 50 cm from the x ray source, but the film is placed further from the source at a distance of 81 cm. The appearance of the star pattern is shown in Figure 16-17b. The magnification is 81/50 = 1.62. This magnification can also be obtained from the radiograph since the pattern with diameter 45 mm appears to have a diameter of 73 mm, yielding a magnification of 73/45 = 1.62. The pattern shown in Figure 16-17b is fuzzy and lacks the detail of the first picture because of the finite size of the focal spot. This fuzzy picture can be used to determine the focal spot size as follows.

Examination of Figure 16-17b shows that there is an interesting loss in definition as one proceeds towards the center of the pattern along one of the spokes and at a certain position the pattern disappears completely. Following the spoke in further towards the center, the pattern reappears but in a reversed way and what was originally a "black" spoke becomes a "white" one. This is commonly referred to as spurious resolution. A little further in, the pattern disappears once more and then reappears reversed back to normal again. The diameters of the first disappearance, D_W and D_L, shown in Figure 16-17c can be used to estimate the width W and length L of the focal spot shown schematically at the bottom of the figure. To see how this is done, consider Figure 16-18.

DOUBLE LINE FOCAL SPOT. Imagine for the moment that the x ray source emits equal amounts of radiation from S_1 and S_2 separated by a distance W. The test pattern is shown at plane O at distance F from the focal spot. If the film is placed *just below* the test pattern it will be irradiated by a square wave intensity pattern O'O", with amplitude h. Each point on the film for this situation always "sees" either both sources or neither. If now the film is moved down to plane P the student may easily see that the pattern disappears completely, since for all points in this plane the film "sees" all of one source or all of the other but never both. The pattern P'P" is drawn with an amplitude h/2. (In doing this we are not taking into account the reduction in intensity due to the larger distance from the source.) Now imagine the film lowered to plane Q. Here, the pattern will reappear with full amplitude. For example, between Q_1 and Q_2 the film still sees both sources, whereas between Q_2 and Q_3 neither source, etc. The intensity is shown as the square wave pattern

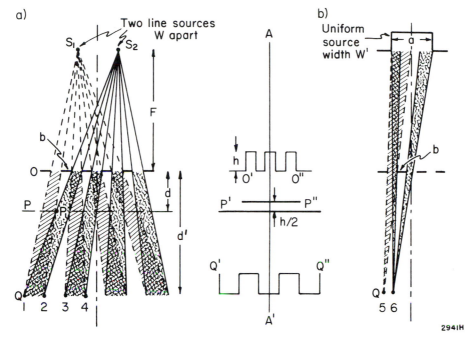

Figure 16-18. (a) Diagram illustrating the way beams from two sources, S_1 and S_2, radiating a test pattern interfere in the region below it. In the plane O there is no distortion and the pattern is perfectly reproduced as the contour O'O". In plane P, distance d below the test object, the pattern completely disappears giving the contour P'P". At distance d' below the test object, plane Q, the pattern reappears as Q'Q" but with phase reversal. (b) Diagram similar to a but for a uniform source.

Q'Q". This pattern, however, is shifted 180° from that of O'O" since along the axis AA' what appeared as a peak in O'O" becomes a valley in Q'Q". This behavior is exactly what we saw in the test pattern of Figure 16-17b.

The condition for the first disappearance may be obtained from Figure 16-18a. It will occur when lines from S_1 and S_2 drawn through the two ends of b (the width of the opaque spoke) intersect at P_1. Since the small triangle with base b and apex P_1 is similar to triangle $S_1S_2P_1$ we obtain:

$$\frac{W}{b} = \frac{F + d}{d} \qquad (16\text{-}9)$$

Now when the film is placed distance d below plane O the pattern is magnified by M where

$$M = (F + d)/F \qquad (16\text{-}10)$$

This magnification is the one usually encountered in radiology, since it is the magnification of the structures being imaged. It should not be confused with the magnification m = d/F (eq. 16-8) of the focal spot as seen in a pinhole picture. These two magnifications are related by

$$m = (M - 1) \qquad (16\text{-}11)$$

Rewriting equation 16-9 we obtain

$$W = b \frac{(F + d)}{F} \cdot \frac{F}{d} = b \frac{M}{m} \qquad (16\text{-}12)$$

Now the quantity bM is the width of the opaque bar (or the transparent part) at the disappearance point as seen in the magnified image. This is equal to $\theta \cdot D_w/2$ where θ is the angular width of the opaque bar in radians,* and D_w is the diameter of the pattern at the first disappearance position as illustrated in Figure 16-17c. Hence,

$$\begin{array}{l}\text{W (width of focal spot} \\ \text{for a double source)}\end{array} = \theta \cdot \frac{D_w}{2} \cdot \frac{1}{(M - 1)} \qquad (16\text{-}13)$$

This is the relation between the width, W, of the focal spot and the diameter, D_w, of the pattern where loss of resolution first occurs.

UNIFORM SOURCE OF WIDTH W′. We now consider the other extreme when the source is considered to be of width W′ emitting the same amount of x rays in each part of this width. The situation is depicted in Figure 16-18b. For this case the first disappearance will occur in plane Q. Point Q_5 "sees" the left half of the source. Point Q_6 "sees" the left quarter and the right quarter of the source, etc. so the pattern will disappear in plane Q. It is easy to see from similar triangles that:

$$\frac{W'}{2b} = \frac{F + d'}{d'} = \frac{F + d'}{F} \cdot \frac{F}{d'} = \frac{M}{m}$$

so that:

$$\begin{array}{l}\text{W′ (width for uniform} \\ \text{source)}\end{array} = \frac{2bM}{m} = \theta \, D_w \cdot \frac{1}{m} = \theta \, D_w \frac{1}{(M - 1)} \qquad (16\text{-}14)$$

This width is twice the value given by equation 16-13.

The locus of points where the pattern first disappears is taken from Figure 16-17b and reproduced in Figure 16-17c. From this contour the diameters D_w and D_L may be measured. Further, from Figure 16-17b the diameter of the circle can be determined and compared with the known diameter, which is stamped on the star pattern, allowing one to determine M. We illustrate with an example.

Example 16-5. From the data presented in Figure 16-17, determine the focal spot size in two directions at right angles.

---

*An angle measured in radians is the arc divided by the radius. The total angle around a point is $2\pi r/r = 2\pi$. Thus 2π radians = 360°.

The test pattern in Figure 16-17b has a diameter of 73 mm, while the actual pattern has a diameter of 45 mm.

$\therefore$ M = 73/45 = 1.62

By measurement, using the scale, D_L = 49 mm; D_w = 46 mm

$$2° = \frac{2\,\pi}{180} \text{ radians} = .0350 \text{ radians}$$

Assuming a double line source (eq. 16-13) $W = \dfrac{46(.0350)}{2(.62)} = 1.3 \text{ mm}$

Assuming uniform source (eq. 16-14) $W = \dfrac{46(.0350)}{(.62)} = 2.6 \text{ mm}$

The actual source will have a width between these extremes, usually closer to the larger.

In direction at right angles (eq. 16-14) $L = \dfrac{49(.0350)}{.62} = 2.8 \text{ mm}$

These answers should be compared with the nominal focal spot of 2.0 × 2.0 mm for that tube.

The size of the focal spot is not a precisely defined quantity. We have already seen that it depends on tube loading. It also depends upon the angle from the beam axis, so every point in a radiograph is really imaged by a differently shaped focal spot. When a thin object is imaged with very little magnification, the size of the focal spot introduces very little loss of detail. On the other hand, when very large magnifications are involved, unless the focal spot is very small, a great deal of detail is lost. Although the resolution test pattern really does not give a precise determination of the focal spot, it does tell us a good deal about the imaging properties of the tube and the detail that may be seen in a radiograph.

It should be noted that if the focal spot has no sharp edges, for example the gaussian distribution shown in Figure 16-26, there will be no place where the pattern suddenly disappears and the star technique will not allow one to determine the focal spot. For this situation the spoke pattern will gradually disappear as one proceeds towards the center.

To describe the imaging properties in a more quantitative manner we will now introduce the modulation transfer function.

16.11   MODULATION TRANSFER FUNCTION

The creation of a diagnostic image in the mind of the radiologist involves a whole series of imaging components, such as the focal spot, the fluorescent screen, the film or image intensifier, and finally the viewing system including the eye and brain of the radiologist. Each of these components produces some degradation of the final image. The modulation transfer function (MTF) was introduced into diagnostic radiology to allow the study of this complex problem in a quantitative way.

BASIC CONCEPTS. The problem is illustrated in Figure 16-19. In panel a is shown an input signal that could be the primary radiological image illustrated in Figure 16-1. We wish to determine how any one of the imaging devices shown in Figure 16-19b might alter this input signal to yield an output signal depicted in panel c. To simplify the problem we assume the input signal is a sinusoidal variation of x ray fluence A'B'C' D'E' that may be represented by:

$$\Psi' = \Psi'_{av} + \Psi'_0 \cos 2\pi fy'$$

where y' is a distance along the horizontal axis; the frequency, f, is the reciprocal of the distance between the peaks of the sine wave and is measured in line pair per millimeter; $2\pi fy'$ is an angle in radians. Frequency in this application should really be called *spatial* frequency to differentiate it from *temporal* frequency. When this x ray fluence is presented to the imaging system, the output signal is ABCDE, shown in panel c. In general, the output pattern for a linear* imaging device will be sinusoidal but changed in frequency by the factor 1/M where M is the magnification of the device. Of more importance is the fact that the amplitude of the output sinusoidal pattern will usually be changed.

MODULATION. The input signal is a sine wave superimposed upon a steady value. The information content in such a signal is described by the modulation M'(f), which is defined by (see V10)

$$M'(f) = \frac{\psi'_0}{\psi'_{av}} = \frac{\psi'_{max} - \psi'_{min}}{\psi'_{max} + \psi'_{min}} \qquad (16\text{-}15a)$$

The student can verify the equivalence of the two expressions for M'. If $\psi'_0 = \psi'_{av}$ the modulation has its maximum value of 1.0 and the maximum information is conveyed. If $\psi'_0 = 0$ the modulation is 0 and no information is carried.

In the same way we determine the modulation of the output signal:

$$M(f) = \frac{\psi_0}{\psi_{av}} = \frac{\psi_{max} - \psi_{min}}{\psi_{max} + \psi_{min}} \qquad (16\text{-}15b)$$

This output modulation is always less than the input value, i.e. there is a loss of information. Of more importance than M and M' is their ratio, called the modulation transfer (MT), since this determines the informa-

---

*The theory that we shall develop assumes that the output of the imaging device is proportional to the input whatever the amplitude—that is, we have a linear system. This is the case for screens and intensifiers but not for films. Despite this reservation, the concepts are still useful since to a first approximation the error involved in assuming linearity is small.

tion *transferred* by the system thus:

$$\text{Modulation Transfer} \quad (MT) = \frac{\text{Modulation of Output Signal}}{\text{Modulation of Input Signal}} = \frac{M}{M'} \qquad (16\text{-}16a)$$

This expression usually has its maximum value when f is small. It is, therefore, common to normalize the function to this value; we represent the normalized MTF by MTF_N, given by:

$$MTF_N(f) = \frac{M(f)}{M'(f)} \cdot \frac{M'(0)}{M(0)} \qquad (16\text{-}16b)$$

where M(0) is the modulation for f = 0. To test the system, we usually have available a whole series of test patterns of different frequencies but the *same* modulation. If this is the case then M'(f) = M'(0) and the MTF_N reduces to:

$$MTF_N(f) = \frac{M(f)}{M(0)} \qquad (16\text{-}16c)$$

In other words we can measure the MTF by looking at the *output* modulation at a series of frequencies and do not need to look at the input pattern.

The MTF is useful because if it is determined for each component in the imaging system, the resultant MTF for the whole system is found by multiplying the individual MTFs together. This is illustrated in Figure

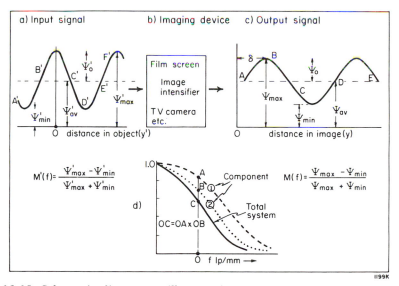

Figure 16-19. Schematic diagram to illustrate how various components in an imaging system alter the input pattern A'B'C'D'E' to yield an output pattern ABCDE. Panel d shows how the MTF of the total system can be calculated from the MTF values for two components of the system.

16-19, where it is assumed that a system has two components whose MTFs are given by curves 1 and 2. The multiplication of the ordinate at each frequency yields the MTF of the system.

PHASE. As well as altering the modulation of the input signal, the imaging device often alters the phase angle, δ, as illustrated in Figure 16-19c where we show $\delta = -90°$, which corresponds to a distance of 1/4 of a wavelength of the output. This phase shift is usually not important in diagnostic radiology—it merely means that the structure is imaged slightly to the left or right of its actual position. In the star pattern of Figure 16-17, this phase shift means the spokes will at certain positions appear bent or reversed, black being converted to white.

Experimental Determination of MTF

The measurement of the MTF experimentally is not easy since we are unable to produce sinusoidal variations of x ray fluence at a variety of spatial frequencies. This means indirect methods of measurement must be used. One approach is to measure the MTF for an imaging device using a square wave test pattern and then correct the response to that which would have been observed had one used a sinusoidal test pattern. To do this requires a detailed knowledge of Fourier transforms. This type of calculation will be dealt with in section 16.13. Another approach is to present the imaging device with a very narrow slit of x rays a few tens of micrometers wide. The interpretation of the observed pattern again requires a detailed knowledge of Fourier transforms. This, too, will be discussed in 16.13.

To determine the MTF we present the input of the imaging device with a signal and examine the output. This is illustrated in Figure 16-20a where a square wave test pattern (or a slit) is placed in contact with a film. For the frequencies occurring in radiology this will give a *perfect* reproduction regardless of the size of the focal spot, and the MTF of the film is close to 1 at all frequencies as illustrated.

If we place a screen next to the film as in b there will be a loss of modulation at higher frequencies because of the spreading of the light before it reaches the film. The image of the square wave test pattern (or a slit) will be blurred.

If we move the test pattern back from the film as in c the image, which was sharp in a, will now appear blurred because of the size of the focal spot. As the frequency is increased the MTF will go to zero, then increase and go to zero again as illustrated. Clearly the MTF is now a function of the magnification, M, as well as the size of the focal spot. The frequencies observed in the image plane will be 1/M times the frequency of the test pattern. It will be shown in section 16.13 that the MTF due to the focal spot is proportional to the Fourier transform of the distribution of emission from the spot.

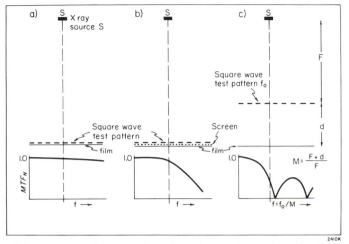

Figure 16-20. Diagrams to illustrate how imaging devices alter the MTF. (a) Square wave test pattern in contact with film. (b) Square wave test pattern in contact with screen, which is in contact with film. (c) Square wave test pattern some distance from the film. The square wave test pattern could equally well be a slit of x ray fluence.

To illustrate these ideas, we shall make an approximate determination of the MTF for a particular focal spot using a bar pattern. Bar patterns are available consisting of three slots in lead whose widths are equal to the opaque regions between them. The test patterns come in a series of some 20 frequencies between 0.6 and 5.0 lp/mm. These are simultaneously imaged on film and then carefully measured with a densitometer. Several density traces are averaged to reduce the random fluctuations due to noise and the densities converted to exposures using the characteristic curve of Figure 16-12. A few of the exposure traces are illustrated in Figure 16-21. The modulation for each of the output patterns can be determined using equation 16-15b. For example the MT for the 1.0 lp/mm pattern can be obtained from Figure 16-21 by measuring ψ_{max} and ψ_{min} to give MT = 0.70.

For the first pattern (0.6 lp/mm), $\psi_{min} = 0$ so that MT = 1.0. The fact that ψ_{min} is close to zero shows that the lead is thick enough to be opaque to the x rays.

The reader should note that as the frequency is increased the modulation decreases rapidly and reaches zero about half way between f = 1.6 and 1.8, at a frequency of about 1.7. It then increases to a maximum at f = 2.8 and decreases to zero at f = 4. Beyond f = 4 the modulation transfer is for all practical purposes zero. The region between f = 1.7 and f = 4 is the region of spurious resolution, since the traces show two peaks when we know that there are in reality three peaks.

The MT values determined in this way are plotted in the insert to Figure 16-21. The frequency scale is the frequency of the test pattern.

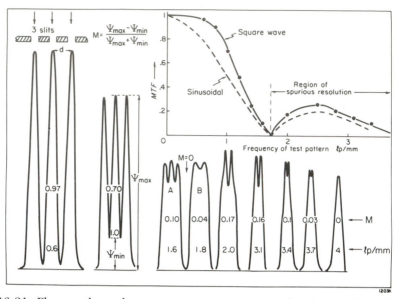

Figure 16-21. Fluence through a square wave test pattern for frequencies of 0.6, 1.0, 1.6, 1.8, 2.0, 3.1, 3.4, 3.7, and 4.0 lp/mm. The magnification was 1.7 so that, for example, the distance d = 1.7(1/0.6) = 2.83 mm.

The actual frequencies one would measure from the densitometer traces are smaller by the factor 1/M. In the next section we will discuss how the MTF for the sinusoidal test pattern can be obtained from the square wave pattern.

16.12 THEORETICAL DETERMINATION OF MTF FOR FOCAL SPOT

Imagine the x ray fluence from the focal spot is the pattern of radiation RR'R" shown in Figure 16-22a. Following a method developed by Morgan (M21) we will now show how one may calculate the MTF of this focal spot. We test the system by placing a sinusoidal test pattern in the object plane Y (distance F from focal spot) and observe the output pattern in the image plane X at a distance (F + d). The test pattern is constructed in such a way that the transmission of x rays is given by:

$$\text{Transmission} = T_{av} + T_0 \cos 2\pi fy$$

where T_{av} is the average transmission of the pattern, $(T_{av} + T_0)$ the maximum transmission, and $(T_{av} - T_0)$ the minimum.

In the absence of the pattern, let $\psi(a)$ represent the energy fluence* reaching 0 from a width, da, of the target at a distance a from the axis

---

*This could be energy fluence, photon fluence, or exposure since calculations with these are linear; it could not be density.

0″0. The total fluence reaching point P is K:

$$\text{where } K = \int_{\text{target}} \psi(a)\,da \qquad (16\text{-}17)$$

If the target is so small that one can consider that all of the radiation comes from a point source at 0″, then the pattern of radiation in the image plane is simply:

$$\psi' = K\{T_{av} + T_0 \cos(2\pi fy/M)\}$$

This is shown as the curve A′B′C′D′ in the image plane. It is the same shape as the test pattern and has its peak value on the axis 00″. Its frequency is reduced from f to f/M where M is the magnification, (F + d)/F. The modulation of this pattern according to equation 16-15a is:

$$M' = T_0/T_{av} \qquad (16\text{-}18)$$

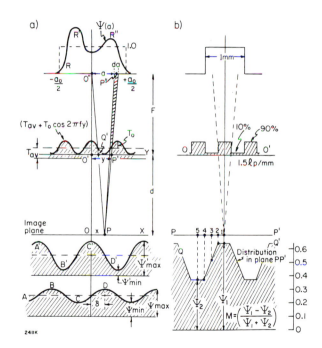

Figure 16-22. (a) Diagram to illustrate how the energy fluence may be calculated at point P in the plane OX, when radiation from the focal spot is used to image a sinusoidal test pattern in plane Y at magnification M = (F + d)/F. (b) To illustrate how the energy fluence distribution in the plane PP′, produced by a square wave test pattern OO′ in the object plane may be calculated. The x ray source is assumed to be uniform, of width 1 mm, the test pattern is 1.5 lp/mm and the magnification = 2.0. The modulation for this case is 0.266.

Consider now the real focal spot, which emits the pattern of radiation RR′R″ as illustrated in Figure 16-22a. The increment of fluence, $d\psi(x)$, at P arising from the emission from da is:

$$d\psi(x) = \{T_{av} + T_0 \cos 2\pi fy\}\,\psi(a)\,da \qquad (16\text{-}19)$$

This expression involves three variables: distances a in the plane of the target, y in the plane of the test pattern, and x in the plane of the detector. We now obtain the relation between these distances. From the similar triangles O″OP and O″O′Q′ we write:

$$O'Q' = x \cdot \frac{F}{F+d} = \frac{x}{M}$$

where M is the magnification $= (F + d)/F$. From the similar triangles PO″P″ and PQ′P′:

$$Q'P' = a \cdot \frac{d}{F+d} = a\frac{d}{F}\frac{F}{F+d} = a\frac{m}{M}$$

where $m = d/F$. This gives

$$y = O'Q' + Q'P' = \frac{x}{M} + \frac{m}{M}a$$

After substituting this value for y in equation 16-19 we add up the contributions from all areas of the emitting target to yield:

$$\psi(x) = KT_{av} + T_0 \int_{-\infty}^{+\infty} \cos(Ax + Ba) \cdot \psi(a)da \qquad (16\text{-}20)$$

where
$$K = \int_{-\infty}^{+\infty} \Psi(a)\,da; \qquad A = \frac{2\pi f}{M}; \qquad B = \frac{2\pi fm}{M} \qquad (16\text{-}20a)$$

Using the relation $\cos(Ax + Ba) = \cos Ax \cos Ba - \sin Ax \sin Ba$ and rearranging, the integral becomes:

$$\Psi(x) = KT_{av} + T_0 \cos(Ax) \int_{-\infty}^{+\infty} \cos(Ba)\Psi(a)da$$

$$- T_0 \sin(Ax) \int_{-\infty}^{+\infty} \sin(Ba)\Psi(a)da \qquad (16\text{-}21)$$

Note the terms $\cos Ax$ and $\sin Ax$ can be taken outside the integral because the integration is with respect to the variable a. It is convenient to represent the two integrals by:

$$R(f) = \int_{-\infty}^{+\infty} \cos(Ba)\Psi(a)da \qquad I(f) = \int_{-\infty}^{+\infty} \sin(Ba)\Psi(a)da \qquad (16\text{-}22)$$

The integrations can always be performed numerically if $\psi(a)$ is known and often mathematically if ψ is of suitable form. Rewriting equation 16-21 we obtain:

$$\Psi(x) = KT_{av} + T_0\left[\cos(Ax) \cdot R(f) - \sin(Ax) \cdot I(f)\right] \quad (16\text{-}23)$$

This expression gives us the distribution of radiation in the image plane. It is the difference between a cosine term and a sine term. The student may easily show that equation 16-23 may be written as:

$$\Psi(x) = KT_{av} + T_0 H(f) \cos (Ax + \delta) \qquad (16\text{-}24)$$

where $H(f)* = \sqrt{\left[R(f)^2 + I(f)^2\right]}$ and $\tan \delta = I(f)/R(f)$

The output of this imaging system is the curve ABCD of Figure 16-22a. The distribution in the image plane is sinusoidal of frequency f/M and shifted in phase by the angle δ. We are primarily interested in the amplitude of the variations in this plane rather than the value at any particular value of x. Since the cosine term fluctuates between 1 and -1 as we move along the x-axis, the maximum and minimum values are:

$$\psi_{max} = KT_{av} + T_0 H(f) \qquad\qquad \psi_{min} = KT_{av} - T_0 H(f)$$

Substituting these values in equation 16-15b we obtain:

$$M(f) = \frac{T_0 H(f)}{KT_{av}} \qquad (16\text{-}25)$$

The modulation that is *transferred* relative to a point focal spot is found by dividing this equation by equation 16-18 to give:

$$MTF = H(f)/K \qquad (16\text{-}26)$$

If we wish to express the MTF relative to its value at $f = 0$, we note that $H(0) = 1.0$ so that:

$$MTF_N = H(f) \qquad (16\text{-}27)$$

These are general expressions for the MTF; to evaluate it requires a knowledge of $\psi(a)$ and the determination of $R(f)$ and $I(f)$ by integration of equation 16-22.

In the next section we will see that $H(f)$ is the Fourier transform of $\psi(a)$.

Special Case—the MTF for Uniformly Emitting Focal Spot of Width a_0

Suppose the focal spot emits uniformly as illustrated by the dotted lines in Figure 16-22a. The energy fluence is 1.0 from $-a_0/2$ to $+a_0/2$ and zero outside these limits. Since the emission from the target is symmetrical about the Y axis, and since sin Ba is an odd function, the integral $I(f)$ vanishes. This means the phase shift δ (see eq. 16-24) is zero and $H(f) = R(f)$. Using equation 16-22 we determine $R(f)$:

$$R(f) = \int_{-a_0/2}^{+a_0/2} \cos Ba \cdot da = \left[\frac{1}{B} \sin Ba\right]_{-a_0/2}^{+a_0/2} = \frac{2}{B} \sin \frac{Ba_0}{2}$$

$$= a_0 \frac{\sin\theta}{\theta} \quad \text{where} \quad \theta = \frac{Ba_0}{2} = \frac{\pi f m a_0}{M}$$

---

*H(f) is the modulus of the function and mathematically is always positive. However, it is often shown as going negative, indicating that peaks and valleys are interchanged, i.e. reversed in phase.

The determination of K is simply $\int_{-a_0/2}^{-a_0/2} da = a_0$; hence, using equation 16-26 we obtain:

$$\text{MTF (uniform source width } a_0) = \frac{\sin \theta}{\theta} \text{ where } \theta = \frac{\pi f m a_0}{M} \qquad (16\text{-}28)$$

This function is plotted against the parameter θ in Figure 16-23. The MTF is equal to 1.0 at $\theta = 0$, drops to zero when $\theta = \pi$, is negative from π to 2π, and then becomes positive again. The MTF can be related to the spatial frequency f provided the width of the uniformly emitting source a_0 and the magnification M are known. Suppose $a_0 = 1$ mm and M = 2.0, then f = 2 line pairs/mm at $\theta = \pi$ thus fixing the frequency scale of Figure 16-23.

The negative values plotted in Figure 16-23 should in fact be positive as they were in Figure 16-21. This occurred because we have plotted $\sin \theta/\theta$ instead of the absolute value of this function according to equation 16-24. The negative values have some advantage since they show where a phase shift occurred.

At f = 2, where the MTF goes negative there is a sudden phase shift from 0 to 180°. At point F where the MTF goes positive, there is a second phase shift from 180° to 360°. The sudden phase shift occurs for a symmetric focal spot. If the focal spot is not symmetric, the phase shift will be more or less continuous as f is increased. The phase shift is seldom of much importance in radiology since it only appears as a small shift in the position of a structure.

Example 16-6. An x ray tube has a uniformly emitting focal spot of width $a_0 = 1.5$ mm. A test object is placed 80 cm from the target and is imaged at a distance of 100 cm from the source. Determine the spatial frequency in the test object for which the MTF will first be zero.

From equation 16-28, the relative MTF will first be zero when $\theta = \pi$ and hence $f m a_0 = M$.

The geometric factors are: M (eq. 16-10) = 100/80 = 1.25
                              m (eq. 16-11) = (M − 1) = .25

The required frequency is $f = \dfrac{M}{m a_0} = \dfrac{1.25}{.25} \times \dfrac{1}{1.5 \text{ mm}} = 3.3$ lp/mm

This theoretical discussion shows us another way to determine the MTF. If one first determines the spatial distribution of radiation from the focal spot, i.e. $\Psi(a)$, by carefully taking a pinhole picture with m = 1, one could then determine the MTF by numerical integration using equation 16-22, 24, and 25. This approach is possible and will be dealt with in the next section after we have introduced the idea of a Fourier transform.

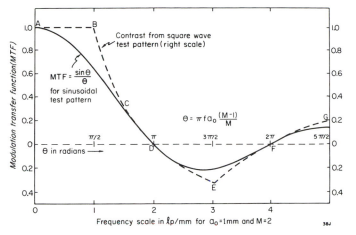

Figure 16-23. The MTF (eq. 16-28) plotted as a function of the parameter $\theta = a_0 \pi f$ $(M - 1)/M$ where a_0 is the width of the uniformly emitting source, f is the frequency in lp/mm, and M is the magnification. The graph also shows the MTF for a square wave test pattern.

MTF from Square Wave Test Pattern

We have seen that the sinusoidal test pattern has some mathematical and conceptual advantages, but since it cannot be made we now analyze what can be learned from a square wave test pattern.

Figure 16-22b shows a uniformly emitting focal spot of 1 mm width irradiating a square wave test pattern in which we have assumed the opaque part transmits 0.1 of the x rays while the transparent part transmits 0.9. The modulation of this step wedge under perfect imaging conditions is simply $(0.9 - 0.1)/(0.9 + 0.1) = 0.8$. Now, consider the modulation that will be observed in the image plane PP' when a test pattern with 1.5 lp/mm is radiographed at magnification 2.0. Consider in turn points P_1, P_2, P_3, P_4, and P_5. Point P_1 "sees" 2/3 of the source through the part of the step wedge that transmits 90% of the radiation and 1/3 through the part that transmits 10%. So, the total fluence at P_1 is .667(.9) + .333(.1) = .663. This locates the corresponding point on the fluence distribution QQ'. From the diagram the student can easily show that P_2 sees the same amount of radiation as P_1. Point P_3 sees 1/2 the source at 90% transmission and the other half of the source at 10%, yielding a fluence of $0.45 + .05 = .50$ locating point Q_3. Finally, point P_5 will yield a fluence of $.9(1/6) + .1(4/6) + .9(1/6) = .366$ represented by Q_5. The variation of fluence in the image plane is shown by QQ'. The modulation in this plane is $(.633 - .366)/(.633 + .366) = 0.266$. It is usual to relate this modulation to that obtained for zero frequency, i.e. under conditions of no loss in modulation. Hence, the 0.266 should be divided by 0.8 to give 0.333. This modulation transfer is plotted as point C in Figure

16-23. Calculations for test patterns of other frequencies may be carried out in the same way to yield the dashed curve. The curve is 1.0 from f = 0 to f = 1, then falls to zero at f = 2 in agreement with our findings in the last section. From f = 2 to 4, the pattern is reversed corresponding to the region of spurious resolution.

One of the difficulties with this analysis arises because the *shape* of the fluence pattern in the image plane is *not* the same as the shape of the square wave test pattern, that is, the pattern QQ' of Figure 16-22b is not the same as OO'. This means that as we proceed along the curve ABCDEFG of Figure 16-23, the shape of the pattern in the image plane continually changes. At A it is a square wave like the test pattern, at B the student may easily show that it becomes a triangular or sawtooth distribution, at C it is trapezoidal as shown in Figure 16-22b, while at D it vanishes, etc. Now, although the modulation at B is the same as at A, the pattern at B would be much harder to see because the sharp edges in it are removed.

It should be noted the square wave and sinusoidal test patterns show zero crossing at the same frequencies and do not differ much except in the region from f = 0 to 1.0 lp/mm. For these reasons, not much error is made by carrying out tests with the square wave pattern but using an analysis based on a sinusoidal pattern. If a more precise calculation is required, it is possible to determine the MTF for a sinusoidal test pattern from the experimental results for the square wave test pattern using a method discussed by Coltman (C14). This involves a relatively simple point-by-point correction. It is left as an exercise for the student to carry out such a correction (see problem 29).

16.13   FOURIER TRANSFORM

The Fourier transform is a powerful mathematical tool that has applications to the imaging process and radiology. (Excellent reference books on Fourier transforms are B29, D10.) Imagine some function $\phi(x)$ that describes a distribution along the x axis of a radiation pattern. It could, for example, be the pattern along a line across a pinhole picture of a focal spot, or across a picture of a slit, or in fact across any radiation pattern. The Fourier transform of this function, $\phi(x)$, is defined by:

$$H(f) = \int_{-\infty}^{+\infty} \phi(x)\, e^{-2\pi ifx}\, dx = \int_{-\infty}^{+\infty} \phi(x)(\cos 2\pi fx - i \sin 2\pi fx)\, dx$$

where i is the square root of -1. Note that the integration is with respect to x, yielding a function of the spatial frequency, f. H(f) is called the Fourier transform of $\phi(x)$. In general, it is a complex quantity made up of a real part, R(f), and an imaginary part, I(f), where:

$$R(f) = \int_{-\infty}^{+\infty} \phi(x) \cos 2\pi fx \ dx \qquad (16\text{-}29)$$

$$I(f) = - \int_{-\infty}^{+\infty} \phi(x) \sin 2\pi fx \ dx$$

The amplitude, $|H(f)|$, and phase angle, δ, are given by:

$$|H(f)| = \sqrt{R(f)^2 + I(f)^2} \qquad \tan \delta = \frac{I(f)}{R(f)} \qquad (16\text{-}30)$$

The student should immediately note that the Fourier transform integrals $R(f)$ and $I(f)$ are the same as $R(f)$ and $I(f)$ (eq. 16-22) except for a factor m/M. This means that to determine an MTF, one merely takes the Fourier transform of the focal spot distribution and changes the frequency scale by the factor $m/M = (M - 1)/M$. This will be dealt with later in this section; in the meantime, we will explore further the meaning of the Fourier transform.

Fourier Transform of a Rectangular Pulse

To clarify these ideas, imagine $\Psi(x)$ is the function illustrated in Figure 16-24a, which is equal to a constant, k, from $-a_0/2$ to $+a_0/2$ and zero outside this range. The Fourier transform of this function is easily obtained by substituting $\phi(x) = k$ in equation 16-29 to yield

$$R(f) = \frac{k \ a_0 \sin (\pi fa_0)}{\pi fa_0} \qquad I(f) = 0 \qquad (16\text{-}31a)$$

$\Psi(x)$ and its Fourier transform are plotted in Figure 16-24a, b. It is the familiar function introduced in the last section. Its height at $f = 0$ is ka_0 and its first zero is at $f = 1/a_0$.

It is important to understand the meaning of the Fourier transform. It really tells us that the rectangular pulse, $\Psi(x)$, can be considered as being the sum of an infinite number of cosine functions with frequencies from $-\infty$ to $+\infty$ with amplitudes given by $R(f)$ of equation 16-31a. Mathematically this means that

$$\Psi(x) = \int_{-\infty}^{+\infty} \frac{k}{\pi f} \sin (\pi fa_0) \cdot \cos (2\pi fx) df$$

where the integration is with respect to f. Often this integration cannot be carried out analytically, so the integral is replaced with a sum, thus:

$$\Psi(x) = 2 \sum_{f_1}^{f_n} \frac{k}{\pi f} \sin (\pi fa_0) \cos(2\pi fx) \ \Delta f \qquad (16\text{-}31b)$$

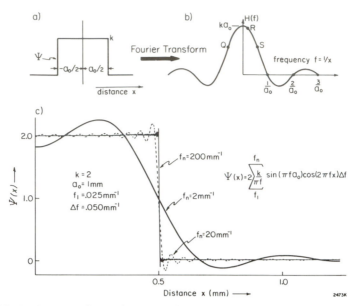

Figure 16-24. (a) Rectangular pulse $\Psi(x)$ of constant value k between $-a_0/2$ and $+a_0/2$ (b) H (f) the Fourier transform of $\Psi(x)$ given by equation 16-31a. (c) Graphs to illustrate the idea that the rectangular pulse $\Psi(x)$ can be considered to be the sum of a series of cosine functions with amplitudes R(f) (eq. 16-31). Graphs plotted for k = 2, a_0 = 1 mm, f_1 = .025 mm^{-1}, Δf = .050 mm^{-1} for f_n = 2, 20, and 200 mm^{-1}.

which may be evaluated with a computer. To obtain a good representation of $\Psi(x)$, the frequency interval (Δf) should be made small, f_1 should be close to zero, and f_n large compared to $1/a_0$. The student may write a computer program to do this summation to yield the graphs of Figure 16-24c. In plotting these we have placed k = 2, a_0 = 1 mm, f_1 = 0.025 mm^{-1}, and Δf = 0.050 mm^{-1} and have drawn graphs for f_n = 40Δf, 400Δf, and 4000Δf. When a small band of frequencies are included, the rectangular pulse is not well described; however, as the number of frequencies is increased the reproduction becomes better and better, and with frequencies from .025 mm^{-1} to 200 mm^{-1} the rectangular pattern is almost perfectly reproduced by the appropriate summation of cosine terms.

Fourier Transform of Very Narrow Slit

Imagine now that the rectangular pulse described above is made very narrow by allowing $a_0/2$ of Figure 16-24a to approach zero. Since the first zero in the transform occurs at f = $1/a_0$ the width of the central region of the transform will become infinitely wide as a_0 approaches zero. This means that the portion QRS of Figure 16-24b will become essentially flat and very wide and in the limit the Fourier transform of the narrow slit will be a line parallel to the x axis, as illustrated in Figure 16-25b. This

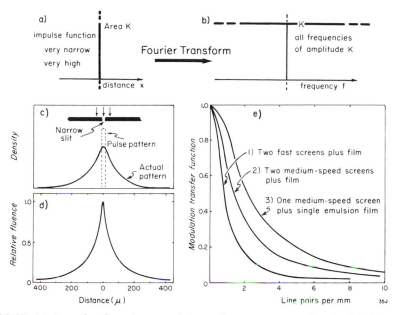

Figure 16-25. (a) Impulse function consisting of a very narrow band of infinite height including an area K. (b) The Fourier transform of a includes all frequencies with the same amplitude K. (c) Observed density produced by x rays passing through a narrow slit. (d) Corresponding relative fluence that would give this density. (e) Typical Fourier transforms of d, yielding the MTF for three screen-film combinations.

means an infinitely narrow slit can be represented by the sum of an infinite number of cosine functions *all with the same amplitude.* We use this idea to develop a practical way to determine the MTF of an imaging system.

LINE SPREAD FUNCTION: Figure 16-25 shows the density of a film exposed to radiation that passes through a 10 μm slit between lead jaws in contact with the film screen combination. If there were no distortion produced by the film, the density would appear as the dotted pulse pattern. The actual pattern of density is broader than this, showing some density at distances up to 500 μm from the center of the slit as if photons were actually hitting the film at these positions. The blackening in regions remote from the slit is due to scattering and diffusion of light when screens are used. When "no-screen" films are used, the x rays are absorbed directly in the film, and the spreading of the image is much smaller and is determined by the range of the electrons set in motion. The spreading due to grain size is smaller still and is usually not seen.

From the characteristics of the film it is possible to calculate the relative fluence that would give rise to this density pattern. This procedure requires great care (H19). Such a pattern is shown in Figure 16-25d. If the imaging system were perfect, the relative fluence would be an impulse pattern that is not shown. The curve shown in Figure 16-25d is called the line spread function. It may be obtained for any system but is particularly useful in dealing with films and film-screen combinations.

We now determine the Fourier transform of this line spread function by numerical integration of equation 16-29. This can be done using fast Fourier transform programs, which are available on most computers. Since the fluence pattern has lost its sharp edges, the Fourier transform would show that the amplitude of the high frequencies is small. Since the narrow slit contains *all* frequencies of *the same amplitude,* to obtain the MTF we would divide each amplitude of the Fourier transform by a constant value *so the MTF is in fact the Fourier transform of the line spread function.* Typical values for the MTF are given in Figure 16-25e for three different screen-film combinations. The fastest combination (curve 1) lacks high frequency response. A film used with two medium-speed screens gives a better response at high frequencies, while a film used with only one screen is even better. A film used with no screens would have the best high frequency response. The gain of picture quality represented by high frequency response is, of course, obtained at the expense of exposure.

FOURIER TRANSFORMS AND FOCAL SPOTS. The insert to Figure 16-26 shows three focal spot distributions. Curve a is the rectangular distribution of width a_0. Curve b is a single gaussian, while curve c is a double gaussian. Most focal spots would have a fluence distribution similar to one of these three. The constants describing these were adjusted so that all three curves pass through P and P'. It is left as an exercise for the student (see problem 19) to find the Fourier transform of these distributions using equation 16-29 and to show that they yield the curves of Figure 16-26. It should be noted that the uniform source and the double gaussian cross zero near $\theta = 3$ radian $\approx 180°$ giving a region of spurious resolution. In contrast the single gaussian shows no region of spurious resolution.

There is no agreement on the best type of focal spot. One could argue that since the MTF for the single gaussian never crosses zero to give a region of spurious resolution it should be best. However, because it has no sharp edges, objects in the image plane will never be sharply delineated and so may be missed by the radiologist. On the other hand, the square pattern or the double gaussian will generate sharp edges in the image plane, which will be easier to observe. If the radiologist is aware of the distortion present in the regions of spurious resolution, he can interpret the false edges he sees. One could conclude that it is better to see a structure in a distorted way than not see it at all. The use of these curves is illustrated by an example.

Example 16-7. A pinhole picture with unit magnification was taken of a focal spot yielding the fluence distribution given by curve c of Figure 16-26 with width PP' = 1.5 mm. The tube was then used to image a struc-

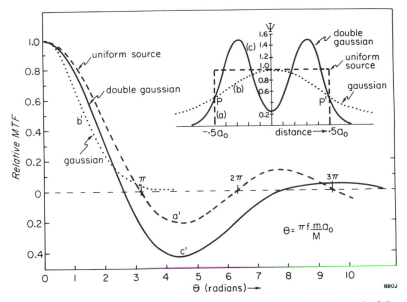

Figure 16-26. The insert shows the intensity distribution across three typical focal spots. (a) Rectangular distribution of height 1.0 and width a_0. (b) A gaussian distribution $y = e^{-\alpha x^2/a_0^2}$ with $\alpha = 2.772$. This passes through P and P' so the full width at half maximum is a_0. (c) A double gaussian to simulate a focal spot with two line like structures. Its equation is $y = k[e^{-\beta(x-\gamma a_0)^2/a_0^2} + e^{-\beta(x+\gamma a_0)^2/a_0^2}]$ where $k = 1.515$, $\beta = 27.72$, $\gamma = .3$. The peaks are separated by 0.6 a_0 and the curves pass through P and P'. The main graph shows the MTF for the three focal spots as a function of the dimensionless variable $\theta = \pi fma_0/M$.

ture with the detecting system 100 cm from the source and the object 85 cm from the source. Assuming the eye can detect a relative MTF of 0.1, determine the limit of resolution in lp/mm.

From curve c' of Figure 16-26 we locate $\theta = 2.4$ radians at an MTF of 0.1

The geometric factors are $M = \dfrac{100}{85} = 1.176$

$$m = \frac{15}{85} = 0.176$$

Substituting these values in $\theta = \pi fma_0/M$ we obtain

$$f = \frac{\theta M}{\pi ma_0} = \frac{2.4(1.176)}{\pi(.176)(1.5)} = 3.4 \text{ lp/mm.}$$

16.14　　　　　　　　**MTF OF IMAGING SYSTEMS**

It was seen in Figure 16-19 that the frequency response of each component of an imaging system is given by the normalized modulation transfer function $(\text{MTF})_N$ and that the response of a complete system can be found by multiplying the ordinates of the normalized MTFs for each component. We now consider the key components for image intensifiers, for screen-film combinations, and for complete imaging systems.

IMAGE INTENSIFIERS. The MTFs of the imaging components in an image intensifier (from K9) are shown in Figure 16-27a. The components arranged in the order in which they cause deterioration of the MTF are (A) the electron optics, (B) the output phosphor, and (C) the input phosphor.

It can be seen that the input phosphor, which absorbs the x rays, is still the major limitation of the MTF of the intensifier, although steady improvement in this phosphor is being made by manufacturers. Recently these improvements have brought the MTF of the intensifier closer to the MTF of the high-speed screen-film combination, which is shown for comparison as curve D. It can be seen that the resultant MTF of the intensifier, curve E, although it is determined mainly by the MTF of the input phosphor, is also affected significantly by the combined MTFs of the electron optics and of the output phosphor. Thus, the latter two components cannot be neglected in future work to improve intensifier performance, and indeed, significant improvements have been made in them in the last few years.

SCREENS AND FILMS. MTF's for typical films and screen-film combinations are shown in Figure 16-27b. When soft x rays are absorbed in a film, the region sensitized is small so that the MTF remains close to 1.0 even at high frequencies. This fact has been exploited in films used for mammography. In contrast, when film is exposed to light from screens, the scattering of light leads to loss of the MTF. The MTF of the film will depend on the thickness of the emulsion, and with the double emulsion films, it will also depend on the thickness of the film base.

Curve C shows the MTF for a DuPont Lo-dose® screen-film combination for mammography. The single screen is placed behind the film so that the x rays pass through the film first. The x rays are thus absorbed in the surface of the screen which is closest to the film, thus reducing the spread of light reaching the film. This maximizes the MTF of both the film and the screen-film combination.

Curve D shows the MTF for a DuPont HiPlus-Cronex 4® screen-film combination, a combination that has a speed typical of that used for most radiography. The deterioration in MTF is a combination of the effects of the double screens, the thickness of the phosphor, the amount of light reflected at the base of the screen, and cross-over of light from one emulsion to the other in the film. The MTF can be improved by preferential absorption of scattered light by incorporating a dye in the phosphor. The components of the MTF are seldom published separately by the manu-

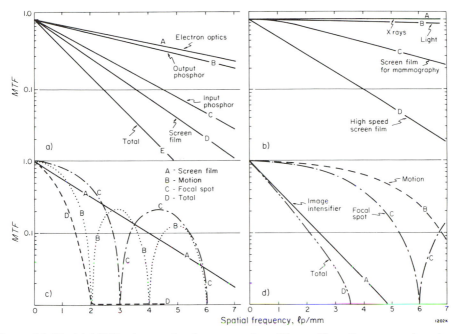

Figure 16-27. (a) MTFs due to A. electron optics of intensifier, B. output phosphor of intensifier, C. input phosphor (X ray screen) of intensifier, D. high speed film-screen combination for comparison, E. total for a 23 cm image intensifier (adapted from K9). (b) MTFs of A. film exposed to x rays only, B. film exposed to light, C. DuPont Lo-dose screen-film combination for mammography, D. typical high speed screens such as 3M-α8, Dupont Hi Plus, and Siemens-Special. (c) MTFs due to A. Screen-film combination, B. motion (1.33 cm/sec with magnification of 1.5, 25 ms exposure time), C. focal spot (1.0 mm square profile, magnification 1.5), D. resultant total MTF. (d) MTFs due to A. 23 cm image intensifier, B. motion (1.33 cm/sec with magnification of 1.5, 6 ms exposure time), C. focal spot (0.5 mm square profile, magnification 1.5), D. resultant total MTF.

facturers since the adjustment of these components to produce a screen-film combination with a commercially acceptable speed and MTF is a trade secret. However, they can and should be measured by the physicist, who needs a complete understanding of the screen-film imaging system in order to suggest ways to their improvement.

IMAGING SYSTEMS. In considering the MTF of a complete imaging system, all the components that produce a deterioration in MTF must be included. Typically, the most important components are the focal spot, motion in the patient, and the image detector. However, a complete analysis should include motion of the x ray tube or of the image detector and the effects of a stationary or moving grid. Further, the analysis should be carried out for different depths in the patient, for different positions in the image field, and for different directions in the image plane, since both focal spot blurring and the MTF of the image detector will vary with position and direction.

Here we will consider only the focal spot, patient motion, and the detector, and only for the axis of the beam. Curve A in Figure 16-27c gives the MTF for a typical high speed screen-film combination. Curve B is the MTF resulting from the blurring caused by an object with a sharp edge moving at 1.33 cm/s during an exposure of 25 ms at magnification 1.5. For this exposure the image of the object moves 0.5 mm. The resultant MTF is similar to the MTF for a focal spot with a square wave distribution of x ray emission. This takes the form $|\sin \theta/\theta|$ as shown in Curve B. There is of course a change of phase when $\sin \theta/\theta$ is negative.

Curve C is the MTF due to the focal spot, which emits x rays uniformly across its width. Curve C is similar in shape to Curve B but the zero crossing points are more widely spaced. Curve D is the resultant MTF for the complete imaging system for a point in the patient that is imaged with a magnification of 1.5 as might be used in radiography of the chest and abdomen. Note that after D reaches zero it does not rise appreciably at any higher frequency so spurious resolution is not present.

In Figure 16-27d is shown a similar set of curves for the same point in the patient but now using an image intensifier as the detector. The MTF of the intensifier, curve A, is not as good as that of the screen-film combination. However, because of the higher sensitivity of the intensifier a shorter exposure time and a smaller focal spot may be used to obtain a fluorographic image. Thus the MTF due to the motion, curve B, is greatly improved and the MTF due to the focal spot, curve C, is significantly improved over those for the screen-film combination. Thus, the resultant MTF, curve D, although it shows roughly the same MTF at a frequency of 1 lp/mm, shows that the intensifier is substantially better than the screen-film combination at frequencies from 1 to 3.5 lp/mm, because motion and focal spot blurring can be minimized.

To design the optimum system it is necessary to know the frequency components of the structures in the patient that need to be visualized. When this information is available, an appropriate choice can be made of focal spot size, time of exposure, and type of receptor. The analysis must also take into account the noise in the system.

16.15   **NOISE AND MOTTLE**

X RAY MOTTLE. We saw in section 16.04 that statistical variation in the number of x ray photons forming each point in the image leads to mottling of the image. When the x ray exposure is very low, for example, when a rare earth screen-film combination is used, this mottle becomes visible to the eye and may affect the ability to see structures that are small or of low contrast. We now calculate the amount of mottle one can expect from a given exposure.

Let us assume that we are dealing with a monochromatic source at 40 keV where the photon fluence per roentgen is 2.17×10^{10} photons/

cm² R (see appendix Table A-2b). Imagine now that the minimum area the radiologist can resolve is .03 cm × .03 cm. After an exposure of 0.1 mR, the number of photons that have passed through this area is:

$$2.17 \times 10^{10} \frac{\text{photons}}{\text{cm}^2 \, \text{R}} \times 9 \times 10^{-4} \, \text{cm}^2 \times 10^{-4} \, \text{R} = 1950$$

If we assume 50% of these are absorbed, then the number that contribute to the image is 975. The statistical fluctuation in this number is $\sqrt{975}$ = 31, and there will be about 3% mottle. If the gamma of the film is 3.0, there will be a 9% variation in the light reaching the eye from spot to spot on the film. This can certainly prove distracting to the radiologist. These ideas are illustrated in Figure 16-28, where enlarged photographs of two films are shown after exposures of 0.07 and 0.35 mR. The films were arranged to have nearly the same density by using a fast screen for radiograph a and a much slower screen for radiograph b. The picture with the small exposure shows considerable mottle.

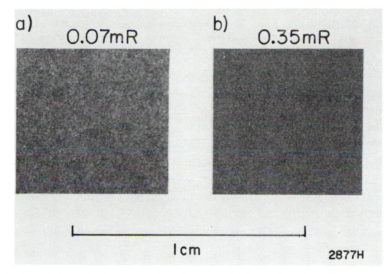

Figure 16-28. Enlarged photographs of exposed film selected to illustrate mottle. (a) Kodak XR film exposed to 0.07 mR with Agfa MR-800 screen. (b) Kodak XR film exposed to .35 mR using Dupont SP screen.

Mottle cannot be completely eliminated. It can be reduced by increasing the number of x ray photons that form the image, by introducing unsharpness in the image receptor and hence blurring the mottle, or by reducing the film contrast and hence making it less visible. Mottle may be rendered invisible by altering the conditions under which the radiologists view the film. For example, if the film is placed far enough from the radiologist's eye, the mottle will disappear.

OTHER SOURCES OF RANDOM NOISE. X ray mottle is just one form of random noise. There are other sources of noise that may affect the image. The film itself may introduce noise due to the finite size of the individual grains of developed silver. This is called film *granularity*. Noise may be introduced by random variations from point to point in the sensitivity of a fluorescent screen; this is called structural noise. In an image intensifier noise may also be caused by random variations in the number of electrons emitted by the photoemissive surface per x ray quantum absorbed in the fluorescent screen. In addition, noise arises in television camera tubes and in electronic circuits. When fluoroscopic images are viewed, the radiologist must contend as well with random variations in *time*, since any given point on the screen will fluctuate in brightness.

The use of the standard deviation gives an incomplete description of image noise. A more complete one is obtained if we describe the noise by its frequency components, that is, we find the Fourier transform of it. It is usual to plot the square of the Fourier transform against frequency, yielding the power spectrum. This is called the Wiener spectrum (D10).

MEASUREMENT OF NOISE. In a radiological system, this is not easy; furthermore, it requires the availability of a good microdensitometer coupled to a computer. The film to be studied is carefully exposed uniformly over an area of some 10 cm^2 and developed. It is then scanned with a microdensitometer having an aperture about 10 μm wide and 0.5 mm high yielding a trace shown in the insert to Figure 16-29. This trace is digitized and stored in the computer. The computer is then programmed to take the Fourier transform of the signal giving the amplitude of the sine waves present in the noise. This scanning procedure is repeated some 10 times and the 10 Fourier transforms are averaged. If enough traces are taken and averaged, a relatively smooth curve of amplitude versus frequency is obtained. The amplitude of the Fourier transform is then squared and plotted against frequency, as illustrated in Figure 16-29.

Wiener spectra often show four rather different regions. The rapid increase in noise at low frequencies (in region A) is due to low frequency variations in the imaging system. These are caused by structural variations in screens and image intensifiers or due to nonuniformity of the x ray beam or film development.

Region B, where the noise is more or less constant, is called "white noise" and is caused by random variations such as x ray quantum mottle or electrical circuit noise. Region C shows a rapid decrease in the power at these particular frequencies caused by the decrease in the transfer function of the imaging system. In other words, the imaging system transmits these frequency components with lower gain.

Finally, region D is again "white noise" of constant power at all frequencies, caused by the microscopic structure of most imaging systems such as the grain in film or screen. Of course, at extremely high frequen-

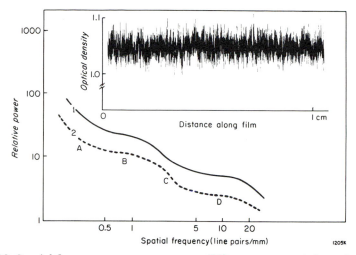

Figure 16-29. Spatial frequency power spectrum (Wiener spectrum) for noise in a radiographic image arising from a screen-film combination. Curve 1—Kodak X-omatic regular screen with XR film with an exposure of ~ 0.35 mR. Curve 2—same screen with XL film at an exposure of 0.7 mR.

cies, even this noise finally disappears since there is no structure in the imaging system capable of giving such frequencies. Figure 16-29 shows two curves using the same screen but different films and exposures. Curve 1 is for a fast high contrast film. The resultant small exposure and the high contrast lead to high noise in the image at all frequencies compared to curve 2, which was obtained using low contrast film with a higher exposure.

The Fourier spectrum is useful since it shows the different frequency components of the noise, giving clues as to how the noise may be reduced. It may also be used in conjunction with the MTF of the imaging system to calculate signal-to-noise ratios at different image planes in the imaging system. In this way the optimization of signal-to-noise ratios in imaging systems may be studied. For a fundamental description of noise, see (D10).

16.16   OPTIMIZATION OF IMAGING SYSTEMS

Oosterkamp (O2) was one of the first to demonstrate quantitatively that the dose to the patient could be reduced and the image quality improved by a careful selection of the x ray beam energy. Villagran (V2) showed experimentally that skin exposure could be reduced by a factor of 2 by use of holmium or tungsten filters, depending on the kV_p used and the thickness of the patient. The selection of more appropriate beam quality has recently been considered theoretically by Motz and Danos (M22). The theory has been complemented by measurements of x ray imaging systems with monochromatic x ray beams in order to provide the fundamental data required to make use of the theory (V11).

The signal-to-noise ratio limits the ability to see a structure in the body. If the signal is hidden in the noise it cannot be seen. Generally it is assumed that a signal-to-noise ratio of 5:1 is required. However, this depends on the size and shape of the structure. Once a satisfactory signal-to-noise ratio is achieved, then the recording medium must be chosen to present the image to the eye in a way that the eye can perceive, i.e. the contrast and density in the image must be appropriate. This may be done in a visual radiographic system by an appropriate choice of screen-film speed, film contrast, and viewing conditions. In a CT scanner it is done by electronic presentation that allows control of contrast and brightness.

Here we will show how the signal-to-noise ratio varies with x ray energy when we image a given structure of the body. The noise is assumed to arise from statistical variations in the number of x ray quanta forming the image. The signal arises from the contrast of the structure relative to its surroundings.

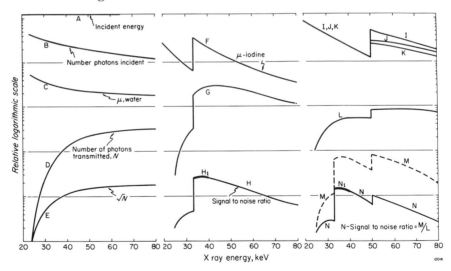

Figure. 16-30. Factors involved in calculating the signal-to-noise ratio when a small concentration of iodine in an artery or kidney is to be imaged.

Figure 16-30 shows the factors that are involved in making the calculation in an example where a low concentration of iodine in an artery or kidney is to be imaged. It is assumed that the energy fluence incident on a 20 cm thick patient at each keV is constant, as illustrated by curve A in Figure 16-30. We have chosen to use a constant energy fluence, since this is perhaps of greatest significance from the point of view of risk. However, the calculation can equally well be done for a constant skin exposure or constant dose to a specific organ. The calculation is first carried out in terms of relative signal and noise levels at each keV to find the relative signal-to-noise ratio. This will tell us the x ray energy to use to obtain the best ratio. The application of scaling factors then allows us to find the incident energy or exposure we must use to obtain a given signal-to-noise ratio. Throughout the calculation we will ignore scattered radiation, although it should be included.

First we calculate the relative noise. To do this we find the number of photons N' incident on the patient by dividing curve A by the photon energy to give curve B. Then we use the mass attenuation coefficient of water, μ_w cm²/g shown in curve C, to calculate the relative number of photons N transmitted through the 20 g/cm² of water at each keV, ($N = N_1 e^{-20\mu_w}$) shown in curve D. We ignore the reduction due to inverse square law since it is the same for each keV. Finally we calculate the relative noise, curve E, by taking the square root of curve D.

Next we calculate the relative signal at each keV. The signal is due to the additional attenuation of a low concentration of iodine present in one area, which is next to an area that contains only water. Curve F is the attenuation coefficient of iodine, μ_i cm²/g. If the amount of iodine is c_i g/cm² the signal is:

$$S = N_1' \left(e^{-20\mu_w} - e^{(-20\mu_w - c_i\mu_i)}\right) = N_1' e^{-20\mu_w} \left(1 - e^{-c_i\mu_i}\right) \approx Nc_i\mu_i \quad (16\text{-}32)$$

The approximation is valid when $c_i\mu_i$ is small compared with 1.0. N is simply the number of photons transmitted through 20 cm of water. Since c_1 is constant, S is proportional to $N\mu_1$, i.e. to the product of the ordinates of curves D and F, yielding curve G.

Finally we divide the relative signal by the relative noise (curve G by curve E) to obtain the signal-to-noise ratio, giving curve H. This is also the product of $\sqrt{N}$ and μ_1 (curve E and curve F). It can be seen that curve H has a flat peak between 33 and 41 keV due to the product of an increasing and a decreasing function, showing that monoenergetic x rays anywhere in this energy band are equally satisfactory to image iodine.

If a spectrum of x rays is used, noise and the signal must be considered separately since signals from x rays at each energy in the spectrum add linearly, while noise adds quadratically.

Energy Required for a Given Signal-to-Noise Ratio

Having established the x ray energy that produces the best signal-to-noise ratio, it is now possible to calculate the minimum energy that must be incident on the patient to produce a given signal-to-noise ratio. Suppose that we wish to image an artery containing 35 mg/ml of iodine and to see a structure that is 1 mm thick over an area of 1 square mm, i.e. 35 × 10^{-4} g/cm² of iodine over 1 mm². We will assume that a signal-to-noise ratio of 5 is necessary to identify this structure. We already know that x rays with energy between 33 and 40 keV are best, so we will redo the calculation at 40 keV using absolute values.

We start by calculating the signal-to-noise ratio for an incident energy of 10^{-7} J/mm^2. Since 1 eV = 1.6×10^{-19} J (Table A-1), a 40 keV quantum has an energy of 6.4×10^{-15} J. Thus 10^{-7} J/mm^2 is carried by 1.56×10^7 quanta per mm^2.

The number of photons transmitted through 20 cm of water is $1.56 \times 10^7 \times 5.2 \times 10^{-3} = 8.11 \times 10^4$ photons/mm^2. The noise ($\sqrt{N}$) will then be 285 photons/mm^2. The signal-to-noise ratio is then $\sqrt{N} \, \mu_1 c_1$ or $285 \times 22.4 \times 35 \times 10^{-4}$, i.e. 22. To meet our criterion of a signal-to-noise ratio of 5:1, we may decrease the incident energy by a factor of $(5/22)^2$ to give 5.2×10^{-9} J/mm^2. This corresponds to an incident exposure of 4 mR (see Table A-2b).

Thus, to identify the structure we must use at least 5.2×10^{-3} J/m^2, or 4 mR, and an x ray energy of 40 keV. It is interesting to note that for the identification of such a structure it is common radiographic practice to use an exposure incident on the patient of 400 mR, indicating that there is much room for the reduction of exposures below those currently used for high speed screen-film combinations. The reductions of up to 8 times achieved with image intensified fluorography go part of the way, but there is clearly room for further reduction.

Sensitivity of Image Sensor

The above calculation of signal-to-noise ratio assumes that all x rays will be detected with equal efficiency. This is, of course, not so. Curve H must now be corrected for the variation with keV in sensitivity of the image sensor. The sensitivity has been calculated by Swank (S26) and has been measured by Vyborny (V11). Figure 16-30 shows the data due to Swank. Curve I is the quantum efficiency for a screen containing 50 mg/cm^2 of Gd_2O_2S. This efficiency is the fraction of incident photons absorbed in the screen. It is found from the attenuation coefficient for Gd_2O_2S or may be measured with monochromatic x rays. The efficiency increases about 5 times at the K-absorption edge for gadolinium, but above the K edge the fate of the fluorescent radiation must be considered.

Above the K-edge, some of the energy of the absorbed x rays will be lost from the screen through K-fluorescence. The pulses of light that come from the absorption of an x ray will now be of two sizes, one corresponding to the total energy of the x ray when the K-fluorescence is reabsorbed in the screen, and the other corresponding to the absorption of the energy of the x ray but not the K-fluorescence. The two sizes of light pulse resulting from similar absorption events alters the statistics, and the variation is no longer as the square root of the number of absorbed quanta. Swank has discussed the effect of this on the noise and has calculated an equivalent coefficient of absorption shown in curve J. If this coefficient is used to calculate the number of x rays absorbed from the number incident on the screen, then the square root of this number correctly predicts the noise in the image. In a similar way, curve K shows the efficiency for the deposition of energy in the screen, and hence for the blackening of the film. It is the coefficient that describes the relative sensitivity of the screens at each keV in order to produce the same optical density on the film.

To find the noise in the image produced by the screens, the relative noise in the x ray beam incident on the screen, curve E, must be multiplied by the square root of curve J. This new relative noise curve is shown as curve L. To find the signal from the screen, we multiply curve G by curve K yielding curve M. Dividing M by L, the relative signal-to-noise ratio for the screen image is found and is seen in curve N. It is a complicated curve involving discontinuities at the K edges of iodine and gadolinium. It indicates that a Gd_2O_2S screen should be used with a narrow band of x ray energies, region N_1, just above the K edge of iodine. Since this is not easy to achieve, this screen may not be optimum for imaging organs containing small amounts of iodine. It would be better to use a screen with an absorption edge closer to that of iodine, such as $BaSrSO_4$, or better still CsI. It is left to the reader to show that a screen of 100 mgm/cm^2 of CsI (220 μm thick) is an excellent absorber for imaging low contrasts of iodine.

CHOICE OF kV_p AND FILTER. It is usually supposed that the exposure to a patient is decreased by increasing the kV_p and filtration. This is too simplistic a point of view and the above calculations show that it may be better to use a lower kV_p, a high atomic number filter such as holmium or gadolinium to produce a narrow x ray spectrum, and an imaging system that will properly absorb the beam and present the image at an appropriate density and contrast. More research on this problem will undoubtedly produce significant improvements in image quality with reduction in patient exposures perhaps by a factor of 10.

MEASUREMENTS WITH MONOENERGETIC X RAYS. In order to check the validity of the above theoretical analysis, and to find the curves I, J, and K for typical screens and intensifiers whose composition is not known, it is necessary to make measurements of the performance of imaging systems with monoenergetic x rays. The method of obtaining beams of x rays that are 90 to 95% monoenergetic has been discussed by Hoffman (H20). The method is illustrated in Figure 16-31. A typical spectrum obtained in our laboratory is shown. An x ray tube operated at a high kV_p and tube current produces an intense fluence, which is used to bombard a sheet of high atomic number material. The sheet emits Kα and Kβ fluorescence together with scattered x rays of a broad range of energies. Kβ radiation and the scattered x rays are largely absorbed by the filter, which is chosen to have an absorption edge just above the Kα fluorescence, leaving a relatively pure Kα fluorescence that can be used for measuring the performance of image sensors or of the total imaging system. The use of a variety of high atomic number elements with appropriate filters enables one to produce "monoenergetic" x rays in the range 8 to 87 keV.

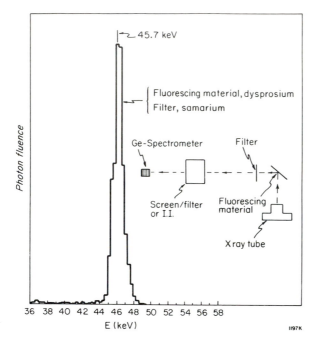

Figure 16-31. Diagram to illustrate how a beam of essentially monochromatic x rays can be isolated from a spectrum using the appropriate fluorescing material and the proper filter.

16.17   ELECTROSTATIC IMAGING

For over 25 years there has been some interest in applying Xerox® techniques to diagnostic radiology. In this technique the film receptor is replaced by a photoconducting selenium plate as illustrated in Figure 16-32. The plate is first charged to about 1500 volts, usually in a positive direction, by moving a fine highly charged wire over its surface so that a corona discharge takes place in the space between the wire and the plate. The selenium plate is a good insulator and will maintain its charge until it is exposed to either light or x rays, which render it partially conducting. The charged selenium plate is loaded into a light-tight cassette and exposed to the x ray beam as illustrated in Figure 16-32b. Where x rays hit the plate the resulting photoconduction discharges the positively charged surface, leaving an image in the form of an invisible charge pattern.

The exposed plate is then transferred to a light-tight box where it is developed by exposure to a cloud of charged particles (often referred to as *toner* particles). The toner particles are charged by friction when they are ejected through a fine nozzle in a stream of air (as illustrated in Fig. 16-32c). The charged toner particles are deposited on the electrostatic image, making it visible. In the Xerox system the blue toner particles are transferred from the selenium plate onto a sheet of special paper and fused into it (as illustrated in Fig. 16-32d and e). The radiologist is thus presented with a sheet of paper with the image in the form of imbedded blue power on it. An alternative way to obtain the visible image is to photograph the powdered Xerox plate using side lighting (as illustrated in Fig. 16-32f). Figure 16-33 shows an image of the breast taken in this way. In the Xerox system this whole process is essentially automatic and is performed in a charging cabinet and a reading cabinet, which may be obtained from the Xerox Corporation. Images may be formed by selecting either positively or negatively charged toner particles using either positively or negatively charged plates.

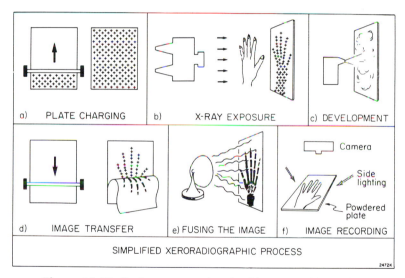

Figure 16-32. Basic processes involved in xeroradiography.

The Xerox system as applied to radiology is called xeroradiography and has been available for many years, but it did not become popular until the early 1970s when Dr. John Wolfe (W10, W11) in collaboration with Xerox Corporation perfected the system and showed that it was an excellent way to radiograph the breast because of the great detail that could be made visible. A little later Boag and collaborators (B30, B31, J15) also investigated the basic problems of xeroradiography and with Johns and his group developed a new electrostatic method for taking pictures called ionography (J16, J17, J18, P15, P16, P17, F6, F7, F8). Concurrently, Xonics developed an almost identical system of electrostatic imaging called electron radiography (P18, S27, S28). In this section we will limit our discussion to the important basic ideas and in particular to the advantages and disadvantages of electrostatic methods of imaging.

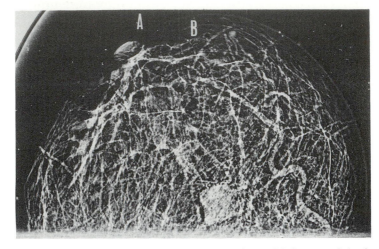

Figure 16-33. Photograph of a powdered selenium plate with image of the breast, courtesy of Boag (B31).

EDGE CONTRAST. The great detail that may be achieved using xeroradiographic techniques is illustrated in Figure 16-33, which shows a photograph of the powder pattern resulting from a xeroradiograph of the breast obtained by Boag (B31). The remarkable detail of this picture is due to edge contrast, which arises from the powder cloud development. At the boundaries between two areas of slightly different exposure, a powder line is drawn making the boundary stand out. For example, point A is just outside the breast, while point B is just inside. These appear to have about the same density while a powder line appears at the boundary between them. Similar powder lines are drawn around each of the internal structures of the breast, leading to the great detail made visible. The student should realize that the system is very nonlinear and includes many artifacts. For example, the density at point B appears the same as A, although in fact the x ray fluence reaching B is considerably less than that reaching A due to the attenuation of several cm of breast tissue. Thus, in the Xerox method the powder density at any point Q is *not* so much determined by the x ray fluence at Q as it is by the small spatial variations of the exposure over small distances near the point Q.

Edge contrast arises from the nature of the electrostatic lines of force near a charge discontinuity. The insert to Figure 16-34 shows a thin block of insulating material in contact with a grounded conductor. The insulator is uniformly charged positively to the right of F_1. These charges will induce negative charges in the grounded conductor. Most of the lines of force from the positive charges will be directed downward into the insulator to terminate on the negative charges on the grounded conductor. However, at the edge of the charge pattern the lines of force will bulge upward and to the left as indicated. These distorted lines of force are called the fringing field.

Figure 16-34. The insert shows the nature of the fringing field at the edges of a charge pattern. The main diagram shows the trajectories of charged toner particles liberated at the top of the diagram and directed by an electric field towards the semiinfinite uniform charged pattern to the right of A. The parameters of the calculations were toner diameter 5 μm; toner charge -8×10^{-17} C per particle; viscosity of air 1.83×10^{-4} poise; driving uniform field 500 V/cm downward; surface charge density 1.0 nC/cm^2; dielectric constant of insulator 3.3. Note the vertical and horizontal distance scales are different.

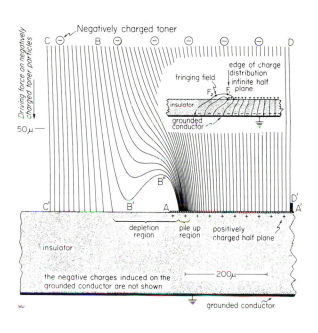

Imagine now that a cloud of negatively charged toner particles were liberated at the top of Figure 16-34 and were directed downwards towards the insulator by a suitable uniform electric field. The surface of the insulator is assumed to be uniformly charged over half of an infinite plane to the right of A. These charges and the induced charges on the grounded conductor will create a complex electric field above the plane C'AA' and will determine the trajectory of the powder particles. Taking into account the viscosity of the air and the charge and size of the toner particles and using the method of images, Plewes (J18) determined the trajectory of the particles (shown in Fig. 16-34). A toner particle starting at B will move along the path BB'B'' to end on the charge pattern just to the right of A. This complex trajectory arises because of the fringing field at the edge of the charge pattern. Note the main distortion in the trajectories occurs in the region 10 to 20 μm above the pattern in a region about 100 μm wide. These distorted trajectories give rise to a depletion region where no powder particles can be deposited and a pile up region just to the right of A, where the particles that should have been deposited in the depletion region are concentrated. Trajectories such as CC' and DD', remote from the charged edge, are almost identical so that as much powder falls on the uncharged region of the plate on the left as on the charged region on the right. Thus, in the powdering process we envisage toner particles falling uniformly towards the charge pattern until they reach a plane about 20 μm above it, at which point they are swept to the left or right to deposit powder just inside each charge discontinuity, thus outlining "edges" in the picture.

IONOGRAPHY. The edge contrast achievable with xeroradiography is certainly a major advantage for certain types of examinations. Unfortunately, Xerox is some 20 times less sensitive than the best screen-film techniques and for this reason its use has been restricted to examinations of the extremities and the breast. During the 1970s a number of people attempted to find ways to make electrostatic imaging more sensitive. One method developed by Boag and Johns, and referred to as ionography, is illustrated in Figure 16-35. The ionography chamber consists of two spherical electrodes whose common center of curvature is the focal spot of the x ray tube. The electrodes are 1 to 5 cm apart and the gap between them is filled with a high atomic number gas such as xenon under a pressure of 5 to 10 atmospheres. A clean insulating foil, on which the image is to be recorded, is placed just under the upper electrode and is held at ground potential, while the lower electrode of the chamber is held at a positive potential of some 10,000 volts. Imagine now a pencil of x rays passing through the object being radiographed along the line FP''. This will give rise to a number of interactions with the gas between P' and P'', and the ejection of high energy electrons in all directions about P'P''. Since the gas is at high pressure and is dense, these electrons will travel only a fraction of a mm from this line. Because of the spherical electrodes the electric lines of force in the chamber are in the same direction as the x ray beam so the high voltage on the lower electrode will drive the positive ions along P''P' to deposit them in circular region on the foil about P'. After the charges are deposited on the foil, the chamber is opened and the charge pattern made visible by powder cloud development. The foil itself with the deposited toner particles becomes the record.

The resolution of the system depends upon the energy of the x ray photons. The higher their energy the greater the range of the electrons set in motion and hence the greater the smearing of the charge pattern on the foil. In principle, either positive or negative ions could be collected. However, it is usually advantageous to collect the heavier positive ions rather than the electrons since the former suffer much less diffusion during the collection process. The higher the pressure of the gas the smaller the range of the electrons set in motion and hence the greater the resolution. The front electrode should be thin and made of low atomic number material in order to minimize the attenuation of the x ray beam in entering the chamber; at the same time it must be strong enough to withstand the forces generated by the high pressure gas. For a 30 cm circular chamber at 5 atmospheres, the front electrode must withstand forces of about 8000 newtons. A curved electrode made of carbon fibers set in resin is one way to achieve strength and minimize attenuation.

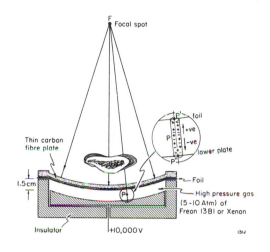

Figure 16-35. Schematic diagram of ionography chamber.

With care, good pictures with resolutions of 5 to 10 lp/mm can be achieved by ionography. Unfortunately, there are a number of difficult engineering problems that must be solved before the system could come into routine use. To create a practical system the following steps would have to be automated: clean the foil, open the chamber, introduce the foil, close the chamber, evacuate the chamber, pressurize the chamber with xenon or some other suitable gas such as Freon®, position the chamber with the center of curvature of the electrodes at the focal spot, turn on the high voltage, expose the chamber to x rays, remove the high voltage, remove the xenon and store it, bring the chamber to atmospheric pressure, open the chamber and remove the charged foil in a dust free environment, powder, and fix the foil. Certainly, with effort all these steps could be automated, but it is a very complex procedure compared with taking a picture with a film-screen combination.

Detailed investigations of the powder cloud method (P15, P16, P17) show that the edge contrast in the image is maximum for short powdering times but gradually decreases as powdering continues and will eventually disappear completely when the charges on the foil are completely neutralized by the powder. The sensitivity of the system thus increases with increase in powdering time. The operator has to balance the advantage of edge contrast against the disadvantage of low sensitivity and hence large exposures. Powder cloud development as used by Xerox employs short development times and is generally far short of completion. Development can also be achieved by liquid toner, which consists of a suspension of charged insulating "spheres" in an insulating liquid. The foil is developed by passing the charged foil through the liquid toner. One passage through the liquid usually gives close to complete development and leads to images with very little edge contrast. Xonics has developed a system called *electron radiography* (XERG), which is essentially the same as ionography. Their system uses liquid toner and produces images with very little edge contrast. They claim sensitivities slightly greater than that achievable with film-screen combinations. At the time of writing, the Xonics system has had limited success in the marketplace. It is partially automated and units are available for breast and lung examinations. The fact that full-sized pictures can be taken on a plastic foil may be a major advantage in an era when films are becoming prohibitively expensive due to their silver content. We have shown (F7) that methods can be designed to get several pictures with different edge contrast from one exposure. There are also ways to read the image on the foil from outside the chamber without ever opening the chamber to the atmosphere. Further, Fenster (F8) has also shown how the high pressure gas can be replaced by an insulating liquid. Some of these ideas may lead to practical imaging methods in radiology.

16.18   TOMOGRAPHY AND STEREORADIOGRAPHY

In an ordinary x ray examination all the structures of the part being examined are superimposed on the radiograph. The multiplicity of the images may at times make it very difficult to interpret the film. The region of interest may be separated from the surrounding structures using body section radiography (illustrated in Fig. 16-36A). During the exposure, the x ray source is moved in one direction from S_1 to S_2 while the film is moved in the opposite direction from P_1 to P_2 at a speed such that a line joining the center of the film to the source passes through P, the center of the region of interest within the patient. From the diagram, it is clear that the image of P will appear at P_1, the center of the film for all positions of the film. On the other hand, structures in some other plane such as Q will produce a blurred image extending from Q_1 near one end of the film to Q_2 at the other end. The greater the distance, or angle of movement of the x ray tube, the narrower is the slice that is in focus and the greater is the blurring of overlying structures. The coupling between the film and the tube is maintained with a rigid rod that is pivoted at a point in the plane of interest. By moving the pivot point to different levels within the patient, a whole series of planes can be radiographed in turn.

Linear motion of the x ray tube and film produces only partial blurring of regions that are out of the focal plane (as illustrated in Fig. 16-36b). A line in the object parallel to the direction of motion is not defocused (as seen in b). For circular motion there is blurring for all lines, but sharp edges appear in the image c. A hypocycloidal or spiral motion gives blurring for all directions in the object and no sharp edges (as seen in d). Most modern tomographs supply all these motions, and the choice of the optimum motion depends upon the study being made.

Stereoradiography

This is used to help visualize x ray images in three dimensions. The patient is held immobilized while two x ray films are taken with a tube shift between exposures. The films are then placed in front of two viewing boxes and arranged so that the right eye sees the film taken with the source in the right-hand position while the left eye sees the other. The films are observed through mirrors adjusted so that the images are superimposed, and the radiologist sees the image in three dimensions. In order to get a proper three-dimensional effect, the angle subtended by the two eyes at the film viewing distance should be equal to the angle subtended by the two positions of the x ray tube at the target-film distance. The relation between these distances may be stated thus:

$$\frac{\text{tube shift}}{\text{target film distance}} = \frac{\text{interpupillary distance}}{\text{viewing distance}} \quad (16\text{-}33)$$

The common viewing distance is about 65 cm, while the average interpupillary distance is 6.5 cm. Hence, the correct tube shift is 1/10 the target film distance.

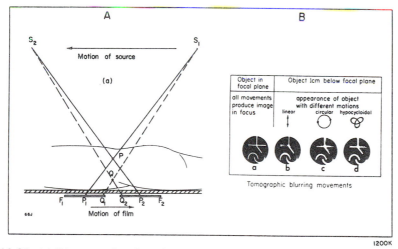

Figure 16-36. (a) Diagram showing the principle of body section radiography. (b) Diagram to illustrate the effects of tomographic motions. The test object in the plane is sharply reproduced in a. The appearance of the same object 1 cm below the plane is shown in b, c, and d for three types of motions. The hypocycloidal motion produces equal blurring in all directions.

Foreign Body Localization

A single radiograph gives no information concerning the relative depths of the various structures. This information is obtained routinely in diagnostic radiology by fluoroscopy from two or more different directions and by obtaining spot films at suitable angles. Such films may be used to guide the surgeon to the foreign object by showing its relationship to significant anatomical structures. Often stereoradiographs are used for the same purpose.

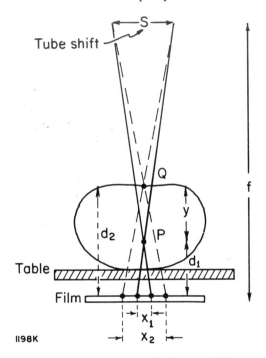

Figure 16-37. Diagram to illustrate the tube shift method to localize a foreign body.

For locating the relative positions of radioactive needles in an implant, two radiographs may be taken exactly at right angles (as described in Chapter 13) or by using the tube shift method illustrated in Figure 16-37. Suppose the object P to be located is at a distance y from the upper surface of the phantom. To determine this distance a radiopaque object such as a coin is placed on the surface of the patient at Q and a double exposure is made with the source shifted a known distance, S, between exposures. The film will show two images for the object at P and two for the object at Q. Suppose the separation in these images is x_1 and x_2. From similar triangles it can be seen that:

$$\frac{x_1}{S} = \frac{d_1}{f - d_1}$$ which may be solved for d_1 to yield $d_1 = \frac{x_1}{x_1 + S} \cdot f$

This expression gives the distance d_1 of the unknown object from the film. If, in addition, the tabletop-to-film distance is known, then the position of the object is determined. When, however, the tabletop-to-film distance is not precisely known, the quantity d_2 is determined from the image shift x_2 for the object at Q as follows:

$$d_2 = \frac{x_2}{x_2 + S} \cdot f$$

and the position of the unknown object calculated from

$$y = d_2 - d_1 = f\left[\frac{x_2}{x_2 + S} - \frac{x_1}{x_1 + S}\right] \qquad (16\text{-}34)$$

All the quantities in equation 16-34 are determined if the tube shift S is known and x_1 and x_2 are the two image shifts that may be measured on the film. This method is capable of considerable precision.

16.19   **CT SCANNING**

INTRODUCTION. The development of computed tomographic scanners has been one of the most explosive phenomena in modern medicine. Since the original invention by Hounsfield (H21) in 1973, many companies have become involved in making machines with ever-increasing sophistication. The first machine was designed to study the head, and it achieved instant clinical success in dealing with neurological problems. Later models were developed to scan any part of the body, enabling the radiologist to visualize organs in cross section and look at such sections on a television screen under different conditions of contrast. Many radiologists consider CT scanning to be the most important development in radiology since the discovery of x rays by Roentgen in 1895. Hounsfield has received many honors for his invention, culminating in the Nobel Prize in Medicine in 1979. This prize was shared with Cormack, who many years ago developed a mathematical method (C15) to deal with the problems of reconstruction that arise in CT scanning.

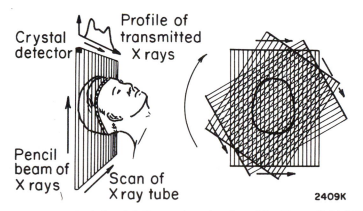

Figure 16-38. Principle of CT scanning developed by Hounsfield (H21).

Basic Concepts. The basic idea of CT scanning is illustrated in Figure 16-38. An x ray tube emitting a pencillike beam is coupled to a radiation detector. The two are moved together on a carriage so that a plane in the head is scanned by a series of parallel rays as the translation takes place. For each ray the fraction of the radiation transmitted is measured and stored in a computer.

In Hounsfield's original scanner 160 measurements of the transmission were made during one translation. The source detector carriage was then rotated by 1° to a new angle and the procedure repeated 180 times. To see how this data can be used to create a CT picture, consider Figure 16-39, which shows a cross-sectional view of the head superimposed upon a rectangular matrix, which for clarity in presentation has been made very coarse. The elements of the matrix are called pixels (picture elements) and our problem is to determine the attenuation coefficient of the head in each picture element and then present these for viewing on a television monitor. Let $\mu(x,y)$ be the average attenuation coefficient of the tissues in the pixel (x,y) for the radiation emitted by the x ray source. The radiation transmitted, I_t, is related to the incident radiation, I_0, by:

$$I_t = I_0 \, e^{-\Sigma \, \mu(x,y) \cdot \Delta l(x,y)} \qquad (16\text{-}35a)$$

where $\Delta l(x,y)$ is the path length through the pixel (x,y) and the summation is carried out along SD from A to B. For the ray shown, 6 pixels $\left[(1,1), (2,1), (3,2), (4,2), (4,3), \text{and } (5,3)\right]$ are involved. If we take the natural logarithm of both sides of equation 16-35a and rearrange we obtain:

$$\ln(I_0/I) = \Sigma \, \mu(x,y) \, \Delta l(x,y) \qquad (16\text{-}35b)$$

The elements of length, $\Delta l(x,y)$, are determined by the geometry of the system and hence can be stored in the computer. The equation thus involves the measured value $\ln(I_0/I)$, 6 length factors, and 6 unknown values for μ.

The ray SD is a typical ray that can be described by the parameter p and the angle θ. In Hounsfield's scanner, p was incremented 160 times for each angle, θ, and θ was incremented by 1° from 0 to 180° to yield $N_T = 160 \times 180 = 28{,}800$ transmission measurements and 28,800 linear equations like equation 16-35b. His picture was reconstructed over a square area containing $N_p = 80 \times 80 = 6400$ pixels. Since N_p is smaller than N_T a solution is possible. Although in principle these equations could be solved by standard matrix inversion techniques, this is impractical because of the large number of unknowns and the fact that the transmission measurements all contain statistical errors making the equations inconsistent. Techniques for the solution of these equations or *reconstruction* will be discussed later. The reconstruction process creates

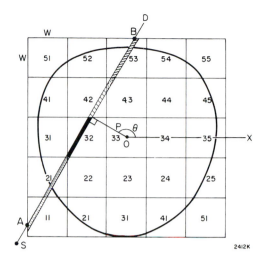

Figure 16-39. Schematic representation of pixels with a cross section of the head superimposed. A typical ray from the source S to the detector D is shown. It can be represented by the parameter p and the angle θ. The path length through each of the pixels is illustrated.

an image that is a map of the x ray attenuation coefficients of the tissue in the plane under examination.

CT NUMBER. Rather than specify the attenuation coefficients, which are determined by the reconstruction procedure, a related quantity the CT number (CTN) is defined by:

$$CTN = \frac{\mu - \mu_w}{\mu_w} \times 1000 \qquad (16\text{-}36)$$

where μ is the attenuation coefficient of the tissue at the pixel position and μ_w is the coefficient for water. When $\mu = \mu_w$ the CT number is zero. On this scale air with negligible attenuation has a CT number of -1000 and dense bone about $+1000$. Most tissues lie in the range -100 to $+100$ with fat slightly negative and muscle slightly positive.

DISPLAY. The image is viewed on a television monitor either as shades of grey or in color. The viewing scale is set by two controls. The LEVEL control selects the CT number corresponding to the middle grey value. This positions the grey scale in the appropriate range of tissue densities of interest. The WINDOW control may then be used to set the slope of the contrast scale. With these two controls the operator can instantly change the display. Increasing the window increases latitude but lowers contrast. Reducing the window too far causes the noise in the image to be emphasized.

Images can be stored permanently on disk or tape in digital form or may be photographed from the television monitor. Multiformat cameras capable of recording 1 to 16 images on a single-emulsion film have been developed for CT.

GENERATIONS OF SCANNERS. Figure 16-40 shows the four generations of scanners that have been developed. Hounsfield's original scanner (Fig. 16-40a) measured 180 projections at 1° intervals with each projection containing 160 points. The reconstructed image was displayed on an 80 × 80 matrix with pixels of about 3 mm on a side. Since the detector viewed an irradiated slice of tissue about 15 mm thick, the attenuation coefficient displayed actually corresponded to volume elements or *voxels* of dimensions 3 × 3 × 15 mm. This machine suffered from two important limitations: long scan times and poor spatial resolution. The scan times were long (about 4 minutes per slice) because a sufficient number of x ray photons needed to be counted in each of the 28,800 measurements to reduce the quantum noise to acceptable levels. Even though the tube was running at maximum output, most of the x rays emitted were rejected by the pencil-beam collimators. This set limits on the shortest scan time that would provide good images. A stationary anode x ray tube was required because a rotating-anode tube that could give higher x ray output would not stand up to the forces imposed on the rotor and bearings by the translate-rotate motion. Machines with such long scan times were only practical for the head, where motion was not a major difficulty.

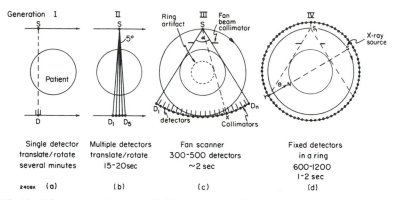

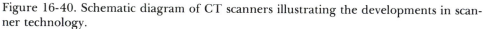

Figure 16-40. Schematic diagram of CT scanners illustrating the developments in scanner technology.

These problems were overcome in part by the introduction of the so-called second generation scanners. These were similar in design to the original machines but used multiple detectors arranged as in Figure 16-40b. The x ray beam was collimated into a narrow fan providing more efficient use of the x ray output and allowing multiple measurements to be made simultaneously.

To illustrate the principle, five detectors are shown in the diagram. After one translation the system can be rotated five degrees instead of one degree, thus yielding a system five times as fast as the original. Scanners with some 40 to 60 detectors, which could do scans in 15 to 20 seconds, soon came on the market. These were still not nearly fast enough to "stop" body motion. Scan speed was still limited by the mechanical constraints of the translate-rotate motion.

The third generation scanner depicted in Figure 16-40c dispensed with translation by collimating the x rays to a wide fan beam, irradiating the entire slice of the patient and using an array of many detectors arranged on an arc that rotates with the x ray source about the patient. Many transmission measurements are made at each angular increment of the x ray source.

The stationary-detector scanner or fourth generation machine eliminated detector motion entirely. Here the detectors are fixed in a large ring surrounding the patient, as in Figure 16-40d, and only the x ray tube rotates about the patient.

Both third and fourth generation scanners can obtain scans in as little as 1 or 2 seconds, although longer scans are frequently used. The greater efficiency of x ray utilization in the fan beam plus the fact that the simpler motion allows rotating anode x ray tubes to be used permits not only fast high quality CT scans of the head but also of the rest of the body, since motion of all but the heart can be controlled over a few seconds. Also, the spatial resolution, which is determined primarily by the number of ray measurements made, can be improved in fast third and fourth generation machines since it is now practical to make many ray measurements quickly. In modern CT machines 5×10^5 or more measurements are made for each slice and the slices can be as thin as 2 mm.

In order to decrease scan times further to "stop" heart motion it is necessary to avoid movement of source or detectors or to use many x ray sources. In 1980 the development of such machines is at the experimental stage.

DETECTORS. Hounsfield's original scanner used one sodium iodide detector coupled to a photomultiplier, as illustrated in Figure 16-41a. The sodium iodide crystal has a rather long decay time and has been replaced in many scanners by crystals of CsI or bismuth germinate. The main disadvantage of these detectors is the expensive photomultiplier and the fact that to date they have not been made smaller than about 1 cm in diameter. In the fan or ring system the detectors must be 2 to 5 mm wide to yield high resolution and must be packed closely together. The crystals can be packed in this way, but the photomultipliers, because of their size, cannot, so light pipes are required to carry the light from the phosphor to the photomultipliers. This certainly complicates the device.

Another type of detector (Y2) is illustrated in Figure 16-41b. It consists of a fan array of high pressure xenon ion chambers about 20 cm long and 1 cm high. Each ion chamber consists of a plane collecting electrode between two tantalum or tungsten plates 2 to 5 mm apart filled with xenon at 5–30 atmospheres. Such a chamber absorbs some 70% of the radiation and produces a current that can be amplified and fed to the computer where the signal is digitized and stored.

Figure 16-41c shows another type of detector consisting of a fluorescing crystal in contact with a photodiode. The x rays are absorbed in the crystal producing light, which in turn produces a current in the diode. The current is amplified, digitized, and fed to the computer. It is clear that a company which can produce a simple, cheap detector of small dimensions will have a major advantage, especially in generation IV scanners, which need more than 1000 detectors for the best image quality. The detectors should have rapid response, be stable, and allow one to make a radiation measurement to a precision of 1/10 of 1% in a few milliseconds—not an easy task. Since the detector array is a major part of the cost of a CT scanner, we can expect development of better and cheaper detectors.

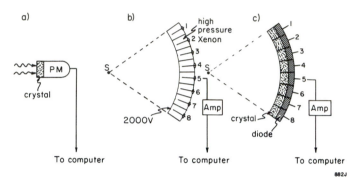

Figure 16-41. (a) Crystal-photomultiplier detector, (b) high pressure xenon detector, (c) crystal diode array.

RING ARTIFACT. In the early days of the fan scanner, images were often troubled by spurious ring artifacts concentric with the center. Imagine a bad detector at position x in Figure 16-40c. In the fan geometry this bad detector will in turn sample rays tangent to the dotted circle. If the bad detector reads too low, then all pixels on the dotted circle will be looked at in turn by this bad detector and so be displayed with too high a density, and a ring will appear. To overcome this problem properly, the detector should be replaced; however, when one realizes there might be 1 or 2 bad detectors in 500 good ones, the replacement of the whole system for 1 bad detector is an impractical solution. In commercial scanners of this type ring artifacts are usually removed by computer programs. The computer could do this by first locating any rings concentric with the center of rotation, thus locating the bad detector(s). For each bad detector the reading from it could be replaced by the average of the readings from the two adjacent detectors. This procedure would remove the ring and in its place introduce some loss in detail in the ring region. In type IV scanners, each detector in the ring eventually samples the radiation through every part of the patient so the system is much less sensitive to the presence of a bad detector.

CALIBRATION OF DETECTORS. The large number of detectors used in a scanner cannot be mass produced to have identical sensitivities. To overcome this they are exposed with no patient in the beam and the readings recorded by the computer, which then determines a calibration factor for each. This procedure is easily carried out in type IV scanners by making the beam wider than the patient so that during one complete rotation every detector will see the source *directly* at least twice—thus allowing for a calibration before and after each scan. In type III scanners calibration must be made before or after the patient is removed from the scanner.

SCATTERED RADIATION. In type III and IV scanners the patient is irradiated by a fan, which will give rise to scattered radiation from the patient to the detectors. In type III such radiation can be almost completely eliminated by collimators, as illustrated in Figure 16-40c. There is no simple way to remove scattered radiation in IV since each detector "looks" at the source at a different angle as the rotation takes place. The normal to the front surface of detector Y is YN. This normal points directly at the x ray source when it is at S but at an angle θ when the source is at S'. This means that there will be more scattered radiation in type IV scanners, but the significance of this for image quality is not yet determined.

X RAY TUBE. In a CT scanner most of the x rays generated in the tube are absorbed in the collimator, allowing the escape of a thin fan of radiation. All rotating anode tubes will easily handle one scan, but in an x ray examination one often requires 20 such scans in rapid sequence on the same patient. Before such a series can be completed the heat loading of the tube may well be beyond design limits and the technician is forced to wait and allow the anode to cool. Many companies are working on the design of high heat capacity x ray tubes for CT application.

PROPERTIES OF THE CT IMAGE. There are several characteristics of CT imaging that distinguish CT from conventional radiological imaging and make it so useful.

1. The CT image is truly tomographic. Only a single slice of the body is irradiated and imaged. Unlike radiography, there is no superposition of unwanted detail from other slices to reduce image contrast and confuse the image as occurs in conventional tomography where the out of slice information is blurred but not removed.

2. Due to the collimation of the radiation to a thin slice both on the source and detector side of the patient, scattered radiation that normally impairs contrast is greatly reduced.

3. Instead of a film-screen combination, a sensitive electronic x ray detector is used. The detector absorbs the x rays efficiently and also can operate with great precision over an extremely wide range of x ray intensity.

4. The image is stored in digital form in a computer with high preci-

sion and is displayed on a television monitor. Viewing contrast can be adjusted to optimize the visualization of clinical detail. One x ray exposure provides an image that can be processed in several ways to extract the maximum diagnostic information from the scan.

5. The image is kept in digital form allowing great potential for the extraction of quantitative information from the scans.

Reconstruction

We have indicated previously that the values of μ for each pixel can in principle be reconstructed from a set of linear equations, but direct solution of this set of equations is impractical. For this reason special algorithms have been developed for CT reconstruction (G15), the most popular of which is the filtered backprojection method. This consists of two steps: convolution followed by back projection.

BACKPROJECTION. Suppose the object to be scanned (Fig. 16-42a) is a cylindrical rod of diameter a_0 and density 1.0 situated in air. Imagine this object being scanned by a vertical pencil of x rays that translates from X to X', and the observer takes measurements spaced a_0 apart. If the object is centered properly, all readings of the transmission will be I_0 except the reading obtained when the beam passes through the center of the object, where we will assume that $\ln(I_0/I) = h$. The profile obtained is thus a delta function of width a_0 and height h. Profiles at any other angle such as θ_n will be identical.

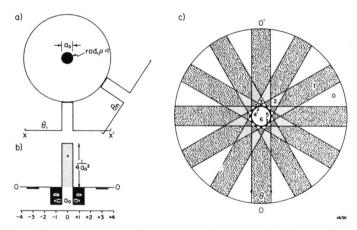

Figure 16-42. (a) Transmission profiles at θ_1 and θ_n for a rod of density 1.0 and diameter a_0 in air. (b) Ramachandran filter function. (c) Back projection of a for $\theta = 0, 30, 60, 90, 120,$ and 150 degrees giving a starlike pattern.

Reconstruction requires that an image of the rod be created at the center of the circle of reconstruction. In Figure 16-42c we have shown the result of simply smearing the projections back along the direction in which they were measured, i.e. backprojection. From the projection at

θ_1 we will, therefore, place a value h in all pixels along the line OO' in the reconstruction circles. Repeating this procedure at all projection angles, we see that the values reinforce at the position of the rod giving a value hN_p where N_p is the number of projections. Our reconstruction is not correct since nonzero values have been placed in the image in regions occupied by air. The result when many projections are taken is that instead of a circle the image of the rod is a star-shaped pattern as illustrated in Figure 16-42c, which shows regions where 6, 5, 4, 3, 2, 1, and 0 beams overlap.

CONVOLUTION. It is apparent that backprojection of the projections can never give a proper solution to the problem. It has been shown by Ramachandran (R13) that if the projections are modified appropriately *before* backprojection then an accurate reconstruction can be achieved. Clearly, negative values must be introduced into the projections so that when backprojection is performed the negative values cancel contributions to the image except at the appropriate locations, e.g. that of the rod in Figure 16-42c. The convolution function, C, that has proved most useful is depicted in Figure 16-42b. It has a positive value at its center and negative or zero values elsewhere:

$$C = \frac{1}{4a_0^2} \text{ for } k = 0$$

$$C = \frac{-1}{\pi^2 a_0^2 k^2} \text{ for } k = \pm 1, \pm 3, \text{ etc.} \qquad (16\text{-}37)$$

$$C = 0 \text{ for } k = \pm 2, \pm 4 \ldots$$

This convolution function is represented in Figure 16-42b. The student may show that if we multiply the profile of Figure 16-42a by the filter function and then backproject, a much improved reconstruction is achieved.

Convolution is a more complex procedure than was implied in the last paragraph. To illustrate this consider the first panel of Figure 16-43 where we show the profile $\ln(I_0/I)$ measured on an elliptical phantom filled with water. The ordinates 1 to 7 are a few of the samples and represent μx. Immediately below this we show the Ramachandran filter function, C. We then multiply each of the ordinates (1, 2, 3, 5, 6, 7) by the corresponding values of the filter function immediately below to yield the values shown in panel 3. We have one positive term and a whole series of negative terms. These positive and negative terms are added to yield 0.22, which is shown in the bottom panel of Figure 16-43 as the ordinate 4' of the convoluted function S'. Thus, to determine *one* ordinate such as 4' on the profile S' we have to multiply *each* ordinate in Figure 16-43 by the corresponding value of the convolution function and integrate. To obtain the next ordinate, 5', we shift the filter function

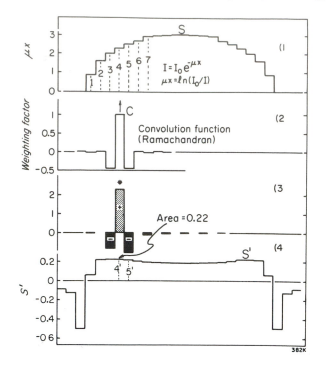

Figure 16-43. Diagram to illustrate convolution. S is a plot of $\ln(I_0/I) = \Sigma\ \mu \cdot \Delta x$ for an elliptical object of density 1.0, sampled with a vertical x ray beam. Curve C is the filter function due to Ramachandran. Panel 3 intermediate step in the convolution process. The area 0.22 gives one ordinate 4' on the convolved profile S'. Panel 4 gives the resultant profile S', which is then backprojected.

one step to the right, again multiply each ordinate (1, 2, 3, . . . 7 . . .) by the corresponding value of the filter function, and add up the contributions. After doing this for each position of the filter function we obtain the profile S'. It is quite different from the profile S with which we started since it has both positive and negative terms. The procedure we have described is referred to as convolving the distributions S with the filter function C to yield the function S'.

The profile S' with its positive and negative values is now backprojected onto the outline of the patient with an appropriate value entered into each pixel in the cross section. These contributions are stored in the computer. The scanner is then moved to its next angular position, a new profile S determined, which is again convolved with the filter function C to yield a new function S'. This is in turn backprojected contributing another set of numbers that are added to the values already present in the computer for each pixel of the patient. This process is continued until all the profiles have been processed and the image is then shown on the television screen for viewing. The procedure we have described lends itself to computer manipulation since it involves multiplications and additions. Many of these operations can be carried out in specialized computer blocks so that the process can be made very fast, yielding an image within seconds after the completion of the scan.

It is instructive to see how the image is built up as backprojection from increasing numbers of angles is carried out. Figure 16-44 shows a se-

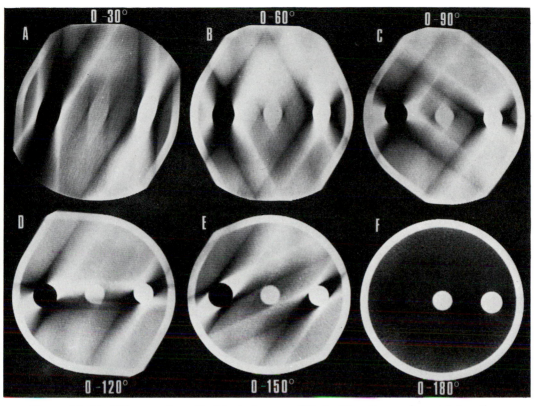

Figure 16-44. CT scan of a cylindrical phantom filled with water and containing three cylinders of Plexiglas® ($\rho \sim 1.1$), Teflon® ($\rho \sim 1.8$), polystyrene ($\rho = 0.95$). Panel A shows the appearance of the image after back-projection from 0 to 30°, B from 0 to 60°, etc. F backprojection over all angles from 0 to 180°.

quence of pictures. The first one, A, shows the image when backprojection has been carried out up to 30°; the next using angles up to 60°, etc. When the backprojection is completed using all angles from zero to 180°, the image suddenly appears showing the cylindrical phantom with its three cylindrical rods.

Artifacts

In an earlier part of this section we discussed the ring artifact due to the malfunction of one or more detectors. There are, however, other artifacts that arise even when everything is operating satisfactorily.

MOTION ARTIFACTS. These often appear in scans of the abdomen due to movement of gas bubbles in the intestines. If an air pocket moves during the scan, inconsistent data is presented to the computer, which then has trouble reconstructing a proper image. The image usually includes extraneous black lines emanating from the region of the gas bubble. These artifacts may at times interfere with a diagnosis. Artifacts of this kind are minimized in the type III and IV generation scanners, which perform scans in 2–3 seconds.

SPECTRAL ARTIFACTS. In writing down equation 16-35 it is implied that the radiation used to scan the patient is monoenergetic and that one can assign a unique value of $\mu(x,y)$ for each pixel in the patient. In actual fact, of course, the beam is heterogeneous and as it passes through the patient the lower energy photons are removed first and the beam becomes harder with depth. If an elliptical shell (as illustrated in Fig. 16-45a) is filled with water and scanned, the edges will be "looked at" by lower energy photons than the center. Thus, pixels near the center will be assigned smaller values of μ than pixels near the edge. A plot of μ across a diameter will thus be a curve concave upwards (Fig. 16-45a). This type of distortion is called the cupping artifact. Unless one is interested in the correct values of μ at different places in the phantom, this type of distortion does not interfere much with the diagnostic quality of the image.

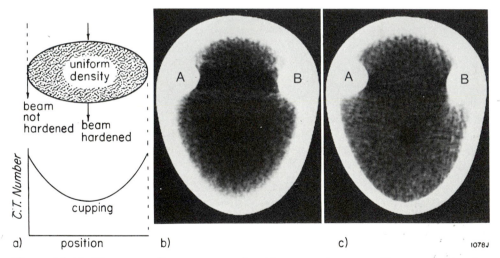

Figure 16-45. Diagram to illustrate spectral artifacts. (a) Diagram to illustrate the hardening of a beam by thick sections of the patient and the resultant distribution of CT numbers giving rise to the "cupping effect." (b) CT scan that shows streaking in the direction AB, which includes a large amount of bone. (c) Same scan as b with most of the artifacts removed by doing a scan with a double detector (F9).

If the phantom contains regions of high density and high atomic number, these will have a large effect on the x ray beam (as illustrated in Fig. 16-45b). Along the line AB the bone removes much of the soft radiation and this region is assigned too low a CT number.

Two ways to remove this type of artifact are either to perform a double scan with two different x ray beams or perform a single scan with two detectors, one behind the other. The front detector will see mostly soft radiation, while the one behind will detect the beam after it has been filtered by the front chamber and so "looks" primarily at the harder radiation. By suitable manipulation of the data from the two detectors it is possible to determine both the atomic number of each pixel and the electron density and in the process overcome most of the spectral artifact as illustrated in Figure 16-45c. (See F9, F10, R14, D11.)

16.20	**MAMMOGRAPHY**

Mammography is a technique for the radiographic examination of the breast. This is a challenging imaging task since connective tissue, glandular tissue, skin, and fat must be visualized but all have very similar attenuation coefficients and thus produce little subject contrast. Furthermore, it is also necessary to image blood vessels, ducts, and microcalcifications as small as 100 μm in diameter.

CONTRAST. The need to visualize structures of low contrast dictates that a low energy spectrum be used to maximize differences in attenuation coefficients of the various tissues. Tube potentials of about 30 kV$_p$ are commonly employed. The use of a molybdenum anode tube with a 30 μm molybdenum filter provides a quasi-monoenergetic beam of 17.5 keV, which is well suited for mammographic imaging with film.

Scattered radiation is an important source of contrast reduction in mammography. Recently a mammographic grid has been introduced by Philips to help remove the scatter. This is a special grid with the space between the lead bars filled with light material to reduce attenuation and thus the dose. Another way to reduce dose is to compress the breast and use a larger field so that less tissue need be traversed by the x rays. This also tends to reduce the amount of scattered radiation incident on the film and so increases the contrast.

RESOLUTION. The requirement of resolving small structures means that fine detail image receptors must be used. In the past a great deal of mammography was performed with direct exposure of "no screen" x ray film giving good resolution but requiring high dose. In the last few years "no-screen" film has been largely replaced by two techniques requiring less radiation: screen-film mammography and xeroradiography.

SCREEN-FILM MAMMOGRAPHY: A single fine detail screen is used to maximize resolution. The screen is placed on the side of the film farthest from the x ray source so that the light, which is produced near the surface of the screen where the x rays enter, has only a short distance to travel back to reach the film. This prevents loss of resolution due to light diffusion in the screen. Screens composed of calcium tungstate or the rare-earth phosphor gadolinium oxysulphide are commonly used. Although the resolution is not as high as with "no-screen" film, the screens enable one to obtain satisfactory images with much smaller exposure.

XERORADIOGRAPHY. This was described in section 16.17. It has a major advantage of edge contrast, which tends to draw powder lines around tumors and other objects of interest. Since contrast is amplified by the development step, less subject contrast can be tolerated in the exposure step and hence higher kilovoltages may be used. Thus, more of the x rays will be transmitted to the detector and the dose to the breast will be lowered. A xeroradiograph of a breast taken on Xerox equipment using blue powder toner that is photographed is shown in Figure 16-33.

DOSES. In mammography, doses must be reduced to the lowest practical level to minimize the risk of cancer induction. Table 16-4 shows measured exposures by Yaffe in our group from a variety of machines in the Toronto area in 1978. The exposures per radiograph at the surface of the breast given in column 8 range from 20 R to 0.2 R, depending on the kV_p, the filtration, the HVL, the type of target in the x ray tube, and the imaging device. Of more interest is the mean dose to the glandular tissues of the breast. This has been studied by Hammerstein (H22) and some of his data are given in column 9. Multiplying entries in column 8 by those in column 9 we obtain the quantity of interest given in column 10. This is the mean dose in mGy to the glandular tissue per radiograph. These doses range from 20 mGy to 0.3 mGy. The low dose techniques at the bottom of the table are in the range 0.3 to 0.5 mGy (0.03 to 0.05 rads).

RISK. With these data and the data given in Table 15-3 we may calculate the risk of death from radiation-induced cancer. The table shows that the risk for breast cancer is 5.0×10^{-3} per Sv.* Multiplying this by 0.4 mGy we obtain $0.4 \text{ mGy} \times 5 \times 10^{-6} \text{ Sv}^{-1} = 2 \times 10^{-6}$ per radiograph. Since two radiographs are usually required, the total risk is 4 per million examinations. In a Toronto breast screening program using mammography Miller† has estimated that such a survey on the high risk group of women (ages 40–49) might find 5000 breast tumors per million. This calculation would suggest that a screening program of this kind would have a net benefit, but there are other factors that must be considered. For example, to yield a benefit one would have to show that an earlier diagnosis would yield a greater cure. In such a study great care would have to be taken to ensure that the doses were kept small, a difficult task since "better" pictures can always be obtained by increasing the dose. Careful monitoring of the units involved would have to be maintained through the study.

---

*This figure is double that shown in Table 15-3 because the latter is the average for men and women.
†A.B. Miller, National Cancer Institute, Toronto, Canada. Personal communication, preliminary results.

TABLE 16-4

Measured Exposures in Mammography

(Typical Values in Ontario 1980)

(1) Manuf.	(2) Absorbing Material	(3) Imaging Material	(4) Anode	(5) Filter (mm)	(6) kV$_p$	(7) HVL mm Al	(8) Exposures Surface of Breast (R)	(9) Mean Dose in mGy per R to Surf.	(10) Mean Dose to Glandular Tissue (mGy)
Kodak	Film	AA film	Mo	.03 Mo	32	.37	20	1.0	20
Kodak	Film	No screen	Mo	.03 Mo	25	.30	4	.9	3.6
Dupont	Lo Dose screen	MRF-31	Mo	.06 Mo	33	.44	.9	1.3	1.2
Xerox	Selenium +ve mode	Selenium	W	2 Al	42	1.1	1.0	2.8	2.8
	−ve mode	Selenium	W	2 Al	42	1.1	.7	2.8	2.0
Kodak	Min R screen	Min R.	W	.5 Al	30	.37	.4	1.0	.4
Kodak	Min R screen	Min R.	Mo	.03 Mo	36	.39	.5	1.1	.5
Dupont	Lo Dose II screen	MRF-31	Mo	.03 Mo	29	.5	.24	1.4	.3
Dupont	Lo Dose II screen	Lo Dose	Mo	.03 Mo	30	.35	.5	1.0	.5
Xonics	Freon at 5 atmos.	Foil	W	.9 Al	36	.83	.2	2.2	.4

*Mean dose to glandular tissue of breast per R to the surface of breast taken from Logan and Muntz (Fig. 6 in L12, H22) but decreased by 20% to allow for backscatter

16.21   **EXPOSURES TO PATIENTS**

Hitherto there has been little concern about radiation exposure to patients during x ray procedures. The concern has been largely for the workers who work with radiation. Indeed the International Commission on Radiological Protection up to 1976 had very little to say about limitation of radiation to patients. During the past few years, there has been growing concern that the quantities of radiation delivered during diagnostic procedures may produce a significant amount of cancer in the population. This was discussed in section 15.03 where we showed that diagnostic radiology contributed a dose equivalent of about 1 mSv per year. Since in this chapter we are concerned with radiations for which the quality factor is close to 1.0 a dose equivalent of 1 mSv is numerically the same as 1 mGy or 100 mrad. In addition, since the conversion factor from exposure in roentgens to dose in rads is close to 1.0, and since we are interested in orders of magnitude only, we may roughly use the same number to specify exposures in roentgens and doses in rads (10^{-2} Gy).

Because of this growing concern the emphasis now is on producing the maximum benefit from radiology for the minimum amount of radiation. Radiologists in the future will have to be concerned with the level of radiation exposure to their patients for each radiograph and each procedure and will have to judge each radiograph not only for its diagnostic quality but also for the penalty in radiation that it has imposed upon the patient. A number of investigations over the last ten years have suggested that the radiation dose to the patient for a given procedure varies from one x ray room to another by a large factor. This was confirmed in a careful study carried out in Ontario where we showed (T10) that for the same procedure the radiation exposure might differ from one room to another by a factor of sixty and that it was a matter of chance whether a patient received a high or low exposure. Some of the results are given in Table 16-5A.

TABLE 16-5

(A) Ranges of Exposures Observed in Toronto in 1978 for Diagnostic Procedures and (B) Important Parameters Giving Rise to These Ranges*

A. Procedure	Range of Exposures (R)	B. Fluoro, exp. rates	
Chest	0.02-.15	Fluoro time	8:1
Barium meal	1.6-90	Beam quality: kV, filter number of phases	12:1
Barium enema	16-128	Screen-film combination	6:1
I.V.P	1.3-41	Density of film	3:1
Gallbladder	4-48	Tabletop attenuation	2:1
		No. exposures/procedure	2.5:1

Note: "B. Fluoro, exp. rates" row has value 20:1.

*From Taylor et al. (T10) and (J14)

In the most extreme case, a barium meal involved a skin exposure of 90 R in one room and 1.6 R in another room for the same examination and for the same diagnostic information. In the "high dose" room the fluoroscopic exposure rate was high because of misadjustment of the automatic exposure rate controls. In addition, in the "high dose" room, an insensitive film-screen combination was used, while in the "low dose" room the radiologist used a 70 mm camera to photograph the output of the image intensifier.

The study also documented the reason for the variations in dose and showed that this was *not* due to faulty equipment but was usually due to the unfortunate choice of factors such as kilovoltage, filtration, and film-screen combination. The work also showed that the high dose could be reduced by a factor of 3 with no loss of diagnostic accuracy. There is ample evidence that this problem occurs in most x ray installations throughout the world and is not just a problem in Ontario.

From Table 16-5b, it can be seen that fluoroscopic exposure rate and fluoroscopic time are the most important parameters. However, the combination of kV, filtration, and number of phases, all of which affect the quality of the beam, also give a factor of 12 in radiation exposure. Another important factor is the screen-film combination, which in this study gave a 6:1 range of speeds. Less important factors are the film density that the radiologists accepted as being reasonable; the attenuation of the tabletop, phototimer, and grid; and the number of radiographic exposures per procedure.

Figure 16-46 shows the distribution of radiation exposures in x ray rooms in Ontario for (a) a single radiograph during an intravenous

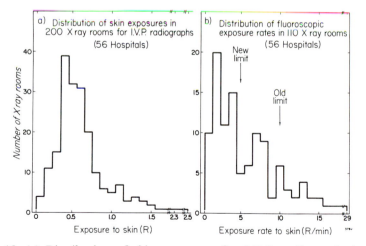

Figure 16-46. (a) Distribution of skin exposures for I.V.P. radiographs in 200 x ray rooms. (b) Distribution of skin exposure rates for fluoroscopic examinations in 110 x ray rooms.

pyelogram and (b) for fluoroscopy for average patients. Note that the most common exposure for an IVP is about 0.4 R but two rooms gave over 5 times this amount, while a number of radiologists used only 0.1R. This demonstrates that if all the hospitals were to be brought down to the minimum radiation levels, the radiation saving would be considerable. The exposure rate during fluoroscopy is particularly interesting because it shows two peaks: one close to the original Canadian Government maximum level of 10 R/min and the other to a newly instituted Ontario Government maximum level of 5 R/min. This demonstrates that if regulatory bodies set maximum levels above which the exposures must not go, then there will be a tendency for service technologists to set their machines to those levels in spite of the fact that it is possible to work with much lower exposure rates. Thus, setting a legal limit may be an unwise step if we are really interested in reducing dose.

RECOMMENDED EXPOSURES IN DIAGNOSTIC RADIOLOGY. With the increasing concern regarding dose in diagnostic radiology, it is useful to have a goal of recommended exposures. These are given in Table 16-6.

Column 5 gives the Canadian Government limits for specific radiographic examinations. These are extreme exposures and must not be exceeded. Column 4 shows the average exposures in Ontario in late 1979. These are less than the Canadian limits and are still decreasing as a result of our dose reduction programs. Column 3 gives the minimum exposures that have been achieved by some radiologists in Ontario. We recommend that radiologists attempt to reduce exposures to the levels of column 3 or lower, keeping in mind that at times higher exposures will be necessary to visualize specific features in the radiograph.

TABLE 16-6
Exposures and Exposure Rates in Diagnostic Radiology

(1) Projection	(2) Patient Thickness	(3) Ontario Minimum Exposure Used mR	(4) Ontario Average Exposure Late 1979 mR	(5) Canadian Federal Gov't. Limit mR
Skull Lateral	15 cm	100	265	300
Cervical Spine A-P	13 cm	90	140	250
Thoracic Spine A-P	23 cm	260	460	900
Chest P-A	23 cm	8	25	30
Lumbar Spine A-P	23 cm	180	620	1000
Lumbar Spine Lat.	32 cm	500	2445	3300
Abdomen A-P	23 cm	190	530	750
I.V.P.	23 cm	150	600	750
Fluoroscopy	20 cm	0.5 R/min	Should not exceed 5 R/min.* (3 R/min, CsI)	Must not exceed 10 R/min.

*The higher values are for the old intensifiers, which used a CdS fluorescent screen.

DIRECTION OF X RAY BEAM. Another factor that influences the dose to specific organs in the patient is the direction in which the beam travels through the patient. There are two possible ways to arrange the x ray tube and image intensifier. The intensifier may be above the table as in Figure 16-47A or below the table as in B, C, and D. The advantage of an overhead tube arises since the tube may be placed further from the patient, thus lowering skin exposures. In addition it makes it easier to manipulate the patient and angle the tube. Furthermore, this configuration can also be used as an excellent general radiographic unit. However, it has the disadvantage that if the radiologist works alongside of it he may receive extra exposure to his head and neck unless he is careful. It also has the disadvantage of increasing the dose to the patient if the absorption of the tabletop is high. We have found absorption of 50% in some cases. Tabletops with high absorption should be replaced.

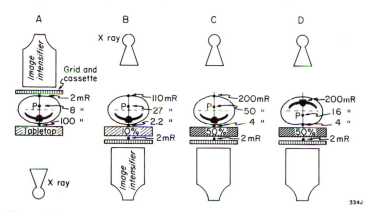

Figure 16-47. Possible arrangements of x ray components that might be used in gastrointestinal examinations and the doses to three points in the patient. Point P is 2 cm anterior to the midline and is the position of a possible pregnancy.

It is also important to consider the organs at risk. The exposures shown in Figure 16-47 are measured values for a typical gastrointestinal examination. All are adjusted to produce an exposure of 2 mR just in front of the grid. This is enough to give a good radiograph. In a female patient the critical tissue that might be exposed is an early pregnancy at point P, 2 cm anterior to the midline. Exposure to P for the same radiograph varies from 8 to 50 mR depending on the orientation of the patient and the orientation of the beam. The best arrangement is A although one like D, with the patient lying prone but with a 10% tabletop attenuation, would be nearly as good. If a male is examined the bone marrow becomes the critical tissue and arrangement B is good, although arrangement A with the patient turned over would be slightly better. If arrangement B is used, the operator should be certain that the tabletop does not absorb more than 10% of the radiation. It is important that the technologist understand these problems so that the patient can be positioned accordingly. They should, of course, provide protection for vital organs that are not part of the diagnostic examination.

FILM DEVELOPMENT AND EXPOSURE. The way the film is developed will affect the exposures required for the examination. Studies in Ontario hospitals (D12) have shown that for films of the same nominal speed the exposure required to produce an optical density of 1.0 may vary by a factor of 3 from one hospital to another depending on the chemistry and conditions used for the processing of the film.

SCREEN-FILM COMBINATIONS. We have already seen that the choice of screen-film combination led to a variation in the required exposure by a factor of 6:1. In fact if one takes the fastest and slowest combination currently available for radiology, the variation in exposure to give density 1.0 is from 7.5 mR to 0.1 mR., i.e. a factor of 75. The combinations requiring less than 0.3 mR give mottled images and so may have limited application. Those requiring 0.35 mR or more are quite satisfactory for general radiography. The use of the slowest combinations with high detail screens is only necessary for examinations requiring great detail, such as visualizing fine structure of bone in the extremities. For such examinations doses to critical organs are small anyway.

As silver rises in price, film manufacturers tend to reduce the quantity of the metal in the emulsion. This may bring about changes in both the characteristic curve and in the exposure required to produce a density of 1.0. To monitor this situation we have developed a simple x ray fluorescent technique to quickly measure silver content (Y5). It may be possible to balance the reduction of silver content by using higher speed rare earth screens.

CHOICE OF FILTER. In the past most radiography has been carried out using aluminum filters to harden the beam. It has been shown (V2) that reduction in exposure by as much as a factor of 2 using rare earth or tungsten filters can be achieved with no significant change in image contrast. It should be noted that the use of such a filter may require the use of two or more times the tube loading.

Summary of Ways of Reducing Radiation Risk in Diagnostic Radiology

a. Reduction of exposure rate and time in fluoroscopy and the replacement of old CdS intensifiers with CsI types.
b. Selection of optimum screen-film combinations with optimization and control of film processing.
c. Selection of appropriate kV_p and filtration for each radiographic view.
d. Acceptance of 70 and 100 mm fluorography in place of full sized spotfilms.

e. Acceptance of mottle in noncritical radiographic and fluoroscopic views.

f. Avoidance of unnecessary examinations and repeat radiographs.

g. Development of new techniques and electronic devices to exploit the gain provided by television systems.

In reducing radiation levels one reduces the risk of cancer from the irradiation. However, dose reduction should not be pressed too far since it may result in inadequate image quality and hence errors in diagnosis. The risk of such errors may be greater than the risk from the radiation. Judgment is required.

16.22   RISKS IN DIAGNOSTIC RADIOLOGY

In order to calculate the risk for a particular organ, one must consider all the types of examinations that may cause irradiation of that organ and the number of such procedures carried out on the population per year. Such a calculation is illustrated in Table 16-7. Three kinds of tissue, the breast, red bone marrow, and the thyroid, are considered. Breasts are irradiated during mammography and during chest radiography. Bone marrow is irradiated during all procedures but particularly during gastrointestinal studies and to some extent during dental radiography. The thyroid is irradiated during dental x ray procedures and during chest radiography, particularly in the taking of lateral views.

Column 2 gives the estimated exposure to the skin in roentgens. The next two columns give our estimate of the average exposure to the organ in roentgens and the corresponding mean dose to the organ in Gy. Column 5 gives the number of examinations per year in Ontario. The next column gives the risk of death per Gy taken from Table 15-3. Note that in Table 15-3 the risk for breast cancer is the average for men and women. Since the risk for men is virtually zero, the risk for women is $5 \times 10^{-3}/$ Gy rather than $2.5 \times 10^{-3}/Gy$. The product of columns 4, 5, and 6 gives the estimated number of deaths per year, which is entered in column 8. Column 7 gives the estimated number of cancers caused by the radiological procedures. It should be noted that in the breast, although the skin dose from a lateral chest is lower than that from mammography, the mean doses to the breast tissue are about the same, and because of the large number of lateral chest films that are taken each year, the relative risk is much higher from lateral chests than it is from mammography. In view of this, the routine indiscriminate use of lateral chest x rays must be critically reexamined (B32).

The total number of deaths expected from all radiological procedures for a given organ is obtained by addition yielding a value of 2.3 for breast, 10 for leukemia, and 0.5 for thyroid.

These numbers should be compared with the number of deaths for

TABLE 16-7
Risks per Year from X ray Examinations in Ontario in 1979—Population 8.5 Million

(1) Organ	(2) Expos. to Skin (R)	(3) Mean Exp. (mR)	(4) Mean Dose To Organ (mGy)	(5) Exam per Year ($\times 10^6$)	(6) Risk Death per Gy ($\times 10^{-3}$)	(7) Canc. per Year	(8) Deaths per Year	(9) Deaths /Year Vital Stats.
Breast								
Lateral Chest	.1	50	.5	0.7	5	3.6	1.8	
P.A. Chest	.03	7	.07	1.2	5	.8	.4	
Mammography	.5	50	.5	.03	5	.16	.08	
Total Breast						4.6	2.3	1269
Leukemia								
G.I.	25	1000	10	0.5	2	10	10	
Dental	.25	.5	.005	10	2	.1	.1	
Total Leukemia						10.1	10.1	565
Thyroid								
Dental	.25	2	.02	10.	.5	2	.1	
Lateral Chest	.10	50	.5	1.4	.5	8	.4	
Total Thyroid						10	.5	38

each site taken from vital statistics for Ontario and entered in column 9. It is seen that the number of deaths due to diagnostic x rays is small (less than 1%) compared to the number of deaths from normal causes. The public should not be alarmed at having a diagnostic x ray examination and yet at the same time the risk is not insignificant. Of course the risk to an individual who may receive many diagnostic examinations over the years is much larger. Suppose, for example, that a person who has a gastrointestinal disease has four examinations at any one time and this is repeated three times over a period of years; the risk of getting leukemia from the x rays is the product of 12, 10 mGy/exam, and 2×10^{-3}/ Gy = 2.4×10^{-4}, or 1 in 4000, which is not insignificant.

Since these risks can be reduced by a program of dose measurement and quality control at relatively little cost, the dose reduction program should be rigorously followed. As of 1980 we have been able to reduce the doses of Table 16-7 by a factor of about 3. As another example, Table 16-4 shows the dose reduction that has been achieved in mammography over the past 10 years to attempt to justify breast screening programs. This table illustrates nicely the dramatic improvement over a period of years that can be attained by the steady application of new technology. Mean doses to glandular tissue have been reduced by 50 to 100 times.

The data presented here are approximate and are included to show how one can attempt a risk benefit analysis. In analyzing the risk to the patient, one must consider the risk of refusing an x ray and thus failing to detect disease. This may well outweigh the risk from the x rays themselves.

16.23   **QUALITY CONTROL**

To check all the variables in an x ray imaging system is a large task. Since x ray machines are often used to capacity by the radiologist, it is important to develop measurement techniques that allow one to check the machine quickly so that the time lost to the radiologist is minimum.

SIMPLE TEST KITS. We have found that a solid state detector similar to that described in section 9.08 used with a special dosimeter (C16, T12) is ideal. The system is illustrated in Figure 16-48. It consists of a storage oscilloscope, an integrator, and 2 diode detectors. With this device one can measure inexpensively and accurately the waveform of the x ray output, check the timer, check the mA linearity, measure the kV_p, and determine the exposure. Since the diodes are sensitive to light the performance of the image intensifier can also be studied. Such kits are now being made commercially,* making it possible for radiology departments to have test equipment to evaluate the performance of their x ray machines and measure radiation exposure. Reduction of exposure cannot be carried out unless exposures can be measured routinely.

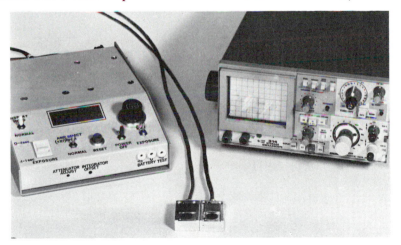

Figure 16-48. Solid state dosimeter for use in a diagnostic x ray department. For details see Campbell and Yaffe (C16).

WAVEFORM. The most powerful single technique for checking the performance of an x ray generator is to visualize the x ray yield as a function of time with a solid state detector that has a fast enough response to follow transients (T12). Ionization chambers are not satisfactory for this

*Optech Inc., Downsview, Ontario.

purpose because of their slow response. Figure 16-49a shows exposures for 1, 2, 3, 4, 6, and 8 pulses in a well-behaved single phase generator; b shows two exceptionally high pulses at the beginning of the exposure due to a switching transient; this may indicate excessive kilovoltage that may lead to premature failure of the tube or HT cables or both (the service technician should correct this condition); c shows the effect of a damaged target that is both warped and cracked, leading to the irregular x ray yield and the sharp spikes of low intensity; d shows the effect of a malfunctioning mA stabilizer that continuously increases the mA; e shows the x ray yield during a long fluoroscopic exposure. This particular trace shows a high initial peak of x rays, followed by a stable region from 1 to 4 s, followed by a slow decay from 4 to 12 s. The initial peak occurred because the filament is preheated to a temperature higher than that necessary for the low fluoroscopic mA. The control circuits reduce the filament temperature during the first second, resulting in a falling x ray output. For this waveform the radiologist terminated the fluoroscopy at 4 seconds but the x ray yield continued and fell slowly to zero at 12 seconds due tò the gradual discharge of the high tension circuit. The initial spike and the long decay should not have been present and more than doubled the dose to the patient. Furthermore, the radiation emitted during the tail could not be seen because the television tube is automatically blanked at the termination of fluoroscopy. Thus the patient was being irradiated without the radiologist's knowledge. Usual methods of quality control that measure steady state conditions do not detect these transients. These transients are commonly found in fluoroscopy but are seldom investigated. The long decay can be eliminated by using higher mA and lower kV or, better, by discharging the high tension circuit with a load resistance that is automatically connected into the circuit at the end of fluoroscopy. Ironically, the conscientious radiologist who might use high kV and a series of 2-second exposures would in fact deliver to the patient three times the radiation in the "off" periods as in the "on" time. This is a serious problem, since half the machines in clinical use studied in our survey had one or both of these faults present.

Such valuable waveforms can be obtained in seconds and a machine can be completely evaluated in an hour. Tests of many machines suggest that often some aspects of a unit were never correct, even at the time of installation.

The waveforms illustrate the difficulty of defining time and kV_p precisely. For example, what is the kV_p in trace b and what is the exposure time in trace e? Regulatory agencies who define these parameters and insist on an unobtainable precision often ignore these problems. Their efforts usually do little to reduce dose and only succeed in increasing costs.

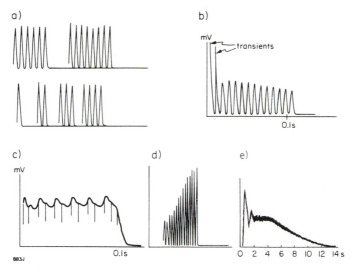

Figure 16-49. Typical x ray wave forms for (a) a correctly set up unit; (b) unit in which transients are present; (c) unit in which target is badly damaged; (d) unit in which mA stabilizer is not working; (e) improperly adjusted fluoroscopic unit giving an initial peak and a long tail.

PEAK KILOVOLTAGE (kV$_p$). The measurement of kV$_p$ has been studied by Ardran and Crooks (A13) and by Jacobson (J19), both of whom used a film to record the transmission of a hardened x ray beam through a Cu step wedge. The degree of transmission is compared visually with the transmission of an optical filter yielding the kV$_p$. A better method developed in our laboratory is demonstrated in Figure 16-50. Two photodiodes are placed side by side in a beam and exposed through filters F$_1$ and F$_2$. The ratio of the signals from the two diodes is a function of the kV$_p$ as seen in the insert. The ratio is easily obtained by adding the inverted signal from detector 1 to a fraction of the signal from detector 2 selected by the potentiometer. With the correct potentiometer setting the two signals can be seen to cancel on the oscilloscope and the kV$_p$ is read from the calibrated potentiometer. This device measures kV instantaneously at any time during an x ray pulse. A single kV measurement can be made in 10 to 20 seconds.

DOSIMETRY. To measure exposure, one of the detectors in Figure 16-50 is connected to a current amplifier and integrator to yield exposure rate or total exposure, which is indicated on a digital display. It is possible to measure down to 1 mR/min or to 0.2 mR with an accuracy of 10%. The device with storage scope is worth about 6,000 dollars and has been invaluable in our dose reduction and quality control program. The device is robust and simple enough to be used by x ray technologists in an in-house quality control program.

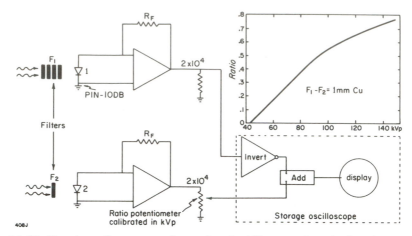

Figure 16-50. Circuit to allow one to determine the kV at any time during the x ray pulse.

Establishing Standards of Attenuation and Sensitivity

To test the sensitivity of the system we need to establish a simple re-producible irradiation condition that can be tested in the laboratory and reproduced quickly with any type of x ray machine encountered in the field. Figure 16-51 shows such a system. The x ray tube is positioned with its target 100 cm from the tabletop. A plastic bucket filled to a depth of 20 cm with water makes a convenient phantom, which is placed on the x ray table. The exposures X_1, X_2, and X_3 are measured for an irradia-tion of 20 mAs with the tube operating at 80 kV_p and a total filtration of 2.8 mm Al. The ratio X_1/X_2 gives the attenuation of 20 cm of water, which varies from 83 to 27 as the voltage is altered from 60 to 120 kV_p (see Fig. 16-51). Over the same kilovoltage range the attenuation of the tabletop, an 8 : 1 grid, and the phototimer X_2/X_3 varies from 11 to 7.

Comparing the Hospital System with the Laboratory Standards

Having established these ratios in our laboratory, any machine in the field can be tested by reproducing the arrangement of Figure 16-51, setting the kV selector to give 80 kV_p and measuring X_1', X_2', X_3'. If X_1'/X_2' and X_2'/X_3' are within 20% of the values given above, we know that the x ray tube is operating properly, the correct filter is in place, and the tabletop, grid, and phototimer give satisfactory transmissions. If, however, the system under test does not give these ratios, the reason for the discrepancy must be determined. If for example X_1'/X_2' is greater than 44, either the filtration is less than 2.8 mm Al or the tube was ac-tually operating at less than 80 kV_p. If the ratio is less than 44, either the filtration is too great or the kV_p is too high. The kV_p and filter should be corrected.

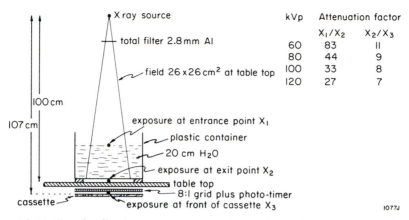

Figure 16-51. Standardization irradiation condition for testing a system in the field.

If the ratio X_2'/X_3' is greater than 9, then we know that the unit under test has components between the patient and the detector that have excess attenuation. The tabletop, grid, and phototimer should be studied and the fault or faults should be corrected.

If the x ray machine is unstable, making it difficult to reproduce the readings X_1, X_2, and X_3, it may be useful to use one of the solid state detectors illustrated in Figure 16-48 as a monitor. The readings X_1, X_2, and X_3 are then corrected to a constant monitor reading.

Testing the Hospital Screen-Film Combinations

Having established the standard irradiation condition we now test the sensitivity of the hospital screen-film combination. We ask the x ray technician to expose their combination in the geometry of Figure 16-51 at 80 kV_p and with an mAs they estimate will give a density 1.0. At the same time we measure the exposure X_3. In general, the film will not have a density of exactly 1.0 so a second exposure is made to bracket density 1.0 in order that the exposure required for density 1.0 may be determined.* Suppose for example, that the hospital uses Kodak® Regular screens and Kodak XRP film, then from laboratory measurements we know that an exposure of 0.58 mR is required to give density 1.0. If in an actual test it required 0.60 mR, then since this is not significantly different from the value of 0.58, we can immediately conclude that the screen, film, and development are *all* satisfactory. If, on the other hand, the exposure required for density 1.0 was 1.6 mR, we know immediately that something is wrong with one or more of the imaging components, i.e. the screen, the film, or the development.

---

*To do these tests accurately one should of course measure the density with a densitometer and this should be done if one is available. A simpler method is to visually compare the test film against pieces of standard film exposed to give suitable density steps from 0.6 to 1.6.

Testing the Screen

The easiest way to test the screen is to repeat the procedure using a screen we know is satisfactory and that is kept as a standard. If the same exposure is required, we know the fault does not lie in the screen. However, if the standard screen required less exposure than the hospital's, their screens must be at fault. This is usually due to yellowing with age and use. Decrease in speed of up to 2 times has been observed, and this can cause a high repeat rate when a department uses a mixture of screens of different ages. If the screens have deteriorated, all screens should be checked in order to decide if all or some should be replaced.

Testing the Film

If the screens are not at fault, the problem must lie with the film or developer. The most likely culprit is the developer, but it is easier to test the film so we do this first. To test the film, one replaces the hospital's film with a film of the same type that has been standardized in the laboratory* and again determine the exposure for a density of 1.0. If the hospital's film is slower by 10–20% one would ignore it because this is within normal manufacturing tolerance. However, if the film were more than 40% slower, one should challenge the manufacturer on their quality control. Since manufacturers are trying to reduce the silver content to minimize increase in costs, it is not surprising that differences in speed for the same type of film of up to 50% have been seen recently. Speeds of film should be specified by the hospital at the time of purchase, and standards should be developed to ensure that these specifications are met. Care should be taken to ensure the proper storage of film.

Testing the Developer

If the films and screens are satisfactory, then the loss of speed must be in the development of the film. First one should check the temperature, the replenishment rate, and the film immersion time. If these are not correct, they should be corrected and the test repeated. Any remaining loss of speed must be due to contaminated or diluted chemicals. To test this, the processor should be emptied, cleaned, and refilled. If the problem still persists, it must be discussed with the supplier, who may be selling the hospital over-diluted chemicals. Once the processing has been brought to an acceptable state it should be monitored daily using standard sensitometric techniques. In one of the simplest systems (G16, L13), the film is exposed to a reproducible light level through a neutral density step wedge and the blackening measured.

---

*This should be the task of the national standards laboratory.

Testing Fluoroscopic and Fluorographic Modes

Measurements by the staff of our laboratories have shown that it is common for fluoroscopic exposure rates and fluorographic exposures to be set incorrectly. If they are set too low, images will be excessively mottled. If they are set too high, the kV_p will often be too high as well, leading to images lacking in contrast. To achieve correct transmission of light, incorrect exposure settings are accompanied by incorrect lens apertures on television and fluorographic cameras, which in turn may lead to further loss of image quality. It is clearly important to set exposures correctly.

Typical values at the front face of the intensifier are for fluoroscopy 25 μR/s; for fluorography with 70 mm camera 70 μR; with a 100 mm camera 100 μR. If values measured in x ray departments differ by more than 50% from these values, the company servicing the equipment should be asked to reset the exposures and lens apertures and carry out any other necessary adjustments, such as refocusing the lenses because of the change of aperture. If then the images are not satisfactory, it may be necessary to check the performance of the intensifier.

The intensifier may be checked with simple equipment as follows:

(a) A 1 cm mesh of copper wire placed in front of the intensifier permits checking the imaged field size. If incorrect potentials are applied to the intensifier the minification will be incorrect and this may affect brightness. Visible field size should be within 10% of the nominal size.

(b) A lead bar resolution test pattern and a telescopic magnifier viewing the output phosphor permits checking that the intensifier is optically focused. At least 3 lp/mm should be visible.

(c) A simple photometer calibrated to measure brightness is then used to measure the conversion factor. This is simply the ratio of the brightness of the output phosphor in candela per square meter (dc/m^2) to the x ray exposure rate in mR/s at the front face of the intensifier. Conversion factors range from 40 to 200 cd m^{-2} mR^{-1}s, the lower values being found for old CdS intensifiers. New CsI intensifiers have factors around 100 cd m^{-2} mR^{-1}s and this is satisfactory for all uses of the intensifier. However, older intensifiers may have factors around 50 cd m^{-2} mR^{-1}s. Even these are satisfactory when they are used just for fluoroscopy and not for fluorography. In a survey of 30 intensifiers where replacement had been suggested because of poor image quality or high exposures, only one 15 year old CdS intensifier really needed to be replaced. In all the others, improper adjustment, dust on lenses or on intensifier output windows, or improper exposure were the cause of the poor image.

(d) With a slightly more complicated photometer the contrast ratio can be measured. This is the ratio of the brightnesses of the central 1% of the intensifier field area with and without a thick lead disc covering the central 10% of the intensifier front surface. It is a measure of the scatter from the periphery of the intensifier to the center portion. This is sometimes referred to as the veiling glare. Typical values for contrast ratios are in the range 4 to 7 for old CdS intensifiers and 6 to 12 for CsI intensifiers. New CsI intensifiers now have contrast ratios up to 20 and 10 should be considered the minimum acceptable. Of course the higher the contrast ratio, the better is the image quality, and this may be a sufficient reason to replace older intensifiers for fluorographic use.

Often the company dealing with a hospital has recommended replacement of an intensifier when in many cases the problem did not lie with it but with the exposure that has been set or with other components in the chain such as the television camera or 100 mm camera. There is a very urgent need for standardization of intensifier and television systems on a routine basis and this standardization should be done regularly by the service technologists when carrying out maintenance on imaging systems. It is common for a technologist servicing equipment not to correct the deficiencies in television systems but instead to turn up the fluoroscopic exposure rate so that the deficiencies are less obvious.

Replacement of image intensifiers is expensive. Rather than replace all the older units it is often satisfactory to use older units of moderate performance in less critical applications and to acquire new units for applications requiring maximum speed, contrast, and resolution.

16.24   CHOICE OF EQUIPMENT

In choosing equipment, it is important to ask questions of the suppliers that will force them to justify the need for expensive and sophisticated add-ons or the provision of more capacity than is really needed for the procedures that are to be carried out. Several components should be evaluated.

GENERATORS. The key question with regard to generators is the amount of power required to carry out the radiological procedures. If angiographic procedures are planned, then 100 kW generators may be necessary to give a rapid sequence of short intense exposures. For general radiography a 70 kW generator is adequate. However, moves toward image intensified fluorography and the use of rare earth screens will lead to lower exposures in the future and generators of half the power may eventually be satisfactory. In general, although three phase generators cost more than single phase, their better performance justifies their purchase.

X ray Tubes: Anode Angle. The choice of the anode angle is the first consideration since it determines the size of the field that can be achieved at a given distance. An angle of 10–12° is a good compromise for most procedures. A smaller angle allows for higher power loading for a given focal spot or a smaller focal spot for a given power. Anodes with 6° angles are useful for small fields and magnification techniques.

Anode Diameter and Rotor Speed. The diameter of the anode determines the loading that can be put upon the target spot, but large diameters increase the time to bring the rotor to full speed and therefore the delay before an exposure. It will also determine to some extent the lifetime of the tubes since heavier anodes may lead to earlier failure. In choosing the speed of the rotor, it is important to consider whether high speed is really necessary. Some manufacturers supply tubes that will run at low speed most of the time and will go to high speed for extreme exposures. This is a desirable feature.

Focal Spot. Nowadays it is possible to obtain a power of 100 kW in a projected focal spot of 1.3 mm, and this is adequate for virtually all purposes. Indeed, many procedures using fast imaging systems can be carried out with a power of 40 kw using a 0.6 mm focal spot, which will lead to improved image detail. This is especially the case with the use of spot filming using an image intensifier. For magnification or for detailed radiography a 0.3 mm focal spot has some advantages. It is possible to obtain a tube with two angles on the target face (see Fig. 2-7) and two focal spot sizes with a high loading on both focal spots. A good compromise in any tube is .6 and 1 mm for normal radiography and .3 and 1 mm for magnification radiography.

Tube Loading. Recently, the introduction of carbon anodes has improved the heat capacity and cooling of the anode, these being the most important limitations of radiographic procedures. In most cases, the target is able to take the instantaneous loading of each exposure but cannot cope with a very busy department making many exposures in a short time. If intensifiers are used, the anode loading may be reduced, saving the department the expense of a carbon anode.

Screens and Films. There are available today some 20 screens and 20 films, which may be combined to produce screen-film combinations of differing speeds and image quality. It is recommended that in any department there should be no more than three types of screens: a detail screen, a high-speed screen, and an ultra-high-speed screen—the detail screen for fine bone work, the high-speed screen for normal radiography, and the ultra-high-speed screen for examinations where poorer image quality can be tolerated, such as pelvimetry and lateral lumbar spines. If possible, only one type of film should be used, in order to avoid mixing films and thus obtaining useless or poor quality pictures that must be repeated, increasing the cost and patient dose. However, in some cases, it is desirable that special films be used for chest radiography in order to record the wide range of exposures involved. Fortunately, the large size of chest films makes them less likely to be confused with the smaller films used for general radiology. In choosing a screen and film it is important to appreciate that there will be mottle in the film if certain very fast types are chosen. In some cases with fast rare earth screens, a radiology department has been sold a slow film in order that the mottle not be visible. The purchase of rare earth screens should be accompanied by the purchase of a high-speed film in order to take full advantage of the more expensive screen.

GRIDS. In choosing a grid, consideration should be given to cost, possible improvement in contrast, and patient dose, all of which increase as the grid ratio is increased. In section 16.09 it was shown that the dose required for a 12:1 grid was about 30% higher than for an 8:1 grid. In addition, 12:1 grids are more expensive than 8:1 grids, and it is doubtful whether they are really justified, especially in an era when dose considerations are of importance. In chest radiography, it is an error of design to use a high ratio grid to greatly increase the contrast and then to use a long latitude underdeveloped film to record the image. It is far better to use a low ratio 5:1 grid and use a normal contrast film to record the image.

IMAGE INTENSIFIER. A choice has to be made concerning the size of the image intensifier. Since the detecting surfaces are curved, and the x ray beam diverges from the focal spot, the size of the region in the patient that can be seen on the intensifier may be some 20% less than the nominal size of the intensifier. Thus, the geometry of the system and the precise size within the patient that is to be seen should be carefully considered.

Currently, large intensifiers of 30 and 35 cm are going into use and these may greatly extend the use of 70 and 100 mm fluorography into general radiography. On the other hand, small 17 cm intensifiers are much better for imaging small organs such as the heart, especially when obliquely angled views are required, since they can be brought much closer to the patient, resulting in sharper images and lower exposures.

Image intensifiers with conversion factors from 60 to 200 cd/m^2 per mR/s are currently available. Conversion factors above 100 cd/cm^2 per mR/s should be specified for image intensified 70 and 100 mm fluorography and for intensifiers viewed directly without television.

PROCESSORS. One of the prime problems with processors in hospitals is the supply of hot water to maintain the processor at a standard temperature. Processors that require only cold water are now available and are to be recommended since they will ultimately lead to much more stable operation. Special care should be taken in choosing the chemistry to be used in the processor since some developers have been shown to seriously underdevelop the film, leading to a 2 to 3 time increase in dose to the patient (D12).

16.25   FUTURE TRENDS

IMAGE RECEPTOR. With the increasing cost of silver-based film, it will be necessary to look at other means of image recording in order to maintain the economic soundness of radiography. Ionography and other means of electrostatic imaging all have a place since they do not use silver but will produce an image on a simple piece of foil or plastic. However, considerable technical problems in using the technique remain to be solved and ways to increase the sensitivity must be found. A good alternative, which is already used to some degree, is the use of films that contain dyes instead of silver as the final product (Section 16.07).

High resolution television systems and recorders are currently under development for the commercial television market and will undoubtedly have a big impact on radiology when they become commercially available. This will enable the electronic recording and recall of radiographic images without loss of detail and without the requirement for expensive recording media such as film, but there will be an increase in the cost of the television components themselves to provide this increase in resolution. Recently, the technique of kinescope recording, or photographing the output of a television monitor, has been revived and extended by Hynes (H17). His group has shown that, using a high resolution television system and a high resolution multiformat camera (Matrix), satisfactory diagnostic images for contrast studies may be obtained with 1/30 the radiation used for a high speed film-screen combination.

Another possible method of electronic recording is digital radiography. In this technique the x rays are absorbed by a line or matrix of small efficient detectors, the signals from each detector being digitized and recorded in a computer for subsequent presentation or image manipulation. Detectors might be solid state fluorescent detectors coupled to solid state diodes. These could be built with high resolution. The ability to change contrast and look for various structures with enhanced edges in the radiographs might make them a very valuable means of image recording. They would, however, require large and fast computers in order to deal with the numbers involved and carry out the computation at high resolution. These are currently under development and in a few years may form the heart of an x ray imaging system.

PATIENT DOSE. The public in 1980 are demanding the use of minimal doses in radiology. Because of this demand there will be a growing acceptance of images that are mottled because of the use of low doses for certain procedures where contrast materials are involved. This will be coupled with the use of special filters and matched kVs and image receptor screens, possibly with push-button selection of the combination of filter, kilovoltage, and screen to minimize dose for each type of examination. The increasing acceptance of standard techniques in radiography and the development of matched systems will lead to a reduction of a factor of 10 in the patient dose over the next few years. With the standardization of techniques and the minimization of doses will come the requirement for quality control in order to maintain the standards. This will require professional responsibility on the part of radiologists and technologists and will require the active participation of physicists in the hospital environment. Finally, it will be necessary to write codes and regulations that do not overregulate the practice of radiology but ensure that certain standards are maintained. The emphasis will change from regulating equipment when it is supplied to specifying the performance of the equipment in the field over a period of time and ensuring that this performance is maintained at an acceptable level.

PROBLEMS

(An asterisk denotes difficult problems.)

1. Determine the fraction of radiation transmitted through (a) 12 cm of tissue plus 1 cm of bone and (b) 13 cm of tissue using radiation generated at 80 kV_p with 2 mm Al filter. Solve the problem using equivalent energies and the attenuation data of Figure 16-2 and Table 16-1. Calculate the fluence contrast produced by the bone.

2. Determine the fluence contrast for the following: (a) 1 cm inclusion of fat in 12 cm soft tissue—use 45 kV_p and 1 mm Al filter; (b) 1 mm artery filled with Hypaque in 13 cm of soft tissue—use 90 kV_p radiation with 2 mm Al filter; (c) 2 cm inclusion of barium mix in 20 cm soft tissue using 90 kV_p with 2 mm Al filter. For these calculations, replace the spectrum of radiation by its equivalent energy and use the data of Figure 16-2 and Table 16-1.

*3. Determine the fluence contrast produced by a 1 cm thick bolus of air in the colon in a patient of 25 cm thickness of soft tissue. Use 105 kV_p, 2 mm Al filter, and the data of Table 16-1. Assume scattered radiation is removed by a grid.

*4. If we assume that a grid is not used, so that in addition to primary there is 3 times as much scattered radiation, calculate the fluence contrast for problem 3.

*5. Convert the spectrum for problem 3 into an exposure spectrum in R/keV interval using the data in the appendix (Table A-2) and repeat problem 3 to calculate the exposure contrast. Should this contrast be exactly the same as in problem 3?

6. If the tube voltage is increased from 70 to 90 kV_p and the focus-to-film distance is decreased from 120 to 100 cm while the tube current is held constant, calculate the factor by which the exposure time should be altered to yield a film with the same density. Assume n = 3.0 in equation 16-2.

7. With a suitable dosimeter verify equation 16-2 for two or three x ray machines in a radiology department. Find the value of n at 60, 80, and 120 kV_p. If the equation is not verified or is different from one machine to another, what checks will you make on the machine to find out why?

8. The input field size imaged on the 2.3 cm output phosphor of an image intensifier

is changed from 23 cm to 13 cm. What will be the change in brightness gain?

9. Calculate from first principles the brightness contrast for adjacent portions of a film with densities 0.50 and 0.55. Repeat the calculations for densities 1.00 and 1.05. Show that the contrast is the same for both cases.

10. A film transmits 0.05 of the light falling on it. Find its density. If two such films are placed together, what fraction of the incident light will be transmitted through the combination? What will be the density of the combination?

11. Using the characteristic curves of Figure 16-12 find and plot the gradients of the film exposed between screens and of the "no-screen" film as a function of density. Compare the plots for the two films.

12. Using Figure 16-12 find the intensification factor for the calcium tungstate screens at density 0.4 and 1.4. The intensification factor is the ratio of the exposure needed to produce a given density when the film is exposed directly to x rays to the exposure needed to produce the same density when the film is exposed between screens.

*13. Determine the characteristic curve of one of the x ray films used in a radiology department.

14. Calculate the minimum bandwidth necessary to transmit by television a chest radiograph 43 × 35 cm with a limiting resolution of 3 lp/mm. How many lines are required?

15. By means of a diagram, discuss what effect will be produced on a film when a focused grid designed for 100 cm is used at 150 cm.

16. Using a diagram, discuss what effect will be produced on a film when a grid focused for 100 cm is exposed with the x ray source in the correct plane but displaced laterally 25 cm. Consider both displacement in the direction of the lead strips and at right angles to this direction.

17. Using a suitable dosimeter, measure with and without the grid in place the x ray exposure to the surface of 20 cm of water required to produce a density of 1.0 on film exposed between screens on two or three x ray machines in a radiology department. Find the grid factors for the grids used in these machines.

18. A chest radiograph is taken at a source-to-film distance of 200 cm. Find the magnification produced in the image of a bone structure 25 cm from the film.

19. A radiograph is made of an object with a width of 3 mm using an x ray tube with a 2 mm focal spot at a source-to-film distance of 100 cm. The part being radiographed is 15 cm from the film. Find the size of the image and the size of the blurred region at its edges.

*20. Obtain a star pattern and determine the size of the focal spot of one of the tubes in the department.

*21. Design a copper sinusoidal test pattern for 60 keV photons with 1.5 line pairs per mm. Construct the test pattern to transmit between 10 and 90%; use the attenuation data in the appendix. Discuss the practicality of this device.

22. Show that equation 16-24 follows from equation 16-23.

23. Draw a diagram like Figure 16-22b for a square wave test pattern of 1.0 line pairs/mm and show that point B of Figure 16-23 is correctly plotted.

*24. Show that the sum of any number of sine curves of frequency f of amplitudes V_1 to V_n, but different phase angles δ_1 to δ_n, yields a sine wave also of frequency f, amplitude V, and phase angle δ where:

$$V = \sqrt{(V_x^2 + V_y^2)}$$
$$\tan \delta = V_y/V_x$$
$$V_x = (V_1 \cos \delta_1 + V_2 \cos \delta_2 \ldots + V_n \cos \delta_n)$$
$$V_y = (V_1 \sin \delta_1 + V_2 \sin \delta_2 + \ldots + V_n \sin \delta_n)$$

*25. Show that the Fourier coefficients for a Fourier series representing a slit that is very narrow compared with its repetition frequency are all the same.

*26. X rays passing through a very narrow slit produce a blackening on a film that corresponds to a triangular distribution of fluences rising from 0 at −0.5 mm to 1.00 at the center of the slit and falling to 0 at +0.5 mm. Determine and plot the modulation transfer function.

*27. X rays passing through a very narrow slit produce a blackening on a film that corresponds in fluence to 1.0 between positions 0.5 mm on either side of the slit center and 0 outside these limits. Calculate and plot the modulation transfer function.

*28. Write a computer program to perform the summation of equation 16-31b and show that a rectangular pulse is given by the sum of cosine terms with amplitude $\sin \pi \, fa_0/\pi fa_0$. Verify the data in Figure 16-24.

29. Using the correction given by Coltman (C14) and the data in Figure 16-23 show that the modulation transfer function for a sinusoidal test pattern may be found by correcting the contrast function for the square wave test pattern.

*30. The mathematical equations describing the focal spots of Figure 16-26 are given in the figure caption. Determine the Fourier transform for these three focal spots and verify the curves of Figure 16-26.

*31. Obtain a pinhole picture of the focal spot of one of the x ray tubes in the department using the film of problem 12. Measure the density of the film with a microdensitometer and convert the density profile to an exposure profile. Take the Fourier transform of this profile and thus determine the MTF of the focal spot.

*32. In a cineradiographic study of the heart, the maximum speed of motion of the coronary arteries is 10 cm s^{-1}. If the heart is imaged with a magnification of 1.3 and an exposure time of 4 ms, calculate the size of a double line focal spot that will give a modulation transfer function at the image intensifier similar to that due to the blurring due to heart motion.

*33. In problem 32, could the focal spot provide enough radiation in 4 ms to image the heart (a) on cine film, (b) on 100 mm film, and (c) directly on to a high speed screen-film combination?

*34. In problem 32, what other factors may lead to a loss of MTF in the intensifier image?

*35. Calculate as a function of energy the relative signal-to-noise ratio for a low level of iodine in a 20 cm patient when the exposure is kept constant for x ray energies from 30 keV to 80 keV.

*36. Repeat the calculation of problem 32 but for a constant dose to a fetus 8 cm deep from the anterior skin of a 20 cm patient with the beam direct in the anterior-posterior direction.

37. Using the assumptions made in the calculations carried out to obtain Figure 16-30, calculate the signal-to-noise ratio when the imaging device is a CsI intensifier with an x ray absorber of 100 mgm cm^{-2}. Use the data for curves I, J, and K given by Swark (S26). Is a CsI intensifier better than a Gd_2O_2S screen for imaging iodine?

38. In stereoradiography, find the correct tube shift for a source-to-film distance of 120 cm and a viewing distance of 60 cm.

39. In locating a foreign object, the tube shift method is used. A coin is placed on top of the patient and a double exposure taken with a tube shift of 30 cm. The source-to-film distance is 100 cm and the 2 image shifts are 5.0 and 7.2 cm. Find the distance of the foreign object below the coin.

40. Using the attenuation coefficients of Figure 16-2 and the relative photon fluence for a 105 kV$_p$ beam in Table 16-1, calculate the attenuation coefficient for a 105 kV$_p$

pencil beam after it has penetrated 5 cm and 20 cm of tissue (beam hardening effect). Neglect the small effect of scatter.

41. Measure the skin exposures to patients or to water phantoms for typical radiographs taken in several radiology departments. Compare these exposures with those in Table 16-6.

42. Measure the fluoroscopic exposure rates to patient or to water phantoms for several fluoroscopic x ray machines in radiology departments. Compare the results to Table 16-6.

43. Using film or TLD dosimeters measure the weekly exposure to the heads, bodies, and forearms of operators carrying out angiographic procedures in radiology departments.

Chapter 17

RADIOBIOLOGY

17.01   **INTRODUCTION**

In the earlier chapters of this book we have been concerned with the mechanisms of energy absorption on a *macroscopic* scale. We have been interested in the amount of energy deposited in tumor volumes consisting of cubic centimeters of material. However, when we come to inquire into basic radiobiological mechanisms, we are interested in amounts of energy absorbed in volumes corresponding to single cells or parts of cells. For such studies, we must know how energy is deposited as the high speed particle (electron, proton, α particle, neutron, etc.) passes through cells. This leads us to a discussion of the energy releases along the track of an ionizing particle. The energy once released gives rise to a variety of highly reactive chemical species which in turn may damage molecules of biological importance such as DNA, and so lead to cell death.

One of the most important cellular functions affected by radiation is the ability of the cell to divide and produce a line of progeny. If a cell retains such an ability following irradiation, it is said to have "survived." The survival of cells after radiation treatment has been extensively studied because of its obvious importance in cancer therapy. We will discuss survival curves in detail. We will then present some of the basic concepts of radiobiology.

Because radiation treatment is usually fractionated, that is, given in a series of daily doses spread over a number of weeks, the four factors that may influence the effect of such fractionated treatment will be discussed. These are the *repair* of sublethal damage, *repopulation* by surviving cells in the irradiated tissues, *redistribution* of cells throughout the division cycle, and *reoxygenation* of hypoxic cells, primarily in tumors. These are often referred to as the "four R's." The important concept of a therapeutic ratio will be described and the equivalence of different fractionation schedules as regards normal tissue or tumor response will be dealt with in terms of isoeffect curves. There will then be a description of some applications of radiobiology to radiotherapy including brief comments on some newer treatment approaches. Finally, we will show how such new radiotherapy techniques can be compared with existing ones by analyzing the survival of patients, and illustrate this with a discussion of the introduction of high energy radiation for treatment of patients with cancer of the cervix.

670

17.02   **INITIAL EVENT—THE PASSAGE OF THE**
CHARGED PARTICLES

EFFICIENCY OF RADIATION DAMAGE. It is important to realize that biological systems are extremely sensitive to radiation. In fact, while a *whole body* dose of 5 Gy will kill many mammals, the rise in temperature resulting from this dose is only 10^{-3} °C (for details regarding this statement, see section 9.12). Since the rise in temperature is so very small, it is clear that if this heat were evenly distributed over the irradiated tissues it could not possibly explain the biological effect. In chapter 6, however, we saw that electrons were set into motion and that the energy deposition was in fact concentrated along these electron tracks. We now examine in greater detail how these electrons (or other particles such as protons or alpha particles) release their energy to a biological system. A large body of evidence suggests that it is the damage done to the genetic material of the cell that determines its survival.

TRACKS OF CHARGED PARTICLES. When a charged particle passes through any material, it leaves a "track" of excited and ionized atoms and molecules. The tracks left by a fast electron and by an α particle in passing through DNA are illustrated in Figure 17-1a. For fast electrons, the energy releases are widely spaced, and even though the track may pass through the DNA, there is a chance that no energy releases will occur in it and no damage be done. The track left by an alpha particle, on the other hand, is so dense that if it passes through the DNA or even near it there will be enough energy released in it to destroy its function.

DISTRIBUTIONS IN SPACE OF ENERGY RELEASES. The energy releases by charged particles are discrete events. Each event gives rise to either an excited or an ionized molecule, along the path of the charged particle.

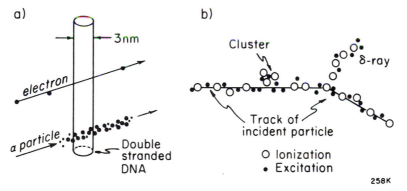

Figure 17-1. (a) Schematic representation of DNA and the tracks of an electron and α particle through it. The fast electron is depicted as depositing energy at 0.25 keV/μm, while the α particle of 5 MeV is shown depositing energy at the rate of 100 keV/μm. (b) Schematic drawing of a charged particle track illustrating the track, ion clusters, and δ ray spurs.

A track with ionization and excitation events is shown schematically in Figure 17-1b. When an atom is ionized, the secondary electron produced may have enough energy to cause several more ionizations or excitations before coming to rest. In a cloud chamber picture, these would appear as a cluster of ionizations near the track. One cluster is shown in Figure 17-1b. In a few cases, the secondary electron may have enough energy to produce a track of its own that will appear as a spur branching off from the main track. Energetic electrons of this kind are known as δ rays; δ rays may have any energy up to 1/2 the energy of the primary particle. The δ rays broaden the effective width of the particle track. This track through the material is tortuous due to the many collisions that occur between the particle and the atoms and molecules of the material. The spacings of the events along it will depend on the energy and type of particle.

LINEAR ENERGY TRANSFER (LET). The way the energy of a high speed particle is dissipated in the medium as the particle is slowed down was discussed in sections 6.12 and 6.17 where methods of calculating LET were developed. The student will remember that LET stands for "linear energy transfer," which in radiobiology is usually expressed in keV/μm of track. LET values encountered in radiobiology are listed in Table 17-1. A typical LET value for the electron tracks set in motion by cobalt 60 gamma rays is 0.25 keV/μm (C17). This would mean that on the average along each micrometer of track 250 eV would be released. In contrast, an alpha particle will lose about 1000 times as much energy in a given length of track, yielding an LET of 250 keV/μm. Table 17-1 also shows typical data for neutrons. Neutrons carry no charge and so do not themselves produce ionization but they do collide with nuclei, in particular with protons, setting them in motion. The LET values for neutrons are thus similar to those of protons.

TABLE 17-1
LET of Ionizing Particles of Radiobiological Interest

Particle	Charge	Energy (MeV)	LET (keV/μm)
Electron	−1	0.001	12.3
		0.010	2.30
		0.100	0.42
		1.00	0.25
		200 kV$_p$ x rays	0.4-36
		cobalt 60 γ rays	0.2-2
Proton	+1	small	92
		2	16
		5	8
		10	4
Alpha	+2	small	260
		5	95
Neutron	0	2.5	15-80 (peak at 20)
		14.1	3-30 (peak at 7)

Spectrum of LET Values. The LET of an ionizing particle depends in a complicated way (I13) on the velocity (energy) and the charge possessed by the particle. The greater the charge and the smaller the velocity, the greater the LET. This was illustrated in Figure 6-16, where LET was plotted as a function of depth for a number of particles. At the surface of the phantom, where the particles have their full energy, LET is small. With increase in depth, the particle loses energy more and more rapidly to reach a maximum rate of energy loss (the Bragg peak) just as it comes to rest. We will see later that the biological effect of radiation depends upon the LET; hence it is important to know the LET at each point in the irradiated volume if one is to predict the biological response.

In most situations that arise in radiotherapy there is a complex spectrum of electrons set into motion, even when the source is monoenergetic, as with cobalt 60. In particular, Table 17-1 shows that cobalt 60 delivers a spectrum of LET values from 0.2 to 2 keV/μm. Approximately the same range of LETs would be produced by x rays in the 4 to 25 MeV range. For these low LET radiations, the LET spectrum is essentially the same at all depths in the irradiated tissue. In contrast, when beams of heavy charged particles are used, the LET varies with depth and great care must be taken to know both *the dose* and *the LET* of the particles at each point in the irradiated volume. This complicates the problem but gives the therapist one more parameter he may be able to manipulate to his advantage in attempting to destroy a tumor and spare normal tissue.

Although the LET gives the average energy loss by a particle per unit length of travel, of still more relevance is the way the energy is deposited in small critical volumes or "targets" in the biological system. This energy deposit on the average is the product of the LET and the path length through the volume. Rossi (R15) has developed an ingenious method to measure the distribution of such energy releases in volumes as small as 1 cubic μm (10^{-18} m^3) demonstrating the large variations in energy depositions from one small volume to another due to statistical fluctuations. The radiobiological implications of these measurements are discussed by Rossi (R16).

17.03   IMMEDIATE RADIOCHEMICAL EFFECTS

Production of Solvated Electrons and Radicals

Following the passage of the charged particle with the production of excited and ionized atoms and molecules, a number of physical and chemical events take place in rapid succession. Since cells are more than 70% water, most of the energy is absorbed by this water, giving rise to the events that are described in the following equations relating to radiation chemistry. We will see later how the reactive species produced in water attack the components of the cell.

$$H_2O \xrightarrow{h\nu} H_2O^+ + e^- \longrightarrow H_2O^+ + e^-_{aq} \qquad (17\text{-}1a)$$

$$H_2O^+ \longrightarrow \cdot OH + H^+ \qquad (17\text{-}1b)$$

$$H_2O \xrightarrow{h\nu} H_2O^* \longrightarrow H \cdot + \cdot OH \qquad (17\text{-}1c)$$

When a water molecule is disrupted by the passage of an ionizing particle, it may be ionized as in equation 17-1a to yield an ionized water molecule, H_2O^+, and an electron. This electron will leave the parent molecule and will become trapped among other water molecules, which because of their polar nature, tend to have their more positively charged hydrogen atoms facing the electron and the more negatively charged oxygen atom away from the electron (as illustrated in Fig. 17-2a). This arrangement of an electron trapped among water molecules is called a solvated or aqueous electron and is represented by e^-_{aq}. It is a transient species with a lifetime of about 1 ms in pure water. It can be detected because it has a strong absorption band at 720 nm (B33).

The fate of the ionized water molecule, H_2O^+, is described by equation 17-1b. It breaks up into a hydrogen ion, H^+, and an hydroxyl radical, $\cdot OH$. The hydrogen ion is just a proton (as illustrated in Fig. 17-2e) and is the normal ion found in any acidic solution. The free radical, $\cdot OH$, is an uncharged species with one electron short of the number required to give stability (see sec. 1.06) and is therefore very reactive. The $\cdot OH$ has a lifetime of about 1 μs in pure water and an absorption band at about 260 nm (A14, T13). The unpaired electron is represented in the diagram by a dot. Its position in the radical is not known.

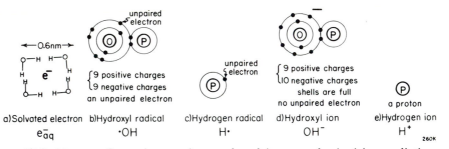

Figure 17-2. Nature of reactive species produced in water by ionizing radiations. (a) Aqueous electron or solvated electron; (b) hydroxyl radical $\cdot OH$; (c) hydrogen radical $H \cdot$; (d) hydroxyl ion OH^-, (e) hydrogen ion H^+.

Finally, water may be excited by the ionizing event to yield an excited water molecule represented by H_2O^*, as indicated by equation 17-1c. H_2O^* breaks apart to give the hydrogen radical $H \cdot$ (Fig. 17-2c) and the hydroxyl radical $\cdot OH$ (Fig. 17-2b). Both have unpaired electrons and are reactive entities. The hydrogen radical has a lifetime of about 1 μsec in pure water and an absorption peak at 200 nm (T14).

The net result of these processes is to produce in water three important reactive species, e_{aq}^-, · OH, and H · with relative yields of about 45%, 45%, and 10% if observed a few μs after the event. The production of these species occurs in about 10^{-6} μs and they remain in pure water for from 1 to 100 μs, and in biological systems for times in the range of 0.1 to 1 μs. These reactive species bring about radiation damage to the biological system by attacking molecules in the cell. It is generally believed that of these species the · OH radical is the most effective in causing biological damage. It is an oxidizing agent and can extract a hydrogen atom from DNA, leaving a radical site on the DNA. Since it is the radiation products from water that attack the cell, the process is called the *indirect mechanism*. Radiation can of course also ionize or excite the cellular macromolecules *directly* and this is called the *direct mechanism*. Both mechanisms can lead to cellular damage. There is good evidence to suggest that damage to DNA is critical for cell survival. Such damage may lead to bases in the DNA being altered or to the sugar phosphate backbone of the molecule being broken. The break can be in one strand or in both. There are also suggestions that damage to membrane or membrane-DNA complexes may be important.

The cell has elaborate mechanisms designed to repair damage so the long-term effects of irradiation will depend on the effectiveness of these repair mechanisms, which in turn may depend on the way the cells are handled *after* the irradiation.

Dependence of Radiation Damage on LET

The effect of radiation on a cell may be strongly dependent on the LET of the ionizing particle involved. If the critical effect can be caused by a single ionization or an ion cluster, then the effect of a given dose will decrease with increase in LET because as the LET increases the spacing between the ionizations decreases and more than one ionization may occur at the critical site. The extra ionizations will be wasted. If, on the other hand, the effect only occurs when a sufficient number of ionizations have been deposited in the radiation sensitive structure, the effect produced by a given dose will increase rapidly with increasing LET. For still higher LET values, ionizations are again wasted. We would expect then that the effect should pass through a maximum and decline. This is illustrated by the work of Skarsgard S29 (see Fig. 17-3a) where the efficiency of radiation in killing cells is plotted as a function of LET. The particles of different LET were obtained using high energy beams of charged nuclei of He, Li, B, C, O, Ne, and A. Clearly, particles with an LET of about 100 keV/μm deposit energy in such a way as to give optimum killing.

Somewhat similar results are illustrated in Figure 17-3b based on data

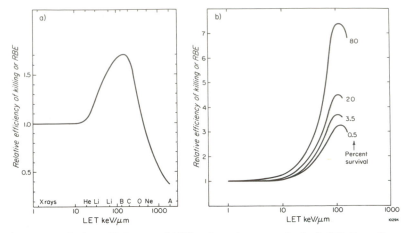

Figure 17-3. (a) Relative efficiency of killing based on survival of CH_2B_2 cells as a function of LET. (Adapted from Skarsgard et al., S29). (b) Data from Elkind and Whitmore (E8) based on the work of Barendsen et al. (B34).

by Barendsen (B34), who used a number of types of ionizing radiation to kill cells. The curves all show a peak sensitivity at about 100 keV/μm. The four curves were obtained for four different levels of survival as indicated. The relative efficiency of killing can be expressed in terms of the radiobiological equivalent (RBE), which will be discussed in section 17.08. The fact that the RBE varies with survival level means the *shape of the survival curves* depends on LET (see Fig. 17-8).

17.04   **ASSAYS FOR PROLIFERATIVE CAPACITY—SURVIVAL CURVES**

One of the most radiosensitive functions of a cell is its ability to retain indefinite proliferative capacity after irradiation. Cells that retain this capacity sufficiently to provide evidence of macroscopic growth are said to have survived the irradiation, while those that do not are regarded as having been killed even though they may undergo a few divisions and still be present in the cell population.

COLONY ASSAY METHOD—IN VITRO. The commonest way to obtain a survival curve is the tissue culture method due originally to Puck (P19). The cells are grown in tissue culture in a defined medium. The number of surviving cells in a suspension is determined by placing a given number of cells on a petri dish with an appropriate medium and incubating them for about 10 days at 37° C. After this time, each surviving cell will have grown into a colony with some 10^3 cells, which can be seen and counted. The appearance of such a petri dish is shown in the insert of Figure 17-4. The number of cells plated is adjusted to give 200 to 400 colonies per plate. To obtain a survival curve, aliquots of the cells are removed after a series of doses and appropriate dilutions performed before plating. The fraction of cells surviving a given dose is directly determined from the number of visible colonies on the plates and the known dilutions. Typical survival curves are shown in Figure 17-4.

IN VIVO ASSAYS. The in vitro method described above has been widely used in radiobiology but it is of crucial importance to study the effect of radiation on cells in their normal environment (in vivo). A number of techniques have been developed over the last 20 years to do this. One of the most elegant is the *spleen-colony method* developed by Till and McCulloch (T15) to determine survival curves for hematopoietic stem cells in the bone marrow. A cell suspension is prepared from the bone marrow of a donor mouse and a known number of these cells are injected intravenously into a heavily irradiated recipient mouse. This irradiation destroys the endogeneous stem cells, allowing the injected ones to grow at a number of sites in the mouse. Cells that lodge in the spleen grow to form discrete colonies, which can be counted just like colonies on a petri dish (see insert of Fig. 17-4). Using this technique, a survival curve for bone marrow stem cells can be established by irradiating the mice donating the cells and determining the number of spleen colonies per injected cell as a function of dose. This technique has also been used by Bush and Bruce (B35) to determine survival curves for leukemic cells, which also form colonies in the spleen. An analogous method that involves counting tumor cell colonies growing in the lungs of recipient mice has been developed for studying the radiation sensitivity of cells in a number of solid animal tumors (H23, H24).

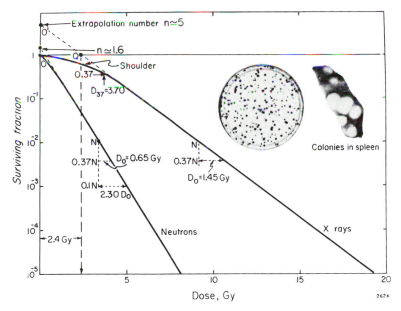

Figure 17-4. Survival curves for hamster fibroblast cells exposed to 280 kV$_p$ x rays and 3 MeV neutrons (adapted from Schneider and Whitmore, S30). The inserts show colonies in a petri dish and on a spleen.

Another of the early techniques for studying leukemic cells was introduced by Hewitt and Wilson (H25) and is called the *limiting dilution assay*. In this method mice with leukemia are irradiated with a series of doses and suspensions of leukemic cells are prepared. Each suspension is then subjected to a series of dilutions and each dilution is injected back into a group of recipient mice. Some mice that receive at least one cell capable of proliferating sufficiently to kill the animal will develop leukemia and die, while those given a sufficiently dilute inoculum will not. By determining the limiting dilution at which a constant fraction of the mice develop leukemia, the number of surviving leukemic cells in the cell suspension can be determined as a function of dose. An analogous method that can be used to study the radiosensitivity of cells in solid tumors is to irradiate the tumor, mince it to produce a cell suspension, and then determine the minimum dilution that will lead to the development of tumors in injected mice (P20).

More recently both of these basic methods have been partially superseded by technical advances that allow both bone marrow and some tumor cells to be grown in vitro, either in semisolid or liquid media. The cells can thus be irradiated in their host animals and their survival determined in vitro using the approach described above (A15, T16).

Finally, a series of ingenious methods have been developed in which cells surviving treatment are allowed to form colonies in situ, i.e. at the site at which they were treated. Such a method is widely used to study the sensitivity of individual crypt stem cells in the small intestine (W12). A series of doses sufficient to reduce the number of surviving crypt cells to a low level are given to mice. The surviving cells grow rapidly to form regenerating crypts, which can be identified on histological sections. By determining the number of regenerating crypts (colonies) as a function of dose, the final slope of the dose-response curve can be obtained. Because the number of stem cells present in each crypt before irradiation is not known, this technique cannot be used to determine the initial part of the survival curve.

17.05   MATHEMATICAL ASPECTS OF SURVIVAL CURVES

Two typical survival curves are shown in Figure 17-4 where the surviving fraction of cells is plotted on a log scale as a function of dose on a linear scale. At large doses these curves become straight showing that in this region the survival decreases exponentially with dose, while at small doses the curves are flattened yielding a shoulder. There are a number of mathematical ways to define the shape of survival curves. All of these are based on the concept of the random nature of energy deposition by radiation. One of the earliest theories is due to Lea (L14) and is often called "target" theory.

SINGLE HIT SURVIVAL CURVE. Suppose a biological sample, which contains N biological entities (such as tumor cells), is given a small dose of radiation dD, which inactivates a small number, dN, of these entities. The number of inactivations, dN, should be proportional to N and dD so that:

$$dN = - \frac{1}{D_0} \cdot N \, dD \qquad (17\text{-}2)$$

where $1/D_0$ is a constant of proportionality and the negative sign indicates that the number of active entities N decreases with increase in dose. This equation was discussed in sections 1.20 to 1.22 and is similar to equations describing the decay of radioactive sources or the attenuation of an x ray beam passing through material. It can be integrated to yield:

$$N = N_0 \, e^{-D/D_0} \qquad \text{(single hit survival curve)} \qquad (17\text{-}3)$$

where N_0 is the number of entities present at zero dose. The curve for neutron inactivation shown in Figure 17-4 is very nearly exponential over the whole dose range and is reasonably well described by this equation, but the curve for x rays is not because of the shoulder.

We now discuss the meaning of D_0. If we place $D = D_0$ in equation 17-3 we find that $N = N_0 e^{-1} = 0.37 \, N_0$. *The mean lethal dose* (D_0) *is the dose required to reduce the population of entities from any value N to 0.37 N* on parts of the survival curve that are exponential. D_0 has another meaning. Equation 17-2 tells us that *initially* a dose ΔD will lead to an inactivation of ΔN entities given by $\Delta N = (\Delta D/D_0)N_0$. If the initial rate of inactivation continued until a dose $\Delta D = D_0$ had been given, the number of inactivations would be $\Delta N = N_0$. Thus, *the mean lethal dose* (D_0) *is the dose that would be required to place one inactivating event ("hit") in each of the biological entities if none were wasted.* Due, however, to the random nature of the energy deposits, some energy will go to cells that have already been destroyed and will be wasted, while some cells will escape altogether so that instead of destroying all the cells, the mean lethal dose (D_0) only destroys 63% of them.

MULTI-TARGET SINGLE HIT SURVIVAL CURVE. The shoulder on the survival curve (Fig. 17-4) cannot be explained by equation 17-3. We can, however, obtain an expression that leads to a shoulder and that fits experimental data quite well. Suppose the cell has "n" targets, each of which must be inactivated to cause cell death. The probability of a single target *not* being hit is e^{-D/D_0} (see eq. 17-3). Therefore, the probability that any individual target will be hit is $(1 - e^{-D/D_0})$. Hence the probability of all of the n targets within one cell being hit is $(1 - e^{-D/D_0})^n$. Thus the probability of survival of a cell that contains n targets is $1 - (1 - e^{-D/D_0})^n$. This leads us to the multi-target single hit equation:

$$N = N_0 \left[1 - (1 - e^{-D/D_0})^n \right] \qquad \text{(multi-target single hit)} \quad (17\text{-}4)$$

For doses large compared with D_0, the student may show that this expression reduces to:

$$N = N_0 \, n e^{-D/D_0} \quad \text{valid for} \quad D \gg D_0 \qquad (17\text{-}5)$$

Since, for large doses, the relation between N and D is exponential it appears as a straight line when plotted on semilog paper. For the x ray curve of Figure 17-4, $D_0 = 1.45$ Gy.

A plot of equation 17-4 will convince the student that this expression leads to a shoulder, which can be described by either the extrapolation number n or the quasithreshold dose, D_q. These parameters are obtained by extrapolating the straight-line section of the survival curve back to zero dose to locate points O' and Q. If we place $D = 0$ in equation 17-5 then $N = n \, N_0$, showing that point O' determines the number of targets n or the extrapolation number. In our example $n \approx 5$. The quasi-threshold dose, D_q, is the distance OQ; it is determined from equation 17-5 by finding the dose D_q that makes $N = N_0$, i.e.

$$1 = n \, e^{-D_q/D_0} \quad \text{or} \quad n = e^{D_q/D_0} \quad \text{or} \quad D_q = D_0 \ln n \qquad (17\text{-}6)$$

This is the relation between n and D_q. For our example, $D_q = 2.40$ Gy so $n = e^{2.40/1.45} = 5.2$ in agreement with the value 5 obtained from the extrapolation number.

OTHER TYPES OF SURVIVAL CURVES. The student may easily show that the survival curve described by equation 17-4 has zero slope at small doses so that the first increment of dose would produce *no* cell killing. Since this is contrary to most observations, a number of more complicated mathematical models have been proposed. One such equation is:

$$\frac{N}{N_0} = e^{-D/D_s}\left[1 - (1 - e^{-D/D_0})^n\right] \qquad (17\text{-}7)$$

The extra parameter D_s is introduced to define the initial slope of the survival curve in the same way as D_0 defines the final slope of the survival curves.*

Another equation that has been proposed by a number of investigators (C18, R16) is:

$$N = N_0 e^{-(\alpha D + \beta D^2)} \qquad (17\text{-}8)$$

This equation defines a survival curve that is concave downwards on a semilog plot and never becomes strictly exponential, although the curvature is small at large doses since β is always much less than α. One way in which this equation can be derived is to assume that two separate sublesions must interact to cause lethality. At the present time the nature of these sublesions is not clear. They might, for example, be

---

*If D_s is large compared with D_0 the final slope of the exponential curve is determined by D_0 and the introduction of D_s does not complicate the expression for large doses. If, however, D_s is comparable to D_0 the final slope is determined by $D_0' = D_0 D_s/(D_0 + D_s)$.

single strand DNA breaks (C18,C19). Such sublesions can be caused by a single ionizing track giving a direct dependence on the first power of the dose, or by two separate tracks producing sublesions independently, giving a dependence on (dose)². The parameters α and β describe the probability of these two mechanisms. These ideas are discussed by Chapman (C20).

In the early days of radiobiology it was usually assumed that if one could fit a survival curve to experimental data one would be able to determine the size and types of targets involved in cell killing. This is no longer believed since survival curves are not precise enough to unequivocally distinguish between various mathematical models, and similar equations can often be developed with very different biological assumptions. For example, the extrapolation number, n, may have nothing to do with the number of targets but might indicate that the cell has repair mechanisms that prevent small amounts of damage from causing cell death. Similarly, equation 17-8 can be derived using assumptions that have nothing to do with the interaction of sublesions (H26).

CALCULATIONS USING SURVIVAL CURVES. Dose calculations using survival curves can often be simplified using D_q and D_0 as illustrated in Figure 17-5. Provided the extrapolated curve and the experimental curve coincide for all doses greater than D_{10} (10% survival), it is easily seen that:

$$D_T = D_q + T(2.30)D_0 \qquad (17\text{-}9)$$

where T is the power of ten by which the surviving fraction is to be reduced and 2.30 is ln (10), so 2.30 D_0 is the dose required to reduce the population by a factor of 10 (see eq. 17-3).

Example 17-1. A tumor contains 10^8 cells. Calculate the dose required to reduce the tumor to 1 surviving cell. Assume $D_0 = 1.45$ Gy and $D_q = 2.40$ Gy.

The population should be reduced by a factor of 10^8 so T = 8.
$D_8 = D_q + 8(2.30) D_0 = (2.40 + 26.7)$ Gy = 29.1 Gy.
The required dose is 29.1 Gy.

Figure 17-5. Simplified survival curve illustrating the calculation of the dose required to reduce the surviving population by various powers of 10.

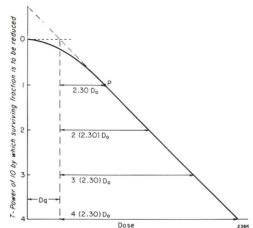

17.06   STATISTICAL NATURE OF RADIATION DAMAGE

In the above example we determined that a dose of 29.1 Gy would reduce the tumor population from 10^8 cells to 1 cell. On the average this is
correct *but* because of the statistical nature of the problem we would expect that, in a group of identical tumors, some would have no surviving
cells, some one, some two, etc. Since radiation damage is random in nature, cell survival follows the Poisson distribution discussed in section
14.05 in dealing with statistical errors in counting a radioactive source.
Let P_n be the probability of finding "n" surviving cells in a tumor when
the expected number is "a"—then the Poisson relation is:

$$P_n = \frac{a^n e^{-a}}{n!} \qquad (17\text{-}10)$$

We illustrate the use of this equation by the following example.

Example 17-2. Imagine that 100 identical tumors with the properties
described in example 17-1 were given 29.1 Gy. Determine the probability of finding tumors with 0, 1, 2, and 3 surviving cells.

For this case the expected number of surviving cells is a = 1.

$$P_0 = \frac{1\,e^{-1}}{0!} = .373 \qquad\qquad P_2 = \frac{1^2\,e^{-1}}{2!} = .186$$

$$P_1 = \frac{1^1\,e^{-1}}{1!} = .373 \qquad\qquad P_3 = \frac{1^3\,e^{-1}}{3!} = .062$$

The sum of these probabilities is 0.994, close to 1.000.

PROBABILITY OF CURE. From this example, we would expect that of the
100 tumors, 37 would be cured, i.e. have no surviving tumor cells, while
the rest would have one or more surviving cells. The important probability is the probability of cure, i.e. the probability, P_0, that no tumor cell
survives. Putting n = 0 in equation 17-10 we obtain a simplified version
of the Poisson distribution:

$$P_0 = \text{probability of cure} = e^{-a} \qquad (17\text{-}11)$$

where "a" is the average or expected number of surviving cells in the
tumor.

It is convenient to plot the percentage of tumors cured on a *linear* scale
as a function of dose, as illustrated in Figure 17-6. The dose scale involves the parameter T, which is the power of ten by which the surviving
fraction is to be reduced. For T = 7 the dose is $D_q + 7(2.30)\,D_0$; for
T = 8 the dose is larger by $(2.30\,D_0)$; etc. The vertical scale gives the percent of tumors cured. For example, for T = 8 we expect that in a tumor
of 10^8 cells "a" = 1, i.e. there is one survivor on the average and according to equation 17-11 the percentage cured is $100\,e^{-1} = 37.3$. This locates

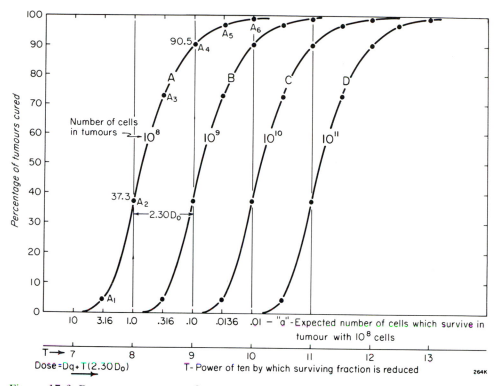

Figure 17-6. Dose response curve for tumors containing 10^8, 10^9, 10^{10}, and 10^{11} cells. T is the power of ten by which the surviving fraction is reduced. The scale "a" gives the expected number of surviving cells for the tumor with 10^8 cells.

point A_2. For a dose 2.30 D_0 larger, T = 9 and "a" = 0.1 leading to point A_4 at 100 $e^{-.1}$ = 90.5. It is left as an exercise for the student to locate points A_1, A_3, A_5, and A_6. Curve A has a sigmoid shape and is often referred to as a *dose response curve*, or in this case a dose cure curve.

Figure 17-6 also shows the cure curves B, C, and D for tumors containing 10^9, 10^{10}, and 10^{11} cells. These curves all have exactly the same shape. Curve B is drawn by shifting curve A to the right by a dose increment of 2.30 · D_0. Curves C and D are located by shifts 2 and 3 times as large respectively.

The calculations we have made in determining the dose cure curve of Figure 17-6 imply a precision that is not achievable by a clinician treating patients, since it is impossible to obtain a group of identical tumors. In the first place, the tumors will not all be of the same size and even if they were they might contain quite different numbers of clonogenic cells (a cell capable of regrowing the tumor). To be specific, a tumor containing 10^{11} cells might contain only 10^8 clonogenic cells, and this is the number that should be used for the calculations above.

In spite of these reservations some basic radiobiological information can be obtained from curves such as Figure 17-6. For example, suppose a study on patients gave a dose cure curve of the same general shape as one of the curves of Figure 17-6. The dose increment required to go from 37% control (point A_2) to 90% control (point A_4) could be read from the graph allowing one to estimate D_0 since $D_0 = (D_{A4} - D_{A2})/2.3$. In most situations, there is no other way to determine D_0 for a tumor growing in a patient. The value of D_0 obtained thus is an upper limit, as illustrated in the following example.

Example 17-3. Plot a dose response curve for a group of 100 patients, half of whom had tumors with 10^8 clonogenic cells and the other half 10^9 cells. Assume $D_0 = 1.45$ Gy and $D_q = 2.40$ Gy.

The solution of this problem can be obtained using equations 17-9 and 17-11. We first enter appropriate values for T in the first column of Table 17-2. We then calculate the corresponding dose using equation 17-9 and enter these in column 2. The expected number of survivors is then determined by dividing 10^8 or 10^9 by 10^T. For example, the first entry is $10^8/10^{7.5} = 3.16$. These are entered in column 3 and 4. In columns 5 and 6 we enter $100\,e^{-a}$, which gives the percent of tumors cured. The last column gives the average of columns 5 and 6, which gives the percentage of patients cured assuming the mixed population.

From the curve generated by the data in columns 2 and 7, the student can determine that the increment in dose required to change the cure rate from 37% to 90% is 4.25 Gy. Thus the effective D_0 is 1.85 Gy. In general, calculations of this kind with tumors in patients will overestimate D_0 because even tumors of the same size are unlikely to have the same number of clonogenic cells.

TABLE 17-2

(1) T	(2) Dose (Gy)	(3) "a"—expected No.	(4)	(5) % cured ($100\,e^{-a}$)	(6)	(7)
	(Gy)	10^8 cells	10^9 cells	10^8 cells	10^9 cells	Mixed
7.5	27.41	3.16	31.6	4.2	0.0	2.1
8.0	29.08	1.00	10.0	36.8	0.0	18.4
8.5	30.74	.316	3.16	72.9	4.2	38.6
9.0	32.41	.100	1.00	90.5	36.8	63.6
9.5	34.08	.0316	.316	96.9	72.9	84.9
10.0	35.75	.0100	.100	99.0	90.5	94.7
10.5	37.42	.00316	.0316	99.7	96.9	98.3

17.07   NORMAL AND TUMOR CELLS—THERAPEUTIC RATIO

The aim of the radiotherapist in treating a patient is to deliver enough radiation to the tumor to destroy it without irradiating normal tissue to a dose that will lead to serious complications. The idea of a compromise between tumor control and the development of complica-

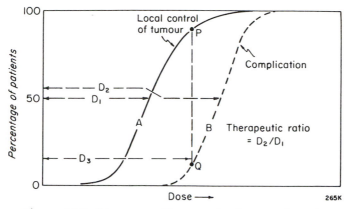

Figure 17-7. Diagram to illustrate the therapeutic ratio.

tions gives rise to the concept of a therapeutic ratio. This is illustrated in Figure 17-7, where curve A is tumor control as a function of dose and curve B represents the percentage of patients who will develop complications as a function of dose. Conceptually curves A and B are meaningful but the precise plotting of them is very difficult because the appropriate data is not available. The situation illustrated in Figure 17-7 is favorable since the dose D_3 is large enough to control the tumor in 90% of patients (point P) while this same dose leads to complications in less than 10% of patients (point Q). The favorable situation arises because curve B is shifted well to the right of curve A. The situation could be described by saying that the therapeutic ratio is large. There is no agreement on how this ratio should be defined; one definition could be D_2/D_1 as illustrated, where D_2 is the dose that leads to serious complications in 50% of the patients and D_1 is the dose that gives tumor control in the same % of patients.

In the early days of radiotherapy it was usually assumed that normal cells were less sensitive to radiation than tumor cells, but the vast majority of radiobiological studies indicate that D_0 values for different mammalian cells irradiated with x or γ rays cluster quite closely around a value of about 1.3 Gy. There seems to be a wider variation in the values of D_q or n that are observed, but there is no evidence that malignant cells generally have different sensitivities to radiation than normal cells. If the skin is the critical normal tissue, i.e. the one whose tolerance dose may limit the radiation dose prescribed, one usually achieves a very good therapeutic ratio, as illustrated in Figure 17-7. For other tumor and critical normal tissue combinations, the curves A and B may be much closer together or even reversed so that the dose required to achieve even a small fraction of cures may result in a significant level of complications. One aim of radiobiology is to find ways of improving the therapeutic ratio. We will deal with this problem in subsequent sections.

17.08 **RADIOBIOLOGICAL EQUIVALENT (RBE)**

Before 1945 most radiotherapy of deep-seated tumors was carried out using 200-400 kV$_p$ x rays. With the widespread introduction of higher energy radiations from cobalt units, betatrons, and linacs it was necessary to compare the effects of these new radiations with the older ones. The easiest comparison is to determine the RBE, defined thus:

$$RBE = \frac{\text{Dose from standard radiation to produce a given biological effect}}{\text{Dose from the test radiation to produce the same biological effect}} \qquad (17\text{-}12)$$

where the standard radiation is usually 200 kV$_p$ x rays.

The determination of RBE is illustrated in Figure 17-8, where neutrons are compared with x rays. These survival curves are the same as those presented in Figure 17-4. The RBE is the ratio of doses that give the same level of survival, for example OX/ON. Because the curves are not the same shape (one has a large shoulder, the other does not) the RBE will depend upon the surviving fraction at which the comparison is made (see insert of Fig. 17-8). In addition, the RBE may depend upon the biological effect being observed. In this case, the end point is survival; other end points could be used, for example, animal death, skin erythema, etc.

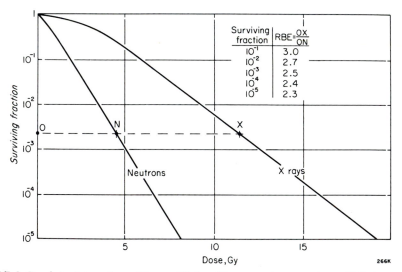

Figure 17-8. Replot of data from Figure 17-4 to illustrate the meaning of RBE. The insert shows the RBE for different surviving fractions.

The RBE of Co-60 radiation or 4–20 MeV radiation relative to 250 kV$_p$ x rays is in the range 0.8 to 0.9, i.e. for the same biological effect a 10 to 20% larger dose of high energy radiation is required to produce the same effect as 250 kV$_p$ x rays. High energy electrons have an RBE in the range 0.7 to 0.8. In contrast to these values, which are close to but *less* than 1.0, heavier particles with their higher LET have RBE values greater than 1.0. For example high energy neutrons have an RBE in the range 1.5 to 3.0 while negative π mesons have RBE values in the range 2 to 3.

An increase in the RBE in itself is of no therapeutic advantage, unless there is a differential effect so that the RBE for normal tissue is smaller than the RBE for the tumor. This would increase the level of tumor cell kill in relation to normal tissue damage, thereby effectively shifting curves A and B of Figure 17-7 farther apart and so increasing the therapeutic ratio.

17.09   CELL CYCLE AND RADIOSENSITIVITY

So far, we have discussed survival curves without regard for the physiological state of the cell during irradiation. The sensitivity of cells is dependent on many factors. One such factor is the position of the cell in its proliferation cycle. The insert to Figure 17-9a shows a typical cell cycle, which depicts the progression of a cell from one division to the next. This cell cycle is marked by two well-defined portions: mitosis, M, where division takes place and the period of DNA synthesis, S. The S and M portions of the cycle are separated by two periods, G_1 (gap 1) and G_2 (gap 2), when DNA is not synthesized but other metabolic processes continue. For mammalian cells growing in culture the S phase is usually in the range 6–8 hours, M less than an hour, G_2 in the range 2–4 hours, and G_1 (which is more variable) lasting from 1–8 hours. The total cell cycle time is usually 10–20 hours.

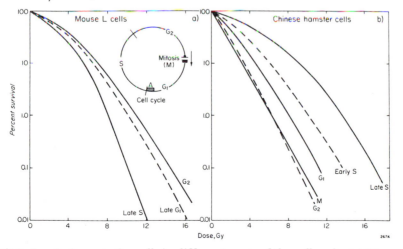

Figure 17-9. Survival curves for cells in different parts of the cell cycle. (a) Mouse L cells synchronized with tritiated thymidine and irradiated with 250 kV$_p$ x rays. (Adapted from Whitmore, W13.) (b) Chinese hamster cells synchronized by shaking from a glass plate at mitosis and irradiated with 50 kV$_p$ x rays. (Adapted from Sinclair, S31.)

In a growing cell population the constituent cells will be asynchronously distributed through all phases of the cycle. It is possible by a number of experimental procedures to select, for examination, groups of cells of similar age (e.g. as illustrated by the group at A in the insert to Fig. 17-9a). When such *synchronous* cell populations are exposed to radiation, we observe a variation in radiosensitivity with cell age as illustrated in Figure 17-9, which shows survival curves for two lines of cells in different phases of their cycle. For mouse L cells, late S-phase appears to be the most sensitive period, while for Chinese hamster cells, the reverse is the case. Other cell lines that have been studied show individual patterns of sensitivity.

Because of this cell-age-specific radiosensitivity, an asynchronous cell population will be partially synchronized by irradiation since those cells in the sensitive portions of the cycle will have a lower probability of survival than those in the resistant phases. Thus when an asynchronous cell population is irradiated, the surviving cells will be partially synchronized into the resistant phase(s). As these cells progress through the cell cycle they will move into the more sensitive phases. It was initially hoped that physicians could take advantage of the increase in sensitivity of a tumor cell population, which results from this partial synchronization. However, practical attempts to exploit such synchronization to improve the therapeutic ratio during the course of a treatment involving 20 to 30 fractions have not proved possible.

REDISTRIBUTION. As a cell population continues to grow following irradiation, the partially synchronized surviving cells are rapidly redistributed throughout the cell cycle, with the result that the cell population will again contain some cells in sensitive phases. This process of redistribution in proliferating cell population will thus tend to increase the cell kill from fractionated treatment relative to that from a single dose. Such an effect will not, of course, occur in nonproliferating cell populations. Consequently, if during a treatment the critical normal tissue is a nonproliferative tissue, redistribution will tend to improve the therapeutic ratio. Redistribution is only one of a number of factors known to influence the response of cell populations to fractionation; two other factors that have the opposite effect are discussed in the next section.

17.10   FRACTIONATION

It has been found empirically, over the 80 years that radiation has been used to treat patients with malignant disease, that fractionating the radiation treatment, so that it is given over a period of weeks, results in a better therapeutic ratio for most tumors than giving the treatment as a single dose. When radiation treatment is fractionated it is found that a much greater total dose is required to achieve a given level of biological damage than when a single dose is used. This indicates that recovery from radiation damage occurs between fractions. This recovery is a complex process involving repair of damage by individual cells and the effects of cell growth during the fractionated course of treatment.

REPAIR. The fact that the survival curves shown in Figure 17-4 have a shoulder (particularly for low LET radiation) suggests that some radiation damage must be accumulated in the cells before they are killed at an exponential rate. Elkind and Sutton (E9) showed that this sublethal damage can be repaired (as illustrated in Fig. 17-10). When the cells were irradiated with single doses, the typical survival curve OO'Q P with a shoulder (n = 5.2) and an exponential portion was obtained. A sample of cells was irradiated with 5.05 Gy to bring them to point O'. At this point the cells were incubated at 37° C for 18 hours to see if some of the damage could be repaired. The cells were then irradiated with a second dose. If no repair had taken place, the curve would follow O'Q.P. The data gave the curve O'Q'P', showing that repair had taken place and that the original shoulder had reappeared.

A variable time was allowed to elapse between the two fractions, and the results are shown in the insert to Figure 17-10. If no repair time was

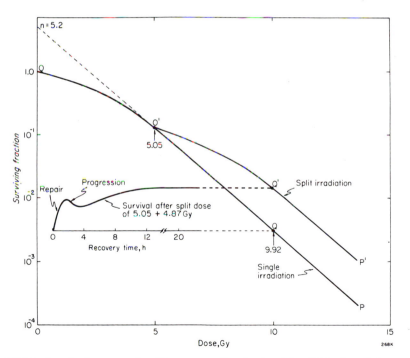

Figure 17-10. Survival curves for Hamster cells obtained by Elkind and Sutton (E9). Curve OO'QP is the survival curve for cells given single exposures. Curve OO'Q'P' is the survival curve when the cells are given 5.05 Gy in one dose, allowed to recover for 18.1 hours, and then given the rest of the radiation. The insert shows the survival of cells given a split dose of 5.05 Gy + 4.87 Gy as a function of the recovery time between the two fractions.

allowed, the surviving fraction after split doses of $5.05 + 4.87 = 9.92$ Gy is read off the graph at point Q. If, on the other hand, 18 hours were allowed to elapse, the surviving fraction corresponds to point Q'. The insert shows that the recovery with time is complicated, rising to about 2/3 of its full value in 1 to 2 hours, showing a slight decrease after about 4 hours, and finally approaching maximum recovery after 12 hours. This complicated recovery process with the dip is probably due to a combination of two processes: a repair process that accounts for the initial rapid rise and the redistribution of the surviving cells that initially tend to be synchronized into the resistant parts of the cell cycle. After 4 hours, a significant portion of this surviving population will have moved into a sensitive portion of the cycle, leading to a reduced survival. Similar results have been obtained by a number of investigators (E8).

SURVIVAL CURVES FOR FRACTIONATED TREATMENT. Suppose the survival curve for a cell line is given by equation 17-7. If we assume that in the time between the end of one fraction and the start of treatment of the next fraction, full repair takes place, so that the surviving cells can be thought of as being in the same state as they were initially, then we can determine the surviving fraction by raising N/N_0 of equation 17-7 to the fth power giving:

$$\frac{N}{N_0} = \left\{ e^{-D/f\, D_s} \left[1 - (1 - e^{-D/f\, D_0})^n \right] \right\}^f \qquad (17\text{-}13)$$

$$= e^{-D/D_s} \left[1 - (1 - e^{-D/f\, D_0})^n \right]^f$$

where D is the total dose given and f is the number of fractions each of value D/f. These ideas are illustrated in Figure 17-11, where the survival curve OACDEFG is obtained when a dose of 12.0 Gy is delivered in 6 fractions each of 2.0 Gy. After these 6 irradiations the surviving fraction is $2 \times 10^2/10^6 = 2 \times 10^{-4}$. In contrast if the treatment had been carried out using a single exposure of 12.0 Gy (curve OB), the surviving fraction would have been about 4×10^{-6}.

REPOPULATION. When a radiation treatment is fractionated over 4 to 6 weeks, as is often the case, the cells in the treated area may proliferate during the course of the treatment. Assuming exponential growth, this can be taken into account by multiplying the expression on the right of equation 17-13 by:

$$e^{+T_i/T_g} \qquad (17\text{-}14)$$

where T_i is the interval in days since the last treatment, i.e. the fractionation interval, and T_g is the parameter describing growth (it is the time in days for a population of cells to increase by the factor e). Cohen (C21) suggests that T_g is about 7 days for human skin. When this regrowth is taken into account the survival curve shows a series of vertical pulses

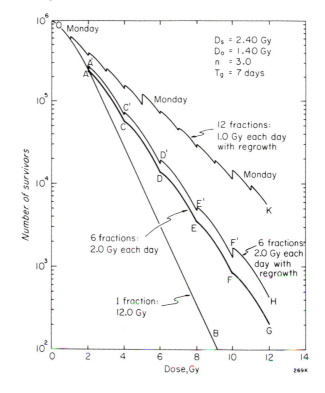

Figure 17-11. Survival of a population of 10^6 cells as a function of dose for a variety of dose fractionations. Curve OAB 1 fraction of 12.0 Gy; curve OACDEFG 6 fractions each of 2.0 Gy; Curve OA' C'D'E'F'H 6 fractions each of 2.0 Gy assuming regrowth; curve OK, 12 fractions each of 1.0 Gy with regrowth. Treatment was started on Monday. The extra regrowth before Monday's treatment is due to regrowth on the weekend.

illustrated by curve OH (Fig. 17-11). After one treatment on Monday the number of survivors is A. One day later (Tuesday) the number of survivors should have increased by the factor 1.15 ($e^{1/7}$). This gives the point A'. For the same reason vertical pulses appear at C', D', E', and F'. The pulse at F' is three times as large because of the extra regrowth during the weekend. It should be noted that when repopulation is taken into account, the fraction of survivors after 6 irradiations each of 2.0 Gy is 4.2×10^{-4}. Finally, Figure 17-11 shows the survival curve when 12.0 Gy is delivered in 12 doses each of 1.0 Gy over a period of 2 weeks plus 2 days. Now the surviving fraction is 5.4×10^{-3}, illustrating that reducing the fraction size decreases the level of cell kill.

Figure 17-11 shows that the fractionation has a major influence on the number of survivors. A meaningful prescription in radiotherapy must obviously include the *total dose,* the *number of fractions,* the *dose per fraction,* and the *overall treatment time.*

17.11   ISORESPONSE CURVES

In Chapters 10, 11, and 12 we developed methods for determining the dose to the tumor region and to normal tissue following the treatment of a tumor by a number of radiation fields. In developing these isodose patterns, it was tactily assumed that there was a direct correspondence

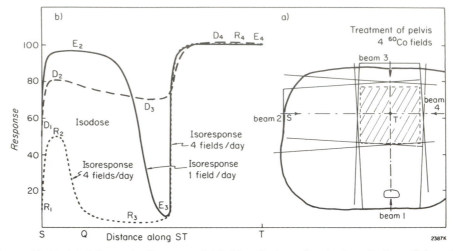

Figure 17-12. (a) Schematic diagram of 4 field technique for the irradiation of the pelvic region with the tumor situated at T. The diagram is symmetrical about the vertical line through T so part of the right hand half of the diagram is omitted. (b) Dose and isoresponse profile along the line ST. Cobalt 60 radiation D_o = 1.30 Gy, D_s = 2.40 Gy extrapolation number n = 3, Tg = 7.0 d. Tumor contains 10^6 cells.

between the dose and the biological effect. From the discussions in this chapter we now know that the time taken to deliver the dose and the way it is fractionated also have an effect. Consider a treatment of the pelvic region with four fields (as illustrated in Fig. 17-12b). The question could be asked, Would it be better to treat with four fields each day or use 4 times the dose and treat only one field each day? The two give the same familiar dose pattern (see section 12.02); along the line ST the *dose* profile starts at about 60% at D_1, rises to a peak at depth 5 mm (D_2), falls to a shallow minimum at D_3, and then rises to a flat plateau at D_4.

To investigate this problem, Niederer and Cunningham (N14) used equations 17-11, 17-13, and 17-14 with suitable radiation parameters to estimate the response in various parts of the pelvis as a result of the fractionated treatment. The response was normalized to 100 at the center of the tumor at T. With *four fields per day* the profile starts near zero at the skin (R_1) rises to a peak at 5 mm depth (R_2), falls to a broad deep minimum at R_3, and then rises rapidly to the plateau at R_4. If only one field is used per day, the profile is quite different, especially in regions outside the tumor volume such as point Q. These regions receive 4 times the dose every fourth day, which we have seen will produce a much larger biological effect than the smaller dose given in daily fractions. Now the response starts at about 60% at S, rises to a broad maximum at E_2 (which is close to 100%), a sharp minimum at E_3, and back up to the plateau at E_4 in the tumor region. It should be noted that these calculations predict that normal tissues outside the tumor volume at Q should be affected by the treatment nearly as much as cells near the center of the tumor at T, suggesting that when multiple fields are used, each field should be treated each day! This will minimize damage to the normal tissues outside the tumor region. In the tumor region, there is not much to choose between the two techniques because, for example, point T receives nearly the same dose each day regardless of whether 1 field is used per day or 4 fields per day with each being given 1/4 the dose. These calculations point to a better therapeutic ratio when all fields are used each day. The technique using 4 fields/day involves little financial penalty since four fields per day can be treated nearly as quickly as 1 per day with a modern unit on an isocentric mount.

The calculations of Niederer et al. (N14) can be used to create isoresponse curves. These exhibit much steeper gradients than isodose patterns, emphasizing the importance of designing the treatment in such a way that the edges of the tumor are adequately covered by the high dose region of the radiation fields.

17.12	THE OXYGEN EFFECT

The presence of oxygen at the time of irradiation acts as a sensitizing agent; the biological effects of the radiation are greater in the presence of oxygen than in its absence. This is illustrated in Figure 17-13, which shows that cells irradiated in the presence of air are about 3 times as sensitive as cells irradiated under conditions of severe hypoxia (very low levels of oxygen). The insert to Figure 17-13 shows how the sensitivity varies with oxygen pressure. As this pressure is increased from zero the sensitivity rises very rapidly, and at 5 kPa (~5% of atmospheric pressure) the sensitivity is about 2.6 times the hypoxic value. As the pressure increases still more, the sensitivity increases very slowly and at 1 atmosphere (101.3 kPa) reaches a value of about 2.7.

The oxygen enhancement ratio (OER) is a convenient parameter to describe the oxygen effect. It can be defined thus:

$$\text{OER} = \frac{\text{Dose to produce a given effect with no } O_2 \text{ present}}{\text{Dose to produce the same effect with 1 atmosphere of air present}} \quad (17\text{-}15)$$

Because the sensitivity curve (insert to Fig. 17-13) is essentially flat above 10 kPa, it does not matter much whether the denominator of equation 17-15 is evaluated at a pressure of 1 atmosphere of oxygen or 1 atmosphere of air. From Figure 17-13 we see that the OER at the 4% survival is AC/AB = 11.0 Gy/4.2 Gy = 2.6. Most investigations of the oxygen effect have shown that the survival curves with and without oxygen are essentially the same shape with the same extrapolation numbers, so the OER is largely independent of the level of survival chosen for the com-

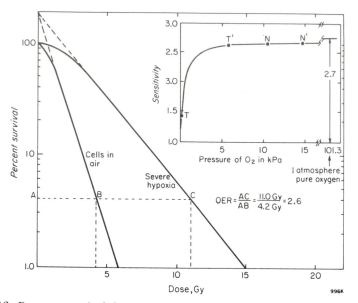

Figure 17-13. Percent survival for cells irradiated in the presence and absence of O_2, illustrating the meaning of the oxygen enhancement ratio (OER). The insert shows the dependence of sensitivity on the partial pressure of oxygen measured in kilopascals. (Adapted from D13, C22.)

parison. Because of this, oxygen can be considered as a dose-modifying agent, and the OER is just the factor by which the dose scale in the presence of O_2 should be multiplied to give the survival curves for hypoxic conditions. The OER values discussed above relate to cells irradiated with low LET radiations such as x or γ rays. Studies show that as the LET increases the OER decreases and reaches a value close to 1.0 for LET values greater than 200 keV/μm (B34).

The oxygen effect is important in radiotherapy because tumors may contain a significant fraction of clonogenic cells, which exist at oxygen tensions low enough to provide full hypoxic radioprotection. In tumors the blood vessels are often poorly formed leading to regions that have an inadequate supply of oxygen. The oxygen tension declines with distance from the capillaries, partly because of the metabolism of the intervening cells that use up oxygen and partly due to diffusion. Taking these two factors into account, calculations suggest that the oxygen tension should fall to near zero at a distance of about 150 μm from the capillary (T17, T18). Such calculations combined with morphological studies suggest that tumor cells can be thought of as being in one of three rather distinct environments (as illustrated in Fig. 17-14) well-oxygenated cells near the capillaries, necrotic cells at zero oxygen tension at distances greater than 100–150 μm from the capillaries, with a layer of hypoxic cells between them. The hypoxic cells are the ones that concern us since they are viable but sufficiently hypoxic to make them resistant to radiation. Such cells may also occur because the blood flow in some tumors may be intermittent, so that for periods of a few minutes or more whole regions of a tumor may be hypoxic.

The importance of a small proportion of hypoxic cells can best be illustrated by constructing a survival curve as illustrated in Figure 17-14. Suppose the tumor of example 17-1 with 10^8 cells ($D_q = 2.40$, $D_0 = 1.45$) contained 1% hypoxic cells with an OER of 2.7. We wish to determine the dose required to reduce the tumor to 1 surviving cell on the average. The easiest way to do this problem is to calculate first the survival curves for each of the populations separately and then add them together. Using 8 cycle log paper we locate P at $D_q + 2.30\ D_0 = 5.73$ Gy and Q at $D_q + 8\ (2.30)\ D_0 = 29.1$ Gy and draw a straight line between them. For the hypoxic fraction we assume the same shaped survival curve with a dose modification of 2.7. We locate R at 2.7 (5.73) = 15.47 Gy and S at $2.7(2.40) + 6(2.30)\ (2.7)D_0 = 60.5$ Gy and draw a straight line between them. The curve APTS shows the sum of these two populations: it follows the well-oxygenated curve down to about 5×10^6 survivors and then follows the hypoxic cell curve from 10^4 to 1 survivor. From the point

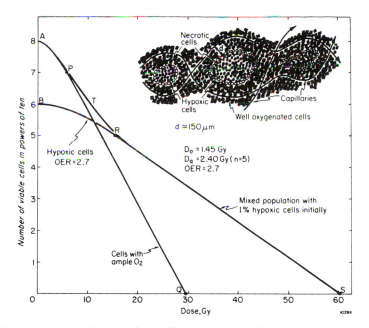

Figure 17-14. APQ, survival curve for well-oxygenated cells with an initial population of 10^8 cells. BRS, survival curve for hypoxic cells with an initial number of 10^6. APTS, survival curve, for a tumor containing 10^8 cells, of which 1% are hypoxic. $D_q = 2.40$ Gy, $D_0 = 1.45$ Gy, OER = 2.7. Insert shows a schematic diagram of a tumor with capillaries wandering through it. Regions more than 150 μm from the capillaries are necrotic. Around each necrotic area is found a layer of hypoxic cells.

of view of cure it is clear that the 1% hypoxic cells determine the dose needed. To reduce the tumor to 1 survivor on the average now requires 60.5 Gy (point S) instead of the value 29.1 Gy (point Q) needed before.

Although the curves of Figure 17-14 are for a model system, there is extensive experimental evidence to suggest that clonogenic hypoxic cells occur in animal tumors. For example, Powers and Tolmach (P20) observed survival curves that were initially steep with a D_0 characteristic of well-oxygenated cells followed by a region with shallower slope characteristic of hypoxic cells. Further studies demonstrated that the cells contributing to the "tail" portion of the survival curve were not intrinsically more radioresistant and that the resistance was caused by a very low oxygen level. Many other animal tumors have been found to exhibit similar breaking survival curves when irradiated in situ, and virtually all solid animal tumors studied to date, even those as small as 1 mm in diameter, have contained a significant fraction of hypoxic cells. Considerable circumstantial evidence (B36, B38) suggests that human tumors also contain hypoxic cells, but it is not yet clear to what degree such cells determine the curability of human tumors treated by fractionated radiation.

REOXYGENATION. The potential problem posed by hypoxic cells in tumors is not as severe for fractionated radiation treatments as it is for single treatments because of a process known as reoxygenation (K10). Studies in animal tumors have shown that not all hypoxic cells remain hypoxic during a fractionated course of radiation. Some of the hypoxic cells gain access to oxygen, becoming reoxygenated, and thereby become more sensitive to subsequent doses of radiation. Thus when a treatment schedule consists of a series of fractions, a tumor that undergoes some reoxygenation will respond as if it contained fewer hypoxic cells. This is illustrated in Figure 17-15.

Curve A shows the survival of cells for 12 fractions of 2.0 Gy, each assuming no hypoxic cells present initially or at any time during the treatment. After 24.0 Gy the surviving fraction is 10^{-5}. Curve B was obtained assuming that initially 10% of the cells are hypoxic. This curve after about 6 Gy is almost completely determined by the hypoxic fraction, since most of the oxygenated cells are now destroyed. Since hypoxic cells probably cannot proliferate between fractions, curve B shows no regrowth after each fraction. After 24 Gy there are some 200 times as many survivors as there were for curve A. Finally curve C was plotted assuming that reoxygenation occurred after each fraction so that at the time of delivery of the next fraction the surviving cell population is the same as the initial one with 10% hypoxic cells. Curve C is not very different from curve A showing that when this amount of reoxygenation occurs during fractionation, hypoxic cells present a smaller problem.

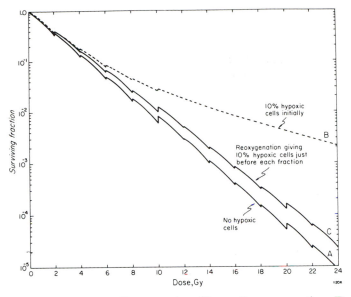

Figure 17-15. Survival curves to illustrate the effects of reoxygenation. $D_q = 2.40$ Gy; $n = 5.2$; $D_0 = 1.45$ Gy; $D_s = 5.0$ Gy, 10 fractions each of 2.0 Gy. (a) No hypoxic cells, (b) 10% hypoxic cells initially and no reoxygenation, (c) 10% hypoxic cells just before each new fraction. Curves calculated using equations 17-13 and 14.

There is no direct evidence that reoxygenation occurs in human tumors but by analogy with animal tumors we can expect that it does. It seems probable that the greater therapeutic effectiveness of fractionated irradiation relative to single treatments is a result of the reoxygenation process. However, studies with a number of animal tumors (K11) indicate that each has its own pattern of reoxygenation, with some tumors showing the maximum extent of reoxygenation within a few hours, while in others the process takes a few days. These findings suggest that present clinical practice may not make the most of reoxygenation for all tumors, since daily fractions are not necessarily optimal. More research in this field is required.

17.13 ISOEFFECT CURVES AND NOMINAL STANDARD DOSE (NSD)

Fractionation has been studied by radiotherapists with no reference to radiobiology, since x rays were first used to treat cancer. Figure 17-16 shows the results of a comprehensive study by Strandqvist (S32). Here the accumulated dose, i.e. the total dose D, used to treat tumors is plotted on a log scale against the overall treatment time, T, on a log scale. In this study, including some 280 carcinomas of the skin and lip, Strandqvist found that if the dose lay above this curve, overdose effects or necrosis of the normal skin occurred, while if the dose lay below this line, underdose effects or tumor recurrences appeared. His results imply that 20 grays in one day is equivalent to 30 in 4 days, 40 in 11 days, 50 in 25 days, or 60 in 45 days.

In addition, the figure also shows the doses that gave similar levels of tumor control for various overall treatment times, as reported by Paterson (P7) for squamous carcinoma of the skin and Friedman (F11) for recurrent cancer of the breast. Considering the complexity of the problem, the agreement between the three sets of data is good.

The curves of Figure 17-16 can be considered as being isoeffect curves since they indicate different treatment schedules that produce essentially the same biological effect. They show that with an increase in the number of fractions and overall time, much larger total doses are required to produce the same effect.

These isoeffect curves arise from the interplay of the four factors (repair, repopulation, redistribution, and reoxygenation) discussed earlier. From the upward slope of the curves it is clear that a great deal of repair of sublethal damage and repopulation must occur during the fractionated treatment. Experimental work with pigs (F12) has indicated, contrary to early expectations, that repair is the most important of these two factors, with repopulation playing a lesser but still significant role. Since repair is related to fraction number while repopulation is more related to overall time it is important to specify both the number of fractions and the overall time when designating a treatment regime. Reoxygenation and redistribution would be expected to reduce the upward slope of an isoeffect curve and it has been suggested that the initial shallower slope of the curve for breast carcinoma is due to reoxygenation partially cancelling out the effect of repair. Experimental studies have demonstrated just such an effect for mammary carcinoma in mice (F13).

NOMINAL STANDARD DOSE. In an attempt to take the number of fractions, the overall number of days, and the total dose into consideration Ellis (E10) has introduced the nominal standard dose (NSD) concept to predict an isoeffect relationship for normal tissue tolerance in clinical radiotherapy. He suggested that the dose, D, normal tissue could tolerate was related to the number of fractions N and the overall time T in days by the relation:

$$D = (NSD) \ T^{0.11} \ N^{0.24} \qquad (17\text{-}16)$$

This is called the Ellis NSD equation. The NSD is a constant that when multiplied by time and number of fractions to the appropriate power yields the total dose in grays. It has been suggested that NSD might be measured in ret (rad equivalent therapy). Since the unit of dose is now the gray, logically the unit should now be get. Neither of these units have

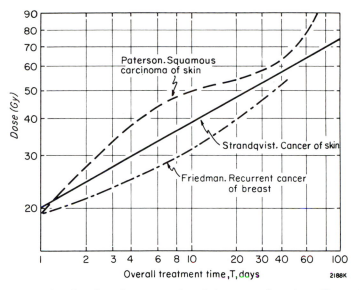

Figure 17-16. Graphs showing the accumulated dose as a function of overall treatment time. Data from Strandqvist (S32) for cancer of the skin, from Paterson (P7) for squamous carcinoma, and Friedman (F11) for recurrent cancer of the breast are plotted.

been made legitimate by the ICRU.

To use the NSD equation, one must determine the numerical value for the NSD. A widely used schedule is 5 treatments per week, each of 2.0 Gy for a 6 weeks period. Assuming the treatment started on Monday morning of the first week and ended on Friday morning of the last week the overall treatment time T is 39 days, the number of fractions N = 30, and the total dose D is 60.0 Gy. Using a calculator the student may determine that $39^{.11} = 1.496$, $30^{.24} = 2.262$, and their product is 3.384. Substituting these values in equation 17-16 and noting that D = 30 × 2 = 60 Gy yields NSD = 17.73. We illustrate the use of this NSD value to determine the dose schedule for other fractionations, as follows.

Example 17-4. A popular prescription in radiotherapy is 5 fractions per week for 4 weeks. What dose per fraction would give an equivalent treatment to the protocol discussed above?

> For this case T = 25, N = 20, $25^{.11} = 1.425$, $20^{.24} = 2.052$
> D = 17.73 × 1.425 × 2.052 = 51.8 Gy
> Dose per fraction = 51.8/20 = 2.59 Gy.
> Thus 20 fractions of 2.59 Gy given in 4 weeks should be equivalent to 30 fractions of 2.0 Gy given in 6 weeks as far as the effect on normal tissues is concerned.

Another example will illustrate how one might predict a reasonable prescription when the fractionation scheme has been rather drastically altered.

Example 17-5. A patient is to be treated with 2 fractions per day, 5 days per week for 4 weeks. Determine the dose per fraction that will yield an equivalent treatment to the one described in example 17-4.

> T = 25, N = 40, $25^{.11}$ = 1.425, $40^{.24}$ = 2.424
> Dose D = 17.73 (1.425) (2.424) = 61.2 Gy
> Dose per fraction = 61.2/40 = 1.53 Gy
> The dose per day is now 2(1.53) = 3.06 Gy compared with 2.59 Gy for the single fraction per day. These doses differ by 18%.

This calculation should be used with caution since the formula was not intended to deal with more than one fraction per day. Furthermore, the fractionated dose of 1.53 Gy is small enough to be on the initial part of the survival curve and less repair may take place than implied by the NSD equation.

Time Dose and Fractionation Factors (TDF)

The NSD formula due to Ellis is not easy to use because of the exponentials, and many mistakes in its use and interpretation have occurred. Another difficulty occurs because the NSD is defined only at the tissue tolerance level, and numbers calculated at intermediate dosages have no clear meaning and *definitely cannot be added together*. To solve this problem the concept of partial tolerance was introduced, and this has been formalized by Orton and Ellis (O3) as a series of time, dose, fractionation (TDF) factors. These TDF factors are independent of the actual value of the NSD and can be added together to compile a treatment regime that reaches a level of normal tissue tolerance. The TDF factors have been tabulated by Orton and Ellis and these tables considerably simplify the use of the NSD concept. A treatment regime known to be at tolerance is looked up in the tables to determine the equivalent TDF factor just as we did earlier to determine NSD. Any combination of treatments that give TDF factors which add up to that defined for tolerance theoretically can then be given, with the same overall normal tissue response. We will use these tables to solve a problem where the dose fractionation scheme is altered part way through the treatment.

Example 17-6. A patient is under a treatment protocol calling for 5 fractions per week each of 2.0 Gy over a 6 week period. After 3 weeks of the treatment external circumstances required that the therapy be completed in 2 weeks. What dose fractions should be used for the remaining treatment?

> Using Table V of Orton and Ellis (O3) we locate under 30 fractions opposite 200 rads (2 Gy) the TDF factor 99. Half this is 49.5. We then look under 10 fractions (the number still to be given) for the

closest number to 49.5. By interpolation we determine the dose fraction is 262 rads. The patient should be treated with 10 fractions of
2.62 Gy over the last two weeks of the treatment.

Orton and Ellis also give a table that allows one to deal with a split
course treatment. The effect of the first part of the treatment is assumed
to partially decay during the rest period.

Considerable experimental work has been done to try to define the
extent to which the NSD formula may predict fractionation schedules
that have equal biological effects. From experiments on pig skin it was
soon recognized that the NSD number could not be used as an equivalent
single dose to a fractionated regime. It was found, however, that over
the range 4 to 30 fractions the formula is reasonably accurate. Recently,
Fowler (F 14) has suggested that this range is only appropriate for acute
reactions and that for late reactions in skin and in other normal tissues
smaller total doses are tolerated, for a few large fractions, than are predicted by the NSD formula. The fraction number exponent is larger
than 0.24 for a few large fractions and smaller than 0.24 for many small
fractions, i.e. the isoeffect curve is not a straight line on a log-log plot
but slightly convex upwards. The time exponent of 0.11 is probably also
too large for late damage that often occurs in nonproliferating or very
slowly proliferating tissues. Overall it is clear that the NSD formula has
limitations but it can be useful as an initial guide for changing the fractionation schedule, at least in the range of 10–30 fractions in a period
up to six weeks. One factor the NSD formula does not consider is the
field size. It is well known that the tolerance of tissue to radiation decreases rapidly with increase in field size (P7); thus calculations comparing treatments can only be made for the same field size. It should also
be emphasized that the NSD formula attempts to predict doses giving
normal tissue tolerance and was not designed to predict doses that would
give the same tumor response, although many workers have tried to do
just that.

17.14 EXAMPLES OF THE APPLICATION OF RADIOBIOLOGY TO RADIOTHERAPY

In the foregoing sections various aspects of our understanding of how
cells respond to radiation have been discussed. It is clear from this discussion that radiobiology studies are not yet at a stage to allow scientific
prediction of the optimum treatment for a given tumor or type of tumor
in patients. Radiobiological studies do, however, provide a scientific
framework within which radiotherapeutic treatments can be generally
understood and potential improvements discussed and their likely benefit evaluated. One example of the use of radiobiological information has

already been presented in the section on isodose and isoresponse curves for multiple field treatments. Further examples of the application of radiobiological information are presented here.

The Oxygen Effect

The demonstration that hypoxic (radioresistant) cells exist in animal tumors and are likely to occur in human tumors has led to a number of approaches to improving the therapeutic ratio by eliminating the protective advantage hypoxic cells might confer on tumors. One such approach is to give patients oxygen or oxygen at high pressure (3-4 atmospheres) to breathe before and during each radiation treatment. If hypoxic cells develop because of oxygen diffusion limitations, then increasing the partial pressure of oxygen in the blood should result in greater diffusion and hence better oxygenation of the hypoxic cells. Extensive studies with animal tumors (S33) have provided evidence that this approach should be effective. Carefully controlled clinical trials run by the Medical Research Council in the United Kingdom (W14, W15, D14, C23) have demonstrated that patients with cancer of the cervix, or with head and neck cancer, may derive some benefit from using high pressure O_2 during radiotherapy while tumors at other sites (e.g. bladder, lung) show little or no overall benefit. Many other *less carefully* controlled trials have given largely negative results. These results combined with the overall difficulty and danger of treating patients in a pressure chamber have meant that this procedure is now used in only a few centers.

Meanwhile, other studies have demonstrated that the physiological state of the patient particularly in relation to anemia can influence prognosis (B38). Retrospective studies showed that patients with cervix or larynx cancer had a poorer prognosis if they were anemic at the time of treatment. A small prospective study with cervix patients has shown that transfusion can alleviate this problem, thus in some centers anemic patients are routinely transfused before treatment. Animal tumor studies have given similar results for transfusion (H27) and have suggested that other physiological factors that can influence tissue oxygenation, e.g. chronic lung disease (S34) and high levels of carboxyhemoglobin in the blood due to heavy smoking (S35), may also influence tumor response to radiation treatment.

High LET Radiation and the Oxygen Effect

We have just discussed ways to try to reduce the number of hypoxic cells by raising the oxygen pressure. Another possible way to deal with hypoxic cells is to use high LET radiation, for which the oxygen effect is smaller, that is, the OER is close to 1.0. Some of the radiations that have been used are neutrons, protons, stripped nuclei such as carbon or neon, and negative π mesons. The production of these particles is very expen-

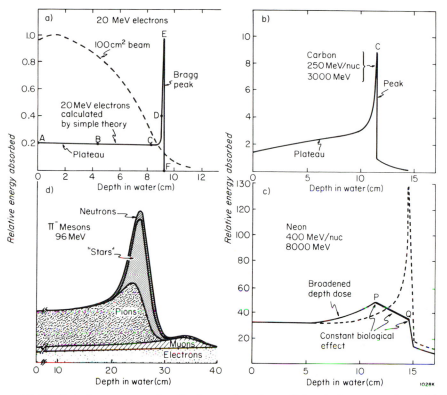

Figure 17-17. Relative energy absorbed as a function of depth for a number of high energy particles. (a) 20 MeV electrons in water. The theoretical curve ABCDEF was determined assuming the electron trajectory was a straight line. With this assumption a Bragg peak will appear. In the real situation the dashed curve is observed. (b) Carbon nuclei with 3000 MeV energy. (c) Dotted curve, neon nuclei with an energy of 8000 MeV. Solid curve, mix of energies to give *constant* biological effect from P to Q. (d) Data for 96 MeV negative pi mesons showing the energy deposited from neutrons, "stars," pions, muons, and electrons, which result when a negative pi meson is stopped.

sive, so experimental work in this field is confined to very few centers. The distribution of energy deposition of some of these particles is illustrated in Figure 17-17.

NEUTRONS. The production of fast neutrons requires a cyclotron as discussed in section 4.09. Such an installation is about ten times the cost of a high energy linac. *Fast neutrons* have an intermediate LET and an OER of about 1.5. They were first used in radiotherapy in 1948 by Stone (S5), but the study was terminated because of the unacceptable late complications in many of the treated patients. The complications often appeared in fatty tissues that were overdosed. At that time it was not fully appreciated that most of the energy absorption took place by collisions between neutrons and hydrogen nuclei. The high concentration of hydrogen in fatty tissues made them the prime target. Recent studies by Sheline (S36) also suggest that these early patients were overdosed because the RBE was underestimated due to an imperfect understanding of the dependence of RBE on fraction size (see sec. 17.08).

Catterall (C24) has treated a significant number of patients with high energy neutrons over a period of about 10 years and claims better results in treating advanced cases than is possible with ^{60}Co gamma rays. It is our impression that workers in a number of other centers are less enthusiastic. One of the problems with fast neutrons is the difficulty of depositing energy at the center of a deep seated tumor because the depth dose achievable is only slightly better than with 250 kV$_p$ x rays.

HEAVY PARTICLES. The inferior depth dose from neutrons has led to the development of facilities to produce protons, negative pi-mesons, or heavy nuclei, e.g. carbon or neon, for cancer treatment (H28, P1, P2). Such particles have the advantage of a significant Bragg peak where the particles come to rest; thus a large dose of high LET radiation can be delivered to deep-seated tumors without giving large doses to overlying tissue. This Bragg peak is usually too narrow to cover most tumors so particles of different energies are combined (as illustrated in Fig. 17-17c) to broaden the high dose region, yielding a *dose* distribution PQ. The slope is adjusted to yield a *constant, biological effect* from P to Q. Particles absorbed at Q have a higher LET than those absorbed at P, so the RBE at Q is larger than at P. The product of the energy absorption and the RBE are designed to give a constant effect from P to Q. The creation of such a tailor-made distribution is not easy since it must take into account the density and atomic number of *all* the tissues between the tumor and the skin surface.

The dose distribution for negative π mesons is illustrated in Figure 17-17d. When these particles come to rest in tissue a large amount of high LET energy is deposited in "stars" when the negative π meson is captured. Pi meson radiotherapy is complicated even more because the beam always contains a mixture of muons, pions, and neutrons. Further the negative π mesons disintegrate with a half-life of about 2×10^{-8}s so the patient must be positioned close to the target where the pions are produced.

The production of stripped nuclei or pi mesons involves immense accelerators that cost hundreds of times that of a 20 MeV linac. These machines may provide a double benefit: improved dose distributions and improved control of hypoxic cells in tumors. If these benefits prove to be great enough, the costs could be justified.

RADIOSENSITIZERS AND HYPOXIC CELLS. A third approach to improving the response of hypoxic cells is the use of oxygen-mimetic radiosensitizers. Many compounds have been identified in cell culture studies as having the potential to specifically sensitize hypoxic cells to radiation treatment while having no effect on well-oxygenated cells, and one particular class of compounds, the nitroimidazoles, have been found to give good radiosensitization of hypoxic cells in in vivo animal tumor studies (F15). Two drugs of this class, metronidazole and misonidazole, are presently undergoing early clinical trials with some encouraging results (B39); it is, however, too early to say how useful the compounds will be. One problem is that there are dose-limiting toxicities that prevent administration of the optimum dose for full sensitization. New drugs that are equally effective radiosensitizers in animal tumors but that may be less toxic are presently under investigation (B39).

CHOICE OF FRACTIONATION. Another possible way to improve the therapeutic ratio could be to alter the fractionation scheme. Here we discuss radiobiological predictions concerning changes in fractionation, an approach that has been widely used by radiotherapists on a largely empirical basis. To focus the discussion, we will compare three possible techniques.

A: 3f of 2.92 Gy/w; for 6w; total dose 52.5 Gy
B: 5f of 2.00 Gy/w; for 6w; total dose 60.0 Gy
C: 4f each of 1 Gy/d, 5d/w; for 3w; total dose 60.0 Gy

Technique B is a well-established conventional treatment used in many centers. Technique A is quite similar involving the same overall time but uses fewer fractions. The total dose is about 12% less than that in B as predicted by the NSD formula. If A was as good as B it would offer an economical advantage in a busy radiotherapy department since more patients could be treated in a given time using it. Technique C is of a more experimental nature involving 4 fractions per day, often referred to as superfractionation. We will now discuss the merits of each technique, considering the effects of repair, repopulation, redistribution, and reoxygenation on both normal and tumor cells.

Consider first *repair;* technique C allows for 59 sessions of repair, each of 6 hours, between each fraction (ignoring weekends), while B allows for 29 sessions of repair, each of 24 hours, and A allows for 17 sessions of repair of 48 hours each. Since from Figure 17-10 we expect repair to be largely complete by 6 hours, technique C will have more repair than B, which in turn will have more repair than A. If tumors do not repair as fast or as completely as normal tissue, then we expect a better therapeutic ratio from technique C. It should be noted, however, that if the individual fraction size is reduced too much, we will eventually lose any advantage because each increment of dose will still be on the single hit portion of the shoulder of the survival curve, where cell killing will be of the nonrepairable single hit type.

For *repopulation,* the important parameter is the overall time of the treatment. Thus we can expect more repopulation to occur in techniques A and B than in C. If the tumor is of the rapidly growing variety while the critical normal tissue shows little proliferation, then we expect technique C to be the better. Alternatively, for a slowly growing tumor in rapidly proliferating normal tissue, A or B would be better.

The effect of *redistribution* is determined by two opposing tendencies. The increase in the number of fractions from A to C will allow for more redistribution sessions to occur, suggesting the greatest response in C; however, the reduction in the time between the individual fractions will reduce the extent to which redistribution can occur in C relative to A. Without a knowledge of the cellular kinetics of the tissues involved and the effect of radiation on them, we cannot choose between C and A.

Since hypoxic cells are largely confined to tumors, *reoxygenation* will affect the response of tumor cells but not normal ones. Consequently, any improvement in therapeutic ratio will depend on the time course of reoxygenation. If reoxygenation is rapid, i.e. occurs in a few hours, C would be no worse than A and could be better, if a reduction in the extent of reoxygenation occurs at later times, as has been observed with some animal tumors. Alternatively, if reoxygenation occurs more slowly, i.e. over days, we can expect A to be the better technique. Studies with experimental tumors support these conclusions. For a rapidly reoxygenating tumor, there was no therapeutic advantage in changing from B to A (P21). On the other hand, for a more slowly reoxygenating tumor, A was found to be more advantageous than B (F13).

An extensive clinical trial in the United Kingdom using head and neck tumors has essentially compared A and B while allowing for individual variations in the total dose from center to center. The most recently published findings (W16) indicate that there is very little difference between the two schedules in terms of normal tissue effects or tumor response.

It is obvious from this discussion that we require more fundamental cellular data to logically predict the effect of altering the fractionation schedule. More basic radiobiological research is required.

HYPERTHERMIA. There is renewed interest in the use of hyperthermia (37 to 50° C) as a treatment for cancer (F16, D15, H29). Fundamental studies with cells in culture have shown that cells are sensitive to a temperature elevation of a few degrees and that animal and human tumors can be made to regress following heating. The heating of cells also increases their sensitivity to radiation and reduces their ability to repair radiation damage; thus, hyperthermia can be used alone or in combination with radiation treatment.

A number of different techniques have been proposed for localized heating of tissue, e.g. ultrasound, radio-frequency electric fields, and microwaves. No one of these techniques is suitable for all parts of the body, hence the development of a number of different techniques is needed. An important aspect of hyperthermia is that a small change in temperature (as little as 0.5° C) can lead to a large change in biological effect, which means that very tight control of the heating is required. Because of differences in heating of different tissues and particularly because of differences in rate of cooling (largely due to blood flow), achieving a controlled rise in temperature in all parts of the heated volume remains a major problem at the present time.

17.15   SURVIVAL OF PATIENTS

In earlier sections of this chapter we have discussed and illustrated survival curves as a function of dose for cells and tumors. However, one of our primary interests is the cure of cancer patients. We need ways to compare the survival as a function of time of groups of patients treated using two different techniques. Further, if there is a difference between the survival times we need to know whether the difference is real or merely a matter of chance. The latter may be a real possibility since often one is tempted to interpret data from a small number of patients where statistical errors are large. After starting a study the investigator often wants to know how well the new technique is working at a time when relatively few patients have entered the study; this also complicates the comparison. Here we will deal with the problem in enough detail to enable an oncologist or physicist to interact effectively with a hospital statistics group in setting up and interpreting a study.

The basic information for such studies must first be obtained, i.e. a group of patients must be followed and their status determined over a period of time. Data of this kind is most easily stored in a computer. To illustrate the procedure we have selected at random 40 patients from our large file of cancer of the cervix patients (over 4,000) and their status is shown in Figure 17-18. Patient 1 was first diagnosed in May, 1961, and died November, 1964. The patient is recorded by a horizontal line starting at B and terminating near the end of 1964. Patient 40 was diagnosed just before the end of 1974 and died April 28, 1977. This history is shown at the bottom of the diagram starting at E. The vertical distance between B and E is immaterial but it is convenient to draw the line BE at approximately 45°. Having drawn this line, the date of diagnosis for the remaining 38 patients locates the starting point of each of their life lines. If *all* patients were followed long enough all lines would end with death, which in this diagram we represent by a small vertical line. In practice some patients are lost to follow up, as for example patient 2. This patient was *last* seen alive near the end of 1969, so this life line is terminated by the letter A to indicate alive. Having drawn in all the life lines, we can now create a survival curve. There are several types of such survival curves.

CRUDE SURVIVAL CURVES. To create these we need to specify an analysis or cut-off date; in our example, we have chosen the end of 1977 and

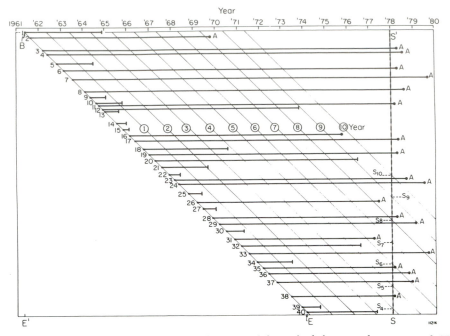

Figure 17-18. Diagram to illustrate how the actuarial survival data can be arranged. The 40 patients used in this chart were taken from our cancer of the cervix files.

drawn a vertical line SS' at this time. The date selected should be the most recent date on which the status of most patients will be known using the usual follow-up procedure. We also draw a series of parallel equally spaced lines, Year 1, Year 2 . . . Year 10, which are 1 year apart measured horizontally. We now count the number of life lines that start along BE and pass through Y1. 40 patients start on BE but only 31 lines reach Y1 so the % survival at 1 year is 31/40 = .775. This value is entered in Table 17-3.

To obtain the survival at 2 years we note that 28 lines cross Y2 so the survival is 28/40 = 0.7. In a similar way the survival at 3 years is 27/40. To obtain the result for 5 years we must take into account the fact that some of the patients (38, 39, and 40) have not been in the study for 5 years at the cut off date and so must be excluded. This idea requires some clarification. In this case, patients 39 and 40 died, so we *do* know their status; however, patient 38's status at five years is unknown. The only way to treat all patients equally requires that we must exclude all three. We therefore locate point S5, the intersection of Y5 and SS' and draw a horizontal dotted line through S5 and consider only those life lines above this line. There are 37 of these lines, of which 23 cross Y5 so the crude survival is 23/37. For year 6, out of 34 patients 19 survive, yielding a crude survival of 19/34. For year 7, 31 patients are at risk, and 17 are

TABLE 17-3
Determination of Crude Survival

Time	Crude S	Time	Crude S
(y)		(y)	
1	31/40 = .775	6	19/34 = .559
2	28/40 = .70	7	17/31 = .548
3	27/40 = .675	8	16/28 = .571
4	24/40 = .600	9	12/25 = .480
5	23/37 = .622	10	8/22 = .364

alive so the crude survival is 17/31. The student should note that patient 31 was alive about 5 months past Y6 but since her status is not known at the end of 1977 we must take the conservative approach and assume she is dead. Of course, the better procedure would be to carry out a search to determine her status. Following this technique we can complete Table 17-3. The results are plotted in Figure 17-19a. It is seen that there are rather large fluctuations in the calculation; for example, the % survival at year 5 is greater than at year 4—clearly an artifact that arises when we start excluding patients.

ACTUARIAL SURVIVAL OR LIFE-TABLE METHOD. A better way to study this problem is to create an actuarial survival curve. This makes use of all the available information and does not require the specification of a cut-off date.

We make the following entries in Table 17-4. In the first column we enter the yearly intervals. The next column gives the number of patients who enter these intervals. From Figure 17-18 we saw that 40 patients enter the first year, 31 the second year (31 life lines cross Y1), 28 the third year, etc. These are entered in column 2.

TABLE 17-4
Calculation of Actuarial Survival

(1) Year Interval	(2) No. Alive Beginning of Year	(3) No. Dying in Interval	(4) No. Last Seen Alive During Interval	(5) No. Exposed To Risk of Dying	(6) Propr. Dying During Year	(7) Propr. Surv. Year	(8) Propr. Surv. to End of Year	(9) Time (y)
							1.000	0
0-1	40	9	0	40	9/40 = .225	.775	.775	1
1-2	31	3	0	31	3/31 = .097	.903	.700	2
2-3	28	1	0	28	1/28 = .036	.964	.675	3
3-4	27	3	0	27	3/27 = .111	.889	.600	4
4-5	24	0	1	23.5	0/23.5 = 0.0	1.000	.600	5
5-6	23	1	1	22.5	1/22.5 = .044	.956	.573	6
6-7	21	0	3	19.5	0/19.5 = 0.0	1.000	.573	7
7-8	18	0	0	18	0/18 = 0.0	1.000	.573	8
8-9	18	1	5	15.5	1/15.5 = 0.65	.935	.536	9
9-10	12	1	1	11.5	1/11.5 = .087	.913	.490	10

In column 3 we enter the number of deaths during each interval. The number is found by counting the life lines that terminate with a death between the sets of parallel lines. For example 3 deaths occur in the interval 1-2 year. In the next column (4) we enter the number of life lines that terminate with an A in each interval. The first A (patient 38) appears between Y4 and Y5. Note that this A is beyond the date of analysis used for the crude survival calculation but it is counted anyway; in fact, we now ignore the vertical line SS′ at the cut-off date.

The next column (5) gives the effective number exposed to risk of dying in each interval. It is based on the assumption that patients last seen alive during any year of follow-up were on the average observed for one half the year. To obtain these numbers we subtract from column 2 half of each entry in column 4 to give the numbers of column 5.

Column 6 gives the proportion dying during the yearly interval. It is found by dividing the entries of column 3 by column 5. We next subtract the entries of 6 from 1.000 to give the proportion of patients surviving each year. These are entered in column 7. To find the probability of surviving to the end of the first year, we multiply 1.00 by 0.775 and enter .775 in column 8 ópposite year one in column 9. To find the probability of surviving to the end of the second year we multiply 0.775 (the 2nd entry of column 8) by 0.903 (the second entry of column 7) to give 0.700. This procedure is followed to give all the entries of column 8. These entries are called the actuarial survival probabilities and are plotted in Figure 17-19b. The actuarial survivals either decrease with time or stay constant but never increase as did the crude survival rates. Actuarial survival rates are in general a better way to represent survival data than are crude survival rates when the data are not complete and some life lines end with an A. If the date of death is known for every patient, the two methods become identical.

KAPLAN-MEIER METHOD (K12). This technique was developed to study survival when small numbers are involved. It is also useful because the calculations are simple and can be done easily without a computer. All patients are first ranked in order of the length of their life lines as illustrated in Table 17-5. For example, the first entry is for patient 15 who died 75 days after entry while the last entry is for patient 4 who is still alive after 5901 days. The table has 40 entries. A convenient way to organize the calculations is to enter the numbers from 40 down to one as shown under B, column 4. In column 5 we enter under C a number one less than B whenever a death occurs, and make no entry when the status is A. This procedure gives rise to the sequence of numbers C from 39 to 24 down to patient number 18; then the numbers 22, 13, and 11 opposite the remaining 3 deaths. We now calculate the survival whenever a death occurs.

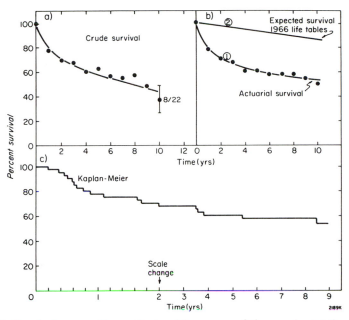

Figure 17-19. Survival curves for patients with cancer of the cervix. (a) Crude survival. (b) Actuarial survival and expected survival of a normal population of women based on 1966 life tables. For a logical comparison these curves should be plotted on a logarithmic scale. (c) Survival determined by the Kaplan-Meier method. Note the change in scale at 2 years.

The survival is constant at 1.00 from zero time to 75 days at which time one patient out of 40 dies so the survival drops to 39/40 = .975; at 134 days the second patient dies so the survival is (38/39)(39/40) = 38/40 = .950. This of course is equivalent to (38/39).975 = .950. Following this procedure we enter the survival values down to .600 for patient 18. These drop by equal steps of 1/40 = .025. Patient 39 is alive so no calculation is made, the survival is still .600. For patient 22 the survival is (22/23).600 = .574. The student can easily verify the rest of the calculations.

The survival calculated by this procedure is shown in Figure 17-19c. It consists of a series of horizontal lines with a step down whenever a death occurs. To illustrate the procedure the time scale was expanded from 0 to 2 years so the graph appears distorted. If it had been plotted on a uniform scale it would appear similar to the actuarial survival curve of panel b.

STATISTICAL ERRORS. The study of patient survival often involves relatively small samples, so statistical errors may often be very large. The determination of the reliability of the data is important. Unfortunately, it is a complex problem, so we will limit our discussion to a few simple calculations and refer the reader to references in the field.

TABLE 17-5
Calculation of Survival by the Kaplan-Meier Method

Patient Number	Time (d)	Status	B	C	Surv
15	75	D	40	39	.975
14	134	D	39	38	.950
22	164	D	38	37	.925
27	187	D	37	36	.900
25	217	D	36	35	.875
10	225	D	35	34	.850
12	237	D	34	33	.825
30	279	D	33	32	.800
38	317	D	32	31	.775
13	396	D	31	30	.750
24	602	D	30	29	.725
5	623	D	29	28	.700
21	749	D	28	27	.675
40	1253	D	27	26	.650
1	1295	D	26	25	.625
18	1377	D	25	24	.600
39	1679	A	24		.600
22	1963	D	23	22	.574
25	2189	A	22		.574
37	2244	A	21		.574
31	2283	A	20		.574
36	2306	A	19		.574
23	2960	A	18		.574
26	2998	A	17		.574
2	3009	A	16		.574
28	3057	A	15		.574
8	3236	D	14	13	.533
29	3236	A	13		.533
20	3339	D	12	11	.488
16	3501	A	11		.488
23	3812	A	10		.488
24	4061	A	9		.488
19	4096	A	8		.488
17	4336	A	7		.488
11	4904	A	6		.488
9	5300	A	5		.488
6	5512	A	4		.488
3	5862	A	3		.488
7	5886	A	2		.488
4	5901	A	1		.488

For a crude survival rate the standard error, σ, in the fraction surviving is calculated using the relation (derived from a binomial distribution):

$$\sigma = \text{standard error} = \sqrt{\frac{p(1-p)}{n}} \qquad (17\text{-}17)$$

where p is the proportion of survivors and $(1 - p)$ is the proportion of deaths in a sample size n (R17). The first entry of Table 17-3 tells us that

31 patients out of 40 survived the first year, giving a survival proportion of 0.775. For this case p = 31/40, (1 − p) = 9/40, and n = 40. Substituting these values in equation 17-17 we obtain:

$$\sigma = \sqrt{\frac{31}{40} \times \frac{9}{40} \times \frac{1}{40}} = 0.066$$

This means that one would expect the true survival to be within the limits of 0.775 ± .066 in 67% of the observation (see Fig. 14-7). From Figure 14-7 we could equally well state that the survival would be in the interval ±2σ = ±0.132 in 96% of the observations.

To indicate the reliability of the data, error bars of length 2σ are often added to the last point on the survival curve where the uncertainty is largest. For example, a calculation similar to the above yields σ = 0.102 for the ten year entry of 0.364. This error bar is plotted in Figure 17-19a.

The extension of the approach to the actuarial survival curve involves calculating the standard error for each of the entries of column 7 in Table 17-4 using the same formula as above and then combining these errors by the established rules for combining standard errors to yield standard errors for the entries in column 8. We illustrate this by a calculation.

Example 17-7. Determine the standard error for the entry 0.700 of Table 17-4.

The entry 0.700 is the product of 0.775 and 0.903. We first determine the standard error for each of these and then the error in their product.

$$\sigma_1 = \sqrt{\frac{31}{40} \times \frac{9}{40} \times \frac{1}{40}} = 0.0660$$

$$\sigma_2 = \sqrt{\frac{28}{31} \times \frac{3}{31} \times \frac{1}{31}} = .0531$$

We now calculate the relative standard error of each

Rel. standard error in .775 is (.0660)/.775 = .0852

Rel. standard error in .903 is (.0531)/.903 = .0588

Relative standard error in .700 is: $= \sqrt{(.0852)^2 + (.0588)^2} = .103$

Standard error in 0.700 = (.103) (.700) = .0725

The procedure is cumbersome but can be simplified using a formula derived by Greenwood (discussed in Gross and Clark, G17). For the comparison of whole survival curves two statistical tests in common use are the Wilcoxon-Gehan test (B40) and the log rank test (P22, P23).

RELATIVE SURVIVAL. In this statistical study of survival we have not yet taken into account the fact that patients will die from other types of disease or "old age" following treatment. Vital statistics (L15) are available giving the probability of death as a function of age. Curve 2 at the top of Figure 17-19b gives the survival curve for a group of women with the same age distribution as those in the study. For this population the 10 year survival is about 85%. One way to take these deaths into account is to divide the observed survival by the expected survival to yield a relative survival. A calculation of this kind would show that the 10 year survival is 52/.85 = 61% rather than 52%. (Other useful references dealing with survival data are C25, R17.)

17.16   EFFECTS OF HIGH ENERGY RADIATION ON CURE RATE

Most of this book has been concerned with the manipulation of radiation to treat patients. We have developed methods of dosimetry that allow precision in physical dose delivery. We have also shown that with high energy radiation one can deliver a higher dose of radiation to the tumor site compared to the surrounding normal tissues. By using high energy radiation we have been able to improve the dose distribution relative to the time when radiation therapy was limited to lower energy machines (200–400 kV). Also, because of the increased bone absorption when low energy photons were used, late complications were a major problem. We now ask ourselves, Has this effort in developing high energy sources, and techniques, produced any change in the cure rate for certain types of cancer? To answer this question the radiation oncologist must subject his clinical results to a critical statistical analysis as discussed in the previous section. Bush (B37) has looked at this problem and some of his results are shown in Figure 17-20. The studies were retrospective and were made possible because there have been in existence in Ontario facilities for following up a very large number of patients for many years. Bush was able to study the cure of cancer of the cervix in two eras: before the introduction of supervoltage, 1935-44, and since the introduction of high energy radiation, 1958-69.

There are two major differences between the eras. First, there was a larger fraction of patients with advanced disease in the earlier era, and this could account for an improvement in survival even if the same therapy techiques were used. Bush (B37) has examined this, and although there were differences in staging, he has estimated that at 5 years approximately half the survival improvement was due to a smaller fraction of advanced cases in the later era. The second difference is the type of radiation used. In the earlier era most patients were treated with 400 kV_p while in the latter they were treated primarily with cobalt 60, or high energy photons from a 22 MeV betatron. This resulted not only in an improvement in 5 year survival, but in a decreased rate of dying over the following years. This difference is illustrated in Figure 17-20. The bottom curve represents the survival of 1336 patients treated for cancer of the cervix in Ontario cancer clinics between the years 1935 and 1944. As can be seen, approximately one-third were alive at 5 years, but only 20% at 14 years. There was no difference in these overall Ontario results from those for a smaller number of patients treated at the Toronto clinic that antedated the Princess Margaret Hospital. Figure 17-20 also shows the survival of 2746 patients treated between 1958 and 1969. When this analysis was done, 2058 patients had been followed 10 years, but only 688 for 14 years or longer. As can be seen 60% of patients were alive at 5 years, and 45% at 14. There was no significant difference in the age of the patients in the two eras, thus the different rates of dying is likely to be due to differences in treatment.

Figure 17-20 also shows that the normal survival of women in the 1944 and 1965 eras was almost identical, so that the patient populations were similar. From the diagram we note that the slope of the survival curves in the recent era is identical to that of the normal population when both are plotted on a semilog scale. This means that, if a woman reaches a point 6 to 8 years after treatment and is still disease free, she will have the same life expectancy as a woman of the same age, in the normal population. In contrast, the survival curve for patients in the

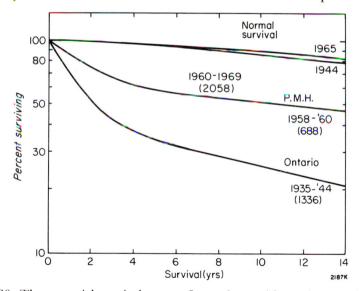

Figure 17-20. The actuarial survival curves for patients with carcinoma of the cervix treated by radiation in two different time periods. The lowest curve is the survival of those patients treated from 1935 to 1944 inclusive in the province of Ontario. The next curve, above, shows the survival of patients treated at the Princess Margaret Hospital between 1958 and 1969 with only the 688 patients between 1958 and 1960 being available for 14-year follow-up at the time of analysis. The upper two curves represent the survival of normal populations of women in Ontario who have the same age distributions as the patients treated. (Taken from Bush, B37.)

earlier era, even after 10 years, shows that patients were dying at a rate greater than the normal population.

This demonstrates that a large fraction of patients have been given the same probability of surviving as women without cancer of the cervix and may be interpreted as evidence for cure. For such cured women, who had a median age of 52 years at the time of diagnosis, an average of an additional 28 years of life has been provided. If they had not had their cancer controlled, the average survival would have been only about 1.5 years.

Because the cost of medical care is a cause for concern in many countries and therapy machines are expensive, it is of value to examine the benefit of treatment for patients with cancer of the cervix, and compare it with what has to be paid by the patient, or the community, to achieve this benefit. Bush (B37) has estimated that for every 100 patients treated, 1463 normal healthy years of life are gained. He also estimated the average direct cost of treatment of a patient with cancer of the cervix to be 3000 dollars (1976) at the Princess Margaret Hospital. This means the cost per year of life is $3000/14.63 = $205. Thus, even though equipment may be expensive, if there is high utilization of it, and the benefits are great, the cost per patient is small.

Which Photon Energy is Best?

During the late 1970s many centers installed linear accelerators in place of cobalt 60 units. The question now is, what energy is optimum? The cobalt 60 unit is essentially equivalent to a 3 to 4 MeV linear accelerator. Should a linear accelerator have an energy of 4, 6, 10, 20, or 25 MeV? In an effort to answer this question, a random study between cobalt 60 and a 22 MeV betatron, in treating patients with stage IIB and III cancer of cervix, was carried out by Allt (A8) and updated by Bush (B37). Some of these results are summarized in Figure 17-21. There is, clearly, a considerable survival advantage in using the betatron. The difference in cure rate was so great that the random study had to be discontinued. Since that time, many types of linear accelerators have come on the market and there are many radiation oncologists who feel that a 6 or 10 MeV linear accelerator is just as good as a betatron. Dose distributions from various types of machines were discussed in Chapter 12. As the energy is increased above 4 MeV it is possible to concentrate more and more energy in the tumor than in the surrounding tissues. If the energy is made too high, the exit dose tends to become excessive and, of course, costs increase. Our analysis showed (sec. 12.11) that an energy of about 25 MeV is optimum. The question is, Can the increase in cost be justified by improved cure rate? In the next decade many centers will gain experience with high energy machines in

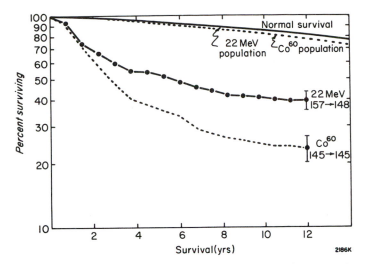

Figure 17-21. The actuarial survival of all patients with advanced Stage IIB and Stage III disease randomized between treatment of ^{60}Co and 22 MV betatron irradiation in a prospective study at the Princess Margaret Hospital. The survival of the normal populations of women with the same age distribution as the patients in each treatment arm are also shown. One standard deviation is shown on each treatment survival curve. (Taken from Bush, B37.)

the 20 MeV range, so this question will be answered. Centers that have had high energy machines will be prevented from studying this problem, because they already know they can do better with high energy radiation.

17.17 SUMMARY OF THE APPLICATION OF RADIOBIOLOGY TO RADIOTHERAPY

The application of radiobiology to the understanding of practical problems in radiotherapy remains to a large extent a qualitative rather than quantitative exercise. From studies with cells in culture and with animal tumors and normal tissues we think we know which factors are important and we have discussed these in the present chapter. At present, radiobiological knowledge provides a framework within which radiotherapeutic successes and failures can be viewed. A brief discussion on how such thinking can be applied to possible changes in fractionation schedules is presented. It is clear from this that a better understanding of the biology of tumors and normal tissues and the kinetics of their response to radiation treatment is required.

The application of radiobiological knowledge to radiotherapeutic practice over the last two decades has had its major impact in relation to the oxygen effect and this remains an area of active interest particularly in the use of hypoxic cell radiosensitizers. We can expect further development of high LET radiations. Further development of radioprotectors as possible therapeutic adjuvants will take place along with greater use of hyperthermia either alone or in combination with radiation and cytotoxic drugs. A greater understanding of isoeffect curves for tumor and normal tissue responses to radiation treatment may also lead to the development of fractionation schedules with better therapeutic ratios.

17.18   SUMMARY OF THE APPLICATION OF PHYSICS TO RADIOLOGY

DIAGNOSTIC RADIOLOGY. Recent applications of physics to the field of imaging have produced ionography and other methods of imaging with ionizing radiation that do not involve film. Developments in the field of both solid state detectors and computers make the storage of images in digital form possible and new methods for processing these images will continue to be investigated. Radiation protection is becoming more of a public concern and imaging techniques that truly minimize dose will be developed.

In recent years other systems for imaging have been explored and very significant results are being obtained with non-ionizing radiation such as ultrasound and NMR. The latter is particularly interesting because it images physiological function in addition to structure.

RADIOTHERAPY. The improved ability to visualize tumors and normal tissues by means of methods developed for diagnostic radiology is a direct aid to radiotherapy. It will reduce the probability of "geographic misses" and facilitate the avoidance of healthy tissues. New methods for dose calculation allow greater precision in the delivery of radiation to a tumor. Our experience with cancer of the cervix leads us to believe that a careful use of high energy beams to other sites should result in further increased cure rates.

If a radiation therapist believes there is an advantage in increasing the dose to the tumor volume relative to normal tissues, high energy radiation (15-25 MeV) must be better than lower radiation (3-6 MeV) for the treatment of patients with deep-seated tumors. We believe that the use of high energy beams and careful treatment planning, including precise dose calculations that take inhomogeneities into account, will result not only in increased cure rates but in reduced complications—this is what much of this book is about.

APPENDICES

The appendices contain resource data used in working through the examples and are required for the solution of many of the problems given at the end of each chapter. They should be useful for the practicing radiation physicist, the radiologist, and the radiation oncologist.

APPENDIX A—BASIC DATA

Table A-1 contains a selection of the physical constants and conversion factors used frequently throughout the text. The numerical values for the physical constants are taken from the *Handbook of Chemistry and Physics*, Vol. 58. The conversion factors are consistent with SI usage.

Table A-2a lists Compton coefficients expressed in units of 10^{-28} m^2/electron (barns per electron). They were calculated using equations 6-12 to 6-15. The electrons are assumed to be at rest and free.

Table A-2b relates energy fluence and photon fluence to exposure calculated using equations 7-42 and 7-43 using the coefficients for air presented in Table A-3a.

Tables A-3 and A-4. Photon interaction coefficients were kindly made available to us on magnetic tape by R. J. Howerton of Lawrence Livermore Laboratory, University of California. This data has also been published in tabular form by Plechaty et al. (P5). Table A-4 contains cross sections for nine elements for coherent scattering (see sec. 6.03) and incoherent (sec. 6.07), photoelectric (sec. 6.01), and pair production (sec. 6.08) processes given in units of 10^{-28} m^2 per atom (barns/at). These have been added to form the mass attenuation coefficients (μ/ρ) listed in units of cm^2/g. The average energy transferred per photon interaction, $\overline{E}_{tr}$, has also been taken from the Plechaty-Howerton data but average energies absorbed, $\overline{E}_{ab}$, were calculated by us (C4). Mass energy transfer and mass energy absorption coefficients have been calculated from $\overline{E}_{tr}$ and $\overline{E}_{ab}$. Included in these tables is an average stopping power, $\overline{S}$, calculated from equation 6-43 using the spectrum of electrons that results from the interaction of photons and the medium. Table A-3 contains photon interaction coefficients for ten mixtures and compounds calculated by the method outlined in example 5-11. The proportions of the components used for each substance are given in the following list.

Composition by weight of materials in Table A-3

1. Air   N(0.755), O(0.232), A(0.013)
2. Water, H_2O H(0.112), O(0.888)
3. Muscle   H(0.1020), C(0.1230), N(0.0350), O(0.7289), Na(0.0008), Mg(0.0002), P(0.0020), S(0.0050), K(0.0030), Ca(0.00007)
4. Bone   H(0.064), C(0.278), N(0.027), O(0.410), Mg(0.002), P(0.070), S(0.002), Ca(0.147)
5. Fat   H(0.1120), C(0.5732), N(0.0110), O(0.3031), S(0.00006)
6. Polystyrene, C_8H_8 H(0.0774), C(0.9226)
7. Lucite, $C_5H_8O_2$ H(0.0805), C(0.5998), O(0.3196)
8. Bakelite, $C_{43}H_{38}O_7$ H(0.0574), C(0.7746), O(0.1680)
9. Lithium fluoride, LiF   Li(0.2675), F(0.7325)
10. Ferrous sulphate solution, $FeSO_4$ in 0.8 N H_2SO_4 H(0.10839), O(0.87894), Na(0.00002) S(0.01255), Cl(0.00004), Fe(0.00006)

Table A-5 gives mass ionizational stopping powers, $S_{ion}(E)$, for electrons in various materials calculated by M. J. Berger and using equation 6-26. The data was extended down to energies of 1 keV by us.

Table A-6 gives ranges and bremsstrahlung yields for electrons slowing down in five materials. The ranges were calculated by numerical integration of equation 6-28; the bremsstrahlung yield by equation 6-31.

Table A-7 gives f_{med} for 8 materials for a range of monoenergetic photon energies. These numbers are determined directly from data in Table A-3 and A-4.

TABLE A-1

Constants, Units, and Conversion Factors

1. PHYSICAL CONSTANTS

speed of light	c	2.997925×10^8 m/s
Avogadro's number	N_A	6.022045×10^{23} mol^{-1}
Planck's constant	h	6.626176×10^{-34} J s
electronic charge	e	1.60218×10^{-19} C
electron mass	m_0	9.109534×10^{-31} kg
proton mass		1.672649×10^{-27} kg
neutron mass		1.674954×10^{-27} kg
average energy deposited in air per liberated charge	W	33.85 J/C = 33.85 eV/ion pair
density of air	ρ	1.293 kg/m^3 at STP (0° C, 101.3 kPa)
		1.205 kg/m^3 at NTP (20° C, 101.3 kPa)

2. RADIATION UNITS

a. by definition   b. by implication

becquerel	1 Bq = 1.0 s^{-1}	1 R = 87.33×10^{-4} J/kg air
gray	1 Gy = 1 J/kg	= 54.51×10^{15} eV/kg air
roentgen	1 R = 2.580×10^{-4} C/kg air	
	3.336×10^{-10} C/cm^3 air at STP	

based on W as above

3. ENERGY CONVERSION FACTORS

electron volt	1 eV = 1.602192×10^{-19} J = 1.602192×10^{-12} erg
	1 MeV = 1.602192×10^{-13} J
calorie	1 cal = 4.18 J
atomic mass unit	1 amu = 931.481 MeV
electron mass	$m_0 = 0.511004$ MeV

4. RADIATION CONVERSION FACTORS

rad	1 rad = $.01$ Gy = 100 erg/g
curie	1 Ci = 3.7000×10^{10} Bq = 3.7000×10^{10} s^{-1}

5. USEFUL RELATIONS

Coulomb's Law $F = k\, q_1\, q_2/r^2$, $k = 8.9875 \times 10^9$ N m^2/C^2

1 esu = 3.336×10^{-10} C = 2.082×10^9 electron charges

Classical radius of electron, $r_0 = \dfrac{ke^2}{m_0 c^2} = 2.81794 \times 10^{-15}$ m

Classical Thomson scattering coef., $\sigma_0 = 8\,\pi\, r_0^2/3 = 66.525 \times 10^{-30}$ m^2

1 day = 1.44×10^3 min = 8.64×10^4 s;   1 y = 5.260×10^5 min = 3.156×10^7 s

curie   1 Ci almost equals the activity of 1 g radium

cumulated activity   1 mCi hr = 1.332×10^{11} Bq s   1 mCi day = 3.197×10^{12} Bq s

6. MATHEMATICAL CONSTANTS AND RELATIONS

$\pi = 3.1416$, $e = 2.7183$, $e^{-1} = .3679$, $e^{-.693} = 0.5$

TABLE A-2a COMPTON COEFFICIENTS FOR FREE ELECTRONS					TABLE A-2b ENERGY AND PHOTON FLUENCE PER ROENTGEN; SPECIFIC GAMMA RAY CONSTANT			

Photon energy $h\nu$	Compton coeff. in 10^{-28} m^2/electron by Klein-Nishina eq.			Average energy transf. (eq. 6-15) $\sigma\overline{E}_{tr}$	Photon energy $h\nu$	Energy fluence per roentgen (for J m^{-2} R^{-1} mult. by 10^{-3})	Photon fluence per roentgen (for m^{-2} R^{-1} mult. by 10^{11})	Specific gamma ray constant Γ in $\dfrac{R\ cm^2}{hr\ mCi}$
	(6-12) σ	(6-14) σ_s	(6-13) σ_{tr}					
(keV)				(keV)	(keV)			
1	.6627	.6614	.0013	.002	1	.0237	1.479	716.0
1.5	.6614	.6594	.0019	.004	1.5	.0709	2.955	358.3
2	.6601	.6575	.0026	.008	2	.1602	5.004	211.6
3	.6576	.6537	.0038	.017	3	.5273	10.98	96.41
4	.6550	.6500	.0050	.031	4	1.125	17.57	60.27
5	.6525	.6463	.0063	.048	5	2.210	27.62	38.34
6	.6501	.6426	.0074	.069	6	3.867	40.28	26.29
8	.6452	.6355	.0098	.121	8	9.479	74.02	14.30
10	.6405	.6285	.0120	.188	10	19.17	119.9	8.839
15	.6290	.6116	.0174	.414	15	69.97	291.5	3.633
20	.6180	.5957	.0223	.721	20	175.8	549.3	1.928
30	.5975	.5664	.0311	1.56	30	622.9	1297.	.8161
40	.5787	.5400	.0387	2.68	40	1390.	2171.	.4877
50	.5615	.5162	.0454	4.04	50	2274.	2842.	.3725
60	.5456	.4946	.0510	5.61	60	3002.	3126.	.3387
80	.5173	.4567	.0606	9.37	80	3687.	2880.	.3677
100	.4927	.4248	.0680	13.8	100	3768.	2355.	.4497
150	.4436	.3631	.0805	27.2	150	3484.	1451.	.7295
200	.4065	.3185	.0879	43.3	200	3250.	1015.	1.043
300	.3534	.2581	.0953	80.9	300	3024.	629.8	1.681
400	.3167	.2186	.0981	124.	400	2945.	460.0	2.302
500	.2892	.1905	.0987	171.	500	2928.	365.9	2.894
600	.2675	.1692	.0983	221.	600	2941.	306.3	3.457
662	.2561	.1584	.0978	253.	662	2953.	278.7	3.799
800	.2350	.1389	.0960	327.	800	3012.	235.3	4.501
(MeV)				(MeV)	(MeV)			
1	.2112	.1183	.0929	.440	1	3114.	194.6	5.442
1.25	.1888	.1000	.0889	.588	1.25	3258.	162.9	6.501
1.5	.1716	.0867	.0849	.742	1.5	3408.	142.0	7.459
2	.1464	.0687	.0777	1.06	2	3701.	115.6	9.157
3	.1151	.0486	.0664	1.73	3	4218.	87.86	12.05
4	.0960	.0377	.0583	2.43				
5	.0829	.0308	.0520	3.14		(eq. 7-42)	(eq. 7-43)	(eq. 7-44)
6	.0732	.0261	.0472	3.86				
8	.0599	.0199	.0400	5.34				
10	.0510	.0161	.0349	6.84				
15	.0377	.0109	.0268	10.7				
20	.0303	.0083	.0220	14.5				
30	.0220	.0056	.0164	22.4				
40	.0175	.0042	.0133	30.4				
50	.0146	.0034	.0112	38.5				
60	.0125	.0028	.0097	46.6				
80	.0099	.0021	.0078	62.9				
100	.0082	.0017	.0065	79.4				

TABLE A-3a - AIR $\bar{Z} = 7.78$

$\rho = 1.205$ kg/m³ (at NTP)

3.006×10^{26} elect./kg

Photon energy $h\nu$ [keV]	Interaction coefficients [cm²/g] $\left(\frac{\mu}{\rho}\right)$	$\left(\frac{\mu_{ab}}{\rho}\right)$	Average energy transf. $\bar{E}_{tr}$ [keV]	abs. $\bar{E}_{ab}$	Average stopping power $\bar{\bar{S}}$ *
1	3673.	3672.	1.00		
1.5	1227.	1226.	1.50		90.1
2	543.7	542.6	2.00		79.9
3	165.6	164.7	2.98		66.1
4	78.80	77.28	3.92		56.6
·5	40.29	39.32	4.88		49.7
6	23.17	22.47	5.82		44.5
8	9.642	9.168	7.61		37.0
10	4.910	4.533	9.23		31.8
15	1.522	1.242	12.2		24.2
20	.7334	.4942	13.5		19.7
30	.3398	.1395	12.3		15.1
40	.2429	.0625	10.3		13.3
50	.2053	.0382	9.31		13.1
60	.1861	.0289	9.33		13.9
80	.1658	.0236	11.4		15.8
100	.1540	.0231	15.0		15.6
150	.1356	.0249	27.6		11.8
200	.1234	.0267	43.4		8.72
300	.1068	.0287	80.8		5.76
400	.0955	.0295	124.		4.46
500	.0871	.0297	171.		3.73
550	.0836	.0296	195.		3.48
662	.0771	.0293	252.		3.07
800	.0707	.0288	327.		2.74
[MeV]			[MeV]		
1	.0636	.0279	.440		2.47
1.25	.0569	.0267	.588	.586	2.25
1.5	.0518	.0255	.741	.739	2.12
2	.0445	.0235	1.06	1.05	1.98
3	.0358	.0206	1.74	1.72	1.86
4	.0308	.0187	2.46	2.43	1.82
5	.0275	.0174	3.22	3.17	1.81
6	.0251	.0164	4.00	3.92	1.81
8	.0221	.0152	5.64	5.48	1.81
10	.0205	.0145	7.37	7.10	1.82
15	.0180	.0135	11.9	11.2	1.86
20	.0171	.0132	16.6	15.5	1.89
30	.0163	.0129	26.3	23.7	1.94
40	.0161	.0127	36.2	31.7	1.98
50	.0161	.0127	46.1	39.3	2.01
60	.0162	.0126	56.1	46.6	2.04
80	.0164	.0124	76.0	60.3	2.08
100	.0168	.0123	96.1	72.9	2.12

TABLE A-3b - WATER $\bar{Z} = 7.51$

$\rho = 1000$ kg/m³

3.343×10^{26} elect./kg

Photon energy $h\nu$ [keV]	Interaction coefficients [cm²/g] $\left(\frac{\mu}{\rho}\right)$	$\left(\frac{\mu_{ab}}{\rho}\right)$	Average energy transf. $\bar{E}_{tr}$ [keV]	abs. $\bar{E}_{ab}$	Average stopping power $\bar{\bar{S}}$ *
1	4083.	4082.	1.00		
1.5	1395.	1394.	1.50		105.
2	627.4	626.1	2.00		92.9
3	194.7	193.8	2.99		76.7
4	82.74	81.92	3.96		65.5
5	42.13	41.46	4.92		57.4
6	24.13	23.55	5.86		51.3
8	9.982	9.532	7.64		42.5
10	5.066	4.684	9.25		36.5
15	1.568	1.269	12.1		27.8
20	.7613	.5016	13.2		22.6
30	.3612	.1411	11.7		17.3
40	.2629	.0637	9.70		15.4
50	.2245	.0396	8.82		15.3
60	.2046	.0305	8.96		16.4
80	.1833	.0255	11.2		18.7
100	.1706	.0253	14.8		18.3
150	.1505	.0276	27.5		13.5
200	.1370	.0297	43.3		9.93
300	.1187	.0320	80.8		6.54
400	.1061	.0328	124.		5.06
500	.0969	.0330	171.		4.22
550	.0930	.0329	195.		3.94
662	.0857	.0326	252.		3.47
800	.0787	.0321	327.		3.10
[MeV]			[MeV]		
1	.0707	.0310	.440		2.79
1.25	.0632	.0297	.588	.586	2.54
1.5	.0575	.0283	.741	.739	2.39
2	.0494	.0261	1.06	1.06	2.22
3	.0397	.0228	1.74	1.73	2.07
4	.0340	.0207	2.46	2.43	2.01
5	.0303	.0192	3.21	3.16	1.98
6	.0276	.0180	3.99	3.91	1.97
8	.0242	.0165	5.62	5.47	1.96
10	.0222	.0157	7.33	7.07	1.95
15	.0193	.0144	11.8	11.2	1.96
20	.0182	.0139	16.5	15.3	1.97
30	.0171	.0134	26.1	23.5	1.99
40	.0167	.0131	36.0	31.3	2.01
50	.0167	.0130	45.9	38.8	2.02
60	.0167	.0128	55.8	45.9	2.03
80	.0169	.0125	75.8	59.2	2.05
100	.0172	.0123	95.8	71.3	2.06

*Av. Stopping Power in [MeV cm²g⁻¹] for the spectrum of electrons produced in the medium by photons of energy $h\nu$

TABLE A-3c - MUSCLE				$\bar{Z}$ = 7.64		TABLE A-3d - BONE				$\bar{Z}$ = 12.31
ρ = 1040 kg/m³						ρ = 1650 kg/m³				
3.312 x 10²⁶ elect./kg						3.192 x 10²⁶ elect./kg				

Photon energy	Interaction coefficients [cm²/g]		Average energy transf. abs.		Average stopping power $\bar{\bar{S}}$ *	Photon energy	Interaction coefficients [cm²/g]		Average energy transf. abs.		Average stopping power $\bar{\bar{S}}$ *
$h\nu$	$\left(\dfrac{\mu}{\rho}\right)$	$\left(\dfrac{\mu_{ab}}{\rho}\right)$	$\bar{E}_{tr}$	$\bar{E}_{ab}$		$h\nu$	$\left(\dfrac{\mu}{\rho}\right)$	$\left(\dfrac{\mu_{ab}}{\rho}\right)$	$\bar{E}_{tr}$	$\bar{E}_{ab}$	
[keV]			[keV]			[keV]			[keV]		
1	3771.	3770.	1.00			1	3464.	3463.	1.00		
1.5	1285.	1284.	1.50		104.	1.5	1181.	1179.	1.50		92.6
2	576.3	575.1	2.00		92.0	2	533.4	531.8	1.99		82.3
3	186.5	185.1	2.98		75.9	3	241.0	236.8	2.95		68.3
4	81.95	80.74	3.94		64.8	4	107.4	105.4	3.92		58.6
5	42.04	41.20	4.90		56.8	5	137.5	126.4	4.60		51.5
6	24.21	23.55	5.84		50.7	6	83.44	77.47	5.57		46.1
8	10.10	9.625	7.62		42.1	8	37.31	34.95	7.49		38.4
10	5.154	4.764	9.24		36.2	10	19.79	18.55	9.37		33.1
15	1.604	1.307	12.2		27.5	15	6.193	5.680	13.8		25.3
20	.7777	.5206	13.4		22.3	20	2.753	2.408	17.5		20.6
30	.3651	.1474	12.1		17.1	30	.9534	.7091	22.3		15.5
40	.2635	.0664	10.1		15.1	40	.5089	.3007	23.6		12.7
50	.2240	.0409	9.13		14.9	50	.3471	.1590	22.9		11.1
60	.2036	.0312	9.20		15.9	60	.2727	.0985	21.7		10.3
80	.1819	.0257	11.3		18.1	80	.2082	.0530	20.4		9.93
100	.1692	.0253	14.9		17.8	100	.1803	.0386	21.4		10.3
150	.1492	.0275	27.6		13.3	150	.1493	.0306	30.7		10.2
200	.1358	.0294	43.4		9.83	200	.1334	.0301	45.2		8.53
300	.1176	.0317	80.8		6.48	300	.1142	.0310	81.6		5.95
400	.1052	.0325	124.		5.01	400	.1018	.0316	124.		4.66
500	.0960	.0327	171.		4.18	500	.0927	.0316	171.		3.90
550	.0921	.0326	195.		3.90	550	.0890	.0315	195.		3.64
662	.0849	.0323	252.		3.44	662	.0820	.0312	253.		3.21
800	.0779	.0318	327.		3.07	800	.0752	.0306	327.		2.87
[MeV]			[MeV]			[MeV]			[MeV]		
1	.0701	.0308	.440		2.76	1	.0676	.0296	.440		2.57
1.25	.0626	.0294	.588	.586	2.51	1.25	.0604	.0283	.588	.586	2.34
1.5	.0570	.0281	.741	.739	2.36	1.5	.0550	.0271	.741	.738	2.20
2	.0490	.0258	1.06	1.06	2.19	2	.0473	.0249	1.06	1.05	2.04
3	.0393	.0226	1.74	1.73	2.04	3	.0383	.0220	1.74	1.72	1.90
4	.0337	.0205	2.46	2.43	1.98	4	.0331	.0201	2.47	2.43	1.85
5	.0300	.0190	3.21	3.16	1.95	5	.0297	.0188	3.23	3.16	1.82
6	.0273	.0178	3.99	3.91	1.93	6	.0273	.0178	4.02	3.92	1.80
8	.0239	.0163	5.61	5.46	1.92	8	.0242	.0166	5.68	5.48	1.79
10	.0220	.0155	7.32	7.07	1.91	10	.0226	.0161	7.43	7.10	1.79
15	.0191	.0142	11.8	11.2	1.92	15	.0202	.0151	12.0	11.2	1.80
20	.0179	.0137	16.5	15.3	1.93	20	.0195	.0149	16.8	15.3	1.81
30	.0169	.0132	26.1	23.5	1.95	30	.0189	.0147	26.5	23.3	1.83
40	.0165	.0129	36.0	31.3	1.97	40	.0189	.0145	36.4	30.8	1.85
50	.0165	.0128	45.9	38.8	1.98	50	.0191	.0145	46.4	37.9	1.86
60	.0165	.0126	55.8	45.9	1.99	60	.0192	.0142	56.4	44.5	1.87
80	.0166	.0123	75.8	59.2	2.01	80	.0196	.0139	76.4	56.8	1.89
100	.0170	.0121	95.8	71.4	2.03	100	.0201	.0137	96.4	67.9	1.91

*Av. Stopping Power in [MeV cm²g⁻¹] for the spectrum of electrons produced in the medium by photons of energy $h\nu$

TABLE A-3e - FAT				$\bar{Z} = 6.46$

$\rho = 916$ kg/m³

3.34 x 10²⁶ elect./kg

TABLE A-3f - POLYSTYRENE, C_8H_8				$\bar{Z} = 5.74$

$\rho = 1044$ kg/m³

3.238 x 10²⁶ elect./kg

Photon energy $h\nu$	Interaction coefficients [cm²/g] $\left(\frac{\mu}{\rho}\right)$	$\left(\frac{\mu_{ab}}{\rho}\right)$	Average energy transf. $\bar{E}_{tr}$	abs. $\bar{E}_{ab}$	Average stopping power $\bar{\bar{S}}$ *	Photon energy $h\nu$	Interaction coefficients [cm²/g] $\left(\frac{\mu}{\rho}\right)$	$\left(\frac{\mu_{ab}}{\rho}\right)$	Average energy transf. $\bar{E}_{tr}$	abs. $\bar{E}_{ab}$	Average stopping power $\bar{\bar{S}}$ *
[keV]			[keV]			[keV]			[keV]		
1	2693.	2692.	1.00			1	2028.	2027.	1.00		
1.5	895.6	895.1	1.50		112.	1.5	654.6	653.7	1.50		108.
2	395.9	394.9	2.00		98.4	2	283.4	282.5	1.99		94.7
3	120.9	120.1	2.98		80.8	3	83.61	82.94	2.98		77.8
4	50.69	50.04	3.95		68.7	4	34.38	33.84	3.94		66.3
5	25.59	25.06	4.90		60.1	5	17.13	16.67	4.87		57.9
6	14.58	14.12	5.81		53.6	6	9.672	9.274	5.75		51.7
8	6.022	5.643	7.50		44.4	8	3.973	3.635	7.32		42.8
10	3.081	2.749	8.92		38.0	10	2.047	1.745	8.52		36.7
15	1.009	.7358	10.9		28.8	15	.7115	.4570	9.64		27.6
20	.5332	.2903	10.9		23.4	20	.4084	.1791	8.77		22.4
30	.2959	.0843	8.55		18.3	30	.2558	.0540	6.33		18.0
40	.2353	.0414	7.04		17.2	40	.2151	.0292	5.44		18.3
50	.2102	.0288	6.85		18.4	50	.1970	.0226	5.73		20.9
60	.1961	.0246	7.51		20.7	60	.1861	.0208	6.72		23.6
80	.1794	.0232	10.3		22.6	80	.1722	.0213	9.89		24.1
100	.1684	.0241	14.3		20.6	100	.1623	.0228	14.1		20.7
150	.1497	.0273	27.4		14.2	150	.1447	.0263	27.3		13.7
200	.1366	.0295	43.3		10.3	200	.1322	.0286	43.2		9.85
300	.1184	.0319	80.8		6.72	300	.1147	.0309	80.8		6.43
400	.1060	.0328	124.		5.19	400	.1027	.0317	124.		4.96
500	.0968	.0330	171.		4.33	500	.0938	.0319	171.		4.14
550	.0929	.0329	195.		4.04	550	.0900	.0319	195.		3.86
662	.0856	.0326	253.		3.55	662	.0830	.0316	253.		3.40
800	.0786	.0321	327.		3.17	800	.0762	.0311	327.		3.04
[MeV]			[MeV]			[MeV]			[MeV]		
1	.0707	.0310	.440		2.84	1	.0685	.0301	.440		2.73
1.25	.0632	.0296	.588	.586	2.58	1.25	.0612	.0287	.588		2.48
1.5	.0575	.0283	.742	.739	2.43	1.5	.0557	.0275	.742	.739	2.33
2	.0493	.0260	1.06	1.05	2.25	2	.0478	.0253	1.06	1.06	2.17
3	.0395	.0227	1.74	1.72	2.09	3	.0382	.0220	1.74	1.73	2.02
4	.0337	.0205	2.45	2.43	2.02	4	.0326	.0198	2.45	2.43	1.96
5	.0299	.0189	3.20	3.15	1.99	5	.0289	.0183	3.20	3.16	1.93
6	.0271	.0176	3.97	3.90	1.97	6	.0262	.0170	3.97	3.91	1.91
8	.0236	.0160	5.58	5.44	1.96	8	.0227	.0154	5.57	5.45	1.90
10	.0215	.0151	7.27	7.04	1.95	10	.0206	.0145	7.26	7.04	1.90
15	.0183	.0136	11.7	11.1	1.96	15	.0175	.0130	11.7	11.1	1.90
20	.0170	.0130	16.3	15.3	1.97	20	.0162	.0124	16.3	15.3	1.91
30	.0158	.0124	25.9	23.5	1.99	30	.0149	.0117	25.8	23.5	1.93
40	.0152	.0120	35.7	31.5	2.00	40	.0144	.0113	35.6	31.5	1.95
50	.0151	.0119	45.6	39.2	2.02	50	.0142	.0112	45.5	39.2	1.96
60	.0150	.0116	55.5	46.6	2.03	60	.0141	.0110	55.4	46.6	1.97
80	.0151	.0114	75.4	60.4	2.05	80	.0141	.0107	75.3	60.5	1.99
100	.0153	.0112	95.4	73.0	2.07	100	.0143	.0105	95.3	73.3	2.00

*Av. Stopping Power in [MeV cm²g⁻¹] for the spectrum of electrons produced in the medium by photons of energy $h\nu$

TABLE A-3g - LUCITE, $C_5H_8O_2$ $\bar{Z} = 6.56$

$\rho = 1180$ kg/m³

3.248×10^{26} elect./kg

Photon energy hν	Interaction coefficients [cm²/g] $\left(\frac{\mu}{\rho}\right)$	$\left(\frac{\mu_{ab}}{\rho}\right)$	Average energy transf. $\bar{E}_{tr}$	abs. $\bar{E}_{ab}$	Average stopping power $\bar{\bar{S}}$ *
[keV]			[keV]		
1	2788.	2787.	1.00		
1.5	927.5	926.9	1.50		106.
2	410.0	409.0	2.00		93.4
3	124.4	123.7	2.98		76.8
4	52.13	51.49	3.95		65.5
5	26.29	25.76	4.90		57.3
6	14.97	14.51	5.82		51.1
8	6.172	5.794	7.51		42.4
10	3.151	2.821	8.95		36.3
15	1.023	.7536	11.1		27.3
20	.5357	.2968	11.1		22.1
30	.2927	.0857	8.78		17.2
40	.2310	.0417	7.22		16.1
50	.2055	.0287	6.97		17.2
60	.1914	.0242	7.60		19.3
80	.1748	.0227	10.4		21.2
100	.1639	.0235	14.4		19.4
150	.1456	.0266	27.4		13.4
200	.1328	.0287	43.3		9.73
300	.1152	.0310	80.8		6.37
400	.1031	.0319	124.		4.92
500	.0941	.0321	171.		4.11
550	.0903	.0320	195.		3.84
662	.0832	.0317	253.		3.38
800	.0764	.0312	327.		3.02
[MeV]			[MeV]		
1	.0687	.0302	.440		2.71
1.25	.0614	.0288	.588		2.47
1.5	.0559	.0275	.741	.739	2.32
2	.0480	.0253	1.06	1.06	2.15
3	.0385	.0221	1.74	1.73	2.01
4	.0329	.0200	2.46	2.43	1.95
5	.0292	.0184	3.20	3.16	1.92
6	.0265	.0173	3.98	3.91	1.91
8	.0231	.0157	5.59	5.45	1.89
10	.0211	.0149	7.29	7.06	1.89
15	.0181	.0134	11.7	11.1	1.90
20	.0169	.0129	16.4	15.3	1.91
30	.0157	.0123	26.0	23.5	1.92
40	.0152	.0120	35.8	31.4	1.94
50	.0151	.0118	45.7	39.0	1.95
60	.0151	.0116	55.6	46.2	1.96
80	.0152	.0113	75.6	59.9	1.98
100	.0154	.0111	95.6	72.4	1.99

TABLE A-3h - BAKELITE, $C_{43}H_{38}O_7$ $\bar{Z} = 6.27$

$\rho = 1400$ kg/m³

3.179×10^{26} elect./kg

Photon energy hν	Interaction coefficients [cm²/g] $\left(\frac{\mu}{\rho}\right)$	$\left(\frac{\mu_{ab}}{\rho}\right)$	Average energy transf. $\bar{E}_{tr}$	abs. $\bar{E}_{ab}$	Average stopping power $\bar{\bar{S}}$ *
[keV]			[keV]		
1	2475.	2474.	1.00		
1.5	813.3	812.2	1.50		103.
2	356.6	355.7	2.00		90.6
3	107.0	106.3	2.98		74.6
4	44.50	43.91	3.95		63.6
5	22.34	21.84	4.89		55.7
6	12.67	12.24	5.80		49.7
8	5.213	4.855	7.45		41.2
10	2.666	2.351	8.82		35.3
15	.8831	.6234	10.6		26.5
20	.4763	.2448	10.3		21.5
30	.2728	.0715	7.86		16.9
40	.2204	.0359	6.52		16.3
50	.1982	.0257	6.48		17.7
60	.1856	.0224	7.24		20.0
80	.1704	.0217	10.2		21.5
100	.1601	.0228	14.2		19.3
150	.1423	.0259	27.3		13.1
200	.1299	.0281	43.2		9.48
300	.1127	.0303	80.8		6.21
400	.1009	.0312	124.		4.80
500	.0921	.0314	171.		4.00
550	.0884	.0313	195.		3.74
662	.0815	.0310	253.		3.29
800	.0748	.0305	327.		2.94
[MeV]			[MeV]		
1	.0672	.0295	.440		2.64
1.25	.0601	.0282	.588		2.41
1.5	.0547	.0270	.742	.739	2.26
2	.0469	.0248	1.06	1.06	2.10
3	.0376	.0216	1.74	1.73	1.96
4	.0322	.0195	2.46	2.43	1.90
5	.0286	.0180	3.20	3.16	1.88
6	.0259	.0169	3.98	3.91	1.86
8	.0225	.0154	5.59	5.45	1.85
10	.0206	.0145	7.28	7.05	1.85
15	.0176	.0131	11.7	11.1	1.85
20	.0164	.0126	16.4	15.3	1.86
30	.0153	.0120	26.0	23.5	1.88
40	.0148	.0116	35.7	31.4	1.90
50	.0147	.0115	45.6	39.0	1.91
60	.0146	.0113	55.6	46.3	1.92
80	.0147	.0110	75.5	59.9	1.94
100	.0150	.0108	95.5	72.4	1.95

*Av. Stopping Power in [MeV cm²g⁻¹] for the spectrum of electrons produced in the medium by photons of energy hν

TABLE A-3i - LITHIUM FLUORIDE, LiF $\bar{Z}$ = 8.31

ρ = 2675 kg/m³

2.786 x 10²⁶ elect./kg

Photon energy $h\nu$	Interaction coefficients $\left(\frac{\mu}{\rho}\right)$ [cm²/g]	$\left(\frac{\mu_{ab}}{\rho}\right)$ [cm²/g]	Average energy transf. $\bar{E}_{tr}$ [keV]	abs. $\bar{E}_{ab}$ [keV]	Average stopping power $\bar{\bar{S}}$ *
[keV]					
1	4216.	4214.	1.00		
1.5	1508.	1507.	1.50		81.6
2	697.4	696.4	2.00		72.4
3	223.7	222.7	2.99		60.1
4	96.76	95.96	3.97		51.5
5	49.84	49.18	4.93		45.3
6	28.75	28.19	5.88		40.5
8	11.99	11.55	7.71		33.8
10	6.076	5.714	9.40		29.1
15	1.833	1.563	12.8		22.1
20	.8480	.6181	14.6		18.0
30	.3613	.1712	14.2		13.7
40	.2440	.0740	12.1		11.8
50	.1998	.0430	10.8		11.3
60	.1780	.0310	10.5		11.7
80	.1560	.0235	12.0		13.2
100	.1440	.0222	15.4		13.5
150	.1261	.0233	27.8		10.6
200	.1145	.0249	43.4		7.92
300	.0990	.0266	80.8		5.26
400	.0885	.0273	124.		4.07
500	.0808	.0275	171.		3.41
550	.0775	.0275	195.		3.18
662	.0714	.0272	253.		2.81
800	.0656	.0267	327.		2.51
[MeV]			[MeV]		
1	.0589	.0259	.440		2.26
1.25	.0527	.0247	.588	.586	2.06
1.5	.0480	.0236	.741	.738	1.93
2	.0412	.0217	1.06	1.05	1.79
3	.0332	.0191	1.74	1.72	1.68
4	.0286	.0174	2.46	2.43	1.63
5	.0256	.0162	3.22	3.16	1.60
6	.0233	.0152	4.00	3.91	1.59
8	.0206	.0141	5.64	5.47	1.58
10	.0190	.0135	7.37	7.09	1.58
15	.0168	.0125	11.9	11.2	1.58
20	.0159	.0122	16.6	15.3	1.59
30	.0152	.0119	26.3	23.4	1.60
40	.0150	.0117	36.2	31.0	1.62
50	.0151	.0116	46.1	38.3	1.63
60	.0152	.0114	56.1	45.2	1.64
80	.0154	.0112	76.1	57.9	1.65
100	.0158	.0110	96.1	69.5	1.66

TABLE A-3j - FERROUS SULPHATE $\bar{Z}$ = 7.83
(sec. 9.)

ρ = 1024 kg/m³

3.342 x 10²⁶ elect./kg

Photon energy $h\nu$	Interaction coefficients $\left(\frac{\mu}{\rho}\right)$ [cm²/g]	$\left(\frac{\mu_{ab}}{\rho}\right)$ [cm²/g]	Average energy transf. $\bar{E}_{tr}$ [keV]	abs. $\bar{E}_{ab}$ [keV]	Average stopping power $\bar{\bar{S}}$ *
[keV]					
1	4074.	4073.	1.00		
1.5	1391.	1390.	1.50		107.
2	626.0	624.7	2.00		94.2
3	209.9	208.0	2.97		77.6
4	89.99	88.84	3.95		66.2
5	46.12	45.31	4.91		58.0
6	26.56	25.90	5.85		51.8
8	11.08	10.59	7.65		42.9
10	5.644	5.244	9.29		36.8
15	1.743	1.440	12.4		27.8
20	.8352	.5733	13.7		22.5
30	.3825	.1616	12.7		17.1
40	.2715	.0721	10.6		15.0
50	.2286	.0437	9.57		14.7
60	.2068	.0329	9.54		15.6
80	.1839	.0264	11.5		17.7
100	.1707	.0257	15.1		17.6
150	.1503	.0277	27.7		13.3
200	.1367	.0297	43.4		9.85
300	.1183	.0319	80.8		6.50
400	.1058	.0327	124.		5.03
500	.0966	.0329	171.		4.20
550	.0927	.0328	195.		3.92
662	.0854	.0325	252.		3.45
800	.0784	.0320	327.		3.09
[MeV]			[MeV]		
1	.0705	.0309	.440		2.77
1.25	.0630	.0296	.588	.586	2.53
1.5	.0574	.0283	.741	.739	2.38
2	.0493	.0260	1.06	1.06	2.21
3	.0396	.0228	1.74	1.73	2.06
4	.0340	.0206	2.46	2.43	2.00
5	.0303	.0192	3.21	3.16	1.97
6	.0276	.0180	3.99	3.91	1.96
8	.0242	.0165	5.62	5.47	1.95
10	.0222	.0157	7.33	7.08	1.95
15	.0193	.0144	11.8	11.2	1.95
20	.0182	.0140	16.5	15.3	1.96
30	.0172	.0135	26.2	23.5	1.98
40	.0169	.0132	36.0	31.3	2.00
50	.0169	.0131	45.9	38.8	2.01
60	.0169	.0129	55.9	45.8	2.02
80	.0171	.0126	75.8	59.0	2.04
100	.0174	.0124	95.9	71.1	2.05

*Av. Stopping Power in [MeV cm²g⁻¹] for the spectrum of electrons produced in the medium by photons of energy $h\nu$

TABLE A-4a   RADIOLOGICAL PROPERTIES OF HYDROGEN

Z=1 ρ = 0.08375 kg/m³ (NTP)   5.974 x 10²⁶ elect./kg   A=1.0080

5.974 x 10²⁶ atom/kg

Photon energy	Basic Coefficients in $\left(10^{-24}\ \frac{cm^2}{atom}\right)$ or $\left(10^{-28}\ \frac{m^2}{atom}\right)$				Interaction coef. in [cm²/g] (To get [m²/kg] divide by 10)			Av. energy transferred or absorbed		Stopping power $\bar{S}$ in $\frac{MeV\ cm^2}{g}$
$h\nu$	σ_{coh} coh.	σ_{inc} incoh.	τ photo	κ pair	$\left(\frac{\mu}{\rho}\right)$	$\left(\frac{\mu_{tr}}{\rho}\right)$	$\left(\frac{\mu_{ab}}{\rho}\right)$	$\bar{E}_{tr}$	$\bar{E}_{ab}$	$=\bar{S}*$
[keV]								**[keV]**		
1	.5805	.0844	11.58		7.316	6.919		.946		
1.5	.4984	.1655	2.957		2.163	1.766		1.23		276.
2	.4141	.2485	1.114		1.061	.6658		1.26		239.
3	.2763	.3832	.2787		.5605	.1682		.900		192.
4	.1881	.4683	.1038		.4542	.0646		.569		161.
5	.1341	.5194	.0481		.4192	.0322		.384		139.
6	.0999	.5508	.0257		.4040	.0196		.291		123.
8	.0613	.5842	.0095		.3913	.0114		.234		101.
10	.0412	.5994	.0044		.3853	.0098		.253		85.5
15	.0194	.6095	.0011		.3764	.0110		.438		63.8
20	.0112	.6068	.0004		.3694	.0135		.733		184.
30	.0051	.5924	.0001		.3570	.0186		1.57		203.
40	.0029	.5759			.3458	.0231		2.68		157.
50	.0018	.5597			.3355	.0271		4.04		122.
60	.0013	.5443			.3260	.0305		5.62		98.6
80	.0007	.5166			.3091	.0362		9.37		69.1
100	.0005	.4923			.2944	.0406		13.8		51.7
150	.0002	.4434			.2651	.0481		27.2		31.1
200	.0001	.4064			.2429	.0526		43.3		21.9
300	.0001	.3535			.2112	.0570		80.9		14.1
400		.3168			.1893	.0586		124.		10.8
500		.2893			.1728	.0590		171.		8.94
550		.2777			.1659	.0589		195.		8.32
662		.2560			.1530	.0584		253.		7.30
800		.2351			.1405	.0574		327.		6.50
[MeV]								**[MeV]**		
1		.2114			.1263	.0556		.440		5.81
1.25		.1890			.1129	.0531		.588		5.28
1.5		.1718			.1027	.0508		.742		4.95
2		.1466		.0002	.0877	.0466		1.06		4.59
3		.1153		.0006	.0692	.0400		1.73		4.29
4		.0962		.0010	.0581	.0353		2.43		4.17
5		.0831		.0014	.0505	.0319	.0317	3.15		4.13
6		.0734		.0018	.0449	.0291	.0290	3.89	3.87	4.11
8		.0601		.0025	.0374	.0253	.0251	5.40	5.37	4.11
10		.0512		.0033	.0325	.0227	.0225	6.97	6.91	4.14
15		.0379		.0045	.0253	.0186	.0183	11.0	10.8	4.21
20		.0304		.0056	.0215	.0164	.0161	15.2	14.9	4.27
30		.0221		.0071	.0175	.0140	.0136	24.0	23.3	4.39
40		.0176		.0081	.0154	.0127	.0122	33.1	31.8	4.48
50		.0147		.0090	.0142	.0120	.0114	42.5	40.4	4.54
60		.0126		.0096	.0133	.0115	.0109	51.9	48.9	4.60
80		.0100		.0107	.0124	.0110	.0102	71.2	65.8	4.69
100		.0083		.0116	.0119	.0108	.0098	90.8	82.5	4.76

*Av. Stopping Power in [MeV cm² g⁻¹] for the spectrum of electrons produced in the medium by photons of energy $h\nu$

TABLE A-4b   RADIOLOGICAL PROPERTIES OF CARBON

Z=6 ρ = 2250 kg/m³   3.008 x 10²⁶ elect./kg   A=12.011
5.014 x 10²⁵ atom/kg

Photon energy hν	Basic Coefficients in $\left(10^{-24}\ \frac{cm^2}{atom}\right)$ or $\left(10^{-28}\ \frac{m^2}{atom}\right)$				Interaction coef. in [cm²/g] (To get [m²/kg] divide by 10)			Av. energy transferred or absorbed		Stopping power $\bar S$ in $\frac{MeV\ cm^2}{g}$ = $\bar{S}*$
	σ_{coh} coh.	σ_{inc} incoh.	τ photo	κ pair	$\left(\frac{\mu}{\rho}\right)$	$\left(\frac{\mu_{tr}}{\rho}\right)$	$\left(\frac{\mu_{ab}}{\rho}\right)$	$\bar E_{tr}$	$\bar E_{ab}$	
[keV]								[keV]		
1	21.57	.2525	43820.		2198.	2197.		1.00		
1.5	19.21	.5016	14130.		709.4	708.5		1.50		93.4
2	16.69	.7730	6107.		307.1	306.2		1.99		82.6
3	12.30	1.283	1793.		90.58	89.89		2.98		68.2
4	9.243	1.690	731.7		37.23	36.68		3.94		58.3
5	7.218	1.990	360.3		18.53	18.07		4.88		51.1
6	5.857	2.208	200.4		10.45	10.05		5.77		45.7
8	4.204	2.503	78.54		4.274	3.940		7.38		37.9
10	3.247	2.704	37.66		2.187	1.891		8.65		32.6
15	1.958	3.023	9.770		.7396	.4945		10.0		24.8
20	1.294	3.192	3.725		.4117	.1930		9.38		20.2
30	.6719	3.307	.9539		.2473	.0570		6.91		16.1
40	.4082	3.300	.3634		.2041	.0297		5.83		16.0
50	.2735	3.252	.1725		.1854	.0222		5.99		17.9
60	.1957	3.188	.0941		.1744	.0200		6.89		20.2
80	.1139	3.054	.0365		.1607	.0200		9.98		21.1
100	.0742	2.924	.0176		.1512	.0213		14.1		18.5
150	.0336	2.647	.0048		.1346	.0245		27.3		12.4
200	.0190	2.431	.0020		.1229	.0266		43.2		8.95
300	.0085	2.117	.0006		.1066	.0287		80.8		5.86
400	.0048	1.899	.0002		.0954	.0295		124.		4.53
500	.0031	1.734	.0001		.0871	.0297		171.		3.78
550	.0025	1.665	.0001		.0836	.0297		195.		3.53
662	.0018	1.535	.0001		.0771	.0294		253.		3.11
800	.0012	1.410			.0708	.0289		327.		2.78
[MeV]								[MeV]		
1	.0008	1.268			.0636	.0280		.440		2.49
1.25	.0005	1.134		.0001	.0569	.0268		.588		2.27
1.5	.0003	1.031		.0016	.0518	.0256		.742	.739	2.13
2	.0002	.8795		.0064	.0444	.0236		1.06	1.06	1.97
3	.0001	.6919		.0186	.0356	.0206		1.74	1.73	1.84
4		.5772		.0308	.0305	.0187	.0185	2.46	2.43	1.78
5		.4984		.0419	.0271	.0174	.0171	3.21	3.16	1.75
6		.4405		.0502	.0246	.0163	.0160	3.98	3.91	1.74
8		.3604		.0670	.0214	.0150	.0146	5.60	5.45	1.72
10		.3069		.0840	.0196	.0143	.0138	7.30	7.06	1.72
15		.2272		.1094	.0169	.0132	.0125	11.7	11.1	1.72
20		.1823		.1321	.0158	.0129	.0121	16.4	15.3	1.73
30		.1327		.1609	.0147	.0128	.0115	26.0	23.5	1.74
40		.1055		.1798	.0143	.0128	.0112	35.8	31.3	1.76
50		.0880		.1962	.0143	.0130	.0111	45.7	38.8	1.77
60		.0759		.2069	.0142	.0132	.0109	55.7	46.0	1.78
80		.0598		.2251	.0143	.0135	.0106	75.6	59.4	1.79
100		.0497		.2404	.0145	.0139	.0104	95.6	71.7	1.81

*Av. Stopping Power in [MeV cm² g⁻¹] for the spectrum of electrons produced in the medium by photons of energy hν

TABLE A-4c   RADIOLOGICAL PROPERTIES OF NITROGEN

Z=7 $\rho = 1.165$ kg/m^3 (NTP) 3.010×10^{26} elect./kg   A=14.007

4.299×10^{25} atom/kg

Photon energy $h\nu$	Basic Coefficients in $\left(10^{-24}\ \frac{cm^2}{atom}\right)$ or $\left(10^{-28}\ \frac{m^2}{atom}\right)$				Interaction coef. in [cm^2/g] (To get [m^2/kg] divide by 10)			Av. energy transferred or absorbed		Stopping power $\overline{S}$ in $\frac{MeV\ cm^2}{g}$ $=\overline{S}*$
	σ_{coh} coh.	σ_{inc} incoh.	τ photo	κ pair	$\left(\frac{\mu}{\rho}\right)$	$\left(\frac{\mu_{tr}}{\rho}\right)$	$\left(\frac{\mu_{ab}}{\rho}\right)$	$\overline{E}_{tr}$	$\overline{E}_{ab}$	
[keV]								[keV]		
1	30.02	.2566	78950.		3396.	3395.		1.00		
1.5	27.35	.5215	26080.		1123.	1122.		1.50		91.8
2	24.33	.8195	11470.		494.2	493.2		2.00		81.3
3	18.61	1.398	3448.		149.1	148.3		2.98		67.2
4	14.21	1.873	1430.		62.17	61.49		3.96		57.5
5	11.10	2.233	713.1		31.23	30.66		4.91		50.4
6	8.925	2.501	400.7		17.72	17.23		5.83		45.1
8	6.243	2.865	159.4		7.245	6.856		7.57		37.5
10	4.722	3.102	77.31		3.660	3.327		9.09		32.2
15	2.802	3.461	20.45		1.149	.8840		11.5		24.5
20	1.867	3.658	7.899		.5771	.3457		12.0		20.0
30	.9810	3.810	2.056		.2944	.0975		9.93		15.5
40	.6015	3.817	.7917		.2240	.0455		8.13		14.1
50	.4043	3.770	.3785		.1957	.0298		7.61		14.6
60	.2903	3.703	.2076		.1806	.0242		8.05		16.1
80	.1698	3.552	.0810		.1635	.0217		10.6		18.1
100	.1111	3.404	.0393		.1528	.0221		14.5		17.0
150	.0506	3.085	.0108		.1353	.0247		27.4		12.1
200	.0287	2.834	.0044		.1233	.0267		43.3		8.85
300	.0128	2.469	.0013		.1068	.0288		80.8		5.82
400	.0072	2.214	.0006		.0955	.0296		124.		4.50
500	.0046	2.023	.0003		.0872	.0297		171.		3.76
550	.0038	1.943	.0002		.0837	.0297		195.		3.51
662	.0026	1.791	.0001		.0771	.0294		252.		3.09
800	.0018	1.645	.0001		.0708	.0289		327.		2.76
[MeV]								[MeV]		
1	.0012	1.479			.0637	.0280		.440		2.48
1.25	.0007	1.323		.0001	.0569	.0268		.588	.586	2.27
1.5	.0005	1.202		.0021	.0518	.0256		.741	.739	2.14
2	.0003	1.026		.0088	.0445	.0236		1.06	1.06	1.99
3	.0001	.8072		.0253	.0358	.0208	.0206	1.74	1.73	1.88
4	.0001	.6733		.0418	.0308	.0189	.0187	2.46	2.43	1.83
5		.5815		.0567	.0274	.0176	.0174	3.21	3.17	1.82
6		.5140		.0678	.0250	.0167	.0163	3.99	3.92	1.82
8		.4204		.0902	.0220	.0155	.0150	5.63	5.48	1.82
10		.3581		.1129	.0203	.0149	.0144	7.35	7.10	1.83
15		.2650		.1466	.0177	.0140	.0133	11.8	11.2	1.87
20		.2127		.1767	.0167	.0139	.0129	16.6	15.4	1.90
30		.1549		.2148	.0159	.0139	.0126	26.2	23.7	1.95
40		.1231		.2400	.0156	.0141	.0124	36.1	31.7	1.99
50		.1027		.2615	.0157	.0144	.0124	46.0	39.4	2.02
60		.0885		.2757	.0157	.0146	.0122	56.0	46.8	2.05
80		.0698		.2996	.0159	.0151	.0120	75.9	60.6	2.09
100		.0579		.3196	.0162	.0156	.0119	96.0	73.4	2.13

*Av. Stopping Power in [MeV cm^2 g^{-1}] for the spectrum of electrons produced in the medium by photons of energy $h\nu$

TABLE A-4d RADIOLOGICAL PROPERTIES OF OXYGEN

Z=8 $\rho = 1.332$ kg/m³ (NTP) 3.011×10^{26} elect./kg   A=15.999
3.764×10^{25} atom/kg

Basic Coefficients in $\left(10^{-24}\ \frac{cm^2}{atom}\right)$ or $\left(10^{-28}\ \frac{m^2}{atom}\right)$

Interaction coef. in $[cm^2/g]$ (To get $[m^2/kg]$ divide by 10)

Av. energy transferred or absorbed $\bar{E}_{tr}$ $\bar{E}_{ab}$ [keV]/[MeV]

Stopping power $\bar{S}$ in $\frac{MeV\ cm^2}{g}$ = S*

$h\nu$	σ_{coh} coh.	σ_{inc} incoh.	τ photo	κ pair	$\left(\frac{\mu}{\rho}\right)$	$\left(\frac{\mu_{tr}}{\rho}\right)$	$\left(\frac{\mu_{ab}}{\rho}\right)$	$\bar{E}_{tr}$	$\bar{E}_{ab}$	S*
[keV]								**[keV]**		
1	39.89	.2268	122100		4597.		4596.	1.00		
1.5	36.97	.4713	41670.		1570.		1569.	1.50		86.4
2	33.55	.7590	18730.		706.2		704.9	2.00		76.8
3	26.61	1.358	5796.		219.2		218.2	2.99		63.8
4	20.79	1.895	2451.		93.11		92.25	3.96		54.8
5	16.40	2.333	1240.		47.38		46.68	4.93		48.2
6	13.20	2.675	704.6		27.12		26.52	5.87		43.2
8	9.143	3.149	285.1		11.19		10.73	7.67		36.0
10	6.804	3.449	140.0		5.656		5.273	9.32		31.0
15	3.941	3.877	37.82		1.718		1.428	12.5		23.7
20	2.622	4.107	14.81		.8107		.5634	13.9		19.3
30	1.389	4.300	3.921		.3617		.1565	13.0		14.7
40	.8552	4.324	1.526		.2524		.0688	10.9		12.9
50	.5761	4.281	.7350		.2105		.0412	9.78		12.5
60	.4144	4.211	.4054		.1893		.0305	9.68		13.2
80	.2432	4.046	.1595		.1674		.0242	11.6		15.0
100	.1595	3.881	.0778		.1550		.0234	15.1		15.0
150	.0729	3.521	.0215		.1361		.0251	27.6		11.5
200	.0414	3.236	.0088		.1237		.0268	43.4		8.55
300	.0186	2.821	.0026		.1070		.0288	80.8		5.67
400	.0105	2.530	.0011		.0957		.0296	124.		4.39
500	.0067	2.312	.0006		.0873		.0298	171.		3.67
550	.0055	2.220	.0004		.0838		.0297	195.		3.43
662	.0038	2.047	.0003		.0772		.0294	252.		3.02
800	.0026	1.880	.0002		.0709		.0289	327.		2.71
[MeV]								**[MeV]**		
1	.0017	1.691	.0001		.0637		.0280	.440		2.43
1.25	.0011	1.512	.0001	.0002	.0570		.0268	.588	.586	2.22
1.5	.0007	1.374		.0028	.0519		.0256	.741	.738	2.10
2	.0004	1.173		.0115	.0446	.0237	.0235	1.06	1.05	1.96
3	.0002	.9225		.0331	.0360	.0209	.0207	1.74	1.72	1.84
4	.0001	.7695		.0544	.0310	.0191	.0189	2.46	2.43	1.80
5	.0001	.6646		.0736	.0278	.0179	.0176	3.22	3.17	1.79
6		.5874		.0880	.0254	.0170	.0166	4.01	3.92	1.79
8		.4804		.1169	.0225	.0159	.0154	5.66	5.49	1.79
10		.4092		.1459	.0209	.0155	.0149	7.40	7.12	1.81
15		.3029		.1892	.0185	.0147	.0139	11.9	11.3	1.84
20		.2431		.2277	.0177	.0148	.0137	16.7	15.4	1.87
30		.1770		.2764	.0171	.0150	.0135	26.4	23.7	1.92
40		.1406		.3085	.0169	.0153	.0133	36.3	31.5	1.96
50		.1174		.3360	.0171	.0158	.0133	46.3	39.1	2.00
60		.1011		.3540	.0171	.0161	.0132	56.2	46.2	2.02
80		.0798		.3843	.0175	.0166	.0130	76.2	59.6	2.07
100		.0662		.4097	.0179	.0172	.0129	96.3	71.9	2.10

*Av. Stopping Power in [MeV cm² g⁻¹] for the spectrum of electrons produced in the medium by photons of energy $h\nu$

TABLE A-4e   RADIOLOGICAL PROPERTIES OF ALUMINUM

Z=13 ρ = 2699 kg/m³   2.902 x 10²⁶ elect./kg   A=26.981
                                          2.232 x 10²⁵ atom/kg

Photon energy	Basic Coefficients in $\left(10^{-24}\ \frac{cm^2}{atom}\right)$ or $\left(10^{-28}\ \frac{m^2}{atom}\right)$				Interaction coef. in [cm²/g] (To get [m²/kg] divide by 10)			Av. energy transferred or absorbed		Stopping power $\bar{S}$ in $\frac{MeV\ cm^2}{g}$
$h\nu$	σ_{coh} coh.	σ_{inc} incoh.	τ photo	κ pair	$\left(\frac{\mu}{\rho}\right)$	$\left(\frac{\mu_{tr}}{\rho}\right)$	$\left(\frac{\mu_{ab}}{\rho}\right)$	$\bar{E}_{tr}$	$\bar{E}_{ab}$	$\overset{=}{S}*$
[keV]								**[keV]**		
1.55	90.07	1.163	15870.		356.2	354.1		1.55		65.4
1.56	90.05	1.164	189900.		4241.	4105.		1.51		65.4
2	82.30	1.515	103200.		2305.	2247.		1.95		59.9
3	68.17	2.125	36080.		806.9	792.1		2.95		50.8
4	57.97	2.611	16490.		369.4	363.6		3.94		44.2
5	49.93	3.054	8814.		197.9	194.8		4.92		39.3
6	43.13	3.465	5224.		117.6	115.6		5.90		35.5
8	32.33	4.186	2246.		50.95	49.83		7.82		29.9
10	24.65	4.767	1151.		26.35	25.57		9.70		26.0
15	14.02	5.695	333.0		7.873	7.411		14.1		20.1
20	9.145	6.169	135.9		3.375	3.031		18.0		16.5
30	4.894	6.588	37.84		1.101	.8514	.8510	23.2		12.5
40	3.067	6.721	15.17		.5571	.3489	.3487	25.1		10.3
50	2.094	6.725	7.453		.3632	.1790	.1789	24.6		9.00
60	1.517	6.663	4.171		.2757	.1076	.1075	23.4		8.27
80	.8974	6.458	1.673		.2015	.0547	.0547	21.7		7.82
100	.5929	6.225	.8266		.1706	.0381	.0381	22.3		8.02
150	.2744	5.680	.2327		.1381	.0285	.0285	31.0		8.13
200	.1571	5.234	.0961		.1225	.0277	.0276	45.2		6.95
300	.0708	4.573	.0284		.1043	.0283	.0283	81.4		4.93
400	.0401	4.105	.0122		.0928	.0287	.0287	124.		3.88
500	.0257	3.752	.0065		.0845	.0288	.0287	171.		3.26
550	.0213	3.604	.0050		.0810	.0287	.0287	195.		3.05
662	.0147	3.324	.0030		.0746	.0284	.0283	252.		2.70
800	.0101	3.053	.0018		.0684	.0279	.0278	327.	325.	2.42
[MeV]								**[MeV]**		
1	.0064	2.746	.0010		.0615	.0270	.0269	.440	.437	2.18
1.25	.0041	2.456	.0007	.0003	.0549	.0258	.0257	.588	.584	1.99
1.5	.0029	2.232	.0005	.0075	.0501	.0247	.0245	.741	.735	1.88
2	.0016	1.905	.0003	.0306	.0433	.0229	.0227	1.06	1.05	1.75
3	.0007	1.499	.0002	.0872	.0354	.0206	.0203	1.75	1.72	1.64
4	.0004	1.250	.0001	.1420	.0311	.0193	.0189	2.48	2.43	1.60
5	.0003	1.080	.0001	.1918	.0284	.0185	.0180	3.27	3.17	1.58
6	.0002	.9545	.0001	.2283	.0264	.0179	.0173	4.08	3.93	1.57
8	.0001	.7808		.3010	.0242	.0175	.0166	5.79	5.51	1.56
10	.0001	.6650		.3734	.0232	.0176	.0166	7.61	7.14	1.56
15		.4922		.4811	.0217	.0178	.0162	12.3	11.2	1.57
20		.3950		.5761	.0217	.0186	.0165	17.2	15.2	1.59
30		.2876		.6961	.0220	.0198	.0167	27.1	22.8	1.61
40		.2285		.7752	.0224	.0207	.0166	37.0	29.7	1.62
50		.1908		.8428	.0231	.0217	.0167	47.0	36.1	1.64
60		.1644		.8858	.0234	.0223	.0164	57.0	42.0	1.65
80		.1296		.9581	.0243	.0234	.0160	77.1	52.8	1.67
100		.1076		1.018	.0251	.0244	.0156	97.1	62.3	1.69

*Av. Stopping Power in [MeV cm² g⁻¹] for the spectrum of electrons produced in the medium by photons of energy hν

TABLE A-4f   RADIOLOGICAL PROPERTIES OF CALCIUM

Z=20 ρ = 1550 kg/m^3 3.005 x 10^{26} elect./kg   A=40.080

1.503 x 10^{25} atom/kg

Photon energy	Basic Coefficients in $\left(10^{-24}\ \frac{cm^2}{atom}\right)$ or $\left(10^{-28}\ \frac{m^2}{atom}\right)$				Interaction coef. in [cm^2/g] (To get [m^2/kg] divide by 10)			Av. energy transferred or absorbed		Stopping power $\overline{S}$ in $\frac{MeV\ cm^2}{g}$ = $\overline{S}$*
hν	σ_{coh} coh.	σ_{inc} incoh.	τ photo	κ pair	$\left(\frac{\mu}{\rho}\right)$	$\left(\frac{\mu_{tr}}{\rho}\right)$	$\left(\frac{\mu_{ab}}{\rho}\right)$	$\overline{E}_{tr}$	$\overline{E}_{ab}$	
[keV]								[keV]		
1.5	216.7	1.571	115300		1736.		1733.	1.50		63.5
2	197.0	2.068	53720.		810.2		807.4	1.99		57.7
3	163.6	2.991	17840.		270.6		268.1	2.97		49.3
4.03	135.2	3.847	7801.		119.3		117.2	3.97		42.9
4.5	124.1	4.193	53680.		808.5		709.7	3.95		40.7
5	114.2	4.540	40880.		616.0		547.7	4.45		38.5
6	97.21	5.161	25200.		380.2		344.5	5.44		34.9
8	74.07	6.132	11490.		173.8		160.9	7.41		29.5
10	59.40	6.845	6147.		93.36		87.38	9.36		25.7
15	37.54	8.076	1911.		29.40		27.68	14.1		19.9
20	25.28	8.855	817.7		12.80		11.96	18.7		16.4
30	13.59	9.627	241.7		3.981	3.575	3.572	26.9		12.4
40	8.614	9.901	100.7		1.791	1.503	1.502	33.6		10.2
50	5.975	9.969	50.85		1.004	.7689	.7679	38.3		8.73
60	4.394	9.933	29.06		.6519	.4474	.4468	41.2		7.76
80	2.650	9.711	12.01		.3662	.1971	.1967	43.1		6.60
100	1.767	9.413	6.061		.2590	.1107	.1105	42.8		6.04
150	.8277	8.651	1.764		.1689	.0505	.0504	44.9		5.78
200	.4779	7.998	.7429		.1385	.0375	.0374	54.2		5.63
300	.2174	7.008	.2244		.1119	.0320	.0319	85.7	85.5	4.66
400	.1235	6.300	.0980		.0980	.0309	.0308	126.	126.	3.83
500	.0794	5.762	.0522		.0886	.0305	.0303	172.	171.	3.27
550	.0657	5.536	.0401		.0848	.0302	.0301	196.	195.	3.07
662	.0455	5.107	.0242		.0778	.0297	.0296	253.	252.	2.73
800	.0312	4.693	.0145		.0712	.0291	.0289	327.	325.	2.45
[MeV]								[MeV]		
1	.0200	4.222	.0081		.0639	.0281	.0279	.440	.436	2.21
1.25	.0128	3.777	.0055	.0005	.0570	.0268	.0266	.588	.582	2.03
1.5	.0089	3.433	.0039	.0185	.0521	.0257	.0254	.740	.732	1.92
2	.0050	2.930	.0024	.0736	.0453	.0240	.0236	1.06	1.04	1.79
3	.0022	2.306	.0013	.2072	.0378	.0221	.0216	1.75	1.71	1.69
4	.0013	1.924	.0009	.3346	.0340	.0213	.0206	2.51	2.43	1.65
5	.0008	1.661	.0007	.4505	.0318	.0211	.0202	3.32	3.18	1.64
6	.0006	1.468	.0005	.5342	.0301	.0209	.0198	4.16	3.95	1.63
8	.0003	1.201	.0004	.6996	.0286	.0212	.0198	5.94	5.54	1.62
10	.0002	1.023	.0003	.8633	.0284	.0222	.0203	7.82	7.17	1.62
15	.0001	.7572	.0002	1.110	.0281	.0236	.0209	12.6	11.2	1.64
20	.0001	.6077	.0001	1.327	.0291	.0256	.0218	17.6	15.0	1.65
30		.4424	.0001	1.598	.0307	.0282	.0225	27.6	22.0	1.68
40		.3516	.0001	1.773	.0319	.0300	.0225	37.6	28.2	1.70
50		.2935	.0001	1.922	.0333	.0317	.0226	47.6	33.9	1.71
60		.2529		2.016	.0341	.0327	.0222	57.6	39.0	1.73
80		.1994		2.175	.0357	.0346	.0215	77.6	48.2	1.75
100		.1655		2.306	.0371	.0363	.0208	97.7	56.0	1.76

*Av. Stopping Power in [MeV cm^2 g^{-1}] for the spectrum of electrons produced in the medium by photons of energy hν

TABLE A-4g   RADIOLOGICAL PROPERTIES OF COPPER

Z=29 $\rho = 8960$ kg/m^3 2.749 x 10^{26} elect./kg   A=63.540

9.478 x 10^{24} atom/kg

Photon energy $h\nu$ [keV]	Basic Coefficients in $\left(10^{-24}\ \frac{cm^2}{atom}\right)$ or $\left(10^{-28}\ \frac{m^2}{atom}\right)$ σ_{coh} coh.	σ_{inc} incoh.	τ photo	κ pair	Interaction coef. in [cm^2/g] (To get [m^2/kg] divide by 10) $\left(\frac{\mu}{\rho}\right)$	$\left(\frac{\mu_{tr}}{\rho}\right)$	$\left(\frac{\mu_{ab}}{\rho}\right)$	Av. energy transferred or absorbed [keV] $\bar{E}_{tr}$	$\bar{E}_{ab}$	Stopping power $\bar{S}$ in $\frac{MeV\ cm^2}{g}$ $\bar{\bar{S}}*$
1.09	526.8	.7259	1036000		9824.		9815.	1.10		45.6
1.1	526.8	.7269	1199000		11370.		11360.	1.10		45.6
2	477.1	1.685	247400.		2349.		2344.	2.00		40.5
4	358.5	3.740	37410.		358.0		354.5	3.96		32.0
5	307.1	4.658	20090.		193.4		190.4	4.92		28.9
6	263.3	5.500	12030.		116.6		114.0	5.87		26.5
8.97	172.5	7.616	3809.		37.81		36.10	8.57		21.4
8.97	172.5	7.617	30300.		288.9		185.9	5.78		21.4
10	152.4	8.214	22970.		219.2		148.7	6.79		20.1
15	92.32	10.37	7785.		74.76	58.21	58.19	11.7		15.8
20	63.47	11.68	3497.		33.86	27.90	27.88	16.5		13.2
30	35.12	13.09	1091.		10.80	9.259	9.248	25.7		10.1
40	22.24	13.69	468.3		4.779	4.097	4.090	34.3		8.32
50	15.34	13.91	241.0		2.561	2.151	2.147	42.0		7.14
60	11.29	13.93	139.6		1.562	1.266	1.263	48.6		6.32
80	6.886	13.72	58.72		.7519	.5506	.5490	58.6	58.4	5.26
100	4.642	13.37	29.98		.4549	.2934	.2924	64.5	64.3	4.63
150	2.202	12.39	8.892		.2226	.1044	.1040	70.4	70.1	3.95
200	1.278	11.50	3.793		.1570	.0594	.0592	75.7	75.4	3.73
300	.5855	10.11	1.169		.1125	.0371	.0370	99.0	98.5	3.43
400	.3340	9.104	.5192		.0944	.0318	.0316	135.	134.	3.04
500	.2153	8.335	.2812		.0837	.0298	.0296	178.	177.	2.68
550	.1783	8.009	.2178		.0797	.0291	.0289	201.	200.	2.54
662	.1236	7.393	.1339		.0725	.0281	.0279	257.	254.	2.29
800	.0848	6.797	.0819		.0660	.0272	.0269	329.	326.	2.07
[MeV]								**[MeV]**		
1	.0544	6.116	.0470		.0589	.0260	.0257	.441	.436	1.88
1.25	.0349	5.473	.0315	.0009	.0525	.0248	.0244	.589	.580	1.73
1.5	.0242	4.976	.0226	.0414	.0480	.0237	.0233	.741	.727	1.64
2	.0136	4.248	.0135	.1598	.0420	.0223	.0217	1.06	1.03	1.54
3	.0061	3.343	.0074	.4393	.0360	.0211	.0204	1.76	1.70	1.45
4	.0034	2.789	.0050	.7031	.0332	.0211	.0200	2.54	2.42	1.42
5	.0022	2.409	.0037	.9345	.0317	.0214	.0201	3.37	3.17	1.40
6	.0015	2.129	.0030	1.107	.0307	.0217	.0202	4.25	3.94	1.39
8	.0009	1.742	.0021	1.447	.0303	.0230	.0208	6.08	5.51	1.38
10	.0005	1.483	.0016	1.783	.0310	.0248	.0220	8.01	7.09	1.39
15	.0002	1.098	.0011	2.281	.0320	.0276	.0232	12.9	10.9	1.39
20	.0001	.8812	.0008	2.717	.0341	.0305	.0246	17.9	14.4	1.41
30	.0001	.6415	.0005	3.268	.0371	.0345	.0255	27.9	20.7	1.43
40		.5098	.0004	3.620	.0391	.0371	.0255	37.9	26.1	1.44
50		.4255	.0003	3.918	.0412	.0395	.0254	48.0	30.8	1.46
60		.3667	.0002	4.107	.0424	.0410	.0248	58.0	35.1	1.47
80		.2892	.0002	4.422	.0447	.0435	.0237	78.0	42.5	1.48
100		.2400	.0001	4.684	.0467	.0458	.0227	98.0	48.7	1.50

*Av. Stopping Power in [MeV cm^2 g^{-1}] for the spectrum of electrons produced in the medium by photons of energy $h\nu$

TABLE A-4h RADIOLOGICAL PROPERTIES OF TIN

Z=50 $\rho = 7298$ kg/m^3 2.537×10^{26} elect./kg A=118.69
5.074×10^{24} atom/kg

Photon energy	Basic Coefficients in $\left(10^{-24}\ \frac{cm^2}{atom}\right)$ or $\left(10^{-28}\ \frac{m^2}{atom}\right)$				Interaction coef. in [cm^2/g] (To get [m^2/kg] divide by 10)			Av. energy transferred or absorbed		Stopping power $\overline{S}$ in $\frac{MeV\ cm^2}{g}$
hν	σ_{coh} coh.	σ_{inc} incoh.	τ photo	κ pair	$\left(\frac{\mu}{\rho}\right)$	$\left(\frac{\mu_{tr}}{\rho}\right)$	$\left(\frac{\mu_{ab}}{\rho}\right)$	$\overline{E}_{tr}$	$\overline{E}_{ab}$	$\overline{\overline{S}}$*
[keV]								[keV]		
2	1395.	2.778	354100.		1804.		1797.	1.99		27.9
3.92	1071.	5.656	62570.		322.9		317.5	3.86		23.8
4	1062.	5.752	183000.		933.9		874.1	3.74		23.7
4.15	1037.	5.955	166400.		849.6		796.8	3.90		23.4
4.46	992.9	6.352	195800.		998.4		941.2	4.21		22.8
4.46	992.8	6.353	227000.		1157.		1091.	4.21		22.8
4.5	988.0	6.397	222500.		1134.		1070.	4.25		22.7
6	811.4	8.171	106400.		544.0		518.8	5.72		20.3
8	636.5	10.25	49950.		256.7		246.0	7.67		17.8
10	516.5	12.05	27420.		141.8	135.9		9.58		15.9
15	339.2	15.36	8958.		47.25	44.73	44.70	14.2		12.8
20	237.7	17.51	3960.		21.39	19.86	19.84	18.6		10.7
30	133.3	20.08	7942.		41.08	14.91	14.88	10.9		8.35
40	86.84	21.44	3734.		19.50	10.00	9.976	20.5		6.93
50	61.28	22.15	2037.		10.76	6.439	6.417	29.9		5.97
60	45.45	22.47	1228.		6.575	4.279	4.262	39.1	38.9	5.30
80	27.69	22.49	544.9		3.019	2.125	2.114	56.3	56.0	4.39
100	18.71	22.13	287.7		1.667	1.200	1.193	72.0	71.5	3.82
150	9.040	20.78	89.60		.6059	.4173	.4136	103.	102.	3.05
200	5.321	19.43	39.36		.3253	.2028	.2007	125.	123.	2.66
300	2.466	17.23	12.63		.1640	.0841	.0830	154.	152.	2.33
400	1.416	15.57	5.796		.1156	.0529	.0521	183.	180.	2.17
500	.9173	14.28	3.234		.0935	.0408	.0401	218.	215.	2.05
550	.7612	13.74	2.542		.0865	.0374	.0368	238.	234.	1.99
662	.5293	12.70	1.612		.0753	.0327	.0321	288.	282.	1.86
800	.3643	11.68	1.021		.0663	.0294	.0288	355.	347.	1.74
[MeV]								[MeV]		
1	.2342	10.52	.6172		.0577	.0267	.0260	.462	.450	1.61
1.25	.1504	9.420	.4096	.0022	.0507	.0246	.0239	.607	.589	1.50
1.5	.1046	8.567	.2930	.1503	.0463	.0233	.0225	.755	.728	1.43
2	.0590	7.317	.1727	.5250	.0410	.0219	.0209	1.07	1.02	1.36
3	.0262	5.761	.0938	1.357	.0367	.0219	.0205	1.79	1.68	1.30
4	.0148	4.807	.0631	2.105	.0355	.0231	.0212	2.60	2.40	1.27
5	.0095	4.152	.0464	2.766	.0354	.0246	.0223	3.48	3.15	1.26
6	.0066	3.670	.0369	3.237	.0353	.0258	.0229	4.39	3.90	1.25
8	.0037	3.002	.0258	4.149	.0364	.0287	.0246	6.29	5.40	1.25
10	.0024	2.557	.0195	5.033	.0386	.0319	.0266	8.26	6.88	1.25
15	.0011	1.893	.0126	6.412	.0422	.0372	.0289	13.2	10.3	1.27
20	.0006	1.519	.0093	7.616	.0464	.0423	.0310	18.2	13.4	1.28
30	.0003	1.106	.0060	9.127	.0520	.0490	.0322	28.3	18.6	1.30
40	.0001	.8789	.0044	10.10	.0557	.0533	.0319	38.3	22.9	1.32
50	.0001	.7337	.0035	10.92	.0592	.0572	.0316	48.3	26.7	1.33
60	.0001	.6321	.0028	11.42	.0612	.0595	.0305	58.3	29.9	1.34
80		.4985	.0021	12.26	.0648	.0634	.0287	78.4	35.4	1.36
100		.4138	.0016	12.95	.0678	.0667	.0271	98.4	40.0	1.37

*Av. Stopping Power in [MeV cm^2 g^{-1}] for the spectrum of electrons produced in the medium by photons of energy hν

TABLE A-4i   RADIOLOGICAL PROPERTIES OF LEAD

Z=82 $\rho = 11360$ kg/m^3 2.383 x 10^{26} elect./kg   A=207.20

2.907 x 10^{24} atom/kg

Photon energy hν	Basic Coefficients in $\left(10^{-24}\ \frac{cm^2}{atom}\right)$ or $\left(10^{-28}\ \frac{m^2}{atom}\right)$				Interaction coef. in [cm^2/g] (To get [m^2/kg] divide by 10)			Av. energy transferred or absorbed		Stopping power $\bar{S}$ in $\frac{MeV\ cm^2}{g}$
	σ_{coh} coh.	σ_{inc} incoh.	τ photo	κ pair	$\left(\frac{\mu}{\rho}\right)$	$\left(\frac{\mu_{tr}}{\rho}\right)$	$\left(\frac{\mu_{ab}}{\rho}\right)$	$\bar{E}_{tr}$	$\bar{E}_{ab}$	$\bar{\bar{S}}*$
[keV]								[keV]		
2.48	3686.	4.278	276000.		812.9		802.1	2.45		14.9
2.48	3686.	4.280	736200.		2151.		2073.	2.39		14.9
2.58	3647.	4.477	663300.		1939.		1870.	2.49		15.0
2.58	3646.	4.479	921300.		2688.		2597.	2.50		15.0
3.06	3475.	5.385	590700.		1727.		1673.	2.97		15.0
3.06	3475.	5.386	793400.		2316.		2247.	2.98		15.0
3.55	3280.	6.262	539600.		1578.		1534.	3.45		15.0
3.55	3280.	6.263	609000.		1780.		1731.	3.46		15.0
3.84	3179.	6.780	494399.		1446.		1408.	3.75		14.9
3.85	3179.	6.782	533600.		1560.		1519.	3.75		14.9
6	2504.	10.28	167200.		493.3		479.7	5.83		13.7
8	2035.	13.20	78790.		235.0		226.8	7.72		12.6
10	1686.	15.75	43960.		132.7		126.8	9.55		11.5
13	1285.	18.87	21980.		67.68	63.52	63.48	12.2		10.3
15.2	1095.	20.72	36270.		108.7	80.52	80.43	11.3		9.60
15.2	1095.	20.72	51139.		151.9	113.5	113.4	11.4		9.60
15.8	1040.	21.23	45730.		136.0	102.8	102.7	12.0		9.39
15.8	1039.	21.23	53030.		157.2	119.2	119.1	12.0		9.39
20	781.5	24.00	28750.		85.91	68.56	68.43	16.0		8.33
30	455.7	28.69	9745.		29.73	24.93	24.85	25.2		6.64
50	213.3	33.03	2441.		7.811	6.594	6.556	42.2	42.0	4.87
60	159.2	33.90	1480.		4.863	4.054	4.026	50.0	49.7	4.35
88	83.99	34.49	512.7		1.835	1.444	1.429	69.2	68.5	3.44
88	83.99	34.49	2456.		7.483	2.118	2.096	24.9	24.7	3.42
100	67.57	34.41	1777.		5.461	1.974	1.952	36.2	35.7	3.17
150	32.81	32.90	620.3		1.994	1.075	1.058	80.9	79.6	2.52
200	19.51	31.03	290.5		.9913	.6027	.5902	122.	119.	2.17
300	9.230	27.77	100.5		.3996	.2540	.2469	191.	185.	1.81
400	5.366	25.22	48.33		.2294	.1419	.1371	247.	239.	1.64
500	3.502	23.21	27.93		.1588	.0945	.0909	298.	286.	1.54
662	2.038	20.68	14.59		.1084	.0616	.0589	376.	360.	1.44
800	1.410	19.06	9.549		.0872	.0485	.0461	444.	423.	1.38
[MeV]								[MeV]		
1	.9111	17.19	6.028		.0701	.0386	.0364	.550	.520	1.32
1.25	.5875	15.40	3.987	.0055	.0581	.0322	.0302	.693	.649	1.26
2	.2317	11.98	1.669	1.701	.0453	.0257	.0235	1.13	1.04	1.18
3	.1034	9.437	.8630	3.944	.0417	.0259	.0231	1.86	1.66	1.14
4	.0583	7.878	.5672	5.782	.0415	.0281	.0244	2.70	2.35	1.12
5	.0373	6.805	.4096	7.288	.0423	.0305	.0258	3.60	3.06	1.11
6	.0259	6.016	.3241	8.380	.0429	.0324	.0268	4.54	3.76	1.11
8	.0146	4.922	.2239	10.45	.0454	.0367	.0291	6.47	5.12	1.11
10	.0093	4.193	.1681	12.40	.0488	.0412	.0313	8.45	6.42	1.12
15	.0042	3.103	.1075	15.66	.0549	.0491	.0342	13.4	9.37	1.13
20	.0023	2.491	.0783	18.48	.0612	.0564	.0366	18.5	12.0	1.15
30	.0010	1.814	.0501	22.23	.0700	.0665	.0378	28.5	16.2	1.17
40	.0006	1.441	.0365	24.56	.0757	.0728	.0371	38.5	19.6	1.19
50	.0004	1.203	.0285	26.54	.0807	.0783	.0363	48.5	22.5	1.20
60	.0003	1.037	.0233	27.77	.0838	.0817	.0348	58.5	24.9	1.21
80	.0001	.8176	.0170	29.83	.0891	.0875	.0324	78.6	29.1	1.23
100	.0001	.6786	.0133	31.53	.0937	.0923	.0304	98.6	32.4	1.24

*Av. Stopping Power in [MeV cm^2 g^{-1}] for the spectrum of electrons produced in the medium by photons of energy hν

TABLE A-5   IONIZATIONAL STOPPING POWERS in [MeV cm^2 g^{-1}]
for electrons in various materials

Electron Energy (MeV)	Air	Water	Muscle	Bone	Fat	Polyst.	Lucite	Bakel.	Carbon	Alumin.
.001	102.3	119.8	118.5	104.9	127.8	122.9	120.9	117.2	104.3	73.63
.0015	78.92	91.79	90.84	81.34	97.09	93.50	92.17	89.47	81.57	59.40
.002	64.93	75.23	74.46	67.10	79.21	76.32	75.34	73.18	66.93	50.08
.003	48.74	56.22	55.65	50.51	58.88	56.76	56.12	54.56	50.07	38.62
.004	39.49	45.44	44.98	41.01	47.44	45.75	45.28	44.04	40.50	31.79
.005	33.45	38.42	38.03	34.77	40.02	38.60	38.23	37.20	34.26	27.20
.006	29.16	33.44	33.11	30.34	34.78	33.56	33.25	32.36	29.84	23.90
.007	25.94	29.72	29.42	27.01	30.87	29.79	29.53	28.74	26.52	21.38
.008	23.42	26.82	26.55	24.40	27.83	26.85	26.63	25.92	23.94	19.40
.009	21.40	24.48	24.24	22.31	25.38	24.50	24.30	23.66	21.86	17.80
.01	19.73	22.56	22.34	20.58	23.38	22.23	21.97	21.35	20.15	16.47
.015	14.43	16.47	16.31	15.07	17.02	16.21	16.03	15.59	14.71	12.19
.02	11.56	13.17	13.05	12.08	13.59	12.96	12.83	12.48	11.78	9.835
.03	8.484	9.652	9.561	8.878	9.941	9.484	9.396	9.145	8.631	7.282
.04	6.844	7.777	7.703	7.164	7.998	7.637	7.569	7.369	6.954	5.905
.05	5.814	6.603	6.540	6.090	6.784	6.481	6.427	6.257	5.907	5.037
.06	5.107	5.797	5.742	5.351	5.952	5.688	5.642	5.494	5.186	4.437
.07	4.590	5.207	5.158	4.811	5.344	5.108	5.068	4.935	4.660	3.998
.08	4.195	4.757	4.712	4.398	4.880	4.665	4.630	4.509	4.258	3.661
.09	3.883	4.412	4.361	4.072	4.514	4.317	4.284	4.173	3.940	3.394
.1	3.631	4.115	4.076	3.808	4.218	4.034	4.005	3.901	3.684	3.179
.15	2.859	3.238	3.207	3.001	3.314	3.172	3.150	3.070	2.899	2.516
.2	2.468	2.793	2.767	2.591	2.857	2.735	2.718	2.648	2.501	2.179
.3	2.083	2.355	2.333	2.181	2.405	2.305	2.291	2.233	2.109	1.848
.4	1.901	2.148	2.128	1.984	2.187	2.102	2.090	2.037	1.924	1.692
.5	1.801	2.033	2.011	1.873	2.064	1.987	1.977	1.927	1.818	1.603
.6	1.742	1.962	1.940	1.805	1.987	1.916	1.906	1.859	1.750	1.548
.7	1.705	1.916	1.894	1.761	1.938	1.870	1.861	1.815	1.705	1.512
.8	1.682	1.886	1.862	1.732	1.904	1.839	1.831	1.786	1.675	1.489
.9	1.668	1.866	1.841	1.712	1.881	1.818	1.810	1.766	1.655	1.473
1	1.660	1.852	1.826	1.698	1.865	1.804	1.796	1.753	1.641	1.464
2	1.684	1.839	1.802	1.679	1.836	1.786	1.780	1.738	1.618	1.463
3	1.739	1.868	1.825	1.705	1.858	1.812	1.807	1.765	1.639	1.493
4	1.789	1.896	1.850	1.731	1.884	1.838	1.833	1.791	1.661	1.522
5	1.832	1.920	1.872	1.755	1.906	1.860	1.855	1.813	1.680	1.546
6	1.869	1.939	1.891	1.775	1.926	1.878	1.874	1.832	1.697	1.567
7	1.902	1.956	1.909	1.793	1.944	1.894	1.890	1.847	1.711	1.584
8	1.930	1.970	1.924	1.808	1.959	1.908	1.904	1.861	1.723	1.599
9	1.955	1.983	1.937	1.822	1.973	1.920	1.916	1.873	1.734	1.613
10	1.979	1.994	1.949	1.834	1.985	1.930	1.926	1.883	1.743	1.624
20	2.134	2.063	2.028	1.912	2.063	1.996	1.992	1.948	1.803	1.699
30	2.226	2.099	2.072	1.953	2.106	2.032	2.028	1.983	1.835	1.739
40	2.281	2.125	2.102	1.981	2.134	2.056	2.053	2.007	1.858	1.766
50	2.318	2.144	2.123	2.002	2.156	2.075	2.071	2.025	1.875	1.787
60	2.346	2.160	2.141	2.018	2.172	2.090	2.087	2.040	1.889	1.803
70	2.371	2.173	2.155	2.032	2.186	2.103	2.099	2.053	1.901	1.815
80	2.391	2.184	2.167	2.043	2.198	2.114	2.110	2.063	1.912	1.827
90	2.408	2.195	2.178	2.054	2.209	2.124	2.120	2.073	1.921	1.837
100	2.432	2.204	2.187	2.063	2.218	2.132	2.129	2.082	1.929	1.846

TABLE A-6   RANGE AND RADIATION YIELD FOR ELECTRONS

Electron Energy (MeV)	AIR		WATER		BONE		CARBON		ALUMINUM	
	R g/cm^2	B fraction	R g/cm^2	B fraction	R g/cm^2	B fraction	R g/cm^2	B fraction	R g/cm^2	B fraction
.01	.0003		.0003		.0003		.0003		.0004	
.015	.0006	.0001	.0005	.0001	.0006	.0001	.0006	.0001	.0007	.0002
.02	.0010	.0001	.0009	.0001	.0009	.0002	.0010	.0001	.0012	.0003
.03	.0020	.0002	.0018	.0002	.0019	.0003	.0020	.0002	.0024	.0005
.04	.0033	.0003	.0029	.0003	.0032	.0004	.0033	.0002	.0039	.0006
.05	.0049	.0004	.0043	.0003	.0047	.0005	.0048	.0003	.0057	.0008
.06	.0067	.0004	.0059	.0004	.0064	.0005	.0066	.0003	.0078	.0009
.07	.0088	.0005	.0078	.0004	.0084	.0006	.0087	.0004	.0102	.0010
.08	.0111	.0005	.0098	.0005	.0106	.0007	.0109	.0004	.0128	.0011
.09	.0136	.0006	.0119	.0005	.0130	.0007	.0134	.0005	.0157	.0012
.1	.0162	.0007	.0143	.0006	.0155	.0008	.0160	.0005	.0187	.0013
.15	.0318	.0009	.0281	.0008	.0304	.0011	.0314	.0007	.0365	.0018
.2	.0507	.0011	.0447	.0010	.0483	.0014	.0500	.0009	.0578	.0022
.3	.0948	.0015	.0838	.0013	.0904	.0018	.0936	.0012	.1076	.0030
.4	.1450	.0019	.1282	.0017	.1384	.0023	.1432	.0015	.1639	.0037
.5	.1989	.0022	.1759	.0020	.1900	.0027	.1965	.0018	.2242	.0043
.6	.2551	.0026	.2258	.0023	.2441	.0032	.2524	.0021	.2871	.0050
.7	.3128	.0029	.2771	.0026	.2999	.0036	.3100	.0024	.3518	.0056
.8	.3715	.0033	.3294	.0029	.3567	.0040	.3689	.0027	.4178	.0063
.9	.4308	.0036	.3824	.0033	.4143	.0045	.4287	.0030	.4845	.0069
1	.4905	.0040	.4359	.0036	.4725	.0049	.4890	.0033	.5517	.0076
2	1.082	.0078	.9720	.0071	1.056	.0096	1.097	.0066	1.220	.0146
3	1.655	.0118	1.502	.0109	1.633	.0147	1.700	.0102	1.872	.0219
4	2.206	.0159	2.019	.0149	2.194	.0199	2.291	.0140	2.501	.0295
5	2.738	.0201	2.524	.0190	2.741	.0253	2.869	.0179	3.109	.0371
6	3.254	.0243	3.020	.0232	3.275	.0307	3.437	.0219	3.698	.0448
7	3.756	.0285	3.506	.0274	3.797	.0362	3.994	.0260	4.270	.0525
8	4.245	.0328	3.984	.0317	4.307	.0417	4.542	.0301	4.827	.0601
9	4.723	.0370	4.454	.0361	4.808	.0472	5.082	.0342	5.370	.0677
10	5.191	.0412	4.917	.0404	5.299	.0527	5.614	.0383	5.900	.0751
20	9.477	.0813	9.237	.0826	9.812	.1044	10.58	.0790	10.66	.1430
30	13.19	.1180	13.08	.1221	13.72	.1514	15.02	.1173	14.63	.2017
40	16.51	.1515	16.55	.1582	17.19	.1932	19.04	.1525	18.04	.2518
50	19.54	.1820	19.73	.1910	20.30	.2304	22.72	.1847	21.04	.2949
60	22.33	.2100	22.65	.2210	23.14	.2638	26.11	.2141	23.71	.3324
70	24.92	.2356	25.36	.2485	25.74	.2938	29.26	.2411	26.13	.3654
80	27.33	.2593	27.88	.2736	28.14	.3209	32.20	.2659	28.33	.3946
90	29.60	.2812	30.25	.2968	30.36	.3457	34.96	.2888	30.35	.4207
100	31.73	.3015	32.47	.3183	32.45	.3683	37.54	.3100	32.22	.4443

Range calculated using eq. 6-28

Radiation yield calculated using eq. 6-31

TABLE A-7 $f_{med} = .873 \dfrac{\left(\dfrac{\mu_{ab}}{\rho}\right)_{med}}{\left(\dfrac{\mu_{ab}}{\rho}\right)_{air}}$ for various materials in [rad/R]

Energy $h\nu$	Water	Muscle	Bone	Fat	Carbon	Polyst.	LiF	Fricke
(keV)								
1	.971	.897	.824	.640	.523	.482	1.00	.969
1.5	.993	.915	.840	.638	.505	.466	1.07	.990
2	1.01	.926	.856	.636	.493	.455	1.12	1.01
3	1.03	.982	1.26	.637	.477	.440	1.18	1.10
4	.926	.912	1.19	.566	.415	.382	1.08	1.00
5	.921	.915	2.81	.557	.401	.370	1.09	1.01
6	.915	.915	3.01	.549	.391	.360	1.10	1.01
8	.908	.917	3.33	.538	.375	.346	1.10	1.01
10	.902	.918	3.57	.530	.364	.336	1.10	1.01
15	.892	.919	3.99	.517	.348	.321	1.10	1.01
20	.886	.920	4.26	.513	.341	.317	1.09	1.01
30	.883	.922	4.44	.528	.357	.338	1.07	1.01
40	.890	.927	4.20	.579	.415	.408	1.03	1.01
50	.905	.935	3.64	.658	.508	.516	.984	1.00
60	.921	.942	2.97	.741	.605	.629	.935	.992
80	.947	.953	1.97	.859	.743	.789	.869	.980
100	.958	.957	1.46	.914	.807	.864	.839	.973
150	.967	.961	1.07	.956	.856	.920	.817	.970
200	.969	.962	.984	.965	.867	.933	.812	.968
300	.971	.962	.943	.968	.872	.938	.810	.968
400	.971	.963	.934	.970	.873	.940	.809	.968
500	.971	.962	.930	.971	.874	.940	.810	.968
600	.971	.962	.930	.971	.874	.941	.809	.968
662	.971	.963	.929	.971	.875	.941	.810	.968
800	.972	.963	.928	.972	.875	.942	.809	.969
(MeV)								
1	.972	.963	.928	.972	.875	.942	.810	.969
1.25	.971	.963	.927	.972	.875	.942	.809	.969
1.5	.971	.963	.927	.972	.874	.941	.809	.968
2	.971	.962	.928	.970	.874	.940	.809	.968
3	.969	.960	.932	.965	.870	.933	.809	.966
4	.965	.956	.937	.957	.864	.926	.810	.963
5	.961	.952	.943	.948	.858	.915	.810	.960
6	.957	.948	.947	.941	.853	.907	.810	.956
8	.951	.940	.957	.925	.842	.890	.810	.952
10	.944	.933	.966	.909	.831	.872	.810	.946
15	.931	.920	.980	.882	.812	.842	.810	.936
20	.922	.910	.990	.863	.798	.821	.808	.928
30	.909	.896	.998	.839	.782	.795	.805	.916
40	.901	.888	.998	.824	.770	.779	.801	.908
50	.895	.882	.997	.816	.763	.770	.798	.904
60	.889	.877	.994	.809	.758	.763	.794	.899
80	.884	.870	.987	.802	.751	.756	.789	.893
100	.878	.865	.978	.797	.746	.751	.783	.888

APPENDIX B—RADIATION THERAPY DATA

These tables are intended to present representative data for making dosage calculations for radiation treatments. They span the range of commonly used functions—backscatter factors, percent depth dose, relative depth doses, tissue-air ratios, tissue phantom ratios, and scatter-air ratios—over an energy range from superficial therapy to 25 MeV. The emphasis is on providing data for examples and problems used in this book rather than being general reference material for radiotherapy departments. This is a change in policy compared with previous editions of this book. We now feel that, with the proliferation of different types of high energy equipment, general data might lead to incorrect dosage. We wish to emphasize that each user of a radiation machine must ensure that the data *he* uses applies to *his* equipment.

Table B-1a contains backscatter factors measured for circular fields in the 100 kV to 400 kV range (J20). The backscatter factors for rectangular fields presented in Table B-1b were obtained from the data for circular fields by the sector integration method described in section 10.04.

Table B-2. Percentage depth doses are presented for the full range of energies from about 70 kV_p to 25 MV. Tables B-2a through d were obtained directly from measurements made in circular beams (J4, J5, J21, J22). Again the square and rectangular field data of Tables B-2e and B-2f are obtained from the circular field data. Table B-2g is taken from BJR Supplement 11 (B13), Table B-2h has been computed from tissue phantom ratio data given by Van Dyk (V7), and Table B-2i is from unpublished data measured by Rawlinson et al. (R1). Numbers in parentheses were obtained by extrapolation.

Table B-3. The relative depth dose data are obtained from tissue-phantom ratios by methods described in Chapter 10.

Table B-4. Tissue phantom ratios for cobalt radiation, Table B-4a, were calculated from tissue-air ratio data of Table B-5c. The tissue phantom ratios presented in Table B-4b for 25 MV x rays were measured by Rawlinson et al. (R1).

Table B-5. The tissue-air ratios given in Tables B-5a, b, and c were measured by Johns et al. (J5). Table B-5d is from Gupta and Cunningham (G10).

The Physics of Radiology

TABLE B-1

(a)

Backscatter Factors for Circular Fields, B(r, hν)

HVL	Area (cm^2)	10	16	20	25	35	50	64	80	100	150	200	300	400
mm Al	radius (cm)	1.78	2.26	2.52	2.82	3.34	3.99	4.51	5.05	5.64	6.77	7.98	9.75	11.3
1.0		1.108	1.128	1.138	1.148	1.164	1.179	1.189	1.197	1.205	1.218	1.229		
2.0		1.118	1.143	1.154	1.168	1.190	1.211	1.225	1.238	1.250	1.266	1.279		
3.0		1.134	1.164	1.179	1.194	1.217	1.240	1.256	1.270	1.283	1.302	1.318		
4.0		1.141	1.174	1.190	1.208	1.236	1.265	1.283	1.299	1.314	1.334	1.350		
mm Cu														
0.25		1.174	1.205	1.220	1.237	1.263	1.292	1.312	1.330	1.348	1.374	1.395	1.424	1.450
0.5		1.186	1.220	1.235	1.254	1.282	1.314	1.336	1.357	1.376	1.406	1.430	1.463	1.492
1.0		1.150	1.184	1.200	1.221	1.252	1.288	1.314	1.338	1.360	1.393	1.420	1.458	1.490
1.5		1.138	1.169	1.184	1.201	1.230	1.262	1.284	1.306	1.327	1.361	1.391	1.428	1.460
2.0		1.119	1.145	1.160	1.176	1.201	1.230	1.250	1.269	1.288	1.320	1.348	1.385	1.418
3.0		1.098	1.120	1.130	1.144	1.164	1.188	1.205	1.222	1.238	1.266	1.289	1.316	1.340
4.0		1.076	1.094	1.104	1.114	1.132	1.152	1.168	1.182	1.197	1.220	1.240	1.264	1.280

(b)

Backscatter Factors for Rectangular Fields

HVL mm Cu	4×4	4×6	4×8	4×10	4×15	4×20	6×6	6×8	6×10	6×15	6×20
					Field Size (cm × cm)						
0.5	1.214	1.244	1.261	1.272	1.285	1.292	1.283	1.306	1.321	1.340	1.350
1.0	1.180	1.211	1.230	1.243	1.258	1.266	1.252	1.279	1.297	1.318	1.330
1.5	1.166	1.193	1.210	1.222	1.237	1.245	1.230	1.253	1.269	1.291	1.303
2.0	1.144	1.169	1.184	1.194	1.208	1.216	1.201	1.222	1.237	1.257	1.269
3.0	1.116	1.137	1.149	1.158	1.170	1.176	1.164	1.182	1.194	1.211	1.221

HVL mm Cu	8×8	8×10	8×15	8×20	10×10	10×15	10×20	15×15	15×20	20×20
0.5	1.334	1.352	1.376	1.390	1.373	1.401	1.418	1.439	1.462	1.489
1.0	1.311	1.333	1.360	1.375	1.357	1.389	1.407	1.430	1.456	1.487
1.5	1.282	1.302	1.330	1.345	1.324	1.357	1.376	1.400	1.426	1.457
2.0	1.248	1.265	1.292	1.307	1.286	1.317	1.335	1.358	1.384	1.415
3.0	1.204	1.219	1.241	1.253	1.237	1.262	1.277	1.296	1.315	1.337

TABLE B-2

Percent Depth Dose for Circular Fields, P(d, r, F, hν)

(a) HVL 1.0 mm Al. (Approximately 70 kvp with Inherent Filtration)

Area (cm^2)	0	3.1	7.0	12.5	28.3	50	100
radius (cm)	0	1.0	1.5	2.0	3.0	4.0	5.64

	d (cm)							
	0	100	100	100	100	100	100	100
	0.5	61	74	79	81	84	86	87
	1	42	56	61	63	65	67	69
FSD	2	23	32	36	39	41	42	44
15 cm	3	13	19	22	24	26	27	29
	4	8	12	13	15	17	19	20
	8	2	2	3	3	4	4	5
	0	100	100	100	100	100	100	100
	0.5	62	75	80	82	84	86	88
	1	44	58	63	65	67	68	70
FSD	2	24	34	38	41	43	44	45
20 cm	3	14	20	23	25	28	29	31
	4	9	13	15	16	18	20	21
	8	2	3	3	4	4	5	6
	0	100	100	100	100	100	100	100
	0.5	63	76	81	83	85	88	89
	1	45	60	64	66	68	70	71
FSD	2	25	36	40	42	44	46	48
30 cm	3	16	22	25	27	30	31	33
	4	10	14	16	18	20	22	23
	8	2	3	4	4	5	6	7

(b) HVL 3.0 mm Al. (Approximately 120 kvp 1 mm Al. Filter)

	d (cm)							
	0	100	100	100	100	100	100	100
	0.5	75	85	87	88	89	90	90
	1.	58	70	74	76	77	78	80
FSD	2	37	48	53	56	59	60	62
15 cm	3	24	33	37	41	45	46	48
	4	17	23	27	30	34	35	37
	8	4	6	8	9	11	13	14
	0	100	100	100	100	100	100	100
	0.5	76	86	88	89	90	91	91
	1	60	72	75	77	79	80	81
FSD	2	39	51	55	58	62	63	65
20 cm	3	27	35	40	43	47	49	51
	4	19	25	29	32	36	38	40
	8	5	7	9	10	12	14	16
	0	100	100	100	100	100	100	100
	0.5	77	86	88	90	91	92	92
	1	62	74	77	79	81	82	83
FSD	2	41	54	58	61	65	66	67
30 cm	3	29	39	43	46	51	53	55
	4	21	28	32	35	40	42	44
	8	6	9	10	12	14	17	19

Percent Depth Dose for Circular Fields, P(d, r, F, hν)

(c)   HVL 2.0 mm Cu   FSD 50 cm

Area (cm^2)	0	20	35	50	80	100	150	200	400
radius (cm)	0	2.52	3.34	3.99	5.05	5.64	6.77	7.98	11.3
d (cm)									
0	100.0	100.0	100.0	100.0	100.0	100.0	100.0	100.0	100.0
1	81.4	95.0	96.9	97.9	99.4	99.9	101.0	101.6	102.4
2	66.5	85.5	88.5	90.3	92.7	93.8	95.4	96.6	99.0
3	54.0	74.3	78.6	81.3	84.8	86.3	88.8	90.5	93.7
4	44.2	68.9	68.7	71.8	75.8	77.6	80.7	82.8	87.0
5	36.2	54.9	59.5	62.8	67.0	68.8	71.9	74.2	79.2
6	29.6	46.5	51.2	54.5	58.8	61.0	64.2	66.5	71.8
7	24.3	39.6	44.0	47.2	51.5	53.4	57.0	59.2	64.8
8	19.9	33.5	37.7	40.8	44.8	46.8	50.3	52.7	58.5
9	16.4	28.4	32.4	35.2	39.2	40.9	44.4	46.5	52.4
10	13.4	24.0	27.7	30.3	33.9	35.7	38.9	41.3	46.7
11	11.1	20.4	23.7	26.0	29.4	31.0	34.0	36.3	41.6
12	9.1	17.2	20.2	22.3	25.4	27.0	29.7	31.8	36.9
13	7.5	14.7	17.3	19.2	21.9	23.4	26.0	28.0	32.7
14	6.2	12.5	14.8	16.5	19.0	20.3	22.8	24.7	28.9
15	5.1	10.6	12.6	14.1	16.4	17.7	19.9	21.7	25.5
16	4.2	8.9	10.8	12.1	14.2	15.3	17.4	19.1	22.6
17	3.5	7.6	9.2	10.4	12.3	13.3	15.2	16.8	20.0
18	2.9	6.5	7.8	8.9	10.7	11.6	13.3	14.8	17.7
19	2.4	5.5	6.7	7.7	9.2	10.0	11.6	13.0	15.6
20	2.0	4.7	5.7	6.6	7.9	8.7	10.2	11.4	13.8

(d)   Cobalt-60   11 mm Pb   SSD 80 cm

Area (cm^2)	0	20	50	100	200	400
radius (cm)	0	2.52	3.99	5.64	7.98	11.3
d (cm)						
0.5	100.0	100.0	100.0	100.0	100.0	100.0
1	95.4	97.0	97.7	98.2	98.4	98.5
2	87.1	91.0	92.5	93.4	93.7	94.0
3	79.5	85.3	87.2	88.4	89.0	89.6
4	72.7	79.6	82.0	83.4	84.4	85.2
5	66.5	74.1	76.9	78.5	79.9	80.8
6	60.8	68.9	71.8	73.7	75.2	76.4
7	55.6	63.8	66.8	68.9	70.7	72.1
8	50.9	58.9	62.1	64.2	66.3	68.0
9	46.6	54.3	57.5	59.8	62.1	64.1
10	42.7	50.1	53.3	55.7	58.1	60.3
11	39.2	46.2	49.4	51.8	54.3	56.7
12	35.9	42.6	45.8	48.2	50.8	53.3
13	32.9	39.3	42.4	44.9	47.6	50.1
14	30.2	36.3	39.3	41.8	44.5	47.1
15	27.7	33.5	36.4	38.9	41.8	44.3
16	25.4	31.0	33.8	36.2	39.0	41.7
17	23.3	28.7	31.3	33.8	36.5	39.2
18	21.4	26.5	29.0	31.4	34.2	36.9
19	19.6	24.5	27.0	29.3	32.0	34.7
20	18.0	22.6	25.0	27.3	30.0	32.7

Percent Depth Dose for Rectangular Fields

(e)   Cobalt-60   11 mm Pb   SSD 80 cm

d (cm)	0×0	4×4	4×6	4×8	4×10	4×15	4×20	6×6	6×8	6×10	6×15
0.5	100.0	100.0	100.0	100.0	100.0	100.0	100.0	100.0	100.0	100.0	100.0
1	95.4	96.8	97.0	97.2	97.3	97.4	97.4	97.4	97.6	97.7	97.8
2	87.1	90.6	91.2	91.5	91.6	91.8	91.8	91.9	92.2	92.5	92.7
3	79.5	84.7	85.5	85.9	86.1	86.4	86.4	86.5	86.9	87.3	87.6
4	72.7	79.0	79.9	80.4	80.6	81.0	81.1	81.1	81.7	82.1	82.5
5	66.5	73.5	74.5	75.1	75.3	75.7	75.9	75.9	76.6	77.0	77.5
6	60.8	68.1	69.2	69.9	70.1	70.5	70.7	70.7	71.5	71.9	72.5
7	55.6	62.9	64.1	64.8	65.1	65.5	65.7	65.7	66.5	67.0	67.6
8	50.9	58.0	59.2	59.9	60.3	60.8	61.0	60.8	61.7	62.2	62.9
9	46.6	53.5	54.7	55.3	55.8	56.3	56.6	56.2	57.1	57.7	58.5
10	42.7	49.3	50.5	51.1	51.6	52.2	52.5	52.0	52.9	53.5	54.4
11	39.2	45.5	46.6	47.3	47.8	48.4	48.6	48.1	49.0	49.6	50.5
12	35.9	41.9	43.0	43.7	44.2	44.8	45.1	44.5	45.4	46.0	46.9
13	32.9	38.6	39.7	40.4	40.9	41.4	41.8	41.1	42.0	42.7	43.6
14	30.2	35.6	36.6	37.3	37.8	38.4	38.7	38.0	38.9	39.6	40.5
15	27.7	32.9	33.8	34.5	35.0	35.6	35.9	35.2	36.1	36.7	37.6
16	25.4	30.4	31.3	32.0	32.4	33.1	33.4	32.6	33.5	34.1	35.0
17	23.3	28.1	29.0	29.6	30.0	30.7	31.0	30.2	31.1	31.6	32.6
18	21.4	26.0	26.9	27.4	27.9	28.5	28.8	28.0	28.8	29.4	30.3
19	19.6	24.0	24.9	25.4	25.9	26.5	26.8	26.0	26.7	27.4	28.2
20	18.0	22.1	22.9	23.5	23.9	24.5	24.8	24.0	24.8	25.4	26.2

d (cm)	6×20	8×8	8×10	8×15	8×20	10×10	10×15	10×20	15×15	15×20	20×20
0.5	100.0	100.0	100.0	100.0	100.0	100.0	100.0	100.0	100.0	100.0	100.0
1	97.8	97.8	98.0	98.1	98.1	98.2	98.3	98.3	98.4	98.4	98.4
2	92.8	92.7	93.0	93.2	93.3	93.3	93.6	93.6	93.9	93.9	94.0
3	87.7	87.6	87.9	88.3	88.5	88.3	88.8	88.9	89.3	89.4	89.6
4	82.7	82.5	82.9	83.4	83.6	83.4	84.0	84.2	84.7	84.9	85.2
5	77.7	77.4	77.9	78.5	78.8	78.5	79.2	79.5	80.1	80.4	80.8
6	72.7	72.4	73.0	73.7	74.0	73.6	74.4	74.7	75.4	75.8	76.4
7	67.9	67.5	68.1	68.9	69.2	68.8	69.8	70.1	70.8	71.4	72.1
8	63.3	62.7	63.4	64.3	64.7	64.1	65.2	65.7	66.5	67.2	68.0
9	58.9	58.2	58.9	59.9	60.4	59.7	60.9	61.4	62.3	63.1	64.0
10	54.8	54.0	54.8	55.8	56.3	55.6	56.9	57.4	58.4	59.2	60.2
11	51.0	50.1	50.9	52.0	52.5	51.7	53.1	53.7	54.7	55.6	56.6
12	47.4	46.5	47.3	48.4	49.0	48.1	49.5	50.2	51.2	52.1	53.2
13	44.1	43.2	44.0	45.1	45.7	44.8	46.2	46.9	47.9	48.8	50.0
14	41.0	40.1	40.9	42.0	42.6	41.8	43.1	43.9	44.9	45.8	47.0
15	38.1	37.2	38.0	39.2	39.8	38.9	40.3	41.0	42.0	43.0	44.2
16	35.5	34.5	35.3	36.5	37.1	36.2	37.6	38.3	39.3	40.3	41.5
17	33.1	32.1	32.8	34.0	34.6	33.7	35.1	35.8	36.8	37.8	39.0
18	30.8	29.8	30.5	31.7	32.3	31.4	32.8	33.5	34.5	35.5	36.7
19	28.7	27.7	28.4	29.6	30.2	29.2	30.7	31.4	32.3	33.4	34.6
20	26.8	25.7	26.4	27.6	28.2	27.2	28.6	29.4	30.3	31.4	32.6

TABLE B-2 (continued)

Percent Depth Dose for Square Fields

(f) Cobalt-60 SSD = 100 cm

side d (cm)	0	4	5	6	7	8	10	12	15	20
0·5	100·0	100·0	100·0	100·0	100·0	100·0	100·0	100·0	100·0	100·0
1	95·9	97·1	97·4	97·7	98·0	98·1	98·6	98·7	98·8	98·9
2	87·9	91·4	92·0	92·6	93·0	93·3	93·9	94·3	94·6	94·7
3	80·7	85·8	86·7	87·5	88·0	88·5	89·3	89·8	90·2	90·5
4	73·8	80·2	81·5	82·4	83·1	83·7	84·7	85·3	85·9	86·3
5	67·8	74·8	76·2	77·3	78·2	78·9	80·1	80·9	81·6	82·2
6	62·3	69·7	71·2	72·4	73·4	74·2	75·5	76·3	77·3	78·1
7	57·3	64·8	66·3	67·6	68·6	69·5	70·9	71·9	73·0	74·0
8	52·7	60·1	61·5	62·9	64·0	64·9	66·4	67·5	68·7	70·0
9	48·5	55·7	57·1	58·4	59·5	60·5	62·0	63·2	64·5	66·1
10	44·7	51·5	52·9	54·2	55·3	56·3	57·8	59·0	60·6	62·3
11	41·2	47·7	49·0	50·3	51·4	52·4	53·9	55·2	56·9	58·7
12	38·0	44·1	45·3	46·7	47·8	48·7	50·3	51·6	53·4	55·3
13	35·0	40·8	42·1	43·3	44·4	45·4	47·0	48·4	50·2	52·1
14	32·2	37·8	39·1	40·2	41·4	42·3	43·9	45·4	47·1	49·1
15	29·6	35·0	36·2	37·4	38·4	39·4	41·0	42·4	44·2	46·2
16	27·2	32·5	33·8	34·8	35·8	36·7	38·3	39·8	41·5	43·5
17	25·0	30·1	31·3	32·3	33·3	34·2	35·8	37·1	39·0	41·0
18	23·0	27·9	29·0	30·0	31·0	31·9	33·5	34·9	36·7	38·6
19	21·2	25·8	26·9	27·9	28·8	29·7	31·3	32·7	34·5	36·4
20	19·5	23·8	24·9	25·9	26·9	27·7	29·3	30·7	32·4	34·4
22	(16·5)	(20·6)	(21·5)	(22·5)	(23·3)	(24·2)	(25·6)	(27·0)	(28·5)	(30·5)
24	(14·0)	(17·7)	(18·5)	(19·4)	(20·2)	(21·0)	(22·3)	(23·6)	(25·2)	(27·1)
26	(11·8)	(15·2)	(16·0)	(16·8)	(17·4)	(18·2)	(19·6)	(20·8)	(22·3)	(24·0)
28	(10·1)	(13·0)	(13·7)	(14·4)	(15·1)	(15·8)	(17·1)	(18·2)	(19·7)	(21·4)
30	(8·5)	(11·2)	(12·0)	(12·5)	(13·2)	(13·8)	(15·0)	(16·0)	(17·3)	(19·0)

(g) 6 MV x rays SSD = 100 cm

side d (cm)	0	3	4	6	8	10	12	15	20	25
0		9·5	10·5	12·5	15·0	17·0	19·0	22·0	27·0	31·0
0·2			51·5	54·0		58·5			67·5	
0·5			81·5	83·5		86·5			91·0	
1·0			98·5	98·5		99·0			99·5	
1·5	100·0	100·0	100·0	100·0	100·0	100·0	100·0	100·0	100·0	100·0
2	(98·0)	98·5	98·5	98·5	99·0	99·0	99·0	99·0	99·0	99·0
3	(92·0)	93·5	94·0	94·0	94·5	95·0	95·0	95·0	95·5	95·5
4	(85·5)	88·0	89·0	90·0	90·5	91·0	91·0	91·5	92·0	92·0
5	(80·0)	83·0	84·0	85·0	86·0	86·5	87·0	87·5	88·0	88·5
6	(74·5)	78·0	79·0	80·5	81·5	82·5	83·0	83·5	84·5	85·0
7	(69·5)	73·5	74·5	76·0	77·5	78·5	79·0	80·0	80·5	81·5
8	(65·0)	69·0	70·0	72·0	73·5	74·5	75·0	76·0	77·0	78·0
10	(56·5)	61·0	62·0	64·0	66·0	67·0	68·0	69·0	70·5	71·5
12	(49·0)	53·5	55·0	57·0	59·0	60·0	61·0	62·5	64·0	65·5
14	(43·0)	47·5	48·5	51·0	52·5	54·0	55·0	56·5	58·5	59·5
16	(37·5)	42·0	43·0	45·0	47·0	48·5	49·5	51·0	53·0	54·0
18	(32·5)	37·0	38·0	40·0	42·0	43·5	44·5	46·0	48·0	49·5
20	(28·5)	32·5	33·5	36·0	37·5	39·0	40·0	41·5	43·5	44·5
22	(25·0)	29·0	30·0	32·0	33·5	35·0	36·0	37·5	39·5	40·5
24	(22·0)	25·5	26·5	28·5	30·0	31·5	32·5	34·0	35·5	37·0
26	(19·0)	22·5	23·5	25·5	27·0	28·0	29·0	30·5	32·5	33·5
28	(16·5)	20·0	21·0	22·5	24·0	25·0	26·0	27·5	29·0	30·5
30	(14·5)	17·5	18·5	20·0	21·5	22·5	23·5	24·5	26·5	27·5

Percent Depth Dose for Square Fields

(h)　　　　　　　10 MV x rays　　　　　　　　SSD = 100 cm

I	0.0	4.0	6.0	8.0	10.0	15.0	20.0	25.0	30.0	35.0
1.0	92.0	89.5	90.5	91.7	93.1	96.1	98.7	100.1	100.7	100.9
2.0	112.4	108.1	108.2	108.4	108.7	109.1	109.0	109.0	109.0	109.0
2.5	114.1	109.5	109.1	109.0	109.0	108.9	108.8	108.7	108.6	108.6
3.0	111.9	108.7	108.3	108.2	108.1	107.9	107.8	107.7	107.6	107.6
4.0	105.8	104.7	104.3	104.2	104.1	104.1	104.1	104.0	104.0	103.9
5.0	100.0	100.0	100.0	100.0	100.0	100.0	100.0	100.0	100.0	100.0
6.0	94.7	95.1	95.4	95.6	95.8	96.0	96.1	96.2	96.3	96.5
7.0	89.5	90.4	90.9	91.3	91.7	92.2	92.4	92.6	92.8	93.1
8.0	84.7	86.1	86.6	87.2	87.7	88.3	88.7	88.9	89.2	89.6
9.0	80.1	81.9	82.6	83.2	83.8	84.6	85.1	85.5	85.8	86.2
10.0	75.9	77.8	78.6	79.4	80.1	81.0	81.7	82.1	82.5	83.0
11.0	71.8	73.9	74.9	75.7	76.5	77.6	78.3	78.8	79.3	79.8
12.0	67.9	70.1	71.2	72.2	73.0	74.2	75.1	75.7	76.2	76.8
13.0	64.3	66.6	67.8	68.8	69.7	71.0	72.0	72.7	73.3	73.9
14.0	61.1	63.3	64.6	65.7	66.6	68.0	69.0	69.8	70.4	71.0
15.0	57.9	60.1	61.5	62.6	63.5	65.1	66.2	66.9	67.6	68.2
16.0	54.9	57.1	58.5	59.6	60.6	62.2	63.4	64.2	64.9	65.5
17.0	52.0	54.1	55.6	56.7	57.7	59.5	60.7	61.6	62.3	62.9
18.0	49.3	51.4	52.9	54.1	55.1	56.9	58.2	59.1	59.8	60.4
19.0	46.8	49.0	50.5	51.7	52.7	54.5	55.8	56.7	57.4	58.1
20.0	44.5	46.7	48.1	49.3	50.3	52.2	53.5	54.4	55.1	55.8
21.0	42.2	44.4	45.9	47.0	48.0	49.9	51.2	52.1	52.9	53.6
22.0	40.0	42.2	43.6	44.8	45.8	47.7	49.0	50.0	50.7	51.4
23.0	37.8	40.1	41.5	42.7	43.7	45.5	46.9	47.9	48.6	49.3
24.0	35.7	38.0	39.4	40.6	41.6	43.5	44.8	45.8	46.6	47.3
25.0	33.7	36.0	37.4	38.6	39.6	41.5	42.8	43.8	44.6	45.3
26.0	32.0	34.4	35.7	36.8	37.8	39.7	41.1	42.0	42.8	43.5
27.0	30.4	32.8	34.0	35.1	36.1	38.0	39.3	40.3	41.0	41.8
28.0	28.9	31.2	32.4	33.5	34.5	36.3	37.7	38.6	39.4	40.1
29.0	27.4	29.7	30.9	31.9	32.9	34.7	36.0	37.0	37.7	38.4
30.0	25.9	28.3	29.3	30.4	31.3	33.1	34.4	35.4	36.1	36.8

(i)　　　　　　　25 MV x rays　　　　　　　　SSD = 100 cm

I	0.0	4.0	6.0	8.0	10.0	15.0	20.0	25.0	30.0	35.0
1.0	60.3	66.6	69.0	72.1	75.3	82.3	87.3	90.3	91.9	92.5
2.0	79.6	83.5	85.1	87.0	89.1	93.5	96.7	98.4	99.2	99.5
3.0	98.2	99.6	100.5	101.3	102.2	104.2	105.5	106.0	106.2	106.2
4.0	101.0	101.2	101.4	101.7	102.0	102.8	103.1	103.2	103.3	103.3
5.0	100.0	100.0	100.0	100.0	100.0	100.0	100.0	100.0	100.0	100.0
6.0	96.4	96.4	96.7	96.7	96.7	96.3	96.2	96.2	96.1	96.1
7.0	92.9	92.9	93.4	93.5	93.4	92.7	92.6	92.4	92.4	92.4
8.0	89.2	89.4	90.0	90.2	90.0	89.2	89.1	88.9	88.9	88.9
9.0	85.4	85.7	86.4	86.6	86.5	85.9	85.8	85.6	85.6	85.7
10.0	81.6	82.1	82.9	83.2	83.2	82.7	82.5	82.4	82.5	82.5
11.0	78.0	78.6	79.4	79.8	79.8	79.6	79.5	79.5	79.5	79.5
12.0	74.4	75.1	76.1	76.5	76.6	76.6	76.6	76.6	76.6	76.6
13.0	71.1	72.0	72.9	73.3	73.5	73.6	73.7	73.8	73.8	73.8
14.0	68.1	69.2	69.8	70.3	70.5	70.7	70.9	71.0	71.1	71.1
15.0	65.2	66.4	66.8	67.4	67.7	68.0	68.2	68.3	68.4	68.5
16.0	62.0	63.3	64.0	64.6	64.9	65.3	65.6	65.8	65.9	65.9
17.0	59.0	60.3	61.4	62.0	62.2	62.7	63.1	63.3	63.5	63.5
18.0	56.2	57.6	58.9	59.4	59.7	60.3	60.7	61.0	61.1	61.2
19.0	53.7	55.1	56.5	57.1	57.4	58.0	58.5	58.8	58.9	58.9
20.0	51.2	52.8	54.1	54.8	55.2	55.8	56.3	56.6	56.8	56.8
21.0	49.0	50.7	51.9	52.6	53.0	53.7	54.3	54.6	54.7	54.8
22.0	46.9	48.6	49.8	50.5	51.0	51.7	52.3	52.6	52.8	52.8
23.0	44.8	46.6	47.8	48.5	49.0	49.8	50.4	50.7	50.9	50.9
24.0	42.8	44.7	45.9	46.6	47.1	48.0	48.5	48.9	49.0	49.0
25.0	40.9	42.8	44.0	44.8	45.2	46.2	46.7	47.1	47.2	47.3
26.0	39.2	41.1	42.3	43.1	43.5	44.5	45.1	45.4	45.6	45.6
27.0	37.5	39.4	40.6	41.4	41.9	42.9	43.5	43.8	43.9	43.9
28.0	35.8	37.8	39.0	39.8	40.3	41.3	41.9	42.2	42.3	42.4
29.0	34.2	36.2	37.4	38.2	38.7	39.7	40.4	40.7	40.8	40.8
30.0	32.6	34.6	35.9	36.7	37.2	38.2	38.9	39.2	39.3	39.3

TABLE B-3
Relative Depth Doses for Square Fields

(a)   Cobalt-60   SSD = 65   SAD = 80

	I	0.0	4.0	6.0	8.0	10.0	15.0	20.0	25.0	30.0	35.0
0.5	I	386.5	333.3	312.9	297.1	284.7	262.5	249.3	240.4	233.2	228.0
1.0	I	367.3	320.3	302.5	288.6	277.6	257.2	244.5	235.9	228.8	223.8
2.0	I	334.3	297.9	283.6	272.0	262.4	244.2	232.5	224.6	218.2	213.6
3.0	I	303.0	275.7	264.0	254.2	246.1	230.3	220.0	212.8	206.9	202.8
4.0	I	275.8	255.2	246.0	237.9	230.8	216.8	207.7	201.3	196.0	192.3
5.0	I	251.1	235.3	228.1	221.8	215.9	203.7	195.8	190.3	185.8	182.5
	I										
6.0	I	228.3	216.6	211.1	205.8	200.8	190.4	183.6	178.7	174.9	172.0
7.0	I	207.9	199.2	194.7	190.4	186.3	177.8	172.1	168.2	165.0	162.7
8.0	I	189.2	182.7	179.1	175.7	172.5	165.6	161.0	157.8	155.2	153.0
9.0	I	172.9	167.9	165.1	162.3	159.8	154.3	150.6	148.0	145.9	144.2
10.0	I	157.4	153.8	151.7	149.5	147.6	143.5	140.8	138.8	137.1	135.8
	I										
11.0	I	144.0	141.2	139.6	138.0	136.6	133.4	131.4	129.9	128.7	127.7
12.0	I	131.2	129.3	128.0	127.1	126.1	123.9	122.6	121.5	120.7	120.0
13.0	I	120.3	119.1	118.2	117.6	117.0	115.5	114.7	114.0	113.5	113.0
14.0	I	109.9	109.3	108.9	108.6	108.3	107.6	107.2	106.9	106.6	106.4
15.0	I	100.0	100.0	100.0	100.0	100.0	100.0	100.0	100.0	100.0	100.0
	I										
16.0	I	92.1	92.6	92.8	92.9	93.1	93.5	93.7	94.0	94.1	94.2
17.0	I	84.5	85.4	85.8	86.2	86.5	87.3	87.8	88.3	88.5	88.7
18.0	I	77.3	78.6	79.2	79.7	80.2	81.3	82.0	82.8	83.2	83.4
19.0	I	70.4	72.1	72.8	73.5	74.2	75.6	76.6	77.5	78.0	78.4
20.0	I	63.8	65.8	66.7	67.6	68.4	70.1	71.4	72.5	73.1	73.5
	I										
21.0	I	58.9	61.0	61.9	62.8	63.7	65.6	67.0	68.3	68.9	69.4
22.0	I	54.2	56.3	57.3	58.3	59.2	61.3	62.8	64.2	64.9	65.4
23.0	I	49.6	51.9	52.9	53.9	54.9	57.1	58.7	60.3	61.0	61.6
24.0	I	45.3	47.6	48.6	49.7	50.8	53.1	54.9	56.5	57.3	58.0
25.0	I	41.1	43.4	44.5	45.7	46.8	49.3	51.2	52.9	53.8	54.5
	I										
26.0	I	38.0	40.3	41.4	42.5	43.7	46.1	48.0	49.7	50.6	51.4
27.0	I	34.9	37.2	38.3	39.5	40.6	43.1	45.0	46.7	47.6	48.4
28.0	I	32.0	34.3	35.4	36.6	37.7	40.2	42.1	43.8	44.7	45.5
29.0	I	29.2	31.5	32.6	33.8	34.9	37.4	39.3	41.0	41.9	42.7
30.0	I	26.5	28.8	29.9	31.1	32.2	34.7	36.6	38.2	39.2	40.1
	I										

(b)   25 MV x rays   SSD = 85   SAD = 100

	I	0.0	4.0	6.0	8.0	10.0	15.0	20.0	25.0	30.0	35.0
1.0	I	96.5	103.6	106.4	109.1	112.7	122.1	129.5	135.0	138.2	140.0
2.0	I	127.0	130.0	131.7	133.0	134.9	140.5	145.0	148.2	149.8	150.7
3.0	I	156.0	155.1	155.8	155.7	155.9	157.8	159.6	160.6	160.8	160.8
4.0	I	160.0	157.4	157.2	156.3	155.7	156.0	156.1	156.1	156.0	155.8
5.0	I	157.9	155.0	154.6	153.4	152.5	151.6	151.2	150.9	150.6	150.4
	I										
6.0	I	151.7	148.9	148.9	147.9	147.0	145.8	145.1	144.7	144.3	144.2
7.0	I	145.8	143.0	143.3	142.6	141.7	140.1	139.2	138.7	138.3	138.1
8.0	I	139.6	137.0	137.6	137.0	136.2	134.5	133.6	133.1	132.7	132.5
9.0	I	133.1	130.9	131.6	131.1	130.5	129.0	128.2	127.7	127.4	127.3
10.0	I	127.0	125.1	125.9	125.5	125.0	123.7	123.1	122.6	122.3	122.2
	I										
11.0	I	120.9	119.3	120.2	120.0	119.5	118.6	118.1	117.8	117.5	117.5
12.0	I	115.0	113.7	114.8	114.7	114.3	113.7	113.4	113.2	113.0	112.9
13.0	I	109.7	108.7	109.6	109.6	109.3	109.0	108.8	108.7	108.5	108.5
14.0	I	104.7	104.3	104.7	104.7	104.6	104.4	104.3	104.2	104.2	104.2
15.0	I	100.0	100.0	100.0	100.0	100.0	100.0	100.0	100.0	100.0	100.0
	I										
16.0	I	94.9	94.8	95.5	95.7	95.7	95.8	95.9	96.0	96.1	96.1
17.0	I	90.0	89.9	91.2	91.5	91.5	91.7	92.0	92.2	92.3	92.3
18.0	I	85.6	85.5	87.2	87.6	87.6	87.9	88.3	88.5	88.7	88.7
19.0	I	81.5	81.6	83.4	83.9	83.9	84.3	84.8	85.0	85.2	85.3
20.0	I	77.6	77.9	79.7	80.2	80.4	80.9	81.4	81.7	81.9	81.9
	I										
21.0	I	74.1	74.6	76.3	76.9	77.1	77.7	78.2	78.6	78.8	78.8
22.0	I	70.7	71.4	73.1	73.6	73.9	74.5	75.2	75.5	75.8	75.8
23.0	I	67.4	68.3	69.9	70.5	70.8	71.5	72.2	72.6	72.9	72.9
24.0	I	64.3	65.3	67.0	67.6	67.9	68.7	69.4	69.8	70.1	70.1
25.0	I	61.3	62.4	64.1	64.7	65.1	66.0	66.7	67.1	67.4	67.4
	I										
26.0	I	58.5	59.7	61.4	62.1	62.5	63.4	64.2	64.6	64.9	64.9
27.0	I	55.9	57.1	58.8	59.6	59.9	60.9	61.8	62.2	62.4	62.4
28.0	I	53.3	54.7	56.3	57.1	57.5	58.6	59.4	59.8	60.1	60.1
29.0	I	50.8	52.3	53.9	54.7	55.1	56.2	57.1	57.5	57.8	57.7
30.0	I	48.3	49.9	51.6	52.4	52.8	54.0	54.8	55.3	55.5	55.5
	I										

TABLE B-4
Tissue Phantom Ratios for Square Fields

(a) Cobalt-60 Reference Depth = 5 cm

I	0.0	4.0	6.0	8.0	10.0	15.0	20.0	25.0	30.0	35.0
0.5	1.348	1.229	1.189	1.163	1.147	1.124	1.112	1.104	1.096	1.090
1.0	1.301	1.202	1.171	1.150	1.139	1.119	1.108	1.099	1.093	1.088
2.0	1.220	1.156	1.135	1.119	1.111	1.095	1.086	1.080	1.075	1.070
3.0	1.139	1.104	1.090	1.080	1.075	1.065	1.059	1.054	1.050	1.047
4.0	1.067	1.054	1.047	1.041	1.038	1.033	1.030	1.027	1.025	1.024
5.0	1.000	1.000	1.000	1.000	1.000	1.000	1.000	1.000	1.000	1.000
6.0	0.935	0.948	0.952	0.954	0.957	0.962	0.964	0.967	0.969	0.970
7.0	0.876	0.896	0.903	0.908	0.913	0.923	0.930	0.936	0.940	0.943
8.0	0.819	0.843	0.853	0.861	0.869	0.884	0.894	0.902	0.908	0.911
9.0	0.770	0.796	0.806	0.816	0.827	0.846	0.859	0.869	0.877	0.882
10.0	0.720	0.748	0.760	0.771	0.784	0.808	0.824	0.836	0.846	0.854
11.0	0.676	0.704	0.717	0.730	0.744	0.770	0.789	0.803	0.815	0.823
12.0	0.632	0.661	0.674	0.689	0.703	0.733	0.754	0.770	0.783	0.793
13.0	0.595	0.623	0.638	0.653	0.668	0.700	0.723	0.740	0.754	0.765
14.0	0.558	0.586	0.601	0.617	0.633	0.667	0.692	0.710	0.725	0.738
15.0	0.520	0.549	0.565	0.581	0.598	0.634	0.660	0.680	0.696	0.710
16.0	0.491	0.520	0.536	0.552	0.569	0.606	0.633	0.653	0.670	0.684
17.0	0.462	0.491	0.507	0.523	0.540	0.577	0.605	0.627	0.644	0.658
18.0	0.433	0.462	0.478	0.494	0.511	0.549	0.578	0.600	0.619	0.633
19.0	0.404	0.433	0.449	0.465	0.483	0.521	0.551	0.574	0.593	0.607
20.0	0.375	0.404	0.420	0.436	0.454	0.493	0.523	0.547	0.567	0.581
21.0	0.354	0.382	0.398	0.414	0.431	0.470	0.501	0.525	0.545	0.560
22.0	0.333	0.360	0.375	0.391	0.408	0.447	0.478	0.503	0.523	0.539
23.0	0.312	0.339	0.353	0.369	0.386	0.425	0.455	0.481	0.502	0.517
24.0	0.292	0.317	0.331	0.346	0.363	0.402	0.433	0.459	0.480	0.496
25.0	0.271	0.295	0.309	0.324	0.340	0.379	0.410	0.437	0.458	0.474
26.0	0.256	0.279	0.292	0.307	0.323	0.361	0.392	0.418	0.439	0.455
27.0	0.240	0.263	0.276	0.290	0.306	0.343	0.373	0.399	0.420	0.436
28.0	0.225	0.247	0.260	0.274	0.289	0.325	0.355	0.380	0.401	0.417
29.0	0.209	0.231	0.243	0.257	0.271	0.307	0.336	0.361	0.382	0.398
30.0	0.194	0.215	0.227	0.240	0.254	0.289	0.318	0.342	0.363	0.379

(b) 25 MV x rays Reference Depth = 5 cm

I	0.0	4.0	6.0	8.0	10.0	15.0	20.0	25.0	30.0	35.0
1.0	0.558	0.616	0.638	0.666	0.695	0.759	0.806	0.834	0.850	0.855
2.0	0.752	0.787	0.802	0.820	0.839	0.880	0.910	0.927	0.936	0.939
3.0	0.945	0.958	0.966	0.974	0.982	1.002	1.014	1.020	1.022	1.022
4.0	0.991	0.993	0.995	0.997	1.000	1.008	1.011	1.012	1.013	1.013
5.0	1.000	1.000	1.000	1.000	1.000	1.000	1.000	1.000	1.000	1.000
6.0	0.982	0.982	0.985	0.986	0.985	0.982	0.981	0.980	0.980	0.980
7.0	0.965	0.964	0.970	0.971	0.971	0.963	0.962	0.960	0.960	0.960
8.0	0.944	0.944	0.951	0.954	0.953	0.945	0.943	0.941	0.940	0.941
9.0	0.920	0.922	0.930	0.933	0.933	0.927	0.925	0.923	0.923	0.923
10.0	0.896	0.900	0.908	0.912	0.913	0.909	0.906	0.905	0.905	0.905
11.0	0.871	0.876	0.885	0.890	0.892	0.890	0.889	0.888	0.888	0.889
12.0	0.846	0.852	0.863	0.869	0.871	0.871	0.871	0.871	0.872	0.872
13.0	0.824	0.832	0.841	0.847	0.850	0.852	0.853	0.854	0.855	0.855
14.0	0.803	0.814	0.820	0.826	0.830	0.833	0.835	0.836	0.837	0.838
15.0	0.782	0.796	0.798	0.805	0.810	0.814	0.816	0.818	0.820	0.821
16.0	0.757	0.770	0.778	0.785	0.790	0.795	0.799	0.801	0.803	0.804
17.0	0.732	0.744	0.757	0.766	0.770	0.776	0.781	0.784	0.787	0.788
18.0	0.710	0.721	0.737	0.747	0.752	0.758	0.764	0.768	0.771	0.772
19.0	0.689	0.701	0.719	0.729	0.734	0.742	0.748	0.752	0.755	0.757
20.0	0.669	0.682	0.700	0.710	0.716	0.725	0.732	0.736	0.739	0.741
21.0	0.651	0.665	0.682	0.693	0.700	0.709	0.716	0.721	0.725	0.727
22.0	0.633	0.648	0.665	0.676	0.683	0.693	0.701	0.706	0.710	0.712
23.0	0.615	0.631	0.648	0.659	0.667	0.677	0.686	0.691	0.695	0.698
24.0	0.598	0.614	0.631	0.643	0.651	0.662	0.671	0.677	0.681	0.684
25.0	0.580	0.597	0.615	0.627	0.635	0.647	0.656	0.662	0.667	0.669
26.0	0.564	0.582	0.599	0.612	0.620	0.633	0.643	0.649	0.653	0.656
27.0	0.548	0.566	0.584	0.597	0.605	0.618	0.629	0.635	0.640	0.642
28.0	0.532	0.551	0.569	0.582	0.590	0.604	0.615	0.622	0.626	0.629
29.0	0.516	0.536	0.553	0.567	0.575	0.590	0.601	0.608	0.613	0.616
30.0	0.500	0.520	0.538	0.552	0.560	0.576	0.587	0.595	0.600	0.602

TABLE B-5

Tissue-Air Ratios for Circular Fields, T_a (d, r, hν)

Radius (cm)	0	2.52	3.34	3.99	5.05	5.64	6.77	7.98	11.3
Area (cm²)	0	20	35	50	80	100	150	200	400
d, (cm)									

(a)

				HVL 1.0 mm Cu					
*0	1.00	1.20	1.25	1.29	1.34	1.37	1.40	1.42	1.49
2	.682	1.08	1.18	1.25	1.33	1.36	1.42	1.48	1.58
4	.472	.844	.948	1.02	1.13	1.18	1.27	1.33	1.43
6	.330	.631	.726	.799	.900	.954	1.04	1.10	1.24
8	.232	.466	.546	.612	.695	.741	.835	.894	1.04
10	.163	.341	.406	.452	.527	.569	.646	.703	.838
12	.114	.246	.294	.339	.400	.432	.499	.549	.675
14	.079	.178	.218	.250	.300	.325	.382	.425	.534
16	.055	.128	.158	.184	.225	.245	.290	.326	.421
18	.039	.093	.116	.135	.167	.183	.219	.248	.327
20	.027	.067	.084	.099	.125	.138	.168	.190	.254

(b)

				HVL 3.0 mm Cu					
*0	1.00	1.13	1.16	1.19	1.23	1.24	1.27	1.29	1.33
2	.736	1.03	1.10	1.15	1.20	1.22	1.27	1.30	1.39
4	.542	.828	.912	.968	1.05	1.08	1.14	1.18	1.29
6	.404	.651	.727	.785	.861	.905	.975	1.03	1.14
8	.296	.500	.565	.617	.694	.738	.800	.855	.974
10	.222	.382	.435	.480	.552	.591	.659	.703	.820
12	.164	.290	.335	.372	.430	.465	.519	.565	.676
14	.123	.220	.256	.284	.332	.364	.410	.455	.552
16	.092	.167	.197	.219	.258	.283	.325	.365	.452
18	.068	.128	.152	.169	.201	.220	.259	.290	.370
20	.051	.098	.116	.130	.157	.171	.204	.232	.299

(c)

				Cobalt 60					
*0.5	1.000	1.016	1.021	1.025	1.032	1.035	1.042	1.048	1.064
2	.905	.956	.961	.975	.985	.998	1.014	1.022	1.041
4	.792	.880	.900	.914	.932	.941	.953	.964	.987
6	.694	.795	.820	.835	.856	.867	.883	.898	.925
8	.608	.708	.734	.752	.776	.787	.805	.824	.858
10	.534	.627	.653	.672	.696	.708	.730	.751	.790
12	.469	.553	.578	.596	.622	.636	.658	.678	.723
14	.412	.489	.513	.531	.557	.571	.595	.616	.662
16	.361	.435	.455	.472	.497	.509	.533	.557	.605
18	.317	.384	.405	.421	.444	.457	.480	.501	.552
20	.278	.339	.359	.375	.399	.411	.431	.454	.503

* This entry is also the backscatter factor.

Cobalt-60

d (cm)	0×0	4×4	4×6	4×8	4×10	4×15	5×5	6×6	6×8	6×10	6×15	7×7	8×8	8×10
*0.5	1.000	1.015	1.018	1.020	1.022	1.025	1.018	1.022	1.025	1.027	1.031	1.025	1.029	1.032
1	.965	.996	1.001	1.005	1.008	1.012	1.003	1.009	1.014	1.018	1.023	1.015	1.021	1.025
2	.905	.956	.965	.970	.973	.978	.967	.976	.983	.988	.994	.985	.992	.997
3	.845	.915	.926	.932	.936	.942	.928	.940	.948	.954	.961	.950	.959	.966
4	.792	.872	.885	.893	.897	.903	.888	.902	.912	.918	.926	.914	.924	.931
5	.742	.829	.843	.852	.856	.863	.847	.862	.873	.880	.889	.875	.887	.895
6	.694	.786	.801	.810	.815	.823	.805	.821	.833	.840	.851	.835	.847	.856
7	.650	.743	.758	.767	.773	.781	.762	.778	.791	.799	.810	.793	.807	.819
8	.608	.700	.715	.725	.731	.740	.719	.736	.749	.757	.769	.751	.765	.775
9	.570	.659	.674	.684	.689	.700	.677	.695	.708	.716	.730	.710	.724	.734
10	.534	.620	.635	.644	.650	.661	.638	.655	.668	.677	.691	.671	.685	.695
11	.501	.581	.596	.606	.612	.623	.600	.616	.630	.639	.652	.632	.647	.658
12	.469	.546	.560	.570	.576	.587	.563	.580	.594	.603	.617	.596	.611	.622
13	.440	.513	.527	.537	.544	.555	.530	.547	.561	.570	.584	.563	.578	.589
14	.412	.482	.496	.505	.512	.523	.499	.515	.528	.538	.552	.531	.545	.557
15	.386	.454	.467	.476	.483	.494	.470	.485	.498	.507	.522	.501	.515	.526
16	.361	.427	.440	.449	.455	.466	.443	.458	.470	.479	.494	.472	.485	.496
17	.338	.402	.414	.423	.429	.440	.417	.431	.443	.452	.467	.445	.458	.469
18	.317	.378	.390	.398	.404	.415	.393	.406	.418	.426	.441	.420	.433	.443
19	.297	.355	.366	.375	.381	.391	.369	.383	.394	.403	.417	.396	.409	.420
20	.278	.333	.344	.353	.358	.369	.347	.361	.372	.380	.394	.374	.386	.396
22	.246	.293	.304	.312	.317	.327	.306	.318	.328	.336	.350	.330	.342	.352
24	.215	.258	.268	.275	.280	.290	.270	.281	.290	.298	.311	.292	.303	.312
26	.187	.228	.236	.243	.248	.257	.238	.249	.258	.264	.277	.259	.270	.278
28	.164	.200	.210	.215	.219	.228	.210	.221	.228	.234	.246	.230	.239	.246
30	.144	.178	.185	.190	.194	.202	.186	.195	.202	.208	.218	.203	.212	.219

d (cm)	8×15	8×20	10×10	10×15	10×20	12×12	15×15	15×20	20×20	20×30	25×25	30×30	35×35
*0.5	1.037	1.041	1.035	1.042	1.046	1.041	1.051	1.056	1.063	1.071	1.073	1.080	1.084
1	1.032	1.035	1.031	1.038	1.043	1.038	1.048	1.054	1.062	1.069	1.072	1.079	1.084
2	1.005	1.009	1.004	1.013	1.018	1.014	1.025	1.032	1.040	1.049	1.052	1.059	1.065
3	.975	.980	.974	.985	.990	.985	.999	1.006	1.016	1.026	1.029	1.038	1.044
4	.942	.947	.940	.952	.959	.953	.968	.977	.987	.999	1.002	1.014	1.021
5	.907	.913	.905	.918	.925	.919	.936	.946	.957	.971	.974	.988	.998
6	.869	.876	.867	.882	.890	.883	.902	.912	.925	.940	.944	.959	.970
7	.830	.837	.827	.844	.853	.845	.866	.878	.893	.909	.913	.929	.941
8	.790	.798	.787	.805	.815	.806	.830	.843	.859	.877	.881	.899	.912
9	.751	.760	.747	.767	.778	.768	.793	.808	.825	.845	.849	.869	.882
10	.713	.722	.709	.729	.741	.730	.756	.771	.790	.811	.816	.837	.852
11	.675	.685	.672	.692	.704	.692	.719	.736	.755	.777	.782	.803	.820
12	.640	.650	.636	.657	.670	.658	.685	.702	.722	.744	.750	.772	.790
13	.607	.618	.603	.625	.638	.626	.653	.670	.690	.713	.720	.743	.762
14	.575	.586	.571	.593	.606	.594	.622	.639	.660	.684	.691	.715	.734
15	.545	.556	.540	.563	.576	.563	.593	.610	.633	.656	.662	.687	.706
16	.516	.527	.510	.533	.547	.533	.564	.582	.605	.628	.634	.660	.679
17	.488	.499	.483	.506	.519	.506	.536	.554	.577	.601	.608	.633	.653
18	.462	.474	.457	.479	.493	.479	.509	.528	.551	.575	.582	.607	.627
19	.438	.449	.433	.455	.469	.455	.485	.503	.526	.550	.557	.583	.603
20	.415	.426	.410	.431	.445	.431	.461	.479	.502	.527	.534	.560	.580
22	.369	.380	.364	.385	.398	.384	.413	.431	.456	.481	.488	.515	.535
24	.329	.340	.324	.345	.358	.345	.373	.390	.412	.438	.446	.471	.492
26	.294	.304	.290	.309	.322	.308	.336	.352	.373	.398	.405	.431	.451
28	.263	.270	.257	.276	.288	.276	.302	.320	.339	.362	.368	.393	.413
30	.233	.242	.228	.245	.257	.244	.268	.286	.305	.328	.335	.358	.377

*This entry is also the backscatter factor.

APPENDIX C—SCATTER-AIR RATIO DATA

Table C-1. The scatter-air ratio data for HVL 1 mm Al presented in Table C-1a were derived from the measured percentage depth dose data given in Table B-2a and backscatter factors from Table B-1a. The method used is discussed in section 10.13. Table C-1b for HVL 2 mm Cu is similarly derived from Table B-2c. Scatter-air ratios for cobalt radiation are taken from Gupta and Cunningham (G10). Scatter-air ratios for high energy radiation, Tables B-2d and B-2e, are derived from tissue phantom ratio data measured by Van Dyk (V7) for 10 MV radiation and by Rawlinson (R4) for 25 MV radiation. To derive scatter-air ratios from tissue-phantom ratio data, it is necessary to assume tissue-air ratio data for the reference depth. This has been done by methods discussed in section 10.13.

TABLE C-1
Scatter-Air Ratios for Circular Fields, S(d, r, hν)

(a)   HVL - 1.0 mm Al

Field radius in cm at depth d

d (cm)	1.0	2.0	3.0	4.0	5.0	6.0	7.0	8.0	10.0	15.0
0.0	.057	.115	.152	.178	.200	.215	.225	.230	.238	.244
0.3	.150	.220	.273	.310	.340	.364	.385	.395	.405	.410
0.5	.177	.268	.335	.379	.410	.435	.450	.460	.470	.485
1.0	.192	.280	.345	.392	.435	.460	.475	.485	.495	.520
1.5	.181	.261	.323	.372	.414	.440	.456	.465	.474	.500
2.0	.142	.215	.200	.323	.355	.380	.393	.400	.407	.425
3.0	.031	.142	.200	.245	.272	.290	.300	.310	.320	.330
4.0	.056	.097	.135	.173	.195	.210	.220	.227	.236	.250
6.0	.023	.045	.065	.082	.095	.106	.116	.120	.127	.141
8.0	.015	.030	.045	.058	.068	.078	.085	.090	.095	.100
10.0	.014	.027	.038	.047	.054	.059	.063	.066	.068	.070

(b)   HVL - 2.0 mm Cu

Field radius in cm at depth d

d (cm)	1	2	3	4	5	6	7	8	9	10	12	14	16*	18*	20*
0	.067	.129	.183	.229	.267	.298	.325	.349	.371	.392	.431	.464	.493	.522	.599
1	.130	.239	.330	.402	.458	.504	.540	.574	.602	.627	.672	.711	.741	.763	.776
2	.147	.274	.382	.469	.539	.593	.635	.677	.713	.746	.804	.855	.901	.945	.994
3	.139	.270	.388	.489	.574	.643	.697	.742	.784	.820	.887	.940	.991	1.039	1.098
4	.129	.255	.373	.479	.568	.643	.704	.756	.803	.844	.916	.975	1.025	1.068	1.109
5	.118	.235	.348	.451	.541	.619	.683	.739	.787	.831	.905	.973	1.029	1.078	1.124
6	.105	.215	.323	.423	.512	.589	.654	.709	.758	.800	.881	.950	1.027	1.122	1.255
7	.094	.193	.291	.385	.471	.547	.613	.670	.718	.762	.846	.918	.978	1.031	1.079
8	.082	.170	.260	.348	.430	.504	.570	.627	.677	.720	.802	.873	.939	.996	1.043
9	.071	.150	.232	.313	.389	.460	.523	.579	.630	.674	.756	.827	.888	.940	.986
10	.061	.132	.206	.281	.353	.420	.480	.535	.584	.627	.706	.773	.831	.881	.924
11	.055	.117	.183	.251	.317	.379	.436	.487	.532	.576	.652	.720	.777	.822	.855
12	.050	.106	.165	.225	.284	.340	.393	.441	.486	.527	.600	.664	.718	.764	.802
13	.045	.093	.145	.199	.253	.304	.354	.399	.441	.478	.548	.611	.660	.704	.739
14	.039	.082	.128	.175	.223	.271	.317	.360	.399	.436	.502	.558	.606	.645	.677
15	.035	.072	.113	.156	.199	.243	.284	.324	.361	.396	.458	.509	.553	.592	.623
16	.028	.061	.097	.135	.175	.215	.253	.290	.325	.358	.416	.466	.506	.539	.569
17	.026	.055	.086	.120	.154	.190	.225	.259	.292	.322	.377	.425	.461	.493	.516
18	.023	.047	.074	.103	.134	.166	.199	.231	.263	.291	.343	.385	.421	.447	.471
19	.019	.040	.064	.090	.118	.148	.178	.207	.236	.263	.312	.352	.383	.408	.426
20	.016	.035	.055	.078	.102	.128	.155	.183	.210	.234	.280	.318	.347	.369	.385

*Extrapolated values which are less accurate

TABLE C-1 (continued)

755

Scatter-Air Ratios for Circular Fields, S(d, r, hν)

(c) Cobalt-60 radiation

Depth d (cm)	1	2	3	4	5	6	7	8	9	10	11	12
				Field radius in cm at depth d								
0.5	.007	.014	.019	.026	.032	.037	.043	.048	.054	.058	.063	.067
1	.013	.025	.037	.048	.058	.066	.073	.078	.084	.089	.094	.098
2	.023	.045	.064	.080	.091	.102	.110	.116	.122	.127	.133	.139
3	.032	.061	.084	.103	.118	.130	.139	.147	.154	.161	.166	.172
4	.038	.071	.099	.121	.137	.151	.162	.170	.179	.186	.191	.197
5	.041	.076	.107	.134	.152	.166	.178	.189	.198	.206	.212	.218
6	.042	.080	.114	.141	.160	.176	.190	.201	.211	.219	.226	.234
7	.042	.081	.115	.143	.164	.181	.196	.209	.220	.229	.239	.246
8	.041	.080	.114	.142	.165	.185	.199	.214	.225	.236	.246	.254
9	.040	.078	.112	.140	.164	.183	.200	.216	.228	.240	.251	.260
10	.038	.075	.109	.136	.161	.181	.199	.215	.229	.242	.252	.262
11	.036	.071	.104	.132	.157	.178	.197	.213	.227	.241	.252	.262
12	.035	.069	.099	.128	.153	.174	.194	.210	.225	.239	.251	.261
13	.034	.066	.095	.124	.149	.170	.190	.207	.223	.237	.249	.260
14	.032	.063	.092	.120	.145	.168	.186	.204	.220	.235	.247	.258
15	.031	.060	.089	.116	.140	.162	.182	.200	.216	.231	.244	.255
16	.030	.058	.086	.112	.136	.157	.177	.196	.212	.227	.240	.252
17	.029	.056	.083	.108	.132	.153	.172	.191	.207	.223	.236	.248
18	.027	.054	.080	.104	.128	.148	.167	.186	.202	.218	.232	.244
19	.026	.052	.077	.101	.124	.144	.162	.181	.197	.213	.226	.239
20	.024	.049	.074	.097	.119	.139	.157	.176	.192	.207	.221	.234
22	.022	.044	.067	.088	.109	.128	.146	.163	.180	.194	.208	.222
24	.020	.040	.060	.080	.099	.118	.136	.152	.168	.182	.196	.208
26	.018	.036	.054	.073	.091	.108	.125	.142	.156	.170	.184	.196
28	.016	.032	.049	.067	.083	.098	.115	.132	.156	.159	.172	.184
30	.015	.030	.045	.061	.076	.089	.105	.121	.134	.146	.159	.170

d (cm)	13	14	15	16	17	18	19	20	21	22	23	24	25
0.5	.070	.073	.076	.078	.080	.082	.084	.085	.086	.087	.088	.088	.089
1	.101	.104	.107	.109	.112	.114	.116	.118	.119	.120	.121	.122	.123
2	.142	.146	.149	.152	.154	.156	.158	.160	.161	.162	.164	.166	.167
3	.176	.180	.184	.187	.190	.193	.195	.198	.200	.202	.203	.204	.205
4	.201	.205	.210	.215	.218	.222	.225	.228	.231	.233	.235	.237	.239
5	.224	.229	.235	.240	.245	.248	.252	.255	.258	.261	.263	.264	.266
6	.241	.246	.252	.257	.262	.265	.269	.272	.275	.278	.280	.282	.284
7	.254	.260	.267	.273	.278	.282	.287	.290	.294	.296	.299	.302	.304
8	.263	.271	.278	.285	.289	.294	.298	.301	.305	.309	.311	.313	.315
9	.269	.277	.284	.292	.298	.303	.308	.312	.316	.319	.322	.324	.327
10	.271	.279	.288	.295	.302	.308	.314	.318	.324	.327	.331	.333	.336
11	.272	.280	.289	.296	.304	.311	.316	.322	.328	.331	.334	.337	.339
12	.272	.281	.290	.297	.305	.312	.318	.324	.330	.333	.337	.340	.342
13	.270	.280	.290	.298	.306	.313	.319	.325	.332	.335	.340	.342	.345
14	.268	.279	.288	.297	.305	.313	.320	.326	.333	.337	.341	.344	.347
15	.266	.277	.286	.295	.303	.311	.318	.325	.331	.336	.340	.344	.347
16	.263	.274	.283	.292	.300	.308	.315	.322	.328	.333	.337	.342	.346
17	.259	.271	.279	.288	.296	.304	.311	.318	.324	.329	.334	.339	.343
18	.255	.266	.275	.284	.292	.300	.307	.313	.320	.325	.330	.335	.339
19	.251	.261	.270	.280	.288	.295	.303	.309	.315	.321	.326	.331	.335
20	.246	.257	.265	.275	.284	.291	.299	.305	.311	.316	.321	.326	.329
22	.233	.246	.255	.264	.273	.280	.288	.295	.301	.306	.311	.316	.319
24	.220	.235	.243	.252	.259	.267	.275	.281	.288	.294	.299	.304	.309
26	.207	.219	.229	.236	.245	.253	.260	.266	.272	.279	.284	.289	.295
28	.194	.205	.214	.222	.230	.238	.245	.251	.258	.264	.269	.274	.279
30	.181	.191	.200	.208	.215	.223	.230	.236	.242	.249	.255	.260	.265

TABLE C-1 (continued)

Scatter-Air Ratios for Circular Fields, S(d, r, hν)

(d)   10 MV x rays

Field radius in cm at depth d

d (cm)	1.0	2.0	3.0	4.0	5.0	6.0	7.0	8.0	10.0	12.0	15.0	20.0	25.
0.0	.004	.015	.032	.055	.085	.120	.156	.193	.252	.298	.342	.377	.40
0.3	.006	.019	.038	.060	.085	.113	.141	.169	.215	.252	.290	.316	.33
0.6	.010	.024	.043	.063	.086	.108	.130	.152	.188	.217	.246	.265	.27
1.0	.013	.029	.048	.067	.086	.103	.120	.137	.163	.182	.200	.214	.22
1.6	.017	.035	.053	.070	.081	.090	.098	.105	.118	.127	.137	.149	.15
2.0	.021	.040	.057	.070	.079	.084	.089	.092	.100	.106	.112	.121	.12
2.3	.023	.042	.057	.066	.072	.076	.079	.082	.088	.093	.099	.107	.11
2.5	.025	.044	.058	.066	.072	.075	.078	.082	.088	.093	.099	.106	.11
2.7	.026	.046	.059	.065	.070	.074	.077	.080	.085	.090	.096	.104	.10
3.0	.029	.049	.061	.070	.076	.080	.084	.088	.095	.101	.107	.115	.12
4.0	.038	.064	.075	.085	.092	.096	.100	.104	.111	.117	.124	.134	.14
5.0	.041	.070	.084	.094	.102	.108	.113	.117	.125	.131	.139	.150	.15
6.0	.043	.073	.090	.102	.109	.116	.122	.128	.137	.144	.153	.163	.17
8.0	.045	.078	.099	.114	.125	.131	.137	.144	.154	.163	.173	.188	.20
10.0	.046	.080	.103	.119	.131	.138	.145	.153	.166	.177	.189	.205	.21
12.0	.045	.080	.104	.121	.134	.143	.152	.160	.174	.187	.201	.218	.22
14.0	.044	.078	.103	.121	.135	.144	.154	.164	.181	.194	.209	.227	.23
16.0	.043	.076	.099	.118	.133	.144	.155	.166	.184	.198	.213	.233	.24
18.0	.041	.072	.095	.115	.130	.142	.154	.165	.184	.198	.212	.236	.25
20.0	.040	.070	.091	.109	.126	.140	.152	.163	.182	.197	.212	.237	.25
25.0	.036	.063	.082	.099	.115	.130	.143	.155	.175	.191	.208	.233	.25
30.0	.032	.057	.075	.094	.109	.121	.133	.144	.163	.178	.194	.219	.23

(e)   25 MV x rays

Field radius at d cm

d (cm)	1.0	2.0	3.0	4.0	5.0	6.0	7.0	8.0	10.0	12.0	15.0	20.0	30.
0.0	.030	.060	.090	.120	.154	.181	.210	.246	.300	.350	.400	.450	.48
1.0	.026	.053	.081	.109	.144	.175	.200	.225	.270	.300	.340	.385	.41
2.0	.020	.042	.063	.081	.103	.122	.142	.160	.185	.205	.230	.255	.27
3.0	.015	.030	.047	.063	.078	.090	.100	.111	.129	.146	.164	.180	.19
4.0	.011	.023	.035	.045	.056	.065	.073	.082	.094	.103	.112	.124	.13
5.0	.009	.019	.028	.036	.043	.048	.053	.057	.065	.072	.080	.090	.11
6.0	.008	.018	.027	.036	.042	.047	.050	.053	.057	.060	.065	.073	.08
7.0	.008	.016	.025	.034	.042	.046	.047	.049	.053	.057	.063	.070	.08
8.0	.008	.017	.026	.036	.046	.050	.052	.055	.059	.063	.068	.075	.08
10.0	.009	.019	.030	.039	.049	.055	.059	.062	.066	.070	.076	.083	.09
12.5	.010	.023	.037	.049	.060	.069	.074	.078	.085	.091	.099	.109	.12
15.0	.011	.023	.038	.052	.065	.076	.082	.086	.092	.097	.105	.116	.13
17.5	.012	.026	.040	.054	.068	.078	.086	.093	.102	.111	.120	.130	.14
20.0	.013	.029	.046	.060	.073	.084	.090	.096	.106	.116	.127	.140	.15
22.5	.014	.030	.048	.062	.075	.085	.095	.101	.112	.120	.132	.145	.15
25.0	.014	.031	.049	.064	.076	.087	.097	.104	.116	.128	.139	.153	.16
30.0	.015	.032	.050	.065	.079	.091	.100	.108	.122	.132	.142	.152	.16
35.0	.014	.032	.051	.066	.080	.091	.100	.109	.122	.137	.150	.164	.17
40.0	.013	.031	.051	.067	.080	.092	.102	.110	.124	.138	.152	.166	.18

ANSWERS TO PROBLEMS

Chapter 1
(1) 1.39 m s^{-2} (2) 50 V   (3) 516 × 10^{-4} C/kg   (4) 40 Gy, 2.50 × 10^{11} MeV/g   (5) 40.7 × 10^{12} Bq, 26.7 GBq   (8) 1000, 88 MeV   (9) 2.224 MeV   (10) 1:100   (11) 333.3 m, 3.72 × 10^{-9} eV   (12) 3 × 10^{9} Hz, 1.24 × 10^{-5} eV   (13) 5.45 × 10^{14} Hz, 2.25 eV   (14) 4.43 pm, 67.7 × 10^{18} Hz   (15) 0.564 pm   (16) 35.4 fm   (17) 50.4 × 10^{30} s^{-1} (18) 18.4 pm   (19) 1.86 GeV   (20) 2.96, 0.941   (22) 66.0 GBq   (24) 22 cm, 1.59 cm   (25) 1.21 × 10^{4} (26) 9.36 × 10^{-8} (27) 17.9 kBq, 48.4 μCi   (29) 1.105, 1.105   (30) 6.93%   (31) 1.16 s^{-1} (32) 0.258 d^{-1}, 3.88 d

Chapter 2
(1) 60 kV, 85 kV$_p$ (3) 32.0 kW, 64.0 kJ, 15.3 kcal   (4) 7.5 kJ s^{-1}, 1.79 kcal s^{-1} (5) 9.7 mm, 3.9   (6) 75:1   (9) 166 V, 105 V   (14) Just barely, yes   (16) 480,000 HU   (17) Yes, 0.4 s, about 180   (20) 37.5 R/min

Chapter 3
(2) 1.37 × 10^{-11} s^{-1}, 36.5 MBq, 0.986 mCi   (3) 6.6 × 10^{13}, 4.12 × 10^{-6} J/s   (4) 11.6 d, 0.086 d^{-1}, 0.89 mCi, 33.0 MBq   (5) 11.63 d, 12.06 × 10^{13} (6) 2.42 × 10^{14} (7) 1.73 × 10^{11} (10) 1.015 MeV   (12) 24.7 MeV   (13) 80.9 MeV   (14) 32.0 MeV   (15) 251 MeV   (16) 9.9 × 10^{-3} (17) No   (18) 140 × 10^{-4} J   (20) 2.37 GBq, 2.6 GBq   (21) 47.5 MW   (22) 91 GBq   (23) 13.7 min   (24) 22.7 GBq, 14.6 GBq, 1.7 × 10^{-4} (27) 3.27 MeV

Chapter 4
(1) 314 km   (2) 4.57 cm   (4) 0.67 cm, 1.0 cm   (5) 13.9 keV   (6) 28.3   (7) 14.9 MHz   (8) 7.56 × 10^{-26} kg, 9.1 m

Chapter 5
(1) 0.985, 0.955, 0.400, 0.985, 0.956, 0.549   (2) 23.1 cm   (3) 99.1, 95.5, 55, 99.1, 95.6, 63.8   (4) 231 kg/m^2 (5) 40.6, 15.2, 1.3, 40.6 kg m^{-2} (6) 30 cm   (7) 0.172 × 10^{-28} m^2/el, 0.0498 cm^2/g, 13.4 m^{-1} (8) 845 m^{-1}, 0.0744 m^2/kg   (9) 903, 253   (10) 71.9, 28.1, 13.8 keV   (12) 6.14 × 10^4, 6.14 × 10^4 MeV, 2.70 × 10^4 MeV, 3.44 × 10^4 MeV   (14) 1630, 86   (15) 6.98 MeV   (16) 3.02 MeV   (18) 30.1 × 10^3 MeV   (23) 7.61 × 10^5, 7.61 × 10^5 MeV, 3.35 × 10^5 MeV, 4.26 × 10^5 MeV   (24) 16.8 × 10^{-9} °C max

Chapter 6
(5)   2.0 × 10^3 (6)   2.9 × 10^2 (10)   7.6   (11)   1700   (19)   127   (20) 4.11 × 10^4, 59.6 × 10^4 MeV, 22.6 × MeV, 2.98 × 10^4, 4.5 × 10^4 MeV, 142 × 10^4 MeV, 116 × 10^4 MeV, 3.0 × 10^4 MeV, 109 × 10^4

757

MeV (21) 1.36×10^4, 1.63×10^4, 18.9×10^4, 2.55×10^3 keV, 0, 18.8×10^5 keV, 135×10^5 keV, 1.63×10^5 keV, 0, 18.9×10^5 keV (26) 1.91×10^3, 376, 31.8 MeV/cm^2, 18.7°

Chapter 7

(1) 6.74×10^6 cm^{-2} s^{-1}, 5.27×10^6 MeV cm^{-2} s^{-1}, 781 keV, 915 keV (2) 2.53×10^{-5} J kg^{-1} s^{-1}, 2.52×10^{-5} Gy/s (3) 1040 keV (4) 96 keV, 12.9 keV (5) 0.051 Gy (7) 2.68 Gy (8) 2.15 Gy (10) 2.43 MeV, 1.2 cm, 10.3 m, 0.8 cm (11) 0.753 Gy/min (12) 1.25 Gy/min (14) 0.0123 Gy

Chapter 8

(5) 7.64×10^8 cm^{-2} s^{-1}, 0.059 R/s (6) 1.46 (9) 0.8 mm Cu (11) 2.0 R, 1.87×10^{-3} J, 4.17×10^{-3}

Chapter 9

(2) 11.6 ms (3) 0.803 (4) 0.0033 (5) 0.998 (6) 0.408 (10) 0.013 (11) 0.027 (14) 102 R/min (15) 88 R/min (16) 29.7 R (19) 1.64×10^{-6} molar, 0.0036 (20) 133 Gy (23) 22.8 Gy (26) 326 J m^{-2} min^{-1}, 1.69×10^{15} m^{-2} min^{-1}

Chapter 10

(1) 2.38 min (2) 5.4×7.3 cm^2, 3.33 Gy (5) 0.643, 0.513, 0.431 Gy/min, 1.06, 1.19, 1.30 Gy/min, 5.4×9.0, 5.1×8.5, 4.9×8.1 cm^2 (6) 3.78 min (7) 1.04, 1.30, 1.55, 3.89 min, 1.23, 1.65, 2.09 Gy (8) 0.839, 0.862, 0.536, 0.396, 0.316 Gy/min, 4.80 min, 1.06, 1.45, 1.82 Gy (9) 0.0653 cm^{-1}, 0.041 cm^{-1} (10) 0.369 (11) 0.20 (12) 0.03 Gy (13) 55.9

Chapter 11

(1) 0.50 Gy/min, 4 min (3) 0.96 (4) 0.95 (5) 0.2 cm (6) 37.4 (9) 2 Gy, no (10) 0.15

Chapter 12

(3) 1.07, 1.06, 0.82, 0.66, 1.27, 1.26, 1.15, 1.09, 1.0, 1.30, 1.68, 1.66 (5) 1.14, 0.99, 0.85, 0.80, 0.80 (6) 17.4, 23.8, 22.2 Gy, 17.8 and 16.6 Gy, (b), 18.3, 15.8 Gy, 21.6, 23.3 Gy (7) 1.04 Gy (9) 44.1 Gy, 37.4, 43.5, 54.5 Gy, 44.1 Gy (12) 1.01 Gy/min (14) 1.04 min

Chapter 13

(1) 4.78×10^{11}, 2.64×10^8, 2.32×10^9 (2) 1.65 R/hr (3) 781 keV, 1040 keV (6) 1.2 (7) 0.10 mg Ra eq. (0.5 mm Pt) (8) 135 hr, 89 Gy, 52 Gy (9) 8.0 mg (13) 2048 hr per mg Ra used (16) 130 hr, 23 Gy

Chapter 14

(2) 21, 15, 29 (3) 100, 1%, 44.7, 2.2% (4) 18,000, 0.75% (5) 90 min, 110 min (6) 5.73%, 5.77% (7) ±79 ml (8) 1000 s^{-1} (9) 63.5 μs, 1063 s^{-1} (10) 0.159 MBq (11) 11.7 h (12) 25.5 h (15) 1.97 μGy

Chapter 15
(1) 4.5 mSv   (5) 60 cm concrete or 11 cm Pb   (6) 10^{-7} Gy/min

Chapter 16
(1) 2.4%, 4.4%, -45.5% (2) 13.9%, -55%, -99% (3) 24.3%   (4) 6.1%
(5) 24.7%   (6) reduce exposure by a factor of 3.1   (8) 0.32 (68% less)
(9) -10.9% (10) 1.3, 1/400, 2.6   (12) 20, 40   (14) 60 MHz, about 1500
(18) 1.14   (19) 3.88 mm, 0.35 mm   (27) $\sin \pi f / \pi f$ where f is in lp/mm
(30) $\sin \theta / \theta$, $\epsilon^{-\theta^2/\alpha}$, $\epsilon^{-\theta^2/\beta} \cos 2\gamma\theta$ (32) 0.87×1.73 mm   (33) yes, only
just, no   (38) 12.7 cm   (39) 5.1 cm   (40) 0.27 cm^{-1}, 0.22 cm^{-1}

REFERENCES

A1. Adams, G.D., G.M. Almy, S.M. Dancoff, A.O. Hanson, D.W. Kerst, H.W. Koch, E.F. Lanzl, L.H. Lanzl, J.S. Laughlin, H. Quastler, D.E. Riesen, C.S. Robinson, L.S. Skaggs: Techniques for application of the betatron to medical therapy, Am J Roentgenol 60:153, 1948.

A2. Attix, F.H.: The partition of kerma to account for bremsstrahlung. Health Phys 36:347, 1979.

A3. Attix, F.H., L. DeLavergne: Plate separation requirements for standard free-air ionization chambers. Radiology 63:853, 1954.

A4. Almond, P.R., H. Svensson: Ionization chamber dosimetry for photon and electron beams. Theoretical considerations. Acta Radiol Ther Phys Biol 16:177, 1977.

A5. Attix, F.H., ed.: Luminescence dosimetry. Proceedings of International Conference on Luminescence Dosimetry. Washington, D.C.: Atomic Energy Commission, 1967.

A6. Andrew, J.W., J. Van Dyk, H.E. Johns: Use of scattered radiation measurements in radiotherapy dose calculations based on computed tomography (CT) images. Proc Soc Photo-Optical Instrum Eng 173:342, 1979.

A7. Aspin, N., H.E. Johns: The absorbed dose in cylindrical cavities within irradiated bone. Br J Radiol 36:350, 1963.

A8. Allt, W.E.C.: Supervoltage radiation treatment in advanced cancer of the uterine cervix. Can Med Assoc J 100:792, 1969.

A9. Attix, F.H., V.H. Ritz: A determination of the gamma-ray emission of radium. J Res Natl Bur Stand 59:293, 1957.

A10. Anger, H.O.: Scintillation camera. Rev Sci Instrum 29:27, 1958.

A11. Anger, H.O.: Survey of radioisotope cameras. Trans Instrum Soc Amer 5:311, 1966.

A12. Adler, H.I., A.M. Weinberg: An approach to setting radiation standards. Health Phys 34:719, 1978.

A13. Ardran, G.M., H.E. Crooks: Checking diagnostic x-ray beam quality. Br J Radiol 41:193, 1968.

A14. Adams, G.E.: The oxidizing species in irradiated water and aqueous solutions. In: G. Silini, ed.: Radiation research. Proceedings of the 3rd International Congress of Radiation Research, Cortina d'Ampezzo, Italy, 1966. Amsterdam: North-Holland, 195, 1969.

A15. Abrahams, S., J.E. Till, E.A. McCulloch, L. Siminovitch: Assessment of viability of frozen bone marrow cells using a cell-culture method. Cell Tissue Kinet 1:255, 1968.

B1. Brookhaven National Laboratory—Neutron Cross Sections, Vol. 1, Resonance Parameters, June 1973 #325/ED3

B2. Brahme, A., G. Hultén, H. Svensson: Electron depth absorbed dose distribution for a 10 MeV clinical microtron. Phys Med Biol 20:39, 1975.

B3. Bewley, D.K.: Fast neutron beams for therapy. Curr Top Radiat Res 6:249, 1970.

B4. Bruce, W.R., H.E. Johns: The spectra of x rays scattered in low atomic number materials. Br J Radiol Suppl. 9, 1960.

B5. Berger, M.J., S.M. Seltzer: Tables of energy losses and ranges of electrons and positrons. NASA SP-3012. Washington, D.C.: National Aeronautics and Space Administration, 1964.
   and
   Berger, M.J., S.M. Seltzer: Additional stopping power and range tables for protons, mesons, and electrons. NASA SP-3036. Washington, D.C.: National Aeronautics and Space Administration, 1966.

B6. Bruce, W.R., H.E. Johns: Experimentally determined electron energy distribution produced by cobalt 60 gamma rays. Br J Radiol 28:443, 1955.

B7. Bruce, W.R., M.L. Pearson, H.E. Johns: Comparison of Monte Carlo calculations and experimental measurements of scattered radiation produced in a water phantom by primary radiations with half value layers from 1.25 mm Cu to 11 mm Pb. Radiat Res 17:543, 1962.

B8. Bentley, R.E., J.C. Jones, S.C. Lillicrap. X ray spectra from accelerators in the range 2 to 6 MeV. Phys Med Biol 12:301, 1967.

B9. Boag, J.W.: Ionization chambers. In: F.H. Attix, W.C. Roesch, eds.: Radiation dosimetry. Vol. II. New York: Academic Press, 1, 1966.

B10. Bewley, D.K., E.C. McCullough, B.C. Page, S. Sakata: Neutron dosimetry with a calorimeter. Phys Med Biol 19:831, 1974.

B11. Bernier, J.P., L.D. Skarsgard, D.V. Cormack, H.E. Johns: A calorimetric determination of the energy required to produce an ion pair in air for cobalt-60 gamma-rays. Radiat Res 5:613, 1956.

B12. Burkell, C.C., T.A. Watson, H.E. Johns, R.J. Horsley: Skin effects of cobalt 60 telecurie therapy. Br J Radiol 27:171, 1954.

B13. Cohen, M., D.E.A. Jones, D. Greene, eds.: Central axis depth dose data for use in radiotherapy. Br J Radiol Suppl. 11, 1972.

B14. Batho, H.F.: Lung corrections in cobalt 60 beam therapy. J Can Ass Radiol 15:79, 1964.

B15. Bush, R.S., H.E. Johns: The measurement of build-up on curved surfaces exposed to Co^{60} and Cs^{137} beams. Amer J Roentgenol 87:89, 1962.

B16. Batho, H.F., M.E.J. Young: Tissue absorption corrections for linear radium sources. Br J Radiol 37:689, 1964.

B17. Baimel, N.H., M.J. Bronskill: Optimization of analog-circuit motion correction for liver scintigraphy. J Nucl Med 19:1059, 1978.

B18. Brownell, G.L., W.H. Sweet: Localization of brain tumors with positron emittors. Nucleonics 11:11, 1953.

B19. The BEIR Report. The effects on populations of exposure to low levels of ionizing radiation. Washington, D.C.: National Academy of Sciences, National Research Council, 1972.

B20. BIER III Report. National Academy of Sciences. Committee on the Biological Effects of Ionizing Radiations. The effects on populations of exposure to low levels of ionizing radiation: 1980. Washington, D.C.: National Academy Press, 1980.

B21. Birch, R., M. Marshall, G.M. Ardran: Catalogue of spectral data for diagnostic x rays. London: The Hospital Physicists' Association, 1979.

B22. Buchanan, R.A., S.I. Finkelstein, K.A. Wickershein: X-ray exposure reduction using rare-earth oxysulfide intensifying screens. Radiology 105:185, 1972.

B23. Boldingh, W.H.: Grids to reduce scattered x-rays in medical radiography. Philips Res Rep Suppl (Netherlands) 1:1, 1964.

B24. Burgess, A.E.: Focal spots: I. MTF separability. II. Models III. Field characteristics. Invst Radiol 12:36, 1977.

B25. Bernstein, H., R.T. Bergeron, D.J. Klein: Routine evaluation of focal spots. Radiology 111:421, 1974.

B26. Brubacher P., B.M. Moores: The modulation transfer function of the focal spot with a twin-peaked intensity distribution. Radiology 107:635, 1973.

B27. Burgess, A.E.: Interpretation of star test pattern images. Med Phys 4:1, 1977.

B28. Burgess, A.E.: Effect of asymmetric focal spots in angiography. Med Phys 4:21, 1977.

B29. Brigham, E.O.: The fast fourier transform. Englewood Cliffs, N.J.: Prentice Hall, 1974.

B30. Boag, J.W.: Xeroradiography. Phys Med Biol 18:3, 1973 **and** Xeroradiography and ionography, a review. In: Proceedings of The Symposium on Advances in Biomedical Dosimetry. Vienna, Austria: IAEA. 475, 1975.

B31. Boag, J.W., A.J. Stacey, R. Davies: Xerographic recording of mammograms. Br J Radiol 45:633, 1972.

B32. BRH—Directed efforts eliminate 160,000 unnecessary chest x rays annually. U.S. Dept. of Health and Human Services Bureau of Radiological Health, Bulletin XV, 4, 1, March 9, 1981.

B33. Boag, J.W., E.J. Hart: Absorption spectrum of "hydrated electron." Nature 197: 45, 1963.

B34. Barendsen, G.W.: The influence of oxygen on damage to the proliferative capacity of cultured human cells produced by radiations of different LET. In: Cellular Radiation Biology. 18th Ann Symp M.D. Anderson Hospital. Baltimore, Williams and Wilkins 331, 1965.

B35. Bush, R.S., W.R. Bruce: The radiation sensitivity of transplanted lymphoma cells as determined by the spleen colony method. Radiat Res 21:612, 1964.

B36. Bush R.S., R.P. Hill: Biologic discussions augmenting radiation effects and model systems. Laryngoscope 85:1119, 1975.

B37. Bush, R.S. Malignancies of the ovary, uterus and cervix. London: Edward Arnold, 1979.

B38. Bush, R.S., R.D.T. Jenkin, W.E.C. Allt, F.A. Beale, H. Bean, A.J. Dembo, J.F. Pringle: Definitive evidence for hypoxic cells influencing cure in cancer therapy. Br J Cancer (Suppl) 37:302, 1978.

B39. Brady, L.W.: Radiation sensitizers: their use in the clinical management of cancer. New York: Masson Publishing, 1980.

B40. Burdette, W.J., E.A. Gehan: Planning and analysis of clinical studies. Springfield, Ill.: Charles C Thomas, 1970.

C1. Cunningham, J.R., W.R. Bruce, H.P. Webb: A convenient ^{137}Cs unit for irradiating cell suspensions and small laboratory animals. Phys Med Biol 10:381, 1965.

C2. Cunningham, J.R., C.L. Ash, H.E. Johns: A double headed cobalt 60 teletherapy unit. Amer J Roentgenol 92:202, 1964.

C3. Cormack, D.V., H.E. Johns: Electron energies and ion densities in water irradiated with 200 keV, 1 MeV and 25 MeV radiation. Br J Radiol 25:369, 1952.

C4. Cunningham, J.R., H.E. Johns: Calculation of the average energy absorbed in photon interactions. Med Phys 1:51, 1980.

C5. Cunningham, J.R., M.R. Sontag: Displacement corrections used in absorbed dose determination. Med Phys 7:672, 1980.

C6. Cameron, J.R., N. Suntharalingam, G.N. Kenney: Thermoluminescent dosimetry. Madison: University of Wisconsin Press, 1968.

C7. Clarkson, J.R.: A note on depth doses in fields of irregular shape. Br J Radiol 14:265, 1941.

C8. Cunningham, J.R.: Scatter-air ratios. Phys Med Biol 17:42, 1972.

C9. Cunningham, J.R., D.J. Wright, H.P. Webb, J.A. Rawlinson, P.M.K. Leung: A semiautomatic cutter for compensating filters. Int J Radiat Oncol Biol Phys 1:355, 1976.

C10. Cunningham, J.R.: Tissue inhomogeneity corrections in photon beam treatment planning. In: Orton C., ed.: Progress in Med Phys. New York: Plenum Publishing, New York (in press).

C11. Cunningham, J.R., D.J. Wright: A simple facility for whole-body irradiation. Radiology 78:941, 1962.

C12. Carling, E.R., B.W. Windeyer, D.W. Smithers. British practice in radiotherapy, London: Butterworth, 1955.

C13. Chaney, E.L., W.R. Hendee: Effects of x ray tube current and voltage on effective focal spot size. Med Phys 1:141, 1974.

C14. Coltman, J.W.: The specification of imaging properties by response to a sine wave input. J Opt Soc of Amer 44:468, 1954.

C15. Cormack, A.M.: Representation of a function by its line integrals, with some radiological applications. J App Phys 34:2722, 1963.

C16. Campbell, C.C.M., M.J. Yaffe, K.W. Taylor: Measurement of time variations of x-ray beam characteristics. Proc Soc Photo-Optical Instrum Eng 173:312, 1979.

C17. Cormack, D.V., H.E. Johns: Electron energies and ion densities in water irradiated with 200 keV, 1 MeV and 25 MeV radiations. Br J Radiol 25:369, 1952.

C18. Chadwick, K.H., H.P. Leenhouts: A molecular theory of cell survival. Phys Med Biol 18:78, 1973.

C19. Chapman, J.D., C.J. Gillespie, A.P. Reuvers, D.L. Dugle: The inactivation of chinese hamster cells by x-rays: the effects of chemical modifiers on single- and double-events. Radiat Res 64:365, 1975.

C20. Chapman, J.D.: Biophysical models of mammalian cell inactivation by radiation. In: R.E. Meyn, H.R. Withers: Radiation Biology in Cancer Research. New York: Raven Press, 21, 1980.

C21. Cohen, L.: Theoretical "iso-survival" formulae for fractionated radiation therapy. Br J Radiol 41:522, 1968.

C22. Chapman, J.D., D.L. Dugle, A.P. Reuvers, B.E. Meeker, J. Borsa: Studies on the radiosensitizing effect of oxygen in chinese hamster cells. Int J Radiat Biol 26:383, 1974.

C23. Cade, I.S., J.B. McEwen, S. Dische, M.I. Saunders, E.R. Watson, K.E. Halnan, G. Wiernik, D.J.D. Perrins, I. Sutherland: Hyperbaric oxygen and radiotherapy: a Medical Research Council trial in carcinoma of the bladder. Br J Radiol 51:876, 1978.

C24. Catterall, M.: The results of randomized and other clinical trials of fast neutrons from the Medical Research Council cyclotron, London. Int J Radiat Oncol Biol Phys 3:247, 1977.

C25. Coldman, A.J., J.M. Elwood: Examining survival data. Can Med Assoc J 121:1065, 1979.

D1. Dillman, L.T., E.C. Von der Lage: Radionuclide decay schemes and nuclear parameters for use in radiation dose estimation. MIRD pamphlet #10. New York: Society of Nuclear Medicine, 1975.

D2. Dixon, W.R., C. Garrett, A. Morrison: Radiation measurements with the Eldorado cobalt 60 teletherapy unit. Br J Radiol 25:314, 1952.

D3. Dutreix J., A. Dutreix, M. Bernard: Étude de la dose au voisinage de l'interface entre deau milieux de composition atomique différente exposes aux rayonnement γ du ^{60}Co. Phys Med Biol 7:69, 1962.

D4. Drost, D.J.: Experimental dual xenon detectors for quantitative CT and spectral artefact correction. M.Sc. Thesis, University of Toronto, 1979.

D5. Dosimetry Protocols:
    a. Hospital Physicists Association (HPA). A code of practice for the dosimetry of 2 to 35 MV x-rays and ^{137}Cs and ^{60}Co gamma ray beams. Phys Med Biol 13:1, 1969.
    b. HPA. A practical guide to electron beam dosimetry below 5 MeV for radiotherapy puposes. 1975; HPA Report Series 13.
    c. HPA. A practical guide to electron dosimetry. 1971; HPA Report Series 4.
    d. American Association of Physicists in Medicine (AAPM), Scientific Committee on Radiation Dosimetry (SCRAD). Protocol for the dosimetry of x- and gamma-ray beams with maximum energies between 0.6 and 50 MeV. Phys Med Biol 16:379, 1971.
    e. AAPM. Code of practice for x ray therapy linear accelerators. Med Phys 2:110, 1975.
    f. Nordic Association of Clinical Physics (NACP). Procedures in external radiation dosimetry with electron and photon beams with maximum energies between 1 and 50 MeV. Acta Radiol [Ther], (Stockh) 19:155, 1980.

D6. Domen, S.R., P.J. Lamperti: A heat-loss compensated calorimeter: theory, design and performance. J Res Natl Bur Stand 78A:595, 1974.

D7. Domen, S.R., P.J. Lamperti: Comparisons of calorimetric and ionometric measurements in graphite irradiated with electrons from 15 to 50 MeV. Med Phys 3:294, 1976.

D8. Dickens, C.W.: A radiotherapy mould room manual. Surrey, England: The Royal Marsden Hospital, 1971.

D9. Dahl, O., K.J. Vikterlöf: Dose distributions in arc therapy in the 200 to 250 kV range. Acta Radiol [Suppl], (Stockh) 171, 1958.

D10. Dainty, J.C., R. Shaw: Image Science. New York: Academic Press, 1974.

D11. Drost, D.J. A. Fenster: Experimental dual xenon detectors for quantitative CT and spectral artifact correction. Med Phys 7:101, 1980.

D12. Daniels, C., K.W. Taylor: Variations with kVp of exposure and attenuation throughout a radiographic system and assessment of the speed of films, screens and processors. Proc Soc Photo-Optical Instrum Eng 273:73, 1981.

D13. Deschner, E.E., L.H. Gray: Influence of oxygen tension on x-ray induced chromosomal damage in Ehrlich ascites tumor cells irradiated in vitro and in vivo. Radiat Res 11:115, 1959.

D14. Dische, S.: Hyperbaric oxygen: the Medical Research Council trials and their clinical significance. Br J Radiol 51:888, 1978.

D15. Dewey, W.C., M.L. Freeman, G.P. Raaphorst, E.P. Clark, R.S.L. Wong, D.P. Highfield, I.J. Spiro, S.P. Tomasovic, D.L. Denman, R.A. Coss: Cell biology of hyperthermia and radiation. In: R.E. Meyn, H.R. Withers, eds.: Radiation Biology in Cancer Research. New York: Raven Press, 589, 1980.

E1. Evans, R.D.: The atomic nucleus. New York: McGraw-Hill, 1955.

E2. Epp, E.R., H. Weiss: Experimental study of the photon energy spectrum of primary diagnostic x rays. Phys Med Biol 11:225, 1966.

E3. Epp, E.R., M.N. Lougheed, J.W. McKay: Ionization build-up in upper respiratory air passages during teletherapy with cobalt 60 radiation. Br J Radiol 31:361, 1958.

E4. Epp, E.R., H. Weiss: Spectral fluence of scattered radiation in a water medium irradiated with diagnostic x rays. Radiat Res 30:129, 1967.

E5. Ehrlich, M.: Photographic dosimetry of x- and gamma rays. National Bureau of Standards Handbook 57. Washington, D.C.: U.S. National Bureau of Standards, 1954.

E6. Ege, G.N., A. Warbick-Cerone, M.J. Bronskill: Radionuclide lymphoscintigraphy —an update. In: V.I. Sodd, D.R. Allen, D.R. Hoogland, R.D. Ice, eds.: Radiopharmaceuticals II: Proceedings of the Second International Symposium on Radiopharmaceuticals. New York: Society of Nuclear Medicine 241, 1979.

E7. Ege, G.N.: Internal mammary lymphoscintigraphy in breast carcinoma: a study of 1072 patients. Int J Radiat Oncol Biol Phys 2:755, 1977.

E8. Elkind, M.M., G.F. Whitmore: The radiobiology of cultured mammalian cells. New York, Gordon and Breach, 1967.

E9. Elkind, M.M., H. Sutton: Radiation response of mammalian cells grown in culture. I. Repair of x-ray damage in surviving chinese hamster cells. Radiat Res 13:556, 1960.

E10. Ellis, F.: Dose, time and fractionation: a clinical hypothesis. Clin Radiol 20:1, 1969.

F1. Fedoruk, S.O., H.E. Johns: Transmission dose measurement for cobalt 60 radiation with special reference to rotation therapy. Br J Radiol 30:190, 1957.

F2. Fitzpatrick, P.J., W.D. Rider: Half body radiotherapy. Int J Radiat Oncol Biol Phys 1:197, 1976.

F3. Farmer, F.T.: A sub-standard x ray dose-meter. Br J Radiol 28:304, 1955.

F4. Fano, U.: Note on the Bragg-Gray cavity principle for measuring energy dissipation. Radiat Res 1:237, 1954.

F5. Friedell, H.L., C.I. Thomas, J.S. Krohmer: An evaluation of the clinical use of a strontium-90 beta ray applicator with a review of the underlying principles. Am J Roentgen 71:25, 1954.

F6. Fenster, A., D. Plewes, H.E. Johns: Efficiency and resolution of ionography in diagnostic radiology. Med Phys 1:1, 1974.

F7. Fenster, A., H.E. Johns: Closed-system ionography for diagnostic radiology. Med Phys 3:379, 1976.

F8. Fenster, A., H.E. Johns: Liquid ionography for diagnostic radiology. Med Phys 1:262, 1974.

F9. Fenster, A.: Split xenon detector for tomochemistry in computed tomography. J Comput Assist Tomogr 2:243, 1978.

F10. Fenster, A., D. Drost, B. Rutt: Correction of spectral artifacts and determination of electron density and atomic number from computed tomographic (CT) scans. Proc Soc Photo-Optical Instrum Eng 173:333, 1979.

F11. Friedman, M., A.W. Pearlman: Time-dose relationship in irradiation of recurrent cancer of the breast; iso-effect curve and tumour lethal dose. Amer J Roentgen 73:986, 1955.

F12. Fowler, J.F., R.L. Morgan, J.A. Silvester, D.K. Bewley, B.A. Turner: Experiments with fractionated x-ray treatment of the skin of pigs. I. Fractionation up to 28 days. Br J Radiol 36:188, 1963.

F13. Fowler, J.F., J. Denekamp, P.W. Sheldon, A.M. Smith, A.C. Begg, S.R. Harris, A.L. Page: Optimum fractionation in x-ray treatment of C_3H mouse mammary tumours. Br J Radiol 47:781, 1974.

F14. Fowler, J.F.: NSD and its clinical relevance (abstract). Br J Radiol 54:170, 1981.

F15. Fowler, J.F., G.E. Adams, J. Denekamp: Radiosensitizers of hypoxic cells in solid tumours. Cancer Treat Rev 3:227, 1976.

F16. Field, S.B., N.M. Bleehen: Hyperthermia in the treatment of cancer. Cancer Treat Rev 6:63, 1979.

G1. General Electric—Chart of the Nuclides. Nuclear Energy Marketing Department, 175 Curtner Avenue, San José, California 95125.

G2. Green, D.T., R.F. Errington: Design of a cobalt 60 beam therapy unit. Br J Radiol 25:309, 1952.

G3. Goldstein H., J.E. Wilkins: Calculations of the penetration of gamma-rays. U.S. Atomic Energy Commission Report NVO-3075. 1954.

G4. Greene, D., J.B. Massey: Letter to the editor, "C_λ values." Phys Med Biol 23:172, 1978.

G5. Greening, J.R.: A compact free-air chamber for use in the range 10-50 kV. Br J Radiol 33:178, 1960.

G6. Greening, J.R.: The derivation of approximate x ray spectral distributions and an analysis of x ray "quality" specifications. Br J Radiol 36:363, 1963.

G7. Greening, J.R.: The determination of x ray energy distributions by the absorption method. Br J Radiol 20:71, 1947.

G8. Greening, J.R.: Saturation characteristics of parallel-plate ionization chambers. Phys Med Biol 9:143, 1964.

G9. Genna, S., J.S. Laughlin: Absolute calibration of a cobalt-60 gamma-ray beam. Radiology 65:394, 1955.

G10. Gupta, S.K., J.R. Cunningham: Measurement of tissue-air ratios and scatter functions for large field sizes, for cobalt 60 gamma radiation. Br J Radiol 39:7, 1966.

G11. Gallaghar, R.G., E.L. Saenger: Radium capsules and their associated hazards. Amer J Roentgenol 77:511, 1957.

G12. Graham, J.B., R.M. Graham, L.S.J. Sotto, N.A. Baily: Spent radon seeds: I. Late effects. Radiology 74:399, 1960.

G13. Gebauer, A., J. Lissner, O. Schott: Roentgen television. New York: Grune, 1967.

G14. Gray, J.E., M. Trefler: Focal spot measurements for quality control purposes using a random object distribution. Opt Eng 15:353, 1976.

G15. Gordon, R., G.T. Herman: Three-dimensional reconstruction from projections: a review of algorithms. Int Rev Cytol 38:111, 1974.

G16. Gray, J.E.: Photographic quality assurance in diagnostic radiology. Nuclear Medicine and Radiation Therapy, Vol. 1 and Vol. 11. U.S. Department of Health and Welfare, Bureau of Radiological Health, HEW Publications (FDA) 76-8043 and 77-8018. Vol. 1 June 1976, Vol. 11 March 1977.

G17. Gross, A.J., and V.A. Clark: Survival distributions: reliability applications in the biomedical sciences. Toronto: Wiley, 1975: 41.

H1. Heitler, W.: The quantum theory of radiation. New York: Oxford University Press, 1954.

H2. Hongerjäger, R.: Untersuchungen uber die azimutale Intensitätsverteilung der Röntgenbremsstrahlung. Ann Physik 38:33, 1940.

H3. Handbook of Chemistry and Physics, 58th edition 1977-78. CRC Press, West Palm Beach, Florida, 1977.

H4. Hoag, J.B.: Electron and nuclear physics. 3rd ed., Princeton, N.J.: D. Van Nostrand Co., 1949.

H5. Health, Education and Welfare. The use of electron linear accelerators in medical radiation therapy: physical characteristics. Overview report #1, February 1976.

H6. Haimson, J., C.J. Karzmark: A new design 6 MeV linear accelerator system for supervoltage radiotherapy. Br J Radiol 36:650, 1963.

H7. Hubbell, J.H.: Photon cross sections, attenuation coefficients, and energy absorption coefficients from 10 keV to 100 GeV. NSRD-NBS 29. Washington, D.C.: U.S. National Bureau of Standards, 1969.

H8. Hubbell, J.H.: Photon mass attenuation and mass energy-absorption coefficients for H, C, N, O, Ar, and seven mixtures from 0.1 keV to 20 MeV. Radiat Res 70:58, 1977.

H9. Hubbell, J.H., W.J. Veigele, E.A. Briggs, R.T. Brown, D.T. Cromer, R.J. Howerton: Atomic form factors, incoherent scattering functions and photon scattering cross sections. J Phys Chem Ref Data 4:471, 1975.

H10. Hettinger, G., N. Starfelt: Energy and angular distribution of scattered radiation in a water tank irradiated by x rays. Ark Fys 14:497, 1959.

H11. The Hospital Physicists' Association. Phantom materials for photons and electrons. Scientific Report Series–20. London: The Hospital Physicists' Association, 1977.

H12. Hall, E.J., R. Oliver: The use of standard isodose distributions with high energy radiation beams—the accuracy of a compensator technique in correcting for body contours. Br J Radiol 34:43, 1961.

H13. Ham, A.W., D.H. Cormack: Histology, 8th ed. Philadelphia: J.B. Lippincott Co., 1979.

H14. Hultberg, S., O. Dahl, R. Thoraeus, K.J. Vikterlöf, R. Walstam: Kilocurie cobalt 60 therapy at the Radiumhemmet. Acta Radiol [Suppl] (Stockh) 179, 1959.

H15. Harrington, E.L.: Radium: radon plants. In Medical Physics. O. Glasser, ed., Chicago, Year Book 1:1193, 1944.

H16. Hall, E.J.: Radiation and life. New York: Pergamon Press, 1976.

H17. Hynes, D.M., E.W. Edmonds, K.R. Krametz, D. Baranoski, T. Hughes: Multi-image camera for spot radiography at fluoroscopic examinations. Radiology 136:213, 1980.

H18. Herz, R.H.: Photographic action of ionizing radiation. Toronto: Wiley, 1969.

H19. Higgins, G.C.: Methods for analyzing the photographic system including the effects of nonlinearity and spatial frequency response. Photograph Sci Eng 15:106, 1971.

H20. Hoffman, E.J., M.E. Phelps: Production of monoenergetic x-rays from 8 to 87 keV. Phys Med Biol 19:35, 1974.

H21. Hounsfield, G.N.: Computerized transverse axial scanning (tomography). Br J Radiol 46:1016, 1973.

H22. Hammerstein, G.R., D.W. Miller, D.R. White, M.E. Masterson, H.Q. Woodard, J.S. Laughlin: Absorbed radiation dose in mammography. Radiology 130:485, 1979.

H23. Hill, R.P., R.S. Bush: A lung-colony assay to determine the radiosensitivity of the cells of a solid tumour. Int J Radiat Biol 15:435, 1969.

H24. Hill, R.P., J.A. Stanley: The lung-colony assay: extension to the Lewis lung tumour and the B16 melanoma-radiosensitivity of B16 Melanoma cells. Int J Radiat Biol 27:377, 1975.

H25. Hewitt, H.B., C.W. Wilson: A survival curve for mammalian leukaemia cells irradiated in vivo (implications for the treatment of mouse leukaemia by whole-body irradiation). Br J Cancer 13:675, 1959.

H26. Haynes, R.H.: The interpretation of microbial inactivation and recovery phenomena. Radiat Res Supp 6:1, 1966.

H27. Hill, R.P., R.S. Bush, P. Leung: The effect of anaemia on the fraction of hypoxic cells in an experimental tumour. Br J Radiol 44:299, 1971.

H28. Heavy Particle Symposium. J Can Assoc Radiol 31:3, 1980.

H29. Hahn, G.M., G.C. Li, J.B. Marmor, D.W. Pounds: Thermal and nonthermal effects of ultrasound. In: R.E. Meyn, H.R. Withers, eds.: Radiation Biology in Cancer Research. New York: Raven Press, 623, 1980.

I1. International Commission on Radiation Units and Measurements. Measurement of absorbed dose in a phantom irradiated by a single beam of x or gamma rays. ICRU Report 23. Washington, D.C.: 1973.

I2. International Commission on Radiation Units and Measurements. Radiation quantities and units. ICRU Report 33. Washington, D.C.: 1980.

I3. International Commission on Radiation Units and Measurements. Average energy required to produce an ion pair. ICRU Report 31. Washington, D.C.: 1979.

I4. International Commission on Radiation Units and Measurements. Linear energy transfer. ICRU Report 16. Washington, D.C.: 1970.

I5. International Commission on Radiation Units and Measurements. Radiation dosimetry: electrons with initial energies between 1 and 50 MeV. ICRU Report 21. Washington, D.C.: 1972.

I6. International Commission on Radiation Units and Measurements. Radiation dosimetry: x rays and gamma rays with maximum photon energies between 0.6 and 50 MeV. ICRU Report 14. Washington, D.C.: 1969.

I7. International Commission on Radiation Units and Measurements. Determination of absorbed dose in a patient irradiated by beams of x or gamma rays in radiotherapy procedures. ICRU Report 24. Washington, D.C.: 1976.

I8. International Commission on Radiation Units and Measurements. Dose specification for reporting external beam therapy with photons and electrons. ICRU Report 29. Washington, D.C.: 1978.

I9. International Commission on Radiological Protection. Recommendations of the International Commission on Radiological Protection. ICRP Publication 26. Oxford: Pergamon Press, 1977.

I10. International Commission on Radiological Protection. Problems involved in developing an index of Harm. ICRP Publication 27. Oxford: Pergamon Press, 1977.

I11. International Commission on Radiological Protection. Protection against ionizing radiation from external sources. ICRP Publication 15. Oxford: Pergamon Press, 1970.

I12. International Electrotechnical Commission (IEC). Draft Document 62C (Central Office), Medical electron accelerators in the range 1-50 MeV. 4 November, 1976.

I13. International Commission on Radiation Units and Measurements. U.S. Nat Bur Standards. Handbook 62. Washington, D.C.: U.S. Department of Commerce, 1957.

J1. Johns, H.E., E.K. Darby, R.N.H. Haslam, L. Katz, E.L. Harrington: Depth dose data and isodose distributions for radiation from a 22 MeV betatron. Amer J Roentgen 62:257, 1949.

J2. Johns, H.E., J.A. Rawlinson, W.B. Taylor: Matrix dosemeter to study the uniformity of high energy x ray beams. Amer J Roentgenol 120:192, 1974.

J3. Johns, H.E., J.A. Rawlinson: Desirable characteristics of high-energy photons and electrons. In: S. Kramer, N. Suntharalingam, G.F. Zinninger, eds.: High energy photons and electrons: clinical applications in cancer management. New York: Wiley, 5, 1976.

J4. Johns, H.E., L.M. Bates, T.A. Watson: 1,000 curie cobalt units for radiation therapy. 1. The Saskatchewan cobalt 60 unit, Br J Radiol 25:296, 1952.

J5. Johns, H.E., E.R. Epp, D.V. Cormack, S.O. Fedoruk: Depth dose data and diaphragm design for the Saskatchewan 1,000 curie cobalt unit. Br J Radiol 25:302, 1952.

J6. Johns, H.E., J.A. MacKay: A collimating device for cobalt 60 teletherapy units. J Fac Radiologists 5:239, 1954.

J7. Johns, H.E., J.R. Cunningham: A precision cobalt 60 unit for fixed field and rotation therapy. Amer J Roentgenol 81:4, 1959.

J8. Johns, H.E., J.E. Till, D.V. Cormack: Electron energy distributions produced by gamma rays. Nucleonics 12:40, 1954.

J9. Johns, H.E.: The physics of radiation therapy. Springfield, Ill: Charles C Thomas, 1953.

J10. Johns, H.E., G.F. Whitmore, T.A. Watson, F.H. Umberg: A system of dosimetry for rotation therapy with typical rotation distributions. J Can Assoc Radiol 4:1, 1953.

J11. Johns, H.E., W.R. Bruce, W.B. Reid: The dependence of depth dose on focal skin distance. Br J Radiol 31:254, 1958.

J12. Johns, H.E., J.R. Cunningham: The physics of radiology. 3rd ed. Springfield, Ill: Charles C Thomas, 1969.

J13. Jones, C.H., K.W. Taylor, J.B.H. Stedeford: Modifications to the Royal Marsden Hospital gold grain implantation gun. Br J Radiol 38:672, 1965.

J14. Johns, H.E.: Impact of physics on therapeutic and diagnostic radiology. The Gordon Richards Memorial Lecture. J Can Assoc Radiol 30:192, 1979.

J15. James, P., H. Baddeley, J.W. Boag, H.E. Johns, A.J. Stacey: Xeroradiography—its use in peripheral contrast medium angiography. Clin Radiol 24:67, 1973.

J16. Johns, H.E., A. Fenster, D. Plewes, J.W. Boag, P.N. Jeffery: Gas ionization methods of electrostatic image formation in radiography. Br J Radiol 47:519, 1974.

J17. Johns, H.E., A. Fenster, D. Plewes: New methods of imaging in diagnostic radiology. Radiology 116:415, 1975.

J18. Johns, H.E.: New methods of imaging in diagnostic radiology. Br J Radiol 49:745, 1976.

J19. Jacobson, A.F., J.R. Cameron, M.P. Siedband, J. Wagner: Test cassette for measuring peak tube potential of diagnostic x-ray machines. Med Phys 3:19, 1976.

J20. Johns, H.E., J.W. Hunt, S.O. Fedoruk: Surface back-scatter in the 100 kV to 400 kV range. BJ Radiol 27:443, 1954.

J21. Johns, H.E., E.R. Epp, S.O. Fedoruk: Depth dose data 75 kV_p to 140 kV_p. B J Radiol 26:32, 1953.

J22. Johns, H.E., S.O. Fedoruk, R.O. Kornelsen, E.R. Epp, E.K. Darby: Depth dose data, 150 kV_p to 400 kV_p. Br J Radiol 25:542, 1952.

K1. Kalsruher Nuklidkarte, Gersbach u. Sohn, Verlag, 8 München 34, Barer Str. 32, West Germany.

K2. Kramer, S., N. Suntharalingam, G. Zinninger: High-energy photons and electrons: clinical applications in cancer management. New York: Wiley, 1976.

K3. Kerst, D.W.: The betatron. Radiology 40:115, 1943.

K4. Karzmark, C.J., N.C. Pering: Electron linear accelerators for radiation therapy: history, principles and contemporary developments. Phys Med Biol 18:321, 1973.

K5. Kemp, L.A.W., B. Barber: Iron as an impurity in colloidal graphite: its effect on thimble ionization chamber performance. Br J Radiol 29:457, 1956.

K6. Karzmark, C.J., A. Deubert, R. Loevinger: Tissue-phantom ratios—an aid to treatment planning. Br J Radiol 38:158, 1965.

K7. Karzmark, C.J., T. Capone: Measurements of 6 MV x-rays. II. Characteristics of secondary radiation. Br J Radiol 41:222, 1968.

K8. Kodak, Image Insight #3, Screen Imaging, Eastman Kodak Company, Rochester, N.Y., 1976.

K9. Kuhl, W., J.E. Schrijvers: Design aspects of x-ray image intensifiers. Acta Electron 20:41, 1977.

K10. Kallman, R.F.: The phenomenon of reoxygenation and its implications for fractionated radiotherapy. Radiology 105:135, 1972.

K11. Kallman, R.F.: Facts and models applied to tumor radiotherapy. Int J Radiat Oncol Biol Phys 5:1103, 1979.

K12. Kaplan, E.L., P. Meier: Non parametric estimation from incomplete observations. J Am Stat Assoc 53:457, 1958.

L1. Loevinger, R., M. Berman: A schema for absorbed dose calculations for biological-distributed radionuclides (MIRD pamphlet #1). Soc. of Nuclear Med 9, Supplement 1, 5, 1968 and revised pamphlet #1.

L2. Leung, P.M.K., H.E. Johns: Use of electron filters to improve the buildup characteristics of large fields from cobalt-60 beams. Med Phys 4:441, 1977.

L3. Levy, L.B., R.G. Waggener, A.E. Wright: Measurement of primary bremsstrahlung spectrum from an 8-MeV linear accelerator. Med Phys 3:173, 1976.

L4. Levy, L.B., R.G. Waggener, W.D. McDavid, W.H. Payne: Experimental and calculated bremsstrahlung spectra from a 25-MeV linear accelerator and a 19-MeV betatron. Med Phys 1:62, 1974.

L5. Loevinger, R.: A formalism for calculation of absorbed dose to a medium from photon and electron beams. Med Phys 8:1, 1981.

L6. Leung, P.M.K., B. Seaman, P. Robinson: Low-density inhomogeneity corrections for 22-MV x ray therapy. Radiology 94:449, 1970.

L7. Laughlin, J.S.: Physical aspects of betatron therapy. Springfield, Ill: Charles C Thomas, 1954.

L8. Leung, P.M.K., J. Van Dyk, J. Robins: A method of large irregular field compensation. Br J Radiol 47:805, 1974.

L9. Legaré, J.M.: Exit-surface dose correction factors for x rays of 1.5 to 4.0 mm Cu half-value layer. Radiology 82:272, 1964.

L10. Leung, P.M.K., W.D. Rider, H.P. Webb, H. Aget, H.E. Johns: A cobalt-60 therapy unit for large field irradiation. Int J Radiat Oncol Biol Phys 7:705, 1981.

L11. Lokan, K.H., N.K. Sherman, R.W. Gellie, W.H. Henry, R. Lévesque, A. Nowak, G.G. Teather, J.R. Lundquist: Bremsstrahlung attenuation measurements in ilmenite loaded concretes. Health Phys 23:193, 1972.

L12. Logan, W.W., E.P. Muntz, eds.: Reduced dose mammography. New York: Masson Pub., 1979.

L13. Lawrence, D.J.: A simple method of processor control. Med Radiogr Photogr 49:2, 1973.

L14. Lea, D.E.: Actions of radiations on living cells, 2nd ed. New York: Cambridge. University Press, 1955.

L15. Life Tables. Canada and Provinces 1975-77. Catalogue No. 84-532. Ottawa: Statistics Canada, 1979.

M1. Moores, B.M., P. Brubacher: Focal spot studies and electron focusing in a demountable x ray tube. Phys Med Biol 19:605, 1974.

M2. Mika, N., K.H. Reiss: Tabellen zur Roentgendiagnostik. Siemens, October, 1973.

M3. Mallinckrodt Nuclear. 2nd Street and Mallinckrodt Street, St. Louis, Missouri, 63160, U.S.A.

M4. Miller, C.W.: Recent developments in linear accelerators for therapy. 1. The continuing evolution of linear accelerators. Br J Radiol 35:182, 1962.

M5. Meulders, J.P., P. LeLeux, P.C. Macq, C. Pirart: Fast neutron yields and spectra with targets of varying atomic number bombarded with deuterons from 16 to 50 MeV. Phys Med Biol 20:235, 1975.

M6. Mayneord, W.V.: The significance of the roentgen. Acta, Union internat contre cancer 2:271, 1937.

M7. McCullough, E.C.: Photon attenuation in computed tomography. Med Phys 2: 307, 1975.

M8. Mak, S., D.V. Cormack: Spectral distributions of scattered x rays at points lying off the beam axis. Br J Radiol 33:362, 1960.

M9. McDonald, J.C., I.C. Ma, J.S. Laughlin: Calorimetric and ionometric dosimetry for cyclotron produced fast neutrons. In: Proceedings of the 3rd Symposium on Neutron Dosimetry for Biology and Medicine, Munich, Germany, May, 1977. Conf—7705106-1. Vienna: International Nuclear Information System, 1977.

M10. McDonald, J.C., J.S. Laughlin, R.E. Freeman: Portable tissue equivalent calorimeter. Med Phys 3:80, 1976.

M11. Mayneord, W.V.: The measurement of radiation for medical purposes. Proc Phys Soc 54:405, 1942.

M12. Meredith, W.J., ed.: Radium dosage, the Manchester system. E. and S. Livingstone, Edinburgh. 1967.

M13. Mallard, J.R., A. McKinnell: Simple techniques to show the distribution of colloidal gold 198 in body cavities. Br J Radiol 30:608, 1957.

M14. Morgan, K.Z.: History of damage and protection from ionizing radiation. In: K.Z. Morgan, J.E. Turner, eds.: Principles of radiation protection. New York: John Wiley and Sons, 1, 1967.

M15. Merriam, G.R., E.F. Focht: A clinical study of radiation cataracts and the relationship to dose. Am J Roentgenol 77:759, 1957.

M16. Moores, B.M., A. Walker: Light output and x-ray attenuation measurements for some commercial intensifying screens. Radiology 128:767, 1978.

M17. Mees, C.E.K., T.H. James: The theory of the photographic process. New York: MacMillan Co, 1966.

M18. Milne, E.N.C.: Characterizing focal spot performance. Radiology 111:483, 1974.

M19. Moores, B.M., W. Roeck: The field characteristics of the focal spot in the radiographic imaging process. Invest Radiol 8:53, 1973.

M20. Milne, E.N.C.: The role and performance of minute focal spots in roentgenology with special reference to magnification. CRC Critical Reviews in Radiological Sciences 2:269, 1971.

M21. Morgan, R.H.: The frequency response function. A valuable means of expressing the informational recording capability of diagnostic x-ray systems. Amer J Roentgen 1:175, 1962.

M22. Motz, J.W., M. Danos: Image information content and patient exposure. Med Phys 5:8, 1978.

N1. Nuclear Data, Section A, Vol. 9. Tables of gamma-gamma directional coefficients. New York: Academic Press, 1971.

N2. Nelms, A.T.: Graphs of the compton energy-angle relationship and the Klein-Nishina formula from 10 keV to 500 MeV. National Bureau of Standards Circular 542, 1953.

N3. Nahum, A.E.: Water/air mass stopping power ratios for megavoltage photon and electron beams. Phys Med Biol 23:24, 1978.

N4. Nahum, A.E.: Calculations of electron flux spectra in water irradiated with mega-voltage electron and photon beams with applications to dosimetry. Ph.D. Thesis, University of Edinburgh, 1976.

N5. Nilsson, B., P.O. Schnell: Build-up studies at air cavities measured with thin thermoluminescent dosimeters. Acta Radiol [Ther] (Stockh) 15:427, 1976.

N6. National and International Standardization of Radiation Dosimetry. 2 vols. Vienna: International Atomic Energy Agency, 1978.

N7. National Council on Radiation Protection and Measurements. Specification of gamma-ray brachytherapy sources. NCRP Report 41. Washington, D.C.: 1974.

N8. National Council on Radiation Protection and Measurements. Natural background radiation in the United States. NCRP Report 45. Washington, D.C.: 1975.

N9. National Council on Radiation Protection and Measurements. Medical x-ray and gamma-ray protection for energies up to 10 MeV. NCRP Report 33. Washington, D.C.: 1968.

N10. National Council on Radiation Protection and Measurements. Structural shielding design and evaluation for medical use of x rays and gamma rays of energies up to 10 MeV. NCRP Report 49. Washington, D.C.: 1976.

N11. National Council on Radiation Protection and Measurements. Radiation protection for medical and allied health personnel. NCRP Report 48. Washington, D.C.: 1976.

N12. National Council on Radiation Protection and Measurements. Radiation protection design guidelines for 0.1-100 MeV particle accelerator facilities. NCRP Report 51. Washington, D.C.: 1977.

N13. NEMA. Measurement of dimensions of focal spots of diagnostic x ray tubes. Standards Publication No. XR5-1974, National Electrical Manufacturers Assoc, 155 East 44th Street, New York.

N14. Niederer, J., J.R. Cunningham: The response of cells in culture to fractionated radiation: a theoretical approach. Phys Med Biol 21:823, 1976.

O1. O'Connor, J.E.: The variation of scattered x-rays with density in an irradiated body. Phys Med Biol 1:352, 1957.

O2. Oosterkamp, I.W.: Monochromatic x-rays for medical fluoroscopy and radiography. Medicamundi 7:68, 1961.

O3. Orton, C.G., F. Ellis: A simplification in the use of the NSD concept in practical radiotherapy. Br J Radiol 46:529, 1973.

P1. Particle Radiation Therapy. Proceedings of an International Workshop, I, October 1975. Key Biscayne, Florida. Amer College of Radiology, 130 South 9th St, Philadelphia.

P2. Particles and Radiation Therapy. Second International Conference, September 1976. Berkeley, California. Int J Radiat Oncol Biol Phys 3:1, 1977.

P3. Podgorsak, E.B., J.A. Rawlinson, M.I. Glavinovic, H.E. Johns: The design of x rays targets for high energy linear accelerators in radiotherapy. Am J Roentgenol 121:873, 1974.

P4. Podgorsak, E.B., J.A. Rawlinson, H.E. Johns: X-ray depth doses from linear accelerators in the energy range from 10 to 32 MeV. Am J Roentgenol 123:182, 1975.

P5. Plechaty, E.F., D.E. Cullen, R.J. Howerton: Tables and graphs of photon interaction cross sections from 1.0 keV to 100 MeV derived from LLL evaluated nuclear data library. UCRL-50400 vol. 6 revision 1. University of California, Lawrence Livermore Laboratory, 1975. Springfield, Va; National Technical Information Service, 1975.

P6. Pages, L., E. Bertel, H. Joffre, L. Sklavenitis: Energy loss, range, and bremsstrahlung yield for 10 keV to 100 MeV electrons in various elements and chemical compounds. Atomic Data 4:1, 1972.

P7. Paterson, R.: The treatment of malignant disease by radium and x-rays. London: Arnold, 1948.

P8. Paterson, R.: A dosage system for gamma ray therapy. Br J Radiol 7:592, 1934.

P9. Paterson, R., H.M. Parker: A dosage system for interstitial radium therapy. Br J Radiol 11:252, 1938.

P10. Paterson, R., H.M. Parker, F.W. Spiers: A system of dosage for cylindrical distributions of radium. Br J Radiol 9:487, 1936.

P11. Pochin, Sir E.E.: Why be quantitative about radiation risk estimates? L.S. Taylor Lecture Series in Radiation Protection and Measurements. Lecture #2. Washington, D.C.: National Council on Radiation Protection and Measurements, 1978.

P12. Philips, Eindhoven: Luminescent screen with pile structure. Philips technical review 33:65, 1973.

P13. Pfeiler, M., J. Haendle: State-of-the-art and development tendencies of x-ray image intensifier television systems. Electromedica 5:148, 1975.

P14. Philips Medical System Division. Methods for determining the imaging characteristics of x-ray tubes. Medicamundi 2:19, 1974.

P15. Plewes, D., A. Fenster, H.E. Johns: Image transfer ionography. J Appl Photogr Eng 1:5, 1975.

P16. Plewes, D., H.E. Johns: Electrostatic fields in ionography. Med Phys 2:61, 1975.

P17. Plewes, D., H.E. Johns: Edge contrast in ionography. Phys Med Biol 23:1060, 1978.

P18. Proudian, A.P., R.L. Carangi, G. Jacobson, E.P. Muntz: Electron radiography: a new method of radiographic imaging: imaging chamber characteristics—a preliminary report. Radiology 110:667, 1974.

P19. Puck, T.T., D. Morkovin, P.I. Marcus, S.J. Cieciura: Action of x-rays on mammalian cells. II. Survival curves of cells from normal human tissues. J Exp Med 106:485, 1957.

P20. Powers, W.E., L.J. Tolmach: Demonstration of an anoxic component in a mouse tumour-cell population by in vivo assay of survival following irradiation. Radiology 83:328, 1964.

P21. Probert, J.C., J.M. Brown: A comparison of three and five times weekly fractionation on the response of normal and malignant tissues of the C_3H mouse. Br J Radiol 47:775, 1974.

P22. Peto, R., M.C. Pike, P. Armitage, N.E. Breslow, D.R. Cox, S.V. Howard, N. Mantel, K. McPherson, J. Peto, P.G. Smith: Design and analysis of randomized clinical trials requiring prolonged observation of each patient. II. Analysis and Exam-Design. Br J Cancer 34:585, 1976.

P23. Peto, R., M.C. Pike, P. Armitage, N.E. Breslow, D.R. Cox, S.V. Howard, N. Mantel, K. McPherson, J. Peto, P.G. Smith: Design and analysis of randomized clinical trials requiring prolonged observation of each patient. II. Analysis and Examples. Br J Cancer 35:1, 1977.

Q1. Quimby, E.H.: Dosage tables for linear radium sources. Radiology 43:572, 1944.

R1. Rawlinson, J.A.: Unpublished data, available on request. Partly included in H.E. Johns and J.A. Rawlinson. Desirable characteristics of high energy photons and electrons in High Energy Photons and Electrons. Simon Kramer, ed. John Wiley and Sons Inc. 1976.

R2. Rockwell, T., ed.: Reactor shielding design manual. Princeton, N.J.: D. Van Nostrand Co. Inc., 1956.

R3. Roesch, W.C.: Dose for nonelectronic equilibrium conditions. Radiat Res 9:399, 1958.

R4. Rawlinson, J.A., H.E. Johns: Percentage depth dose for high energy x-ray beams in radiotherapy. Am J Roentgenol 118:919, 1973.

R5. Rider, W.D., J. Van Dyk: Total and partial body irradiation. In: N.M. Bleehen, E. Glatstein, J. Haybittle, eds.: Radiation Therapy Planning. New York: Marcel Dekker Inc. (in press).

R6. Rawlinson, J.A.: Radium leak testing using scintillating fluid. Internal report. Ontario Cancer Institute. Toronto, Canada, 1967.

R7. Richardson, R.L.: Anger scintillation camera. Chapt 6 in Nuclear medicine physics, instrumentation and agents. The CV Mosby Co., St. Louis, 1977.

R8. Roeck, W.W., E.N.C. Milne: A highly accurate focal spot camera—laboratory and field model. Radiology 127:779, 1978.

R9. Rao, G.U.V., L.M. Bates: The modulation transfer functions of x-ray focal spots. Phys Med Biol 14:93, 1969.

R10. Rao, G.U.V., L.M. Bates: Effective dimensions of roentgen tube focal spots based on measurement of the modulation transfer function. Acta Radiol [Ther] (Stockh) 9:362, 1970.

R11. Rao, G.U.V.: A new method to determine the focal spot size of x-ray tubes. Am J Roentgenol Radium Ther Nuc Med 111:628, 1971.

R12. Robinson, A., G.M. Grimshaw: Measurement of the focal spot size of diagnostic x-ray tubes—a comparison of pinhole and resolution methods. Br J Radiol 48:572, 1975.

R13. Ramachandran, G.N., A.V. Lakshminarayanan: Three-dimensional reconstruction from radiographs and electron micrographs: application of convolutions instead of Fourier transforms. Proc Nath Acad Sci USA 68:2236, 1971.

R14. Rutt, B., A. Fenster: Split-filter computed tomography: a simple technique for dual energy scanning. J Comput Assist Tomogr 4:501, 1980.

R15. Rossi, H.H.: Distribution of radiation energy in the cell. Radiology 78:530, 1962.

R16. Rossi, H.H.: The role of microdosimetry in radiobiology. Radiat Environ Biophys 17:29, 1979.

R17. Reporting of cancer survival and end results. The Executive Secretary, American Joint Committee, 55 East Erie Street, Chicago, Ill. 60611, 1979.

S1. Storm, E., H.I. Israel: Photon cross sections from 1 keV to 100 MeV. Nuclear Data Tables A7:565, 1970.

S2. Schiff, L.I.: Energy-angle distribution of betatron target radiation. Phys Rev. 70: 87, 1946.

S3. Schulz, M.D.: The supervoltage story. Am J Roentgenol 124:541, 1975.

S4. Skaggs, L.S., D.M. Almy, D.W. Kerst, L.H. Lanzl: Development of betatron for electron therapy, with introduction on the therapeutic principles of fast electrons. Radiology 50:167, 1948.

S5. Stone, R.S.: Neutron therapy and specific ionization. Am J Roentgenol 59:771, 1948.

S6. Sternheimer, R.M., R.F. Peierls: General expression for the density effect for the ionization loss of charged particles. Phys Rev B 3:3681, 1971.

S7. Spencer, L.V., F.H. Attix: A theory of cavity ionization. Radiat Res 3:239, 1955.

S8. Skarsgard, L.D., H.E. Johns: Spectral flux density of scattered and primary radiation generated at 250 kV. Radiat Res 14:231, 1961.

S9. Sherman, N.K., K.H. Lokan, R.M. Hutcheon, L.W. Funk, W.R. Brown, P. Brown: Bremsstrahlung radiators and beam filters for 25-MeV cancer therapy. Med Phys 1:185, 1974.

S10. Spiers, F.W.: Effective atomic number and energy absorption in tissues. Br J Radiol 19:52, 1946 **and** Dosage in irradiated soft tissue and bone. Br J Radiol 24:365, 1951.

S11. Skarsgard, L.D., H.E. Johns, L.E.S. Green: Iterative response correction for a scintillation spectrometer. Radiat Res 14:261, 1961.

S12. Scrimger, J.W., D.V. Cormack: Spectrum of the radiation from a cobalt 60 teletherapy unit. Br J Radiol 36:514, 1963.

S13. Spiers, F.W.: Materials for depth dose measurement. Br J Radiol 16:90, 1943.

S14. Sterling, T.D., H. Perry, L. Katz: Automation of radiation treatment planning. Br J Radiol 37:544, 1964.

S15. Sundbom, L.: Individually designed filters in cobalt 60 teletherapy. Acta Radiol [Ther] (Stockh) 2:189, 1964.

S16. Sontag, M.R., J.R. Cunningham: Corrections to absorbed dose calculations for tissue inhomogeneities. Med Phys 4:431, 1977.

S17. Sontag, M.R., J.R. Cunningham: The equivalent tissue-air ratio method for making absorbed dose calculations in a heterogeneous medium. Radiology 129:787, 1978.

S18. Sontag, M.R.: Photon beam dose calculations in regions of tissue heterogeneity using computed tomography. Ph.D. Thesis, University of Toronto, 1979.

S19. Sievert, R.M.: Die Gamma-Strahlungsintensität an der Oberfläche und in der nächsten Umgebung von Radium Nadeln. Acta Radiol 11:249, 1930.

S20. Sinclair, W.K., N.G. Trott: The construction and measurement of beta-ray applicators for use in ophthalmology. Br J Radiol 29:15, 1956.

S21. Supe, S.J., J.R. Cunningham: A physical study of a strontium-90 β-ray applicator. Am J Roentgen 89:570, 1963.

S22. Snyder, W.S., M.R. Ford, G.G. Warner, H.L. Fisher: Estimates of absorbed fractions for monoenergetic photon sources uniformly distributed in various organs of a heterogeneous phantom. MIRD pamphlet #5. New York: Society of Nuclear Medicine, 1969.
and
Snyder, W.S., M.R. Ford, G.G. Warner, S.B. Watson: Absorbed dose per unit cumulated activity for selected radio nuclides and organs. MIRD pamphlet #11, 1975.

S23. SPSE handbook of photographic science and engineering. W. Thomas, ed. New York: Wiley, 1973.

S24. Stevels, A.L.N.: New phosphors for x-ray screens. Medicamundi 20:12, 1975.

S25. Spiegler, P., W.C. Breckinridge: Imaging of focal spots by means of the star test pattern. Radiology 102:679, 1972.

S26. Swank, R.K.: Absorption and noise in x-ray phosphors. J Appl Phys 44:4199, 1973.

S27. Stanton, L., L.W. Brady, F.L. Szarko, J.L. Day, D.A. Lightfoot: Electron radiography: a new x-ray imaging system. Appl Radiol 2:53, 1973.

S28. Stanton, L., D.A. Lightfoot, J.L. Day, L.W. Brady: Edge sharpness and enhancement of electron radiographs (ERGs) produced with powder cloud development. Med Phys 2:22, 1975.

S29. Skarsgard, L.D., B.A. Kihlman, L. Parker, C.M. Pujara, S. Richardson: Survival, chromosome abnormalities, and recovery in heavy-ion- and x-irradiated mammalian cells. Radiat Res Suppl 7:208, 1967.

S30. Schneider, D.O., G.F. Whitmore: Comparative effects of neutrons and x-rays on mammalian cells. Radiat Res 18:286, 1963.

S31. Sinclair, W.K.: Cyclic x-ray responses in mammalian cells in-vitro. Radiat Res 33:620, 1968.

S32. Strandqvist, M.: Studien über die kumulative Wirkung der Röntgenstrahlen bei Fraktionierung. Acta Radiol [suppl] (Stockh) 55, 1944.

S33. Suit, H.D., A.E. Howes, N. Hunter: Dependence of response of a C_3H mammary carcinoma to fractionated irradiation on fractionation number and intertreatment interval. Radiat Res 72:440, 1977.

S34. Siemann, D.W., R.P. Hill, R.S. Bush: The effect of chronic reductions in the arterial partial pressure of oxygen on the radiation response of an experimental tumour. Br J Radiol 51:992, 1978.

S35. Siemann, D.W., R.P. Hill, R.S. Bush: Smoking: the influence of carboxyhemoglobin (HbCO) on tumor oxygenation and response to radiation. Int J Radiat Oncol Biol Phys 4:657, 1978.

S36. Sheline, G.E., T.L. Phillips, S.B. Field, J.T. Brennan, A. Raventos: Effects of fast neutrons on human skin. Am J Roentgenol 111:31, 1971.

S37. Stovall, M., R.J. Shalek: The M.D. Anderson method for computation of isodose curves around interstitial and intercavity radiation sources. Am. J Roentgenol 102:677, 1968.

T1. Trefler, M., J.E. Gray, E.N.C. Milne, W.W. Roeck, G. Gillan: The production of apparent image bifurcation. Radiology 119:451, 1976.

T2. Thoraeus, R.: A study of the ionization method for measuring the intensity and absorption of roentgen rays and of the efficiency of different filters used in therapy. Acta Radiol [Suppl] (Stockh) 15, 1932.

T3. Trout, E.D., J.P. Kelley, A.C. Lucas: Evaluation of Thoraeus filters. Amer J Roentgenol 85:933, 1961.

T4. Thomas, R.L., J.E. Shaw: Radiation measurements with diode detectors. Phys Med Biol (letter) 23:519, 1978.

T5. Tobias, C.A., H.O. Anger, J.H. Lawrence: Radiological use of high energy deuterons and alpha particles. Am J Roentgenol 67:1, 1952.

T6. Tsien, K.C., J.R. Cunningham, D.J. Wright, D.E.A. Jones, P.M. Pfalzner: Atlas of radiation dose distributions. Vol. III, International Atomic Energy Agency, Vienna; 1967.

T7. Tsien, K.C., J.R. Cunningham, D.J. Wright: Effects of different parameters on dose distributions in cobalt 60 planar rotation. Acta Radiol [Ther] (Stockh) 4:129, 1966.

T8. Tod, M., W.J. Meredith: Treatment of cancer of the cervix uteri—a revised "Manchester Method." Br J Radiol 26:252, 1953.

T9. Ter-Pogossian, M.M., N.A. Mullani, D.C. Ficke, J. Markham, D.L. Snyder: Photon time-of-flight-assisted positron emission tomography. J Comput Assist Tomogr 5:227, 1981.

T10. Taylor, K.W., N.L. Patt, H.E. Johns: Variations in x-ray exposures to patients. J Can Assoc Radiol 30:6, 1979.

T11. Toy, A.J., F.E. Hoecker.: Calculating teletherapy room shielding using albedos: a method of predicting exposure rates at, and shielding required in, maze-protected doors. Phys Med Biol 18:452, 1973.

T12. Taylor, K.W.: Quality control in a large teaching hospital. Proc Soc Photo-Optical Instrum Eng 70:146, 1975.

T13. Thomas, J.K., J. Rabani, M.S. Matheson, E.J. Hart, S. Gordon: Absorption spectrum of the hydroxyl radical. J Phys Chem 70:2409, 1966.

T14. Thomas, J.K.: The hydrated electron and the H atom in the radiolysis of water. In: G. Silini, ed.: Radiation Research, Proc 3rd Int Congress of Rad Res 1966 ed. Amsterdam, North-Holland Pub Co 179, 1967.

T15. Till, J.E., E.A. McCulloch: A direct measurement of the radiation sensitivity of normal mouse bone marrow cells. Radiat Res 14:213, 1961.

T16. Thomson, J.E., A.M. Rauth: An in vitro assay to measure the viability of KHT tumor cells not previously exposed to culture conditions. Radiat Res 58:262, 1974.

T17. Thomlinson, R.H., L.H. Gray: The histological structure of some human lung cancers and the possible implications for radiotherapy. Br J Canc 9:539, 1955.

T18. Tannock, I.F.: The relation between cell proliferation and the vascular system in a transplanted mouse mammary tumour. Br J Canc 22:258, 1968.

V1. Van Dyk, J., P.M.K. Leung, B. Taylor, J. Webb, H.E. Johns: A technique for the treatment of large irregular fields. Radiology 134:543, 1980.

V2. Villagran, J.E., B.B. Hobbs, K.W. Taylor: Reduction of patient exposure by use of heavy elements as radiation filters in diagnostic radiology. Radiology 127:249, 1978.

V3. Van Dyk, J., P.M.K. Leung: Thermoluminescent dosimetry: practical considerations for use in radiotherapy. Internal Report. Ontario Cancer Institute, Toronto, Canada. 1979.

V4. Van der Giessen, P.H.: A method of calculating the isodose shift in correcting for oblique incidence in radiotherapy. Br J Radiol 46:978, 1973.

V5. Van de Geijn, J.: The construction of individualized intensity modifying filters in cobalt 60 teletherapy. Br J Radiol 38:865, 1965.

V6. Van Dyk, J., P.M.K. Leung, J.R. Cunningham: Dosimetric considerations of very large cobalt-60 fields. Int J Radiat Oncol Biol Phys 6:753, 1980.

V7. Van Dyk, J.: Practical dosimetric considerations of a 10-MV photon beam. Med Phys 4:145, 1977.

V8. Van Dyk, J., J.J. Battista, J.R. Cunningham, W.D. Rider, M.R. Sontag: On the impact of CT scanning on radiotherapy planning. Comput Tomogr 4:55, 1980.

V9. Vosburgh, K.G., R.K. Swank, J.M. Houston: X-ray image intensifiers. Adv Electron Phys 43:205, 1977.

V10. de Vrijer, F.W.: Modulation. Philips tech rev 36:305, 1976.

V11. Vyborny, C.J., C.E. Metz, K. Doi: Relative efficiencies of energy to photographic density conversions in typical screen-film systems. Radiology 136:465, 1980.

W1. Wyckoff, H.O., A. Allisy, K. Lidén: The new special names of SI units in the field of ionizing radiations. Am J Roentgenol 125:492, 1975.

W2. Whitmore, G.F., H.E. Johns: A 250-curie caesium 137 unit designed for low dosage rates at short source to skin distances. Br J Radiol 32:533, 1959.

W3. Whyte, G.N.: Density effect in γ-ray measurements. Nucleonics 12:18, 1954.

W4. Wyckoff, H.O., F.H. Attix: Design of free-air ionization chambers. National Bureau of Standards Handbook 64. Washington, D.C.: U.S. National Bureau of Standards, 1957.

W5. Weber, J., D.J. van den Berge: The effective atomic number and the calculation of the composition of phantom materials. Br J Radiol 42:378, 1969.

W6. White, D.R.: An analysis of the Z-dependence of photon and electron interactions, Phys Med Biol 22:219, 1977.

W7. White, D.R.: Tissue substitutes in experimental radiation physics. Med Phys 5:467, 1978.

W8. Webb, H.P.: An improved radium safe. Br J Radiol 33:654, 1960.

W9. Wallace, D.M., ed.: Tumours of the bladder. E and S Livingstone, Edinburgh 1959, p. 257.

W10. Wolfe, J.N.: Xeroradiography of the bones, joints, and soft tissues. Radiology 93: 583, 1969.

W11. Wolfe, J.N., R.P. Dooley, L.E. Harkins: Xeroradiography of the breast: a comparative study with conventional film mammography. Cancer 28:1569, 1971.

W12. Withers, H.R., M.M. Elkind: Microcolony survival assay for cells of mouse intestinal mucosa exposed to radiation. Int J Radiat Biol 17:261, 1970.

W13. Whitmore, G.F., S. Gulyas: Recovery processes in x-irradiated mammalian cells. Can Cancer Conf 7th, 1966. Oxford, Pergamon, 1967, p. 370.

W14. Windeyer, Sir B.: Hyperbaric oxygen and radiotherapy. The Medical Research Council's Working Party. Br J Radiol 51:875, 1978.

W15. Watson, E.R., K.E. Halnan, S. Dische, M.I. Saunders, I.S. Cade, J.B. McEwen, G. Wiernik, D.J.D. Perrins, I. Sutherland: Hyperbaric oxygen and radiotherapy: a Medical Research Council trial in carcinoma of the cervix. Br J Radiol 51:879, 1978.

W16. Wiernik, G., N.M. Bleehen, J. Brindle, J. Bullimore, I.F.J. Churchill-Davidson, J. Davidson, J.F. Fowler, P. Francis, R.C.M. Hadden, J.L. Haybittle, N. Howard, I.F. Lansley, R. Lindup, D.L. Phillips, D. Skeggs: Sixth Interim Progress Report of the Br I of Radiol fractionation study of 3 F/week versus 5 F/week in radiotherapy of the laryngo-pharynx. Br J Radiol 51:241, 1978.

W17. Watson, T.A., H.E. Johns, C.C. Burkell. The Saskatchewan 1000 curie cobalt 60 unit. Radiology 62:165, 1954.

Y1. Yaffe, M., K.W. Taylor, H.E. Johns: Spectroscopy of diagnostic x-rays by a Compton-scatter method. Med Phys 3:328, 1976.

Y2. Yaffe, M., A. Fenster, H.E. Johns: Xenon ionization detectors for fan beam computed tomography scanners. J Comput Ass Tomog 1:419, 1977.

Y3. Young, M.E.J., J.D. Gaylord: Experimental tests of corrections for tissue inhomogeneities in radiotherapy. Br J Radiol 43:349, 1970.

Y4. Young, M.E.J., H.F. Batho: Dose tables for linear radium sources calculated by an electronic computer. Br J Radiol 37:38, 1964.

Y5. Yaffe, M.J., G.E. Maudsley: Quantification of silver in radiographic film. Proc Soc Photo-Optical Instrum Eng 273:80, 1981.

Z1. Zworykin, V.K., G.A. Morton: Television. New York: Wiley, 1954.

NAME INDEX

All references used in this book are listed alphabetically, starting on page 760. Each reference has been assigned a letter and a number. The letter is the first letter of the name of the senior author, and the number gives the order of appearance of the citation in the text.

Use of the author index is explained by two examples: Abrahams, S. is senior author in reference A15, which is cited on page 678. Adams, G.E. is senior author in reference A14, cited on page 674 and is a co-author in reference F15, which is cited on page 704.

779

SUBJECT INDEX